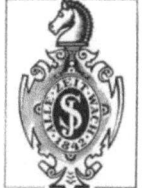

Calcium-Antagonismus

Herausgegeben von
A. Fleckenstein H. Roskamm

Mit 223 Abbildungen

Springer-Verlag
Berlin Heidelberg New York 1980

Internationales Symposium
8. – 9. Dezember 1978, Frankfurt/Main

Herausgeber:
Professor Dr. med. Albrecht Fleckenstein
I. Physiologischer Lehrstuhl der Universität Freiburg, Hermann-Herder-Straße 7, D-7800 Freiburg

Professor Dr. med. Helmut Roskamm
Benedikt-Kreutz Rehabilitationszentrum für Herz- und Kreislaufkranke e.V., Südring 15, D-7812 Bad Krozingen

ISBN-13: 978-3-642-67596-6   e-ISBN-13: 978-3-642-67595-9
DOI: 10.1007/978-3-642-67595-9

CIP-Kurztitelaufnahme der Deutschen Bibliothek
Calcium-Antagonismus / hrsg. von A. Fleckenstein; H. Roskamm. – Berlin, Heidelberg, New York: Springer, 1980

NE: Fleckenstein, Albrecht [Hrsg.]

2127/3140-543210

Table of Contents

List of Contributors

AMENDE, I., Abteilung für Kardiologie, Medizinische Hochschule Hannover, Karl-Wiechert-Allee 9, D-3000 Hannover 61

APPEL, E., Zentrum der Inneren Medizin, Abteilung für Kardiologie der Johann Wolfgang Goethe-Universität, Theodor-Stern-Kai 7, D-6000 Frankfurt/Main

BACHOUR, G., Karlstraße 4, D-4730 Ahlen/Westf.

BECKER, H.-J., Medizinische Klinik, Stadtkrankenhaus Hanau, Akademisches Lehrkrankenhaus, Leimenstraße 20, D-6450 Hanau 1

BEHRENBECK, D. W., Medizinische Klinik und Poliklinik, Lehrstuhl Innere Medizin III − Kardiologie, Universität Köln, Joseph-Stelzmann-Straße 9, D-5000 Köln 41

BELARDINELLI, L., Department of Physiology, University of Virginia School of Medicine, USA-Charlottesville, VA 22908

BENDER, F., Medizinische Klinik und Poliklinik, Abteilung Innere Medizin C, Westfälische Wilhelms-Universität, Westring 3, D-4400 Münster/Westfalen

BERNE, R. M., Department of Physiology, University of Virginia School of Medicine, USA-Charlottesville, VA 22908

BIAGINI, A., C.N.R. Laboratory of Clinical Physiology and University of Pisa, I-Pisa

BOINK, A. B. T. J., Department of Cardiology, University Hospital, Catharijnesingel 101, NL-3500 CG Utrecht

VD BRAND, M., Academisch Ziekenhuis Rotterdam, Dr. Molewaterplein 40, NL-Rotterdam 3002

BREITHARDT, G., Medizinische Klinik B, Universität Düsseldorf, Moorenstraße 5, D-4000 Düsseldorf

BROBMANN, G. F., Chirurgische Universitäts-Klinik, Hugstetter Straße 55, D-7800 Freiburg i.Br.

BROWER, R. W., Cardiovascular Research, Erasmus University, POB 1738, NL-Rotterdam

BUBENHEIMER, P., Benedikt Kreutz Rehabilitationszentrum für Herz- und Kreislaufkranke e.V., Südring 15, D-7812 Bad Krozingen

CLARK, R. E., Division of Cardiology, Washington University School of Medicine, USA-St. Louis, MO 63111

DISTANTE, A., C.N.R. Laboratory of Clinical Physiology and University of Pisa, I-Pisa

EKELUND, L.-G., Department of Clinical Physiology, Karolinska Hospital, S-10401 Stockholm

ENENKEL, W., 4. Medizinische Abteilung mit Kardiologie, Krankenhaus der Stadt Wien-Lainz, Wolkersbergenstraße 1, A-1130 Wien

ENGEL, H.-J., Abteilung für Kardiologie, Medizinische Hochschule Hannover, Karl-Wiechert-Allee 9, D-3000 Hannover 61

FERRARI, F., Cardiothoracic Institute, University of London, 2 Beaumont Street, GB-London W1N 2DX

FLECKENSTEIN, A., Physiologisches Institut der Universität Freiburg, Hermann-Herder-Straße 7, D-7800 Freiburg i.Br.

FLECKENSTEIN-GRÜN, G., Physiologisches Institut der Universität Freiburg, Hermann-Herder-Straße 7, D-7800 Freiburg i.Br.

FREY, M., Physiologisches Institut der Universität Freiburg, Hermann-Herder-Straße 7, D-7800 Freiburg i.Br.

GABRIEL, J., Benedikt Kreutz Rehbilitationszentrum für Herz- und Kreislaufkranke e.V., Südring 15, D-7812 Bad Krozingen

GRADAUS, D., Kurklinik Bad Waldliesborn, Funktionsdiagnostische Abteilung, Quellenstraße 54, D-4780 Lippstadt

GRIMM, W., Chirurgische Universitäts-Klinik, Hugstetter Straße 55, D-7800 Freiburg i.Br.

HAMAMOTO, H., Division of Cardiology, Department of Medicine, Cedars-Sinai Medical Center and UCLA School of Medicine, USA-Los Angeles, CA

HARDER, D. R., Department of Physiology, College of Medicine, East Tennessee State University, USA-Johnson City, TN 37061

HASHIMOTO, K., Hatano Research Institute, Food and Drug Safety Center, J-Hadano, Kanagawa 257

HENRY, P. D., Division of Cardiology, Washington University School of Medicine, USA-St. Louis, MO 63111

HILGER, H. H., Medizinische Klinik und Poliklinik, Lehrstuhl Innere Medizin III − Kardiologie, Universität Köln, Joseph-Stelzmann-Straße 9, D-5000 Köln 41

MEIJLER, F. L., Department of Cardiology, University Hospital, Catharijnesingel 101, NL-3500 CG Utrecht

HOPF, R., Zentrum der Inneren Medizin, Abteilung für Kardiologie, Klinikum der Johann Wolfgang Goethe-Universität, Theodor-Stern-Kai 7, D-6000 Frankfurt/Main

JAKOB, M., Medizinische Klinik der Bundesknappschaft Sulzbach, Akademisches Lehrkrankenhaus der Universität des Saarlandes, D-6603 Sulzbach

JASMIN, G., Département de pathologie, Faculté de médicine, Université de Montréal, CDN-Montéal

KALTENBACH, M., Zentrum der Inneren Medizin, Abteilung für Kardiologie, Klinikum der Johann Wolfgang Goethe-Universität, Theodor-Stern-Kai 7, D-6000 Frankfurt/Main

KALUSCHE, D., Benedikt Kreutz Rehabilitationszentrum für Herz- und Kreislaufkranke e.V., Südring 15, D-7812 Bad Krozingen

TEN KATEN, H. J., Academisch Ziekenhuis Rotterdam, Dr. Molewaterplein 40, NL-Rotterdam 3002

KEIDEL, J., Physiologisches Institut der Universität Freiburg, Hermann-Herder-Straße 7, D-7800 Freiburg i.Br.

KISHIDA, H., Department of Internal Medicine, Nippon Medical School, 1-1-5 Sendagi, Bunkyo-ku, J-Tokyo 113

KOBER, G., Zentrum der Inneren Medizin, Abteilung für Kardiologie, Klinikum der Johann Wolfgang Goethe-Universität, Theodor-Stern-Kai 7, D-6000 Frankfurt/Main

KONRAD, A., Medizinische Klinik der Bundesknappschaft Sulzbach, Akademisches Lehrkrankenhaus der Universität des Saarlandes, D-6603 Sulzbach

KRAIS, T., Kardiologische Abteilung, Medizinische Klinik und Poliklinik, Universitätsklinikum Charlottenburg, Spandauer Damm 130, D-1000 Berlin 19

KREHAN, L., Zentrum der Inneren Medizin, Abteilung für Kardiologie, Klinikum der Johann Wolfgang Goethe-Universität, Theodor-Stern-Kai 7, D-6000 Frankfurt/Main

KRIKLER, D. M., Division of Cardiovascular Medicine, Royal Postgraduate Medical School, Hammersmith Hospital, GB-London W12 0HS

LEMKE, R., Zentrum der Inneren Medizin, Abteilung für Kardiologie, Klinikum der Johann Wolfgang Goethe-Universität, Theodor-Stern-Kai 7, D-6000 Frankfurt/Main

LICHTLEN, P. R., Abteilung für Kardiologie, Medizinische Hochschule Hannover, Karl-Wiechert-Allee 9, D-3000 Hannover 61

LOSSNITZER, K., Medizinische Klinik der Bundesknappschaft Sulzbach, Akademisches Lehrkrankenhaus der Universität des Saarlandes, D-6603 Sulzbach

MANDEL, W. J., Division of Cardiology, Department of Medicine, Cedars-Sinai Medical Center and UCLA School of Medicine, USA-Los Angeles, CA

MASERI, A., C.N.R. Laboratory of Clinical Physiology and University of Pisa, I-Pisa

MAYER, M., Chirurgische Universitäts-Klinik, Hugstetter Straße 55, D-7800 Freiburg i.Br.

MCCULLEN, A., Division of Cardiology, Department of Medicine, Cedars-Sinai Medical Center and UCLA School of Medicine, USA-Los Angeles, CA

MITROVIĆ, V., Kerckhoff-Klinik der Max Planck Gesellschaft, Benekestraße 6 – 8, D-6350 Bad Nauheim

MOTOMURA, S., Department of Pharmacology, Tohoku University School of Medicine, J-Sendai

NARIMATSU, A., Department of Pharmacology, Tohoku University School of Medicine, J-Sendai

NAYLER, W. G., Cardiothoracic Institute, University of London, 2 Beaumont Street, GB-London W1N 2DX

NEUSS, H., Kerckhoff-Klinik der Max Planck Gesellschaft, Benekestraße 6 – 8, D-6350 Bad Nauheim

NIEHUES, B., Medizinische Klinik und Poliklinik, Lehrstuhl Innere Medizin III – Kardiologie, Universität Köln, Joseph-Stelzmann-Straße 9, D-5000 Köln 41

O'HARA, N., Hatano Research Institute, Food and Drug Safety Center, J-Hadano, Kanagawa 257

ONO, H., Hatano Research Institute, Food and Drug Safety Center, J-Hadano, Kanagawa 257

PARODI, O., C.N.R. Laboratory of Clinical Physiology and University of Pisa, I-Pisa

PETER, Th., Division of Cardiology, Department of Medicine, Cedars-Sinai Medical Center and UCLA School of Medicine, USA-Los Angeles, CA

PROSCHEK, L., Département de pathologie, Faculté de médecine, Université de Montréal, CDN-Montréal

REITERER, W., I. Medizinische Abteilung, Allgemeine Poliklinik Wien, A-1000 Wien

ROSKAMM, H., Benedikt Kreutz Rehabilitationszentrum für Herz- und Kreislaufkranke e.V., Südring 15, D-7812 Bad Krozingen

ROWLAND, E., Division of Cardiovascular Medicine, Royal Postgraduate Medical School, Hammersmith Hospital, GB-London W12 0HS

RUBIO, R., Department of Physiology, University of Virginia School of Medicine, USA-Charlottesville, VA 22908

RUIGROK, T. J. C., Department of Cardiology, University Hospital, Catharijnesingel 101, NL-3500 CG Utrecht

RUTSCH, W., Kardiologische Abteilung, Medizinische Klinik und Poliklinik, Universitätsklinikum Charlottenburg, Spandauer Damm 130, D-1000 Berlin 19

SAFER, A., Abteilung Biometrie, Knoll-AG, D-6700 Ludwigshafen/Rh.

SATOH, K., Department of Pharmacology, Tohoku University School of Medicine, J-Sendai

SCHARTL, M., Kardiologische Abteilung, Medizinische Klinik und Poliklinik, Universitätsklinikum Charlottenburg, Spandauer Damm 130, D-1000 Berlin 19

SCHLEPPER, M., Kerckhoff-Klinik der Max Planck Gesellschaft, Benekestraße 6 – 8, D-6350 Bad Nauheim

SCHMUTZLER, H., Kardiologische Abteilung, Medizinische Klinik und Poliklinik, Universitätsklinikum Charlottenburg, Spandauer Damm 130, D-1000 Berlin

SCHNELLBACHER, K., Benedikt Kreutz Rehabilitationszentrum für Herz- und Kreislaufkranke e.V., Südring 15, D-7812 Bad Krozingen

SCHULZ, W., Zentrum der Inneren Medizin, Abteilung für Kardiologie der Johann Wolfgang Goethe-Universität, Theodor-Stern-Kai 7, D-6000 Frankfurt/Main

SEIPEL, L., Medizinische Klinik B, Universität Düsseldorf, Moorenstraße 5, D-4000 Düsseldorf

SERRUYS, P. W., Academisch Ziekenhuis Rotterdam, Dr. Molewaterplein 40, NL-Rotterdam 3002

SEVERI, S., C.N.R. Laboratory of Clinical Physiology and University of Pisa, I-Pisa

SLADE, A., Cardiothoracic Institute, University of London, 2 Beaumont Street, GB-London W1N 2DX

SPÄH, F., Physiologisches Institut der Universität Freiburg, Hermann-Herder-Straße 7, D-7800 Freiburg i.Br.

SPERELAKIS, N., Department of Physiology, University of Virginia School of Medicine, USA-Charlottesville, VA 22908

SPIEL, R., 4. Medizinische Abteilung mit Kardiologie, Krankenhaus der Stadt Wien-Lainz, Wolkersbergenstraße 1, A-1130 Wien

SPIES, H. F., Zentrum der Inneren Medizin, Abteilung für Kardiologie der Johann Wolfgang Goethe-Universität, Theodor-Stern-Kai 7, D-6000 Frankfurt/Main

TAIRA, N., Department of Pharmacology, Tohoku University School of Medicine, J-Sendai

TAUCHERT, M., Medizinische Klinik und Poliklinik, Lehrstuhl Innere Medizin III − Kardiologie, Universität Köln, Joseph-Stelzmann-Straße 9, D-5000 Köln 41

THORMANN, J., Kerckhoff-Klinik der Max Planck Gesellschaft, Beneckestraße 6 − 8, D-6350 Bad Nauheim

TRITTHART, H. A., Institut für Medizinische Physik und Biophysik, Universität Graz, Harrachgasse 21, A-8010 Graz

VAUGHAN WILLIAMS, E. M., Department of Pharmacology, University of Oxford, South Parks Road, GB-Oxford

WATANABE, Y., Cardiovascular Institute, Fujita Gakuen University School of Medicine, Toyoake, J-Aichi 470-11

WERNER, H., Zentrum der Inneren Medizin, Abteilung für Kardiologie, Klinikum der Johann Wolfgang Goethe-Universität, Theodor-Stern-Kai 7, D-6000 Frankfurt/Main

WILLIAMSON, J. R., Division of Cardiology, Washington University School of Medicine, USA-St. Louis, MO 63111

WOLF, R., Abteilung für Kardiologie, Medizinische Hochschule Hannover, Karl-Wiechert-Allee 9, D-3000 Hannover 61

YAMAGUCHI, I., Division of Cardiology, Department of Medicine, Cedars-Sinai Medical Center and UCLA School of Medicine, USA-Los Angeles, CA

YANAGISAWA, T., Department of Pharmacology, Tohoku University School of Medicine, J-Sendai

ZIMMERMANN, A. N. E., Department of Cardiology, University Hospital, Catharijnesingel 101, NL-3500 CG Utrecht

Steuerung der myocardialen Kontraktilität, ATP-Spaltung, Atmungsintensität und Schrittmacher-Funktion durch Calcium-Ionen – Wirkungsmechanismus der Calcium-Antagonisten[1]

A. Fleckenstein

Zur Physiologie und Biochemie der elektro-mechanischen Koppelungsprozesse

Der Erregungsprozeß der Myocardfaser läuft bekanntlich an der äußeren Grenzmembran, der sog. Sarkolemm-Membran ab, die den extrazellulären Raum vom Faserinnern trennt. Die Kontraktion ist dagegen ein intrazellulärer Vorgang. Die zeitliche Koppelung der bioelektrischen und mechanischen Phänomene setzt daher die Existenz eines Systems der Informationsvermittlung von der Zelloberfläche ins Innere der kontraktilen Fasern voraus. Die Natur hat dieses schwierige Problem bekanntlich dadurch gelöst, daß sie sich der Ca^{++}-Ionen als Mittlersubstanz zwischen Membran-Erregung und intrazellulärer Myofibrillen-Verkürzung bedient.

Abspaltung der terminalen Phosphat-Gruppe von Adenosintriphosphat (ATP) durch

Ca^{++}-aktivierte Myofibrillen-ATPase

$$
\begin{array}{ccccccc}
 & O & & O & & O & \\
 & \| & & \| & & \| & \\
Adenosin-O-P-O-P & & O-P-OH \\
 & | & & | & & | & \\
 & OH & & OH & & OH &
\end{array}
$$

Gewinnbare Kontraktions-Energie $\approx 10\,000$ cal/Mol gespaltenes ATP

Entscheidend für die Freisetzung der Kontraktionsenergie ist dabei – in einfachster Weise summarisch dargestellt – die Ca^{++}-bedingte Aktivierung der Myofibrillen-ATPase. Dieses Ferment ist für die Überführung der in ATP gestapelten Energie in mechanische Arbeit verantwortlich. Die Ca^{++}-abhängige Aktivierung der Myofibrillen-ATPase ist jedoch bereits der letzte Schritt in einer Kette von vorgeschalteten Reaktionen, die in ihrer Gesamtheit als sog. „elektro-mechanische Koppelung" imponieren. Diese elektromechanische Koppelung koordiniert mit Hilfe der Ca^{++}-Ionen den Kontraktionsakt zeitlich mit dem Erregungsprozeß. Darüber hinaus regulieren die elektro-mechanischen Koppelungsprozesse mit Hilfe der Ca^{++}-Ionen jedoch auch in quantitativer Hinsicht die Freisetzung der Kontraktionsenergie, indem sie die Menge an ATP bestimmen, die im kontraktilen System utilisiert wird. Ein Ca^{++}-Entzug im Extrazellulärraum führt daher zu einem Verlust der Myocard-Kontraktilität, während das normalerweise Na^+-abhängige Aktionspotential kaum verändert wird (vgl. Abb. 1). Umgekehrt steigt die Kontraktionskraft nach Zusatz von Extra-Ca^{++} über die Ausgangswerte an.

---

1 Zusammenfassende Darstellungen der Myocardeffekte von Ca^{++}-Antagonisten sind in folgenden Publikationen gegeben worden: Fleckenstein [1–5], Fleckenstein u. Mitarb. [6–7]

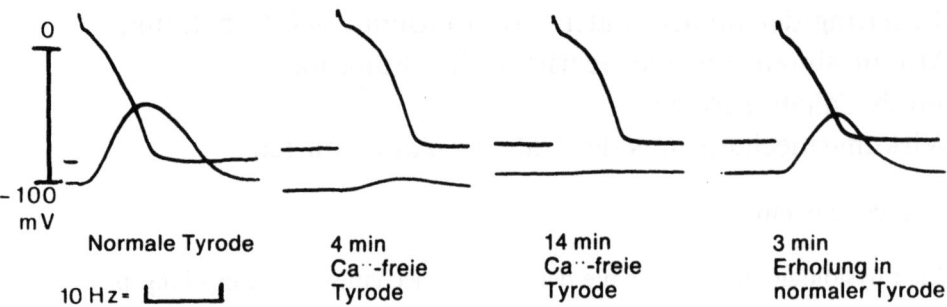

Abb. 1. Selektive Aufhebung der Kontraktilität eines isolierten Kaninchen-Papillarmuskels in einer Ca^{++}-freien Tyrode-Lösung ohne wesentliche Beeinflussung des elektrischen Erregungsprozesses („elektro-mechanische Entkoppelung"). Gleichzeitige Registrierung des Aktionspotentials (oben) mittels einer intrazellulären Mikroelektrode und des Mechanogramms (unten) unter Verwendung einer mechano-elektronischen Transducer-Röhre

Der erste Schritt im Zuge der elektro-mechanischen Koppelungsreaktionen besteht – wie zahlreiche Versuche mit den verschiedensten Methoden ergeben haben – in einer Steigerung der Ca^{++}-Permeabilität der Sarkolemm-Membran im Augenblick der Erregung. Ca^{++}-Ionen dringen dementsprechend während der Dauer des Aktionspotentials ins Innere der Myocardfasern ein und lösen damit die letztlich zur Kontraktion führenden Kettenreaktionen aus. Der Einstrom der Ca^{++}-Ionen erfolgt durch die sog. „langsamen Ca^{++}-Kanäle", die sich bei Depolarisation oder Umpolarisation der erregten Sarkolemm-Membran öffnen (vgl. Abb. 2). Dabei besteht im Regelfall eine strenge Korrelation zwischen der einströmenden Ca^{++}-Menge und der entwickelten mechanischen Spannung. Die langsamen Kanäle entnehmen allerdings das zu transportierende Calcium wahrscheinlich nicht direkt dem Extrazellulärraum; denn in den oberflächlichen Schichten der Sarkolemm-Membran ist offenbar ein eigener Pool von locker gebundenen Ca^{++}-Ionen zur Versorgung der langsamen Kanäle vorhanden.

Der Wirkungsmechanismus positiv oder negativ inotroper Agentien scheint vorzugsweise darauf zu beruhen, daß sie die Kapazität dieser oberflächlichen Ca^{++}-Speicher oder die Leistung des transmembranären Ca^{++}-Transport-Systems steigern oder senken. Adrenalin, Noradrenalin und andere Sympathomimetika mit β-Rezeptoren-stimulierender Wirkung vergrößern offenbar in der Membran-Oberfläche die Pool-Kapazität oder die Bindungs-Affinität für Calcium, so daß sich dieser den langsamen Kanälen vorgeschaltete Ca^{++}-Speicher stärker mit Ca^{++}-Ionen belädt. Unter dem Einfluß von sympathischen Catecholaminen werden dann mehr Ca^{++}-Ionen für den Einstrom durch die langsamen Kanäle – und damit für die Aktivierung des kontraktilen Systems – zur Verfügung gestellt. β-Mimetika bewirken offenbar auf dem Umweg über die Bildung von zyklischem AMP eine verstärkte Phosphorylierung von Membran-Proteinen. Auf diese Weise entstehen unter dem Einfluß der β-Mimetika in den oberflächlichen Schichten der Myocardfaser-Membran mehr Struktur-gebundene, negativ geladene Phosphat-Gruppen, an denen dann zusätzliche Ca^{++}-Ionen locker angelagert bzw. angereichert werden können. Mit Butyryl-Cyclo-AMP kann man übrigens die gleiche Phosphorylierung von Membran-Proteinen herbeiführen und damit die Effekte von Adrenalin, Nor-

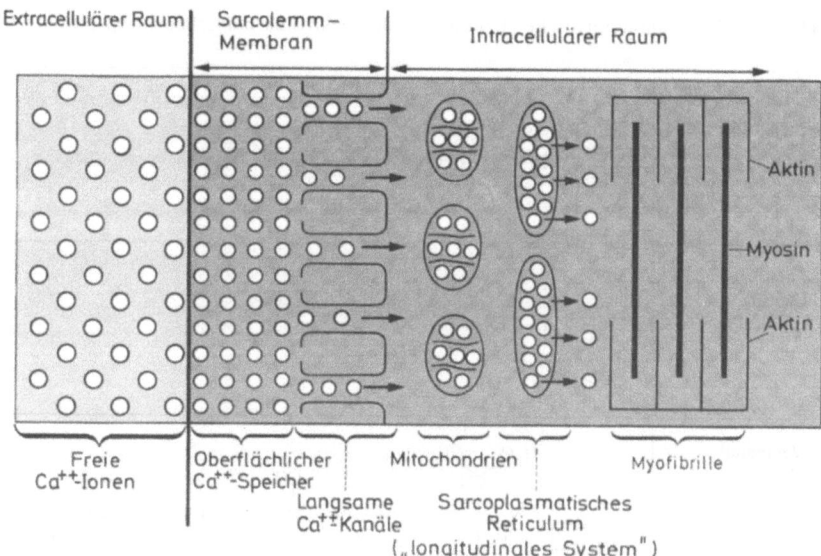

Extracellulärer Raum | Sarcolemm – Membran | Intracellulärer Raum

Aktin
Myosin
Aktin

Freie Ca⁺⁺-Ionen | Oberflächlicher Ca⁺⁺-Speicher | Mitochondrien | Myofibrille

Langsame Ca⁺⁺ Kanäle | Sarcoplasmatisches Reticulum ("longitudinales System")

Abb. 2. Schema der Ca^{++}-abhängigen elektro-mechanischen Koppelungsprozesse in der Myocardfaser und der daran beteiligten zellulären Strukturen. Da die Aktivierung des kontraktilen Systems von den transversalen Tubuli ausgeht, dürften die im Schema dargestellten oberflächlichen Ca^{++}-Speicher und die langsamen Kanäle speziell an den Kontaktstellen zwischen dem transversalen und longitudinalen System, d. h. an der invaginierten Sarkolemm-Membran in der Tiefe der transversalen Tubuli lokalisiert sein

adrenalin oder Isoproterenol auf Ca^{++}-Influx, ATP-Spaltung und mechanische Spannungsentwicklung simulieren.

Hemmung der elektro-mechanischen Koppelungsprozesse durch Ca^{++}-Antagonisten

Eine spezifische Hemmung der elektro-mechanischen Koppelungsprozesse im Warmblütermyocard läßt sich mit Hilfe der in Tabelle 1 aufgeführten Ca^{++}-Antagonisten erreichen. Der Wirkungsmechanismus dieser neuen Gruppe hochpotenter Pharmaka wurde im wesentlichen im Physiologischen Institut Freiburg in den Jahren zwischen 1963 und 1969 aufgeklärt. Gemeinsam ist den Ca^{++}-Antagonisten eine spezifische – den β-adrenergen Catecholaminen entgegengerichtete – Dämpfung der Myocard-Kontraktilität. „Spezifität" bedeutet, daß bei diesen Stoffen die Ca^{++}-antagonistische Hemmung der elektro-mechanischen Koppelung so sehr im Vordergrund steht, daß alle anderen pharmakologischen Effekte deutlich dahinter zurücktreten. Verapamil (Isoptin) und Prenylamin (Segontin) waren die ersten Substanzen dieser Art, die wir schon Ende 1963 prüften. Dabei ergab sich (vgl. [8, 9]), daß diese Stoffe die Wirkungen eines einfachen Ca^{++}-Mangels insofern imitieren, als sie

a) die myocardiale Kontraktionskraft dämpfen, ohne das Aktionspotential stärker zu beeinträchtigen („elektro-mechanische Entkoppelung"),

b) die Utilisation von energiereichem Phosphat im kontraktilen System vermindern,

c) den oxydativen Tätigkeitsstoffwechsel (Extra-Sauerstoff-Verbrauch pro Systole) senken, und

Tabelle 1. Ca^{++}-antagonistische Hemmstoffe der elektromechanischen Koppelung

Prenylamin (Segontin)	$CH-CH_2-CH_2-NH-\underset{CH_3}{CH}-CH_2-$
Fendilin (Sensit)	$CH-CH_2-CH_2-NH-\underset{CH_3}{CH}-$
Verapamil (Isoptin)	CH_3O- CH_3O- $\underset{\underset{C\equiv N}{\mid}}{C}-CH_2-CH_2-CH_2-\underset{CH_3}{N}-CH_2-CH_2-$ $-OCH_3$ $-OCH_3$, $\underset{CH}{\overset{H_3C\quad CH_3}{}}$
Substanz D600	CH_3O- CH_3O- CH_3O- $\underset{\underset{C\equiv N}{\mid}}{C}-CH_2-CH_2-CH_2-\underset{CH_3}{N}-CH_2-CH_2-$ $-OCH_3$ $-OCH_3$, $\underset{CH}{\overset{H_3C\quad CH_3}{}}$
Nifedipin (Adalat. Bay a 1040)	H_3COOC- $-COOCH_3$; H_3C- $-CH_3$; $-NO_2$; $-H$; N–H
Diltiazem (Herbesser)	S; $-OCH_3$; $-OCOCH_3$; $=O$; $CH_2CH_2N\overset{CH_3}{\underset{CH_3}{}}$ HCl
Perhexilin–Maleat (Pexid)	$\underset{H}{N}-CH_2-CH-$; $\underset{\parallel}{\overset{CHCOOH}{CHCOOH}}$

d) durch Gabe geeigneter Dosen von Ca^{++}-Salzen, β-adrenergen Catecholaminen oder Herzglykosiden in vitro und in vivo hinsichtlich ihrer Myocard-Effekte prompt neutralisierbar sind.

Als noch bedeutend wirksamer erwiesen sich im Zuge weiterer Untersuchungen die Verbindung D 600, ein Methoxy-Derivat von Verapamil sowie Nifedipin (Bay a 1040, Adalat), auf deren Ca^{++}-antagonistische Potenzen zuerst von Fleckenstein u. Mitarb. [6, 10] hingewiesen wurde. Die negativ-inotropen Effekte von Prenylamin (Lindner [11], Verapamil (Haas und Härtfelder [12], D 600 (Haas und Busch [13]) sowie Nifedipin (Vater u. Mitarb. [14]) waren zwar bei der pharmakologischen Prüfung dieser Stoffe durch die Herstellerfirmen schon vorher erkannt worden. Klarheit über den Wirkungsmechanismus erbrachte jedoch erst die physiologische Analyse. In den letzten Jahren sind dann noch Fendilin, d. h. Sensit [15] (Fleckenstein u. Mitarb. [15]) und Perhexilin-Maleat, d. h. Pexid (Fleckenstein-Grün u. Mitarb. [16]) hinzugekommen. Diltiazem wurde von japanischen Pharmakologen als Ca^{++}-Antagonist introduziert (vgl. Nakajima u. Mitarb. [17]). Über das Wirkungsspektrum von Niludipin, einem weiteren hoch-aktiven Ca^{++}-Antagonisten aus der Nifedipin-Reihe, haben wir erst kürzlich berichtet (Fleckenstein u. Mitarb. [18]).

Als Beispiel für die Selektivität, mit der diese Stoffe die mechanische Aktivität des Säugetiermyocards zu blockieren vermögen, ist in Abb. 3 ein Experiment mit Verapamil aus einer früheren Publikation [19] wiedergegeben. Hierbei wurde die Kontraktilität eines isolierten Meerschweinchen-Papillarmuskels durch eine hohe Dosis von Verapamil total unterdrückt, während die intrazellulär registrierten Einzelfaser-Aktionspotentiale praktisch unverändert blieben. Das Bild gleicht im Prinzip vollständig dem Verhalten eines Papillarmuskels in Ca^{++}-freier Lösung (vgl. Abb. 1). Extra-Ca^{++}, Herzglykoside oder β-Mimetika (in dem vorliegenden Versuch Isoproterenol) können die Kontraktilität rasch restituieren. Als weiteres Beispiel für die selektive Dämpfung der mechanischen Myocardfunktion durch Ca^{++}-Antagonisten ist in Abb. 4 ein Experiment mit Fendilin wiedergegeben.

Welcher Mechanismus liegt der Wirkung dieser hochaktiven Ca^{++}-Antagonisten zugrunde, die an der elektro-mechanischen Koppelung der Warmblüter-Myocardfaser etwa so spezifisch angreifen wie Curare an den motorischen Endplatten? Die Antwort hierauf ist heute experimentell gut abgesichert: Tracer-Experimente mit Radiocalcium sowie direkte Messungen des transmembranären Ca^{++}-Einstroms in sog. Voltage-Clamp-Versuchen haben nämlich übereinstimmend gezeigt, daß der entscheidende Angriffspunkt der Ca^{++}-Antagonisten an der Membran der Myocardfaser liegt. Tatsächlich können die Ca^{++}-Antagonisten den transmembranären Ca^{++}-Influx in die erregten Myocardfasern selektiv hemmen, ohne die gleichzeitigen Na^{+}-Bewegungen, die der Entstehung der Aktionspotentiale zugrunde liegen, deutlich zu beeinflussen [20]. Dabei sind im Prinzip zwei Angriffspunkte der Ca^{++}-Antagonisten möglich

a) eine direkte Blockierung des transmembranären Ca^{++}-Transportsystems, d. h. der langsamen Kanäle, oder

b) eine Verdrängung von Ca^{++}-Ionen aus den vorgeschalteten Ca^{++}-Speichern in den oberflächlichen Schichten der Sarkolemm-Membran. Hierdurch würde die Pool-Kapazität oder die Bindungs-Affinität für Ca^{++}-Ionen herabgesetzt und die Ca^{++}-Versorgung der langsamen Kanäle mehr oder weniger stark reduziert.

Nayler und Szeto [21] haben gewichtige Argumente für eine Verdrängung von Ca^{++}-Ionen aus dem oberflächlichen Membran-Pool durch Verapamil geliefert. Nach neueren Befunden aus unserem Laboratorium sinkt die Intensität des transmembranären Ca^{++}-Influx − und damit die Kontraktionskraft − besonders rasch

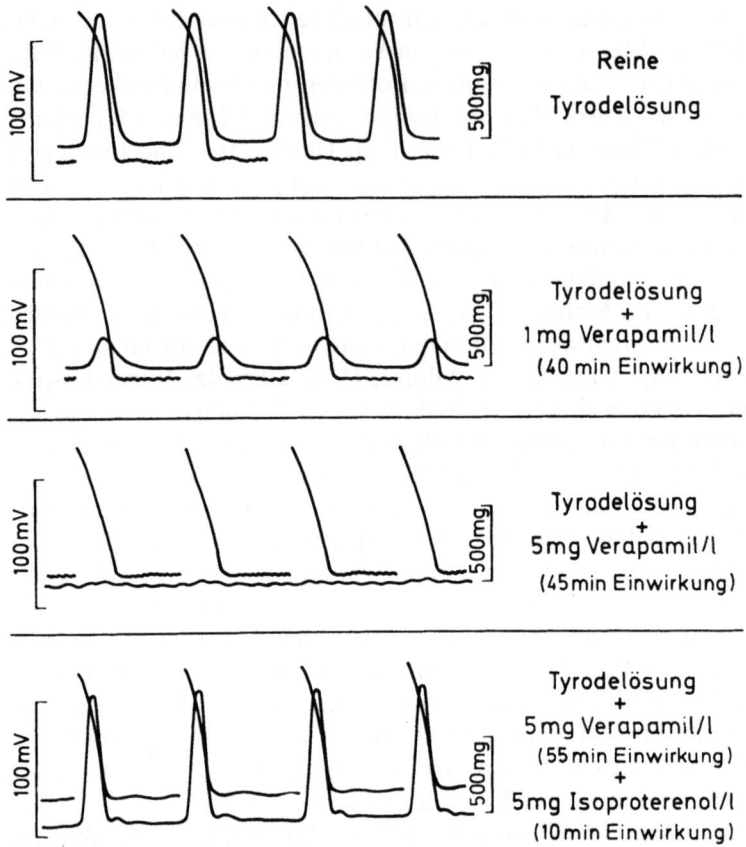

Abb. 3. Selektive Hemmung der Kontraktilität eines elektrisch gereizten isolierten Papillarmuskels vom Meerschweinchen bei Anwendung exzessiv hoher Konzentrationen von Verapamil. Ähnlich wie nach Ca^{++}-Entzug kommt es dabei zu einer kompletten elektromechanischen Entkoppelung mit maximaler Einschränkung der Ca^{++}-abhängigen Spaltung von energiereichem Phosphat. Isoproterenol restituiert die metabolischen und mechanischen Myocardfunktionen vollkommen, da es den gehemmten Ca^{++}-Influx in die erregten Myocardfasern wieder in Gang bringt (nach Fleckenstein [19])

ab, wenn man mit Ca^{++}-Antagonisten behandelte Myocardfasern mit höheren Frequenzen reizt. In dieser Situation kommt es offenbar innerhalb kurzer Zeit zu einer vollständigen Erschöpfung der − unter dem Einfluß von Ca^{++}-Antagonisten stark reduzierten − Ca^{++}-Vorräte in der Membranoberfläche. Mit Hilfe eines Überangebots an extrazellulären Ca^{++}-Ionen läßt sich jedoch die Wirkung der Ca^{++}-Antagonisten auch bei hohen Erregungsfrequenzen überspielen und die Kontraktilität restituieren. Ebenso brauchbar sind β-Mimetika, speziell Isoproterenol, das selbst am Herzen in situ innerhalb von 10−20 sec die Effekte einer Überdosierung von Ca^{++}-Antagonisten wieder aufhebt. β-Mimetika erhöhen offenbar die Kapazität des oberflächlichen Ca^{++}-Pools selbst in Anwesenheit von Ca^{++}-Antagonisten, so daß der transmembranäre Ca^{++}-Influx wieder ausreichend in Gang kommt.

Dagegen haben sich keinerlei Hinweise dafür ergeben, daß Verapamil und andere Ca^{++}-Antagonisten auch intrazelluläre Angriffspunkte besitzen. Die Ca^{++}-abhängige Myofibrillen-ATPase wird z. B. durch Ca^{++}-Antagonisten nicht direkt

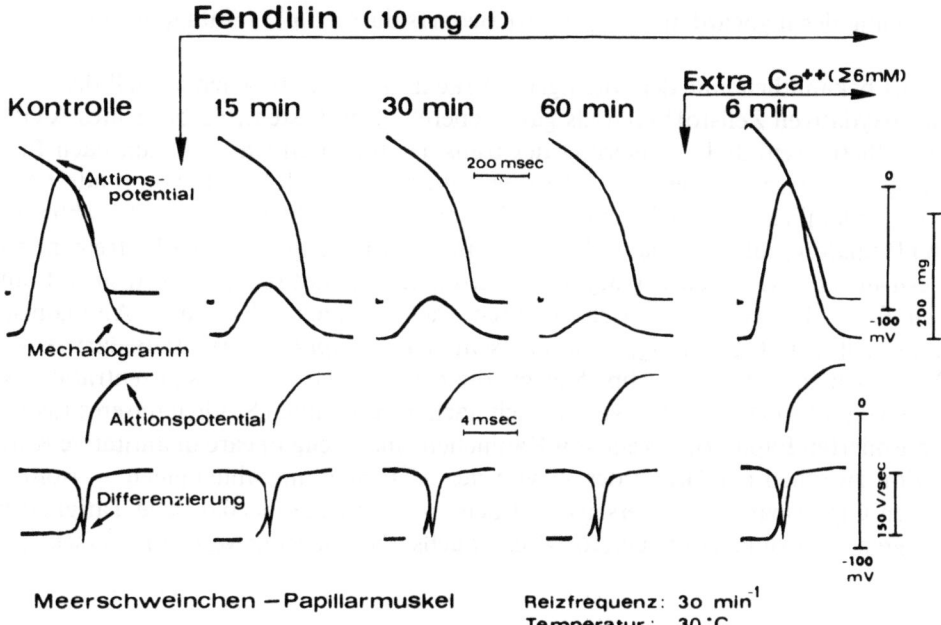

Abb. 4. Selektive Hemmung der Kontraktilität eines elektrisch gereizten Papillarmuskels vom Meerschweinchen unter dem Einfluß von Fendilin (10 mg/l) in Tyrode-Lösung mit 2 mM Ca^{++}/l. Die isometrische Kontraktionsamplitude sinkt hier innerhalb von 60 min auf etwa 25% des Ausgangswertes ab. Trotzdem werden die Aktionspotential-Parameter (Aufstrichsgeschwindigkeit, Overshoot-Höhe, Aktionspotentialdauer (bei 90% Repolarisation gemessen) ebenso wie das Ruhepotential kaum verändert. Anschließend rasche Restitution der Kontraktilität durch Zusatz von Extra-Calcium (Steigerung des Ca^{++}-Gehalts auf 6 mM/l). Die Differenzierungskurve (Ausschlag nach unten) zeigt die maximale Aufstrichsgeschwindigkeit des Aktionspotentials (etwa 175 V/sec) direkt an. Dieser Na^+-abhängige Parameter wird offensichtlich durch Fendilin in der angewandten Konzentration nicht beeinflußt. Intrazelluläre Mikroelektroden-Ableitung von einer einzigen Myocardfaser während eines 90 min dauernden Einstichs [15]

gehemmt. Isolierte Myofibrillen-Bündel, die man nach Zerstörung der Sarkolemm-Membran (an sog. skinned fibres) durch Zusatz von ATP und Ca^{++} zur Verkürzung bringen kann, reagieren auf Ca^{++}-Antagonisten überhaupt nicht. Wir haben diese Versuche 1973 in Zusammenarbeit mit dem Institut von Professor Rüegg durchgeführt. Auch das sarkoplasmatische Reticulum wird offenbar durch Ca^{++}-Antagonisten nicht direkt tangiert: Verapamil konnte hier z. B. nach übereinstimmenden Beobachtungen aus verschiedenen Laboratorien weder die Bindung und Akkumulation, noch die Freisetzung von Ca^{++}-Ionen deutlich beeinflussen [21 – 23]. Schließlich wurde in unserem Institut von Frey und Janke [24] auch die Möglichkeit eines Eingriffs von Ca^{++}-Antagonisten in den Ca^{++}-Stoffwechsel der Herz-Mitochondrien geprüft. Hierbei ergab sich jedoch in Studien an isolierten Mitochondrien, daß z. B. Verapamil erst in einer solchen Konzentration zu einer Veränderung der Ca^{++}-Aufnahme und Ca^{++}-Abgabe führt, die über 1000mal höher liegt als diejenige, welche für die Ausschaltung der Myocard-Kontraktilität erforderlich ist. Die bisher bekannten Ca^{++}-Antagonisten sind also nur spezifische Inhibitoren des transmembranären Ca^{++}-Influx und in dieser Hinsicht den Herzwirkungen der β-adrenergen Sympathomimetika diametral entgegengesetzt.

Senkung des myocardialen Sauerstoff-Bedarfs durch Ca^{++}-Antagonisten

Es ist bekanntlich eine der wichtigsten Erkenntnisse der Biochemie, daß der Zweck des oxydativen Zellstoffwechsels ganz generell darin besteht, verbrauchtes ATP zu resynthetisieren. Jede Steigerung des transmembranären Ca^{++}-Influx nach Erhöhung der extrazellulären Ca^{++}-Konzentration oder nach Zusatz von β-adrenergen Catecholaminen wird daher in den Myocardfasern nicht nur die Ca^{++}-abhängige ATP-Spaltung und mechanische Spannungsentwicklung in die Höhe treiben, sondern auch den O_2-Bedarf. Umgekehrt wird jede Einschränkung des transmembranären Ca^{++}-Influx durch extrazellulären Ca^{++}-Entzug oder Ca^{++}-Antagonisten gleichzeitig ATP-Spaltung, Spannungsentwicklung *und* Sauerstoff-Bedarf senken. Variiert man z. B., wie Abb. 5 zeigt, die extrazelluläre Ca^{++}-Konzentration zwischen 0 und 8 mM Ca^{++}, so ergibt sich nach ausgedehnten Studien unseres Instituts an isolierten Papillarmuskeln von Kaninchen eine streng lineare quantitative Korrelation zwischen der Größe der − von der ATP-Spaltung abhängigen − isometrischen Gipfelspannung einerseits und dem − durch die mechanische Tätigkeit bedingten − Anstieg des Sauerstoff-Verbrauchs über die Ruhewerte andererseits [25].

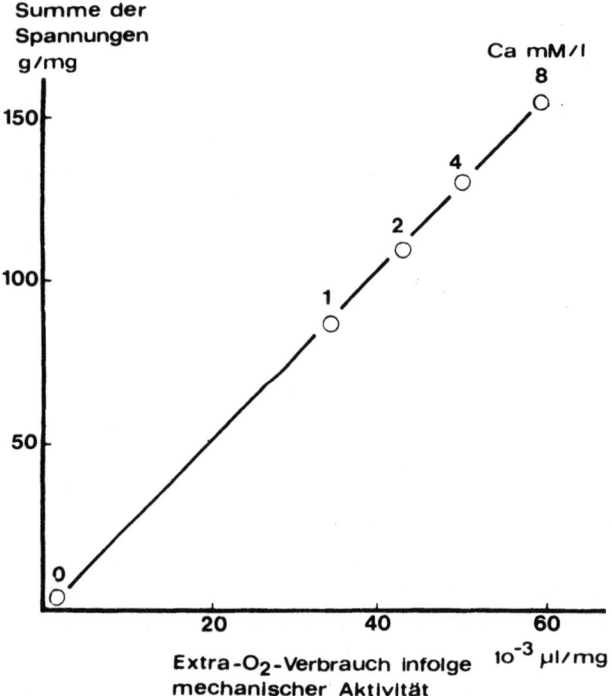

Abb. 5. Lineare Abhängigkeit des Extra-O_2-Verbrauchs infolge mechanischer Aktivität von der Summe der isometrischen Gipfelspannungen von 180 Einzelkontraktionen eines isolierten Kaninchen-Papillarmuskels bei Variation des extrazellulären Ca^{++}-Gehalts zwischen 0 und 8 mM. Die Spannungsmessung erfolgte mit einem induktiven Wegaufnehmer jeweils während 3 min bei einer Reizfrequenz von 60/min. Hierbei wurden die Gipfelpunkte der isometrischen Kontraktionen aufgezeichnet. Die Bestimmung des O_2-Verbrauchs wurde mit einer Platinelektrode während der gesamten Versuchszeit vorgenommen. Die Einwirkungsdauer der Lösungen mit verschiedenem Ca^{++}-Gehalt vor Beginn der Reizung betrug jeweils 15 min. Versuchstemperatur 30 °C [25]

Auch unter dem Einfluß von Ca^{++}-Antagonisten sinkt die isometrische Gipfel-spannung isolierter Papillarmuskeln immer linear zum Tätigkeits-bedingten Extra-Sauerstoff-Verbrauch. Als Beispiele sind in den Abb. 6 – 8 Experimente mit Verapa-mil, Fendilin und Nifedipin wiedergegeben. Die Proportionalität zwischen Span-nungsentwicklung und Extra-Sauerstoff-Verbrauch ist offensichtlich ein Gesetz, das nach unseren Messungen auch für β-Rezeptoren-Blocker gilt. Tatsächlich reduzie-ren die β-Rezeptoren-Blocker und die Ca^{++}-Antagonisten im tätigen Myocard ATP-Spaltung, Kontraktilität und Sauerstoff-Verbrauch letzten Endes nach dem gleichen Grundprinzip, d. h. durch Einschränkung der Ca^{++}-Versorgung des kon-traktilen Systems: Die Ca^{++}-Antagonisten bewirken dies durch direkte Hemmung des Ca^{++}-Transports, die β-Rezeptoren-Blocker auf indirektem Weg, indem sie den fördernden Einfluß der β-adrenergen Catecholamine auf die Ca^{++}-Aufnahme in die erregten Myocardfasern neutralisieren. Der oxydative Basalstoffwechsel des nicht-schlagenden Myocards wird dagegen durch Ca^{++}-Antagonisten und β-Rezep-toren-Blocker innerhalb eines weiten Konzentrationsbereichs nicht beeinflußt. Die Senkung des myocardialen O_2-Bedarfs durch Ca^{++}-Antagonisten und β-Rezeptoren-Blocker ist demnach auch insofern wesensgleich, als sie niemals losge-löst von einer gleichzeitigen Dämpfung der Ca^{++}-abhängigen mechanischen Myo-card-Aktivität zustande kommen kann.

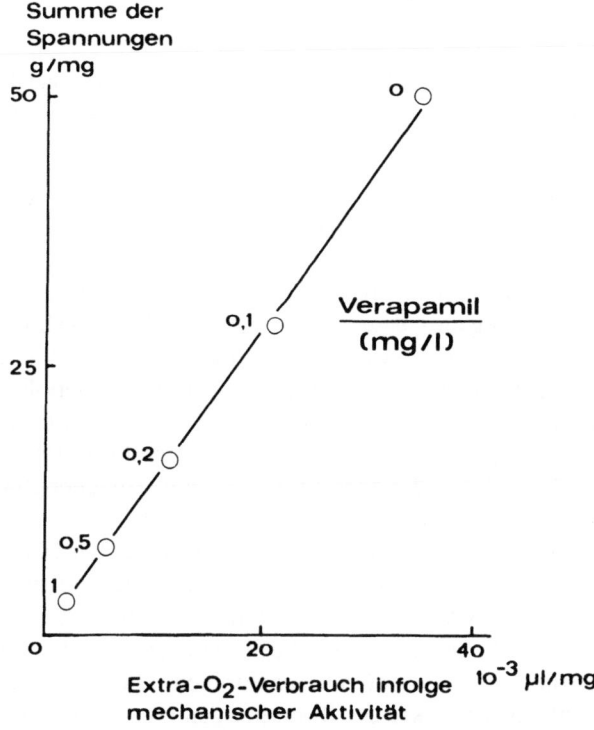

Abb. 6. Lineare Senkung der Summe der isometrischen Gipfelspannungen und des Extra-O_2-Verbrauchs infolge mechanischer Aktivität bei einem Kaninchen-Papillarmuskel (1,5 mg Feuchtgewicht) unter dem Einfluß steigender Konzentrationen von Verapamil (0 mg, 0,1 mg, 0,2 mg, 0,5 mg und 1,0 mg/l Tyrode-Lösung). Ca^{++}-Gehalt 2 mM/l, Temp. 30 °C, Reizfrequenz 60/min während 3 min [25]

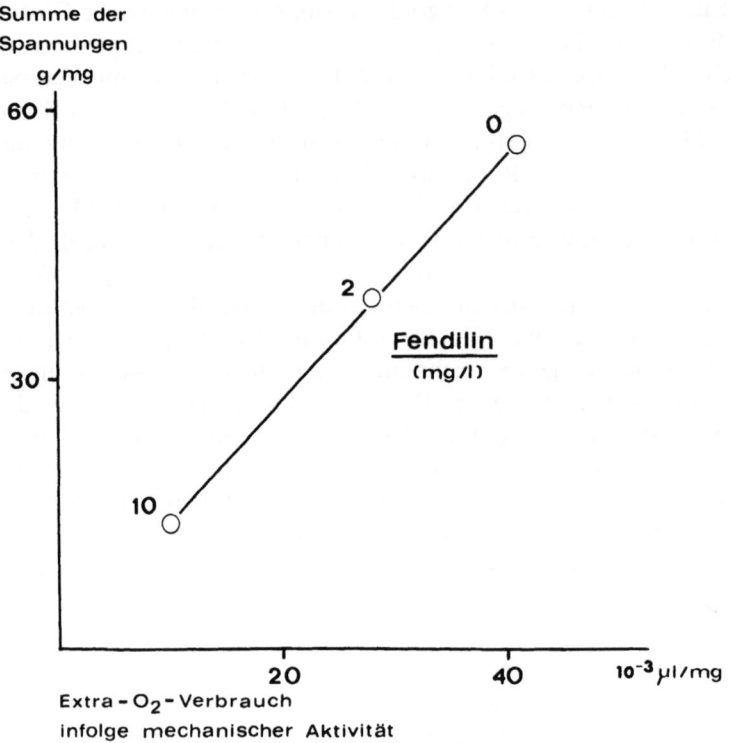

Abb. 7. Lineare Herabsetzung des Extra-O_2-Verbrauchs und der Summe der isometrischen Gipfelspannungen durch Fendilin (2,0 und 10,0 mg/l). Versuchsanordnung wie in Abb. 6 [15]

Dämpfung der Ca^{++}-abhängigen Aktivität nomotoper und ektoper Automatie-Zentren durch Ca^{++}-Antagonisten

Es ist seit langem bekannt, daß Ca^{++}-Mangel nicht nur die elektromechanischen Koppelungsprozesse im Vorhof- und Ventrikelmyocard zum Erliegen bringt, sondern auch die Automatie-Funktion der cardialen Schrittmacher hemmt (vgl. Abb. 9): Sowohl die langsame diastolische Depolarisation der Schrittmacher-Zellen als auch der anschließende Aufstrich der Schrittmacher-Aktionspotentiale ist offenbar obligatorisch mit einem transmembranären Einstrom von Ca^{++}-Ionen verknüpft. Auch die Membran der Schrittmacher-Zellen des Sinus- und AV-Knotens verfügt daher über ein Ca^{++}-Transportsystem, das in völliger Analogie zu den langsamen Kanälen in der Membran gewöhnlicher Myocardfasern auf β-adrenerge Sympathomimetika und Ca^{++}-Antagonisten konträr reagiert. Dies bedeutet, daß β-adrenerge Catecholamine durch Förderung des Ca^{++}-Influx nicht nur die Kontraktionskraft, sondern auch die Sinus-Frequenz steigern und gleichzeitig die Erregungsleitung im AV-Knoten beschleunigen. Die positiv inotropen, chronotropen und dromotropen Effekte der β-adrenergen Catecholamine sind demnach nur verschiedene Manifestationen der gleichen Grundwirkung, d. h. einer Optimierung der transmembranären Ca^{++}-Versorgung von Arbeitsmyocard und Schrittmacherzellen.

Ca^{++}-Antagonisten wie Verapamil, D 600, Diltiazem oder Nifedipin unterdrücken dagegen die automatische Impulsbildung in isoliertem Schrittmacher-

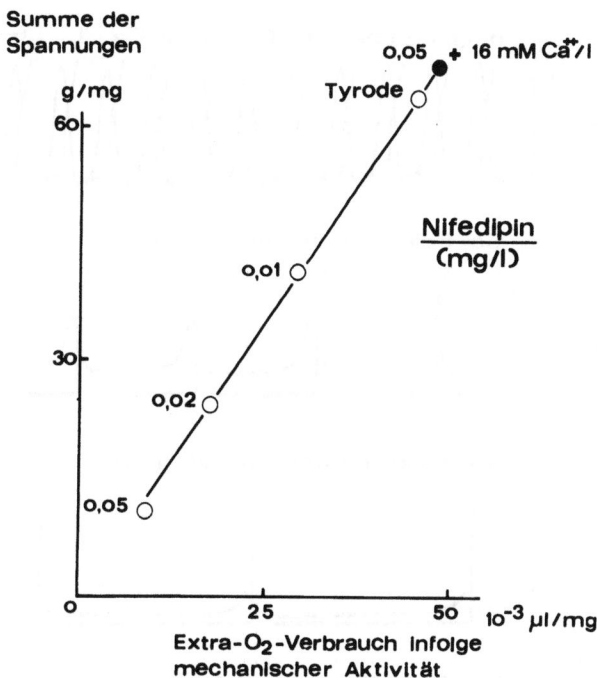

Abb. 8. Lineare Senkung der isometrischen Spannungsentwicklung und des Extra-O_2-Verbrauchs eines isolierten Kaninchen-Papillarmuskels durch wachsende Konzentrationen von Nifedipin (0,01, 0,02 und 0,05 mg/l) in Tyrode-Lösung mit normalem extrazellulärem Ca^{++}-Gehalt von 2 mM. Nach Steigerung der Ca^{++}-Konzentration auf 16 mM/l kommt es in Anwesenheit von 0,05 mg Nifedipin/l zu einer überschießenden Restitution der mechanischen Aktivität und des damit zusammenhängenden Extra-O_2-Verbrauchs [6]

gewebe aus dem Sinus- oder AV-Knoten von Kaninchen, Ratten und Meerschweinchen etwa im gleichen Dosierungsbereich wie die Kontraktilität von Vorhof und Ventrikelmuskulatur [26, 27]. Umgekehrt lassen sich Kontraktilität und Sinusfrequenz sowie die AV-Überleitung mit Hilfe β-adrenerger Catecholamine – speziell Isoproterenol – auch in Anwesenheit der Ca^{++}-Antagonisten prompt restituieren [8, 9,28]. Die Gabe von Extra-Calcium ist weniger wirksam. Bei der speziellen elektrophysiologischen Analyse des Einflusses von Verapamil auf die spontanen Schrittmacher-Aktionspotentiale des Sinusknotens und der zentralen Zone (N-Zone) des AV-Knotens kamen mehrere Arbeitsgruppen zu einem fast identischen Ergebnis [29 – 31]: Verapamil reduziert die Steilheit der langsamen diastolischen Depolarisation, so daß die Frequenz der spontanen Impulsbildung drastisch absinkt. Darüber hinaus werden jedoch auch die Anstiegssteilheit und der Overshoot der Schrittmacher-Aktionspotentiale Dosis-abhängig vermindert (vgl. Abb. 10). Dies führt natürlich zu einer Verlangsamung der Erregungsausbreitung innerhalb des Sinusknotens und zu einer Verlängerung der Überleitungszeit im AV-Knoten – ein Effekt, der durch β-adrenerge Catecholamine wiederum sofort behoben werden kann. Dagegen reagiert der normalerweise Na^+-abhängige Erregungsablauf im Hisschen Bündel, in den Purkinje-Fasern und im Ventrikelmyocard weder auf Ca^{++}-Antagonisten noch auf β-Mimetika. Eine wesentliche Veränderung des QRS-Komplexes – als Ausdruck der intraventrikulären Erregungsausbreitung tritt daher

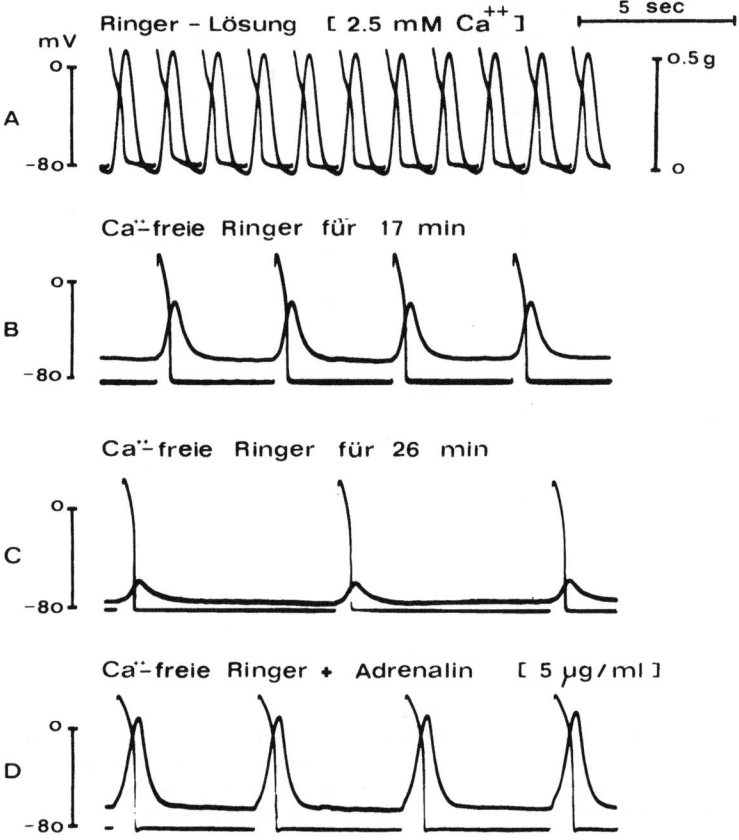

Abb. 9. Gleichzeitige Abnahme der isometrischen Kontraktionsamplitude und der Schlagfrequenz eines spontan tätigen Frosch-Ventrikels nach Überführung aus einer Ca^{++}-haltigen Ringer-Lösung (2,5 mM Ca^{++}) in eine Lösung ohne Ca^{++}. Offensichtlich wird die Schrittmacher-Aktivität in dem Ca^{++}-freien Milieu etwa im gleichen Umfang reduziert wie die mechanische Spannungsentwicklung. Durch Zusatz von Adrenalin lassen sich die spontane Erregungsbildung und die isometrische Kontraktionsamplitude wenigstens vorübergehend reaktivieren, solange noch Spuren von extrazellulärem oder Membrangebundenem Ca^{++} verfügbar sind [56]

unter dem Einfluß dieser Pharmaka nicht ein (vgl. Abb. 11 – 13). Nur überwiegend Na^+-antagonistische Stoffe mit Erregungs-hemmender, lokalanästhetischer Grundwirkung wie z. B. Xylocain (Lidocain) verlängern den QRS-Komplex beträchtlich (vgl. Abb. 13).

Die Automatie-hemmende Wirkung von Ca^{++}-Antagonisten beschränkt sich offensichtlich nicht auf nomotope supraventrikuläre Schrittmacher. Vielmehr wird vor allem Verapamil auch zur Therapie und Prophylaxe ektopischer Erregungsbildung – hauptsächlich im supraventrikulären Bereich – verwendet (Bender [32]; Schamroth u. Mitarb. [33]); Spurell u. Mitarb. [34]; Härtel u. Hartikainen [35]). Schon frühzeitig wurden daher aufgrund pharmakologischer Untersuchungen von Singh und Vaughan-Williams [36] die Ca^{++}-Antagonisten als eigenständige Gruppe von anderen Antiarrhythmika abgegrenzt. Allerdings bieten die Ca^{++}-Antagonisten in dieser Hinsicht bei verschiedenen Tierspezies kein ganz einheitliches Bild. So ist z. B. Verapamil beim Hund (Taira und Narimatsu [37]) und beim Men-

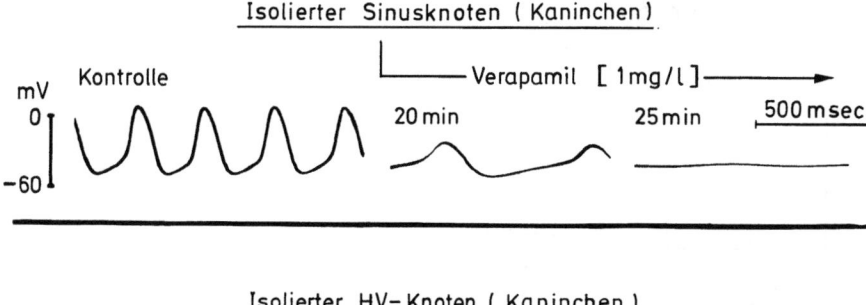

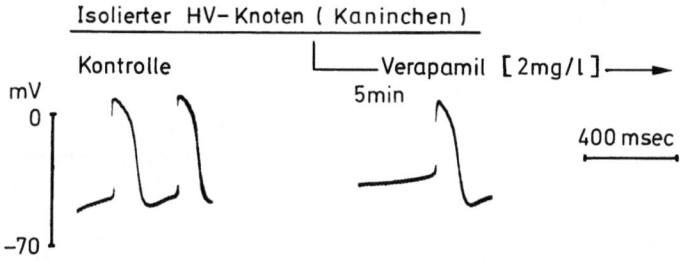

Abb. 10. Hemmung der Schrittmacher-Aktionspotentiale des isolierten, spontan schlagenden Sinus- und AV-Knotens von Kaninchen durch Verapamil. Die Ableitung der Schrittmacher-Potentiale mit intrazellulär eingestochenen Mikroelektroden zeigt besonders im oberen Bildabschnitt, daß Verapamil nicht nur die Steilheit der langsamen diastolischen Depolarisation reduziert, sondern auch den anschließenden Aktionspotential-Aufstrich beträchtlich abflacht, bis es schließlich zu einer völligen Unterdrückung der automatischen Impulsbildung kommt. Auch am isoliert schlagenden AV-Knoten im unteren Bildabschnitt ist die Hemmung der langsamen diastolischen Depolarisation besonders auffällig [29, 31]

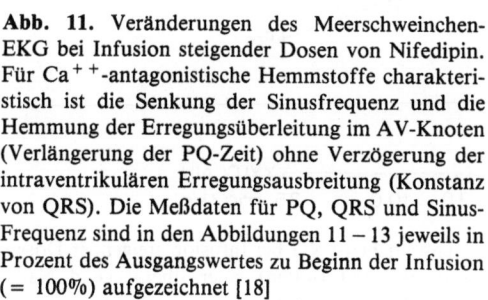

Abb. 11. Veränderungen des Meerschweinchen-EKG bei Infusion steigender Dosen von Nifedipin. Für Ca^{++}-antagonistische Hemmstoffe charakteristisch ist die Senkung der Sinusfrequenz und die Hemmung der Erregungsüberleitung im AV-Knoten (Verlängerung der PQ-Zeit) ohne Verzögerung der intraventrikulären Erregungsausbreitung (Konstanz von QRS). Die Meßdaten für PQ, QRS und Sinus-Frequenz sind in den Abbildungen 11 – 13 jeweils in Prozent des Ausgangswertes zu Beginn der Infusion (= 100%) aufgezeichnet [18]

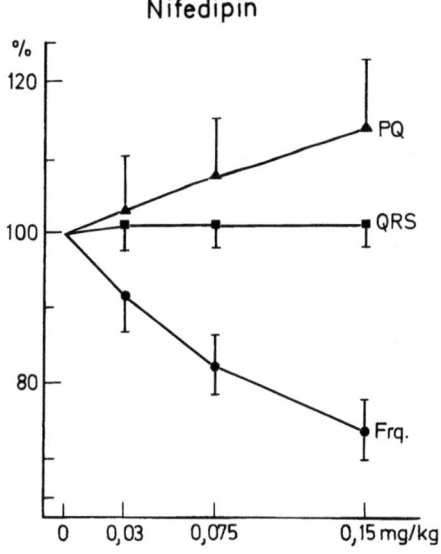

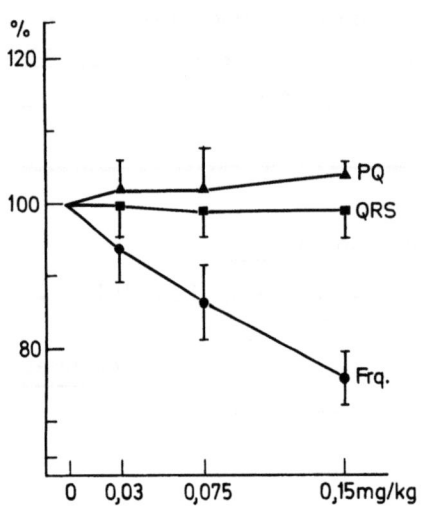

Abb. 12. Meerschweinchen-EKG unter dem Einfluß steigender Dosen von D 600. Ebenso wie bei Nifedipin beschränkt sich die Wirkung des Ca^{++}-Antagonisten D 600 auf die Hemmung des Sinus- und AV-Knotens ohne gleichzeitige Verzögerung des QRS-Komplexes [18]

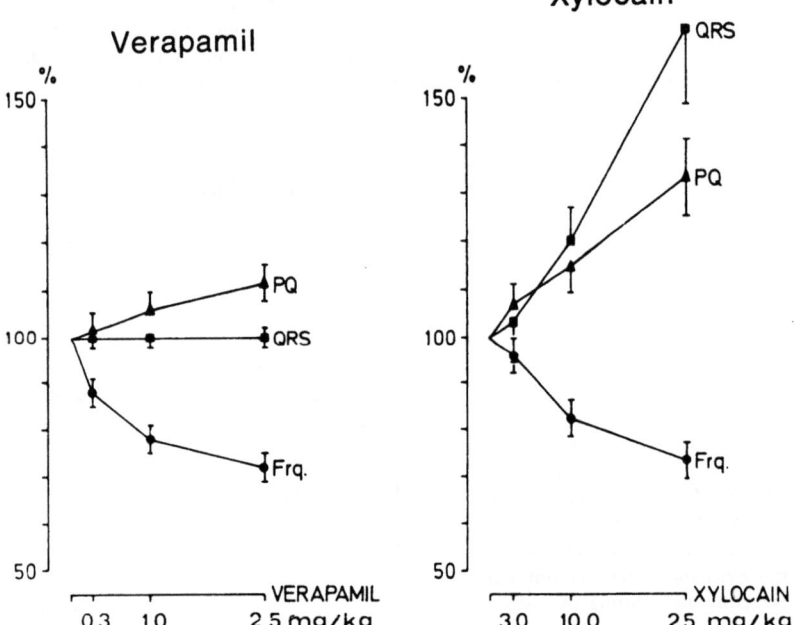

Abb. 13. Unterschiede in der Beeinflussung des Meerschweinchen-EKG bei Infusion steigender Dosen (oben) einer Ca^{++}-antagonistischen Substanz (Verapamil) und (unten) einer überwiegend Na^{+}-antagonistischen Verbindung (Xylocain). Im Gegensatz zu der Ca^{++}-antagonistischen Substanz (Verapamil) ist die Hemm-Wirkung der Na^{+}-antagonistischen Verbindung (Xylocain) nicht auf den Sinus- und AV-Knoten beschränkt. Xylocain und andere überwiegend Na^{+}-antagonistische Erregungs-Inhibitoren wirken vielmehr auch am Ventrikelmyocard im Sinne einer Verzögerung des Aktionspotential-Aufstrichs und dementsprechend der Aktionspotential-Fortleitung. Diese Verlangsamung der intraventrikulären Erregungsausbreitung manifestiert sich im EKG in einer beträchtlichen Zunahme der Dauer des QRS-Komplexes [18]

schen (Bender [32, 38] ein auffällig starker Inhibitor nomotoper und ektoper supra-ventrikulärer Schrittmacher, während Nifedipin in Praxis-üblichen Dosen in dieser Hinsicht auffällig wenig wirkt. Ratten (Refsum [39]) und Meerschweinchen (Fleckenstein u. Mitarb. [18] lassen dagegen keine solchen Unterschiede zwischen Nifedipin und Verapamil erkennen. Das Tierexperiment bedarf daher − was die an-tiarrhythmischen Wirkungen von Ca^{++}-Antagonisten betrifft − dringend einer Er-gänzung und Vertiefung durch klinische Studien am Menschen, die den folgenden Referaten vorbehalten sind.

Die intrazelluläre Ca^{++}-Überladung als pathogenetisches Grundprinzip
bei der Entstehung von Myocardnekrosen −
Cardioprotektion durch Ca^{++}-Antagonisten

Beim Studium der molekularen Wirkungsmechanismen von β-adrenergen Catechol-aminen und Ca^{++}-Antagonisten wendete sich unser Interesse schon frühzeitig auch den Entstehungbedingungen von Myocardnekrosen zu, die im Tierexperiment durch exzessive sympathische Stimulation hervorgerufen werden. Dabei konnten wir erst-mals 1968 aufgrund von Versuchen an Ratten auf zwei wichtige Ergebnisse hinwei-sen (vgl. Fleckenstein [40]):

a) auf die Tatsache, daß die Myocardnekrosen nach hohen Dosen von β-adrenergen Catecholaminen − speziell Isoproterenol − infolge einer deletären Überladung der Myocardfasern mit Ca^{++}-Ionen zustandekommen, und

b) auf die Tatsache, daß Ca^{++}-Antagonisten diese pathologische Ca^{++}-Überladung verhüten können und damit auch die zur Nekrose-Entstehung füh-rende Reaktionskette blockieren.

Zum Verständnis der pathogenetischen Zusammenhänge ist folgendes zu sagen: Die physiologische Grundwirkung β-adrenerger Catecholamine am Myocard, d. h. die Intensivierung von Ca^{++}-Influx, ATP-Spaltung und mechanischer Spannungs-entwicklung, läßt sich offenbar bei höherer Dosierung leicht ins Pathologische stei-gern. Dabei erreicht sowohl der transmembranäre Ca^{++}-Einstrom als auch der Ab-bau von energiereichem Phosphat durch Ca^{++}-aktivierbare ATPasen in den Myofi-brillen, Mitochondrien und im sarkoplasmatischen Reticulum ein extremes Ausmaß (vgl. Abb. 14). Andererseits ließ sich zeigen, daß die intrazelluläre Ca^{++}-Überladung auch schwere Schädigungen der Mitochondrien verursacht (vgl. Abb. 15a, b). Die überhöhte Ca^{++}-Konzentration im Cytoplasma veranlaßt nämlich in den Mitochondrien eine exzessive Ca^{++}-Stapelung, die zu einer Selbst-Zerstörung führt. Nach Überladung mit Ca^{++}-Ionen treten sofort tiefgreifende Veränderungen der Mitochondrien-Struktur (Schwellung, Cristolyse, Vakuolisierung, Verkalkung u.a.) ein, begleitet von einem Verlust der Funktion (Aufhebung der Atmungskon-trolle, Stillstand der oxydativen Phosphorylierung). Dies bedeutet, daß sich bei Ca^{++}-Überladung des Faserinnern die Effekte (a) einer massiven Steigerung des ATP-Verbrauchs und (b) einer gleichzeitigen Hemmung der ATP-Synthese in den Mitochondrien in dramatischer Weise addieren. Aus dieser Koinzidenz resultiert dann ein für die Myocardfaser unter Umständen tödliches Defizit an energiereichen Phosphaten. Letzten Endes beruhen also die Myocardnekrosen infolge Ca^{++}-Überladung ebenso auf einer Erschöpfung der Vorräte an ATP und Kreatin-

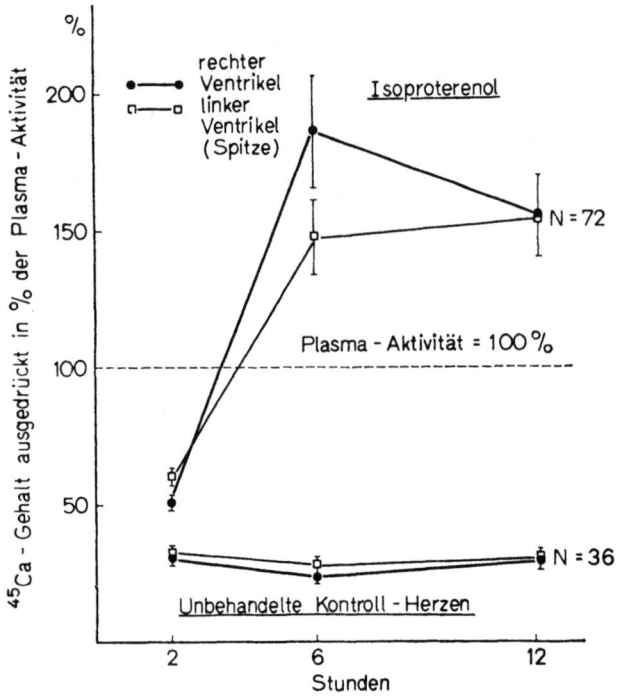

Abb. 14. Steigerung der ^{45}Ca-Netto-Aufnahme ins Myocard des rechten und linken Ventrikels von Ratten nach subkutaner Injektion von 30 mg/kg Isoproterenol. Die ^{45}Ca-Inkorporation in 1 g Myocardgewebe (Frischgewicht) ist jeweils in Prozent bezogen auf die jeweilige ^{45}Ca-Aktivität von 1 ml Plasma während einer Beobachtungszeit von 12 Stunden nach intraperitonealer Verabreichung von 10 μCi ^{45}Ca/kg Körpergewicht angegeben [1, 2, 7]

phosphat, wie dies für die Myocardnekrosen nach Hypoxie und Ischämie gilt (vgl. Abb. 16).

Die Schwere, Ausdehnung und Lokalisation der Catecholamin-bedingten histologischen Veränderungen in der Ventrikelmuskulatur geht dabei jeweils dem Ausmaß der regionalen Ca^{++}-Akkumulation bzw. dem Grad der dadurch verursachten ATP- und Kreatinphosphat-Verarmung in auffälliger Weise parallel. Auch die Sensibilisierung des Myocards für Nekrosen, die nach früheren Beobachtungen von Selye [41], Bajusz [42], Rona, Chappel und Kahn [43] unter dem Einfluß bestimmter Pharmaka (Fluorierte Corticosteroide, Dihydrotachysterol (AT 10), NaH$_2$PO$_4$ u.a.) eintritt, fügt sich in dieses Konzept ohne Schwierigkeit ein; denn unsere Analysen haben gezeigt, daß schon eine kurze Vorbehandlung der Tiere mit diesen Stoffen die Catecholamin-bedingte Radiocalcium-Inkorporation und die intramyocardiale Ca^{++}-Konzentration in einem bisher nicht vermuteten Ausmaß, d. h. auf das 20–30fache erhöhen kann (Abb. 17). Gleichzeitig sinken die ATP- und Kreatinphosphat-Werte auf ein Minimum ab. Eine Überdosierung von Vitamin D$_3$ wirkt nach unseren Befunden ähnlich.

Das wichtigste Ergebnis unserer tierexperimentellen Studien bestand jedoch zweifellos in dem Nachweis, daß organische Ca^{++}-Antagonisten wie z. B. Verapamil, D 600, Nifedipin, Prenylamin und Fendilin bei geeigneter Dosierung die gefährliche Überladung der Myocardfasern mit Ca^{++}-Ionen verhindern können (vgl.

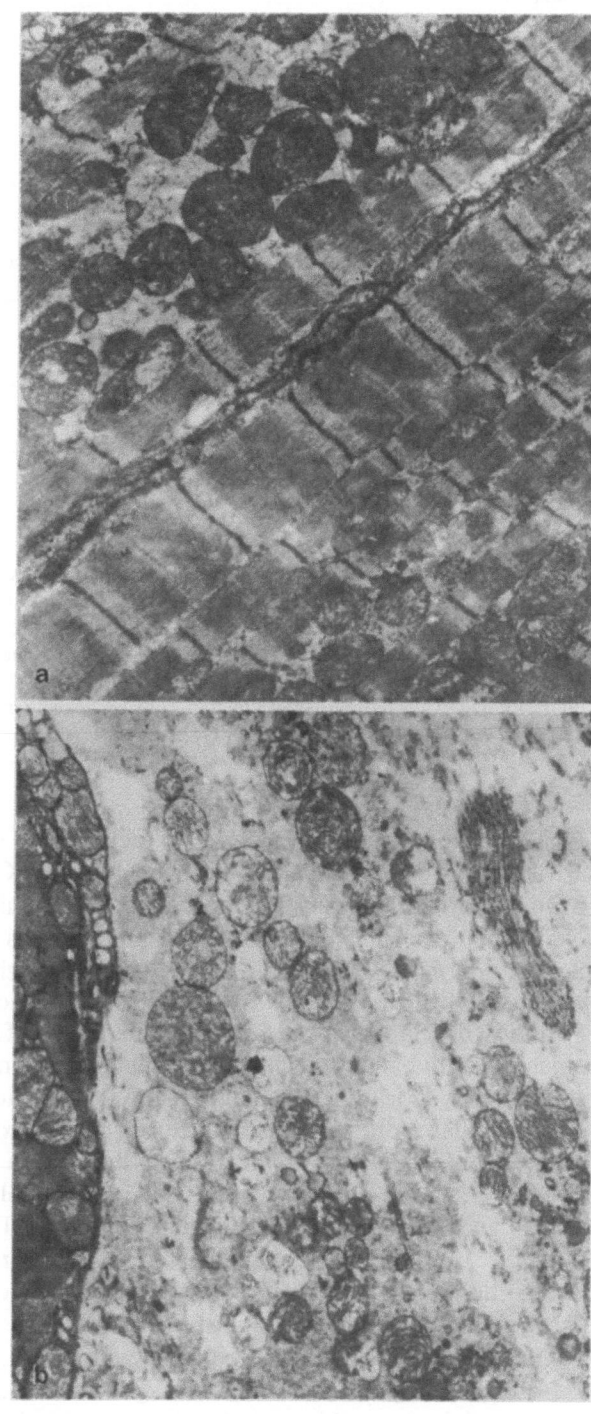

Abb. 15. a Normale Ultrastruktur einer Myocardfaser aus dem rechten Ventrikel einer Kontroll-Ratte [48] **b** Schwere Zerstörungen der Ultrastruktur einer Myocardfaser aus dem rechten Ventrikel einer Ratte 6 Stunden nach subkutaner Injektion der Nekrose-erzeugenden Dosis von 30 mg/kg Isoproterenol. Neben einer Auflösung der Myofibrillen fällt die Schwellung, Cristolyse, Vakuolisierung und Verkalkung der Mitochondrien besonders auf [48]

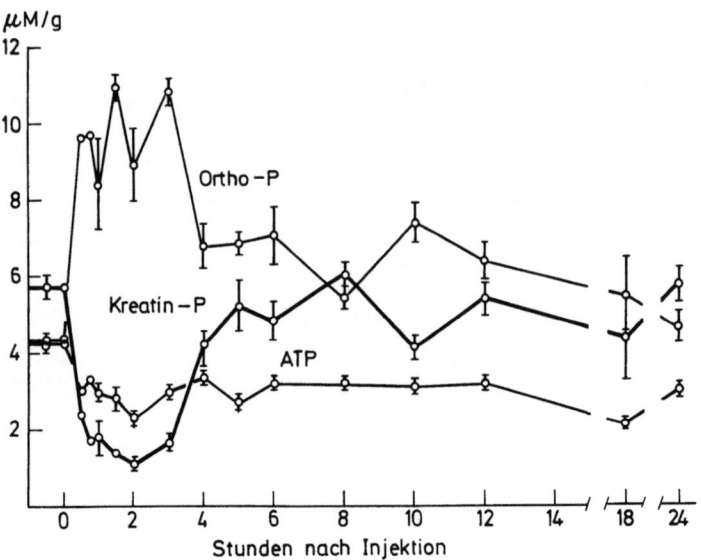

Abb. 16. Beeinflussung der stationären Konzentrationen an ATP, Kreatinphosphat und Orthophosphat im Myocard des linken Ventrikels von 90 Ratten nach subkutaner Injektion von 30 mg Isoproterenol/kg. Der Kreatinphosphat-Gehalt des Myocards wird offensichtlich für die Dauer von 1 – 3 Stunden auf so niedrige Werte gesenkt, wie man sie sonst nur im hypoxischen oder ischämischen Herzen findet. Der ATP-Gehalt fällt im Laufe von 2 Stunden auf fast die Hälfte der Norm ab und regeneriert sich auch während 24 Stunden nur partiell. Spiegelbildlich zum Verhalten der energiereichen Phosphate sind die Veränderungen der Orthophosphat-Fraktion [45]

Abb. 18 – 20). Hierdurch wird der Verbrauch an energiereichem Phosphat auf ein erträgliches Maß reduziert und auch eine Ca^{++}-bedingte Schädigung der Mitochondrien-Struktur und Mitochondrien-Funktion verhütet (Abb. 21 u. 22). Der Gehalt an ATP und Kreatinphosphat stabilisiert sich infolgedessen unter dem Schutz von Ca^{++}-Antagonisten auf einem ausreichend hohen Niveau. Die Myocardfaser wird so in ihrer Gesamtheit, d. h. auch hinsichtlich der Struktur und Funktion der Sarkolemm-Membran und der Myofibrillen, vor den deletären Folgen einer hochgradigen Verarmung an energiereichen Phosphaten bewahrt. Fleckenstein, Janke, Döring u. Pachinger [44] haben in diesem Zusammenhang darauf hingewiesen, daß Verapamil auch die durch cardiotoxische Isoproterenol-Dosen verursachte Freisetzung von myocardialen Fermenten wie z. B. Laktatdehydrogenase (LDH), Laktat-1-Isoenzym (α-HBDH) und Glutamat-oxalacetat-Transaminase (GOT) an Rattenherzen weitgehend unterdrückt. Die cardioprotektiven Wirkungen von Ca^{++}-Antagonisten manifestieren sich dabei nicht nur gegenüber β-adrenergen Sympathomimetika; denn nach unseren Ergebnissen lassen sich z. B. auch die Myocardläsionen infolge Überdosierung von Vitamin D_3 oder Dihydrotachysterol (AT 10) mit Hilfe von Ca^{++}-Antagonisten verhindern.

Neben den organischen Ca^{++}-Antagonisten sind bekanntlich auch höher dosierte perorale Gaben von K^+- und Mg^{++}-Salzen durch cardioprotektive Wirkungen ausgezeichnet (vgl. Abb. 23). Hierbei ließ sich zeigen, daß die K^+- und Mg^{++}-Ionen offenbar mit Ca^{++}-Ionen um intrazelluläre Bindungsstellen konkurrieren und so in kompetitiver Weise eine übermäßige Ca^{++}-Akkumulation verhüten. Auch eine ein-

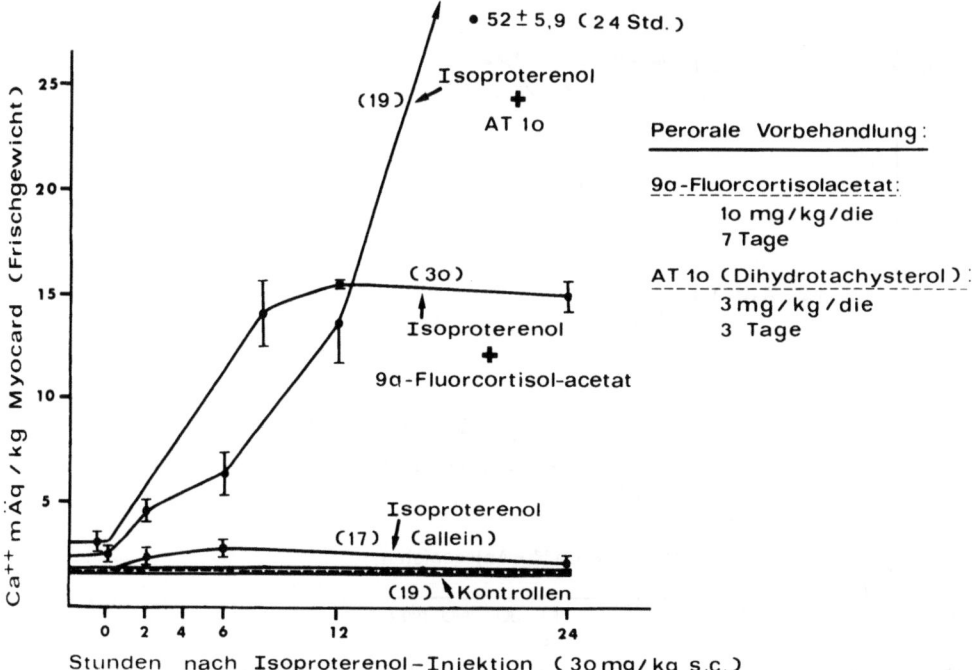

Abb. 17. Exzessive myocardiale Ca^{++}-Anreicherung nach einmaliger Isoproterenol-Injektion (30 mg/kg s.c.) bei AT 10- und 9α-Fluorcortisolacetat-vorbehandelten Ratten. Bei Vorbehandlung mit Dihydrotachysterol (AT 10) wurden 3 Tage lang 3 mg/kg pro die peroral verabreicht. Die Vorbehandlung mit 9α-Fluorcortisolacetat erstreckte sich auf 7 Tage (10 mg/kg s.c. pro die). Der Ca^{++}-Gehalt wurde jeweils im Myocard des ganzen linken Ventrikels bestimmt [46]

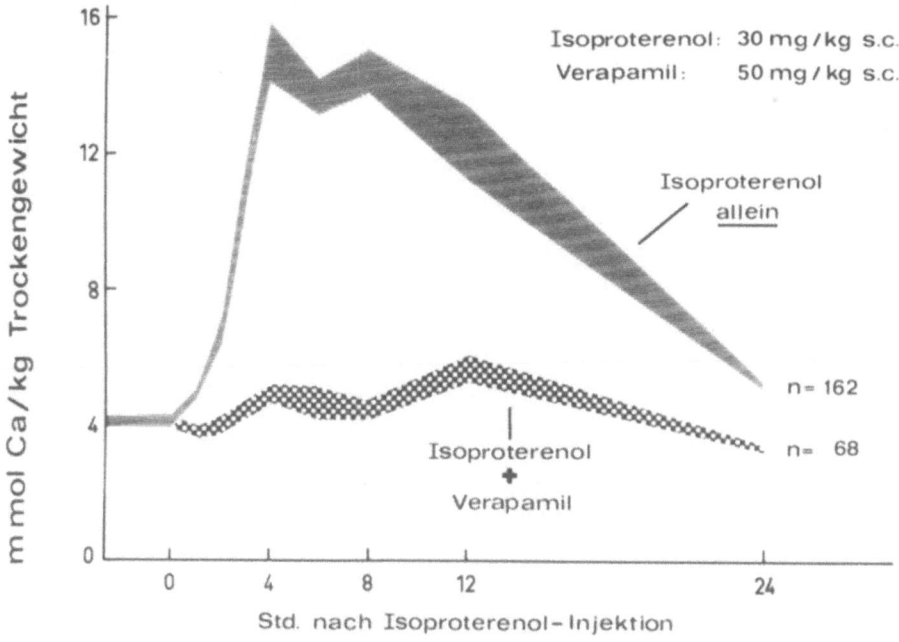

Abb. 18. Hemmung der Isoproterenol-induzierten Ca^{++}-Überladung des Ratten-Myocards durch gleichzeitige subkutane Injektion von Verapamil. Während der Absolut-Gehalt an Ca^{++} nach alleiniger Gabe von Isoproterenol innerhalb von 4 Stunden auf das 4fache der Norm ansteigt, bewegt sich der Ca^{++}-Gehalt der Ventrikelwand nach kombinierter Verabreichung von Isoproterenol und Verapamil nur wenig über dem Kontrollbereich (nach Janke u. Mitarb., 1970, unveröffentlicht)

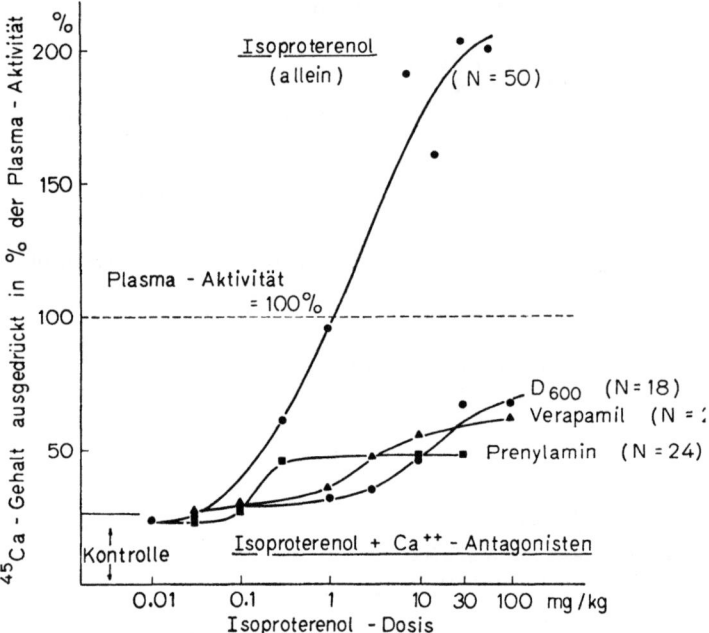

Abb. 19. Schutz des Myocards vor der − durch wachsende Dosen von Isoproterenol verursachten − Überladung mit Radiocalcium durch prophylaktische Verabreichung von Verapamil, D 600 oder Prenylamin. ^{45}Ca-Netto-Aufnahme in das Myocard des rechten Ventrikels von Ratten innerhalb von 6 Stunden nach Applikation von Radiocalcium (10 µCi ^{45}Ca/kg intraperitoneal) unter dem Einfluß von 0,01 − 100 mg Isoproterenol allein bzw. von 0,01 − 100 mg Isoproterenol + Ca^{++}-Antagonisten (Verapamil: 17 mg/kg s.c.; D 600: 10 mg/kg s.c. oder Prenylamin: 250 mg/kg s.c.) [1, 2, 7]

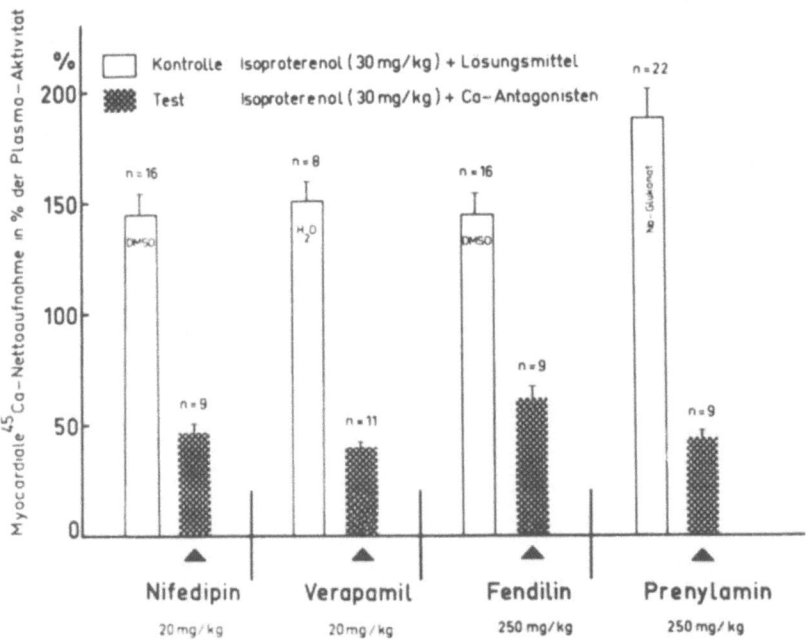

Abb. 20. Hemmung der Isoproterenol-bedingten ^{45}Ca-Überladung des rechten Ventrikelmyocards von Ratten durch gleichzeitige subkutane Verabreichung der Ca^{++}-Antagonisten Nifedipin, Verapamil, Fendilin oder Prenylamin. Die Ca^{++}-Antagonisten wurden jeweils 24 Std und $\frac{1}{2}$ Std vor der Isoproterenol-Gabe in der angegebenen Dosis appliziert. Messung der ^{45}Ca-Inkorporation 6 Std nach der Isoproterenol-Injektion

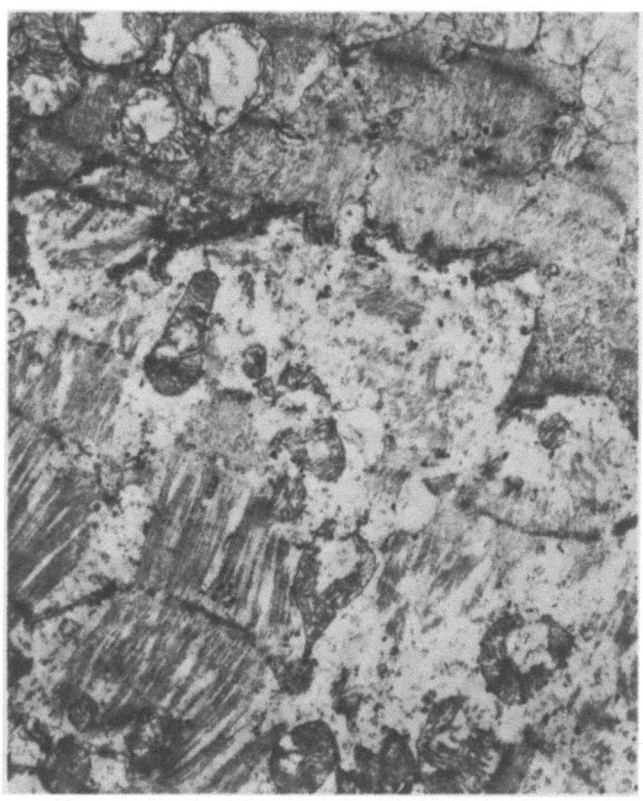

Abb. 21. Schwere Zerstörungen der Myofibrillen-Struktur und der Mitochondrien in einer Faser aus dem rechten Ventrikelmyocard einer Ratte. Abriß der teilweise zerfallenen Myofilamente vom Z-Streifen 6 Std nach alleiniger Injektion von 30 mg/kg Isoproterenol [48]

fache Reduktion des Ca^{++}-Angebots (Senkung der extrazellulären Ca^{++}-Konzentration mittels Calcitonin) wirkt einer Ca^{++}-Überladung des Myocards − und damit der Nekrose-Entstehung − entgegen. Umgekehrt erfährt die Cardiotoxizität hoher Dosen von Catecholaminen, Vitamin D_3 und Dihydrotachysterol eine beträchtliche Potenzierung, wenn infolge eines erhöhten extrazellulären Ca^{++}-Spiegels oder aufgrund eines gleichzeitig bestehenden alimentären K^+- bzw. Mg^{++}-Defizits die intrazelluläre Bindung von Ca^{++} begünstigt wird (Abb. 24).

Wir haben diese Kausalzusammenhänge zwischen Ca^{++}-Überladung des Myocards und Nekrose-Entstehung sowie die entgegengerichteten cardioprotektiven Grundwirkungen der Ca^{++}-Antagonisten in den letzten 10 Jahren in einer größeren Reihe von Experimentalarbeiten hinreichend begründet (Fleckenstein [1, 2, 40]; Fleckenstein, Döring u. Leder [45]; Fleckenstein, Janke, Döring u. Leder [46 − 48]; Fleckenstein, Janke, Döring u. Pachinger [44]; Janke, Fleckenstein, Hein, Leder u. Sigel [49]). Eine nochmalige detaillierte Wiedergabe unserer eigenen Befunde erübrigt sich daher. Dagegen erscheint es wichtig, auf neuere Ergebnisse einiger anderer Arbeitsgruppen hinzuweisen, bei denen die Nekrose-Entstehung aufgrund einer intrazellulären Ca^{++}-Akkumulation ebenfalls als pathogenetisches Prinzip zutage getreten ist. So konnte Lossnitzer − teilweise in Zusammenarbeit mit unserem In-

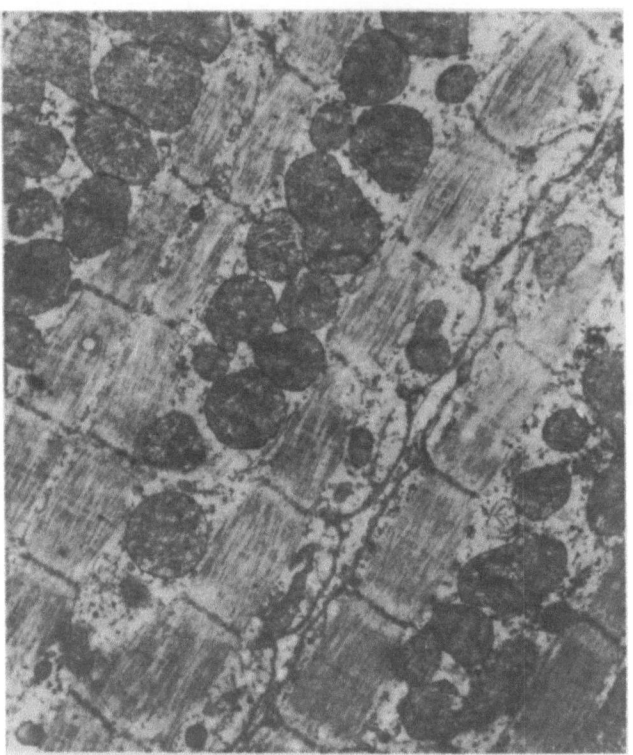

Abb. 22. Verhütung der Isoproterenol-bedingten Faser-Nekrosen bei gleichzeitiger Injektion von 30 mg/kg Isoproterenol *und* 50 mg/kg Verapamil. Das elektronenoptische Bild wurde ebenfalls nach 6 Std Einwirkung von Isoproterenol gewonnen – jedoch unter dem Schutz von Verapamil [48]

stitut (vgl. Lossnitzer u. Mitarb. [50]) – den Nachweis führen, daß die spontan einsetzende Entwicklung von Myocardnekrosen bei hereditär cardiomyopathischen syrischen Hamstern schon in der prä-nekrotischen Phase an einer intrazellulären Ca^{++}-Anreicherung erkennbar ist. Daher war es in den Experimenten von Lossnitzer [51] sowie von Jasmin und Bajusz [52] bzw. Jasmin und Solymoss [53] möglich, mit Hilfe einer länger dauernden prophylaktischen Verabreichung von Verapamil und anderen Ca^{++}-Antagonisten die exzessive Ca^{++}-Akkumulation bereits im pränekrotischen Stadium zu verhindern. Dementsprechend blieben die Herzen der cardiomyopathischen Hamster auch im späteren Verlauf völlig frei von Nekrosen. Auf der gleichen Basis lassen sich schließlich auch die cardioprotektiven Effekte von Verapamil bzw. Nifedipin an hypoxischen und ischämischen Herzen erklären, die neuerdings von Nayler u. Mitarb. [54], sowie von Henry u. Mitarb. [55] beschrieben worden sind. Offenbar ist das pathogenetische Prinzip der intrazellulären Ca^{++}-Überladung mit seinen schweren Konsequenzen für die Mitochondrien-Funktion und Mitochondrien-Struktur selbst bei der Produktion ischämischer Myocardläsionen im Spiel. Ca^{++}-Antagonisten besitzen daher sogar bei Myocard-Ischämie cardioprotektive Potenzen. Frau Professor Winifred Nayler und die Herren Kollegen Lossnitzer, Jasmin und Henry haben es in dankenswerter Weise selbst übernom-

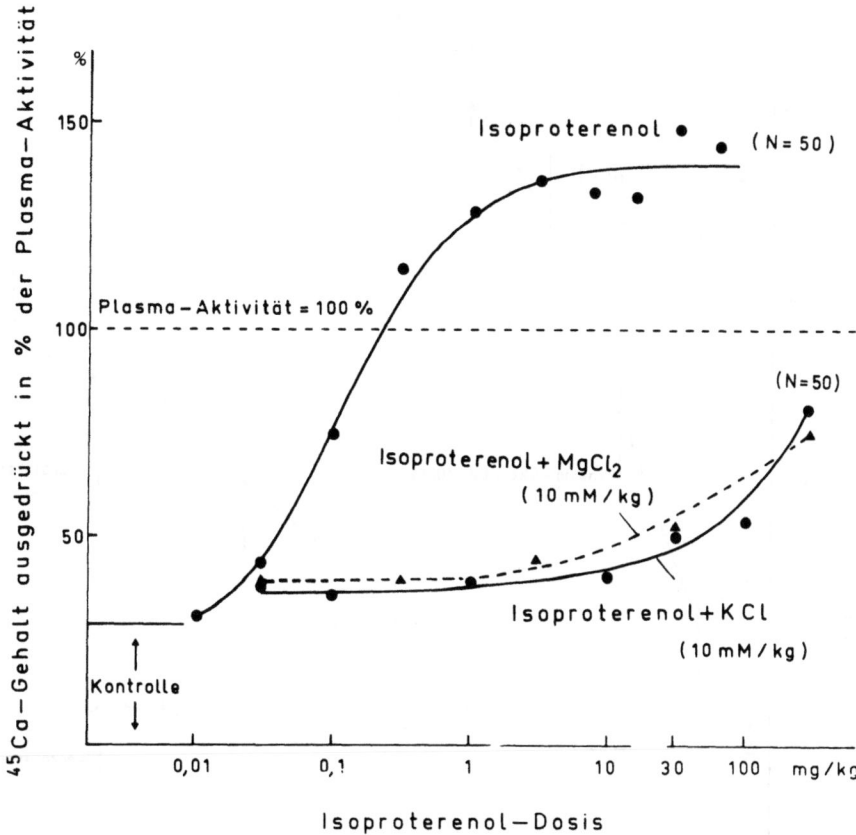

Abb. 23. Schutz des Ratten-Myocards (Innenschicht des linken Ventrikels im Bereich der Herzspitze) vor der Isoproterenol-induzierten Überladung mit Radiocalcium durch einmalige orale Verabreichung von jeweils 10 mM/kg KCl bzw. MgCl$_2$ mit der Schlundsonde. Kalium- und Magnesium-Salze können offenbar als physiologische Ca^{++}-Antagonisten die Isoproterenol-bedingte Ca^{++}-Akkumulation in den Myocardfasern im Bereich niedriger Isoproterenol-Dosen vollständig verhindern [1, 2, 7]

men, ihre diesbezüglichen Forschungsergebnisse im Rahmen dieses Symposiums zu präsentieren.

Die Ergebnisse der Tierexperimente liefern eine rationelle Grundlage für die weitgefächerte Anwendung der Ca^{++}-Antagonisten in der Klinik. Auch beim Einsatz als cardiovaskuläre Therapeutika lassen die Ca^{++}-Antagonisten bekanntlich ein breites Wirkungsspektrum erkennen; sie sind antianginös, antiarrhythmisch, antihypertensiv und cardioprotektiv. Neben Gemeinsamkeiten im klinischen Wirkungs-Profil sind dabei auch gewisse Besonderheiten einzelner Ca^{++}-Antagonisten zu diskutieren. Die Ca^{++}-Antagonisten sind sicherlich keine ein-eiigen Zwillinge – weder im Hinblick auf chemische Struktur, noch hinsichtlich aller ihrer pharmakologischen Eigenschaften. Trotzdem sind die in Tabelle 1 aufgeführten Ca^{++}-Antagonisten als Mitglieder einer neuen pharmakologischen Familie im Grunde eng verwandt. Der Sinn des vorliegenden Referats ist, diese fundamentalen Gemeinsamkeiten im Wirkungsmechanismus am Beispiel der Herz-Effekte von Ca^{++}-Antagonisten darzulegen.

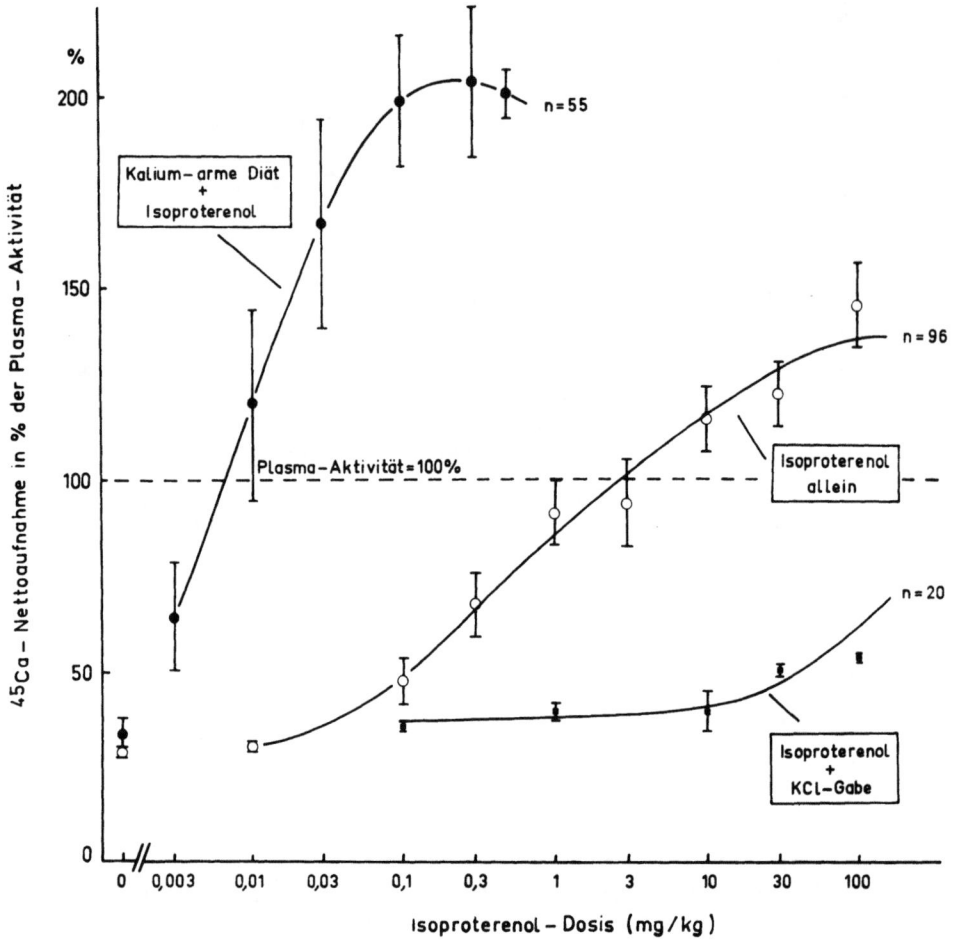

Abb. 24. Abhängigkeit der Isoproterenol-induzierten Radiocalcium-Inkorporation in die Innenschicht des linken Ventrikels von der alimentären Kalium-Zufuhr: Nach 14tägiger Verabreichung einer K^+-armen Diät konnte der K^+-Gehalt des Plasmas bei 55 Ratten auf etwa die Hälfte der Norm gesenkt werden. Bei diesen Tieren führen schon kleinste – normalerweise unwirksame Isoproterenol-Dosen – zu einer extremen Steigerung der Radiocalcium-Inkorporation. Umgekehrt wird, wie bereits in Abb. 23 dargestellt, die Isoproterenol-bedingte Radiocalcium-Aufnahme ins Ratten-Myocard durch zusätzliche Gaben von Kalium-Salzen weitgehend blockiert. Die Radiocalcium-Inkorporation nach Isoproterenol-Gaben bei Normal-Diät zeigt einen intermediären Verlauf. Am linken Ventrikel von Ratten läßt sich die Wirkungsstärke von Isoproterenol – gemessen an der Radiocalcium-Inkorporation – durch alimentäre Kalium-Verarmung oder Kalium-Beladung annähernd im Verhältnis 1:1000 modifizieren (Fleckenstein, Janke u. Frey, unveröffentlicht)

Zusammenfassung

Nach unseren seit 1963 laufenden Untersuchungen sind die Coronartherapeutika Verapamil, D 600, Prenylamin, Nifedipin, Niludipin, Fendilin, Perhexilin u.a. als Repräsentanten einer neuen pharmakologischen Stoffklasse anzusehen, deren molekularer Wirkungsmechanismus auf einem Ca^{++}-antagonistischen Eingriff in die elektro-mechanischen Koppelungsprozesse der Myocardfasern und der glatten Gefäßmuskelzellen beruht. Zur Kennzeichnung des gemeinsamen Wirkungsmodus von Stoffen dieser Art haben wir daher 1969 die Gruppenbezeichnung „Calcium-Antagonisten" introduziert. Das Wirkungsspektrum der Ca^{++}-Antagonisten als cardiovaskuläre Therapeutika ist breit und erstreckt sich auf alle physiologischen und pathophysiologischen Prozesse in den Myocardfasern, Schrittmacher-Zentren und glatten Gefäßmuskelzellen, bei denen Ca^{++}-Ionen eine Schlüsselrolle spielen.

Der entscheidende Eingriff der Ca^{++}-Antagonisten in die elektromechanischen Koppelungsprozesse der erregten Myocardfasern besteht in einer Dosis-abhängigen Reduktion des transmembranären Ca^{++}-Einstroms durch die sog. „langsamen Kanäle". Hierdurch bedingt, transformiert die Ca^{++}-aktivierbare Myofibrillen-ATPase im Augenblick der Erregung weniger Phosphat-gebundene Energie in mechanische Arbeit. Die Reduktion der ATP-Spaltung führt dabei zu einer Zügelung der kontraktilen Funktion und zu einer Dämpfung des für die ATP-Resynthese benötigten oxidativen Tätigkeitsstoffwechsels. Dabei ließ sich im Experiment an isolierten Papillarmuskeln unter dem Einfluß von Ca^{++}-Antagonisten zeigen, daß zwischen der Verminderung a) des transmembranären Ca^{++}-Influx, b) der ATP-Spaltung am kontraktilen System, c) der isometrischen Gipfelspannung und d) des Tätigkeits-bedingten O_2-Verbrauchs eine weitgehend lineare Beziehung besteht. Extra-Calcium, β-adrenerge Sympathomimetika und Herzglykoside heben diese Effekte der Ca^{++}-Antagonisten durch Verbesserung der Ca^{++}-Versorgung des kontraktilen Systems wieder auf. Der oxidative Ruhestoffwechsel des nicht-schlagenden Herzens wird dagegen von den Ca^{++}-Antagonisten nicht betroffen.

Die Aktionspotentiale des Vorhof- und Ventrikelmyocards sowie des Hisschen Bündels und der Purkinje-Fasern sind im wesentlichen Na^+-abhängig und infolgedessen gegenüber Ca^{++}-Antagonisten weitgehend resistent. Im Gegensatz dazu werden für die Elektrogenese der automatischen Schrittmacher-Potentiale im Sinus- und AV-Knoten sowie für die AV-Überleitung Ca^{++}-Ionen obligatorisch als transmembranäre Ladungsträger benötigt. Ca^{++}-Antagonisten können daher in geeigneter Konzentration durch Reduktion des transmembranären Ca^{++}-Influx auch die Automatie-Funktion der supraventrikulären Schrittmacher ebenso wie die Erregungsleitung im AV-Knoten hemmen. Auf ektopische Automatie-Zentren im supraventrikulären Bereich wirken Ca^{++}-Antagonisten offenbar in analoger Weise dämpfend.

Darüber hinaus besitzen Ca^{++}-Antagonisten direkte cardioprotektive Effekte, indem sie einer pathologischen Anreicherung von Ca^{++}-Ionen im Faserinnern entgegenwirken. Zahlreiche zu Myocardnekrosen führende Noxen (sympathische Überstimulation, Stress-Belastung; Überdosierung von Vitamin D_3, Dihydrotachysterol (AT 10), 9α-Fluorcortisolacetat; alimentärer K^+- und Mg^{++}-Mangel; genetische Defekte wie z. B. bei der hereditären Cardiomyopathie des syrischen Hamsters) können die Ca^{++}-Aufnahme ins Faserinnere extrem potenzieren. Hierdurch wird a) eine exzessive Aktivierung intrazellulärer ATPasen und b) eine Ca^{++}-bedingte Schädigung der Mitochondrien verursacht. Hieraus resultiert dann eine deletäre Erschöpfung der ATP- und Kreatinphosphat-Bestände, die schließlich – ähnlich wie nach Hypoxie oder Ischämie – zu Myocardnekrosen führt. Mit Hilfe von Ca^{++}-Antagonisten läßt sich auch diese fatale Ca^{++}-Überladung – und damit der energetische und strukturelle Zusammenbruch der Myocardfasern – verhindern.

Literatur

1. Fleckenstein A (1971) Specific inhibitors and promoters of calcium action in the excitation-contraction coupling of heart muscle and their role in the prevention or production of myocardial lesions. In: Harris P, Opie L (eds) Calcium and the Heart, Proceedings of the meeting of the European Section of the International Study Group for Research in Cardiac Metabolism, held in the Institute of Cardiology, London, on Sept. 6, 1970. Academic Press, London New York, pp 135 – 188
2. Fleckenstein A (1971) Neuere Ergebnisse zur Physiologie, Pharmakologie und Pathologie der elektro-mechanischen Koppelungsprozesse im Warmblütermyokard. In: Keidel WD, Plattig, K-H (Hrsg) Vorträge der Erlanger Physiologentagung 1970. Springer, Berlin Heidelberg New York, S 13 – 52
3. Fleckenstein A (1972) Physiologie und Pharmakologie der transmembranären Natrium-, Kalium- und Calcium-Bewegungen. Arzneimittel-Forsch. (Drug Res.) 22:2019 – 2028
4. Fleckenstein A (1975) Fundamentale Herz- und Gefäßwirkungen Ca^{++}-antagonistischer Koronar-therapeutika. Med Klin 70:1665 – 1674
5. Fleckenstein A (1977) Specific pharmacology of calcium in myocardium, cardiac pacemakers, and vascular smooth muscle. Ann Rev Pharmacol Toxicol 17:149 – 166
6. Fleckenstein A, Tritthart H, Döring HJ, Byon YK (1972) Bay a 1040 – ein hochaktiver Ca^{++}-antagonistischer Inhibitor der elektro-mechanischen Koppelungsprozesse im Warmblütermyokard. Arzneim Forsch 22:22 – 33
7. Fleckenstein A, Döring HJ, Janke J, Byon YK (1975) Basic actions of ions and drugs on myocardial high-energy phosphate metabolism and contractility. In: Schmier J, Eichler O (Hrsg) Heart and Circulation. Springer, Berlin Heidelberg New York (Handbuch der experimentellen Pharmakologie, vol XVI/3, pp 345 – 405)
8. Fleckenstein A (1964) Die Bedeutung der energiereichen Phosphate für Kontraktilität und Tonus des Myokards. Verh Dtsch Ges Inn Med 70:81 – 99
9. Fleckenstein A, Kammermeier H, Döring HJ, Freund HJ (1967) Zum Wirkungsmechanismus neu-artiger Koronardilatatoren mit gleichzeitig Sauerstoff-einsparenden Myokard-Effekten, Prenylamin und Iproveratril. Z Kreislaufforsch 56:716 – 744,839 – 858
10. Fleckenstein A, Tritthart H, Fleckenstein B Jr, Herbst A, Grün G (1969) A new group of competitive Ca-antagonists (Iproveratril, D 600, prenylamine) with highly potent inhibitory effects on excitation-contraction coupling in mammalian myocardium. Pfluegers Arch 307:R25
11. Lindner E (1960) Phenyl-propyl-diphenyl-propyl-amin, eine neue Substanz mit coronargefäßerwei-ternder Wirkung. Arzneim Forsch 10:569 – 573
12. Haas H, Härtfelder G (1962) α-Isopropyl-α-(N-methyl-homoveratryl)-γ-aminopropyl-3,4-dimeth-oxy-phenylacetonitril, eine Substanz mit coronargefäßerweiternden Eigenschaften. Arzneim Forsch 12:549 – 558
13. Haas H, Busch E (1967) Vergleichende Untersuchungen der Wirkung von α-Isopropyl-α-(N-methyl-N-homoveratryl)-γ-aminopropyl)-3,4-dimethoxy-phenyl-acetonitril, seiner Derivate sowie einiger anderer Coronardilatatoren und β-Receptor-affiner Substanzen. Arzneim Forsch 17:257 – 271
14. Vater W, Kroneberg G, Hoffmeister F, Kaller H, Meng K, Oberdorf A, Puls, W, Schloßmann K, Stoepel K (1972) Zur Pharmakologie von 4-(2′ Nitrophenyl)-2,6-dimethyl-1,4-dihydropyridin-3,5-dicarbonsäuredimethylester (Nifedipin, Bay a 1040). Arzneim Forsch 22:1 – 14
15. Fleckenstein A, Fleckenstein-Grün G, Byon YK (1977) Fundamentale Herz- und Gefäßwirkungen des Ca^{++}-antagonistischen Koronartherapeutikums Fendilin (Sensit®). Arzneim Forsch 27:562 – 571
16. Fleckenstein-Grün G, Fleckenstein A, Byon YK, Kim KW (1978) Mechanism of action of Ca-antagonists in the treatment of coronary disease with special reference to perhexiline maleate. In: Proc. of a Symposium on Perhexiline Maleate, Strasbourg, France, Sept. 18, 1976. Excerpta Medica, Amsterdam, pp 1 – 22
17. Nakajima H, Hoshiyama M, Yamashita K, Kiyomoto A (1975) Effect of diltiazem on electrical and mechanical activity of isolated cardiac ventricular muscle of guinea pig. Japan J Pharmacol 25:383 – 392
18. Fleckenstein A, Fleckenstein-Grün G, Byon YK, Haastert HP, Späh F (1979) Vergleichende Untersuchungen über die Ca^{++}-antagonistischen Grundwirkungen von Niludipin (Bay a 7168) und Nifedipin (Bay a 1040) auf Myokard, Myometrium und glatte Gefäßmuskulatur. Arzneim Forsch 29:230 – 246
19. Fleckenstein A (1968a) Experimental heart failure due to disturbances in high-energy phosphate metabolism. Proc. Vth Eur. Congr. Cardiol. Athens, Sept. 1968, pp 255 – 269

20. Kohlhardt M, Bauer B, Krause H, Fleckenstein A (1972) Differentiation of the transmembrane Na and Ca channels in mammalian cardiac fibres by the use of specific inhibitors. Pfluegers Arch 335:309–322

21 Nayler WG, Szeto J (1972) Effect of verapamil on contractility, oxygen utilization and calcium exchangeability in mammalian heart muscle. Cardiovasc Res 6:120–128

22. Entman ML, Allen JC, Bornet EP, Gillette PC, Wallick ET, Schwartz A (1972) Mechanisms of calcium accumulation and transport in cardiac relaxing system (sarcoplasmic reticulum membranes): Effects of verapamil, D 600, X537A and A23187. J Mol Cell Cardiol 4:681–687

23. Watanabe AM, Besch HR (1974) Subcellular myocardial effects of verapamil and D 600: comparison with propranolol. J Pharmacol Exp Ther 191:241–251

24. Frey M, Janke J (1975) The effect of organic Ca-antagonists (verapamil, prenylamine) on the calcium transport system in isolated mitochondria of rat cardiac muscle. Pfluegers Arch 359:R26

25. Byon YK, Fleckenstein A (1969) Parallele Beeinflussung von isometrischer Spannungsentwicklung und O_2-Verbrauch isolierter Papillarmuskeln unter dem Einfluß von Ca^{++}-Ionen, Adrenalin, Isoproterenol und organischen Ca^{++}-Antagonisten (Iproveratril, D 600, Prenylamin). Pfluegers Arch 312:R8/9

26. Haastert HP, Fleckenstein A (1975) Ca-dependence of supraventricular pacemaker activity and its responsiveness to Ca-antagonistic compounds (verapamil, D 600, nifedipine). Naunyn-Schmiedebergs Arch Pharmacol [Suppl]:287R39

27. Refsum H, Landmark K (1975) The effect of a calcium-antagonistic drug, nifedipine, on the mechanical and electrical activity of the isolated rat atrium. Acta Pharmacol Toxicol (Kbh) 37:369–376

28. Zipes DP, Fischer JC (1974) Effects of agents which inhibit the slow channel on sinus node automaticity and atrioventricular conduction in the dog. Circ Res 34:184–192

29. Tritthart H, Fleckenstein B Jr, Fleckenstein A (1970) Some fundamental actions of antiarrhythmic drugs on the excitability and the contractility of single myocardial fibres. Naunyn Schmiedebergs Arch Pharmacol 269:212–219

30. Wit AL, Cranefield PF (1974) Effect of verapamil on the sinoatrial and atrioventricular nodes of the rabbit and the mechanism by which it arrests reentrant atrioventricular nodal tachycardia. Circ Res 35:413–425

31. Kohlhardt M, Figulla H-R, Tripathi O (1976) The slow membrane channel as the predominant mediator of the excitation process of the sinoatrial pacemaker cell. Basic Res Cardiol 71:17–26

32. Bender F (1967) Isoptin® zur Behandlung der tachykarden Form des Vorhofflatterns. Med Klin 62:634–636

33. Schamroth L, Krikler DM, Garrett C (1972) Immediate effects of intravenous verapamil in cardiac arrhythmias. Br Med J I:660–662

34. Spurrell RAJ, Krikler DM, Sowton E (1974) Effects of verapamil on electrophysiological properties of anomalous atrioventricular connexion in Wolf-Parkinson-White syndrome. Br Heart J 36:256–264

35. Härtel G, Hartikainen M (1976) Comparison of verapamil and practolol in paroxysmal supraventricular tachycardia. Eur J Cardiol 4:87–90

36. Singh BN, Vaughan-Williams EM (1972) A fourth class of anti-dysrhythmic action? Effect of verapamil on ouabain toxicity, on atrial and ventricular and intracellular potentials and on other features of cardiac function. Cardiovasc Res 6:109–119

37. Taira N, Narimatsu A (1975) Effects of nifedipine, a potent calcium-antagonistic coronary vasodilator, on atrioventricular conduction and blood flow in the isolated atrioventricular node preparation of the dog. Naunyn Schmiedebergs Arch Pharmacol 290:107–112

38. Bender F (1970) Die Behandlung der tachykarden Arrythmien und der arteriellen Hypertonie mit Verapamil. Arzneim Forsch 20:1310–1316

39. Refsum H (1975) Calcium-antagonistic and anti-arrhythmic effects of nifedipine on the isolated rat atrium. Acta Pharmacol Toxicol (Kbh) 37:377–386

40. Fleckenstein A (1968b) Myokardstoffwechsel und Nekrose. Referat anläßlich des VI. Symposiums der Deutschen Gesellschaft für Fortschritte auf dem Gebiet der Inneren Medizin, Freiburg, 8.–9. Nov. 1968. In: Heilmeyer L, Holtmeier HJ (Hrsg) Herzinfarkt und Schock. Thieme, Stuttgart, S 94–109

41. Selye H (1960) Elektrolyte, Stress und Herznekrose. Benno Schwabe, Basel

42. Bajusz E (1963) Conditioning factors for cardiac necroses. Karger, Basel New York

43. Rona G, Chappel CI, Kahn DS (1963) The significance of factors modifying the development of isoproterenol-induced myocardial necrosis. Amer Heart J 66:389–395

44. Fleckenstein A, Janke J, Döring HJ, Pachinger O (1973) Ca overload as the determinant factor in the production of catecholamine-induced myocardial lesions. In: Cardiomyopathies. Recent advances in studies on cardiac structure and metabolism, vol 2. Bajusz E, Rona G (eds). University Park Press, Baltimore London Tokyo, pp 455 – 466

45. Fleckenstein A, Döring HJ, Leder O (1969) The significance of high-energy phosphate exhaustion in the etiology of isoproterenol-induced cardiac necroses and its prevention by iproveratril, compound D 600 of prenylamine. In: Lamarche M, Royer R (eds) Symposium international on drugs and metabolism of myocardium and striated muscle. Nancy, pp 11 – 22

46. Fleckenstein A, Janke J, Döring HJ, Leder O (1971) Die intrazelluläre Überladung mit Kalzium als entscheidender Kausalfaktor bei der Entstehung nicht-coronarogener Myokard-Nekrosen. Verh Dtsch Ges Kreislaufforsch 37:345 – 353

47. Fleckenstein A, Janke J, Döring HJ, Leder O (1974) Myocardial fibre necrosis due to intracellular Ca overload – a new principle in cardiac pathophysiology. In: Dhalla NS (eds) Myocardial biology. Recent advances in studies on cardiac structure and metabolism, vol 4. University Park Press, Baltimore London Tokyo, pp 563 – 579

48. Fleckenstein A, Janke J, Döring HJ, Leder O (1975) The key-role of Ca in the production of non-coronarogenic myocardial necroses. In: Fleckenstein A a. Rona G (eds) Pathophysiology and morphology of myocardial cell alterations. Recent advances in studies on cardiac structure and metabolism, vol 6. University Park Press, Baltimore London Tokyo, pp 21 – 32

49. Janke J, Fleckenstein A, Hein B, Leder O, Sigel H (1975) Prevention of myocardial Ca overload and necrotization by Mg and K salts or acidosis. In: Fleckenstein A a. Rona G (eds) Pathophysiology and morphology of myocardial cell alterations. Recent advances in studies on cardiac structure and metabolism, vol 6. University Park Press, Baltimore London Tokyo, pp 33 – 42

50. Lossnitzer K, Janke H, Hein B, Stauch M, Fleckenstein A (1975) Disturbed myocardial calcium metabolism: A possible pathogenetic factor in the hereditary cardiomyopathy of the Syrian hamster. In: Fleckenstein A a. Rona G (eds) Pathophysiology and morphology of myocardial cell alterations. Recent advances in studies on cardiac structure and metabolism, vol 6. University Park Press, Baltimore London Tokyo, pp 207 – 218

51. Lossnitzer K (1975) Genetic induction of a cardiomyopathy. In: Schmier J, Eicher O (eds) Heart and Circulation. Springer, Berlin Heidelberg New York. Handbuch der experimentellen Pharmakologie, vol XVI/3 pp 309 – 344

52. Jasmin G, Bajusz E (1973) Polymyopathie et cardiomyopathie héréditaire chez le hamster de Syrie. Inhibition sélective des lésion du myocarde. Ann Anat Pathol 18:49

53. Jasmin G, Solymoss B (1975) Prevention of hereditary cardiomyopathy in the hamster by Verapamil and other agents. Proc Soc Exp Biol Med 149:193

54. Nayler WG, Grau A, Slade A (1976) A protective effect of verapamil on hypoxic heart muscle. Cardiovasc Res 10:650 – 662

55. Henry PD, Shuchleib R, Borda LJ, Roberts R, Williamson JR, Sobel BE (1978) Effects of nifedipine on myocardial perfusion and ischemic injury in dogs. Circ Res 43:372 – 380

56. Antoni H, Engstfeld G, Fleckenstein A (1960) Inotrope Effekte von ATP und Adrenalin am hypo-dynamen Froschmyokard nach elektro-mechanischer Entkoppelung durch Ca^{++}-Entzug. Pfluegers Arch 272:91 – 106

Nachweis einer strengen quantitativen Korrelation zwischen Hemmung des transmembranären Calcium-Influx und der mechanischen Spannungsentwicklung des Myocards unter dem Einfluß verschiedener Calcium-Antagonisten[1]

F. Späh und A. Fleckenstein

Das Aktionspotential einer Säugetier-Myocardfaser wird bekanntlich unter Normalbedingungen durch den raschen transmembranären Einstrom von Na^+-Ionen eingeleitet, während der anschließende Influx von Ca^{++}-Ionen durch den sog. „langsamen Kanal" den mechanischen Akt der Kontraktion in Gang bringt. Im Experiment läßt sich jedoch diese klare Arbeitsteilung zwischen den Na^+- und Ca^{++}-Ionen dadurch wieder beseitigen, daß man die Myocardfaser partiell depolarisiert. Durch diese Maßnahme wird das rasche Carriersystem für Na^+ inaktiviert, während der langsame Transportmechanismus für die Ca^{++}-Ionen seine Funktion beibehält. Solche partiell depolarisierten Myocardfasern sind trotz eines Membranpotentials von nur noch $40-45$ mV weiterhin zur Bildung von fortgeleiteten Aktionspotentialen befähigt. Anstelle der Na^+-Ionen fungieren jetzt jedoch die Ca^{++}-Ionen als elektrische Ladungsträger des transmembranären Einwärtsstroms. Daher kommt es bei solchen partiell depolarisierten Myocardfasern nach Überführung in ein Ca^{++}-armes Milieu nicht nur zu einem Verlust der Kontraktilität, sondern auch zu einem Zusammenbruch der bioelektrischen Aktivität (vgl. hierzu [1-3]).

Es ist nach diesen Ergebnissen nicht überraschend, daß Ca^{++}-Antagonisten, die den transmembranären Ca^{++}-Einstrom in die erregten Myocardfasern blockieren, auch an partiell depolarisierten Myocardfasern die Effekte eines einfachen Ca^{++}-Entzugs täuschend ähnlich imitieren können. Tatsächlich verlieren partiell depolarisierte Myocardfasern unter dem Einfluß von Ca^{++}-Antagonisten gleichzeitig mit der Fähigkeit zur Kontraktion auch diejenige zur Bildung von fortgeleiteten Aktionspotentialen − genau so wie nach einfachem Ca^{++}-Entzug. Tritthart u. Mitarb. [4], sowie Kohlhardt u. Fleckenstein [5] haben hierauf schon früher unter Verwendung von Verapamil, D 600 und Nifedipin aufmerksam gemacht.

Die Untersuchungen, über die im folgenden berichtet wird, waren dazu bestimmt, die bisher vorliegenden Ergebnisse weiter zu präzisieren und dabei zu klären:

1. ob auch andere Ca^{++}-Antagonisten (Diltiazem, Prenylamin, Fendilin, Perhexilin maleat u.a.) nach dem gleichen prinzipiellen Schema wie Verapamil, D 600 und Nifedipin wirken, und

2. ob dabei eine bestimmte quantitative Hemmung des transmembranären Ca^{++}-Einstroms (jeweils am Ca^{++}-Aktionspotential ablesbar) stets auch eine ganz bestimmte Abnahme der mechanischen Spannungsentwicklung zur Folge hat − unabhängig davon, welcher spezielle Ca^{++}-Antagonist verwendet wird.

---

1 Eine vorläufige Mitteilung der vorliegenden Ergebnisse erfolgte anläßlich der 50. Tagung (Herbsttagung) der Deutsch. Physiol. Ges. (3.−6. Oktober 1978) in Göttingen, vgl. Pfluegers Arch − Eur J Physiol, Suppl to vol 377, R4 (1978)

Methodik

Papillarmuskeln (Durchmesser: 0,6 mm; Länge: 4−6 mm) wurden aus dem rechten Ventrikel von Meerschweinchen-Herzen exzidiert. Die Basis der Papillarmuskeln wurde am Boden einer kleinen Perfusions-Kammer (Gesamtvolumen: 0,6 ml) befestigt, während das sehnige Ende für isometrische Spannungsmessungen mit einer mechano-elektrischen Transducer-Röhre (Typ: SS 201, Collins Corp., Long Beach, California, USA) verbunden wurde. Die Perfusionslösungen wurden mit 97% O_2 und 3% CO_2 durchperlt. Das Durchströmungsvolumen betrug das 10fache der Perfusions-Kammer, d. h. 6 ml/min. Die Papillarmuskeln wurden mit Rechteck-Impulsen fortlaufend gereizt (Impuls-Dauer: 3−4 msec; Impuls-Frequenz: 30/min). Nach einer Equilibrierungs-Periode von 30 min bei 30°C und einem pH-Wert von 7,4 in normaler Tyrode-Lösung (NaCl: 155 mM; KCl: 4 mM; $CaCl_2$: 2 mM; $MgCl_2$: 1 mM; Glukose: 6 mM; $NaHCO_3$: 11,4 mM; NaH_2PO_4: 0,38 mM) wurde der optimale Dehnungsgrad bestimmt, bei dem die Kontraktionskraft ein Maximum erreichte. Anschließend wurden flexibel montierte Glas-Mikroelektroden von konventioneller Bauart eingestochen und die bioelektrischen Phänomene zusammen mit der mechanischen Aktivität auf einem Oszilloskop (TEKTRONIX 205A) fortlaufend verfolgt. Zusätzlich wurde ein Speicher-Oszilloskop (TEKTRONIX 5115) intermittierend eingesetzt, um die einzelnen Phasen des Versuchsablaufs für die spätere Auswertung fotografisch festzuhalten. Gleichzeitig wurde die Aufstrichsgeschwindigkeit (dV/dt_{max}) des Aktionspotentials durch Differenzierung mit einem Analogrechner fortlaufend mitgeschrieben (möglicher Fehler im Bereich zwischen 1 und 1000 V/sec weniger als 1%). Wenn sich die elektrischen Parameter der angestochenen Myocardfasern in normaler Ringer-Lösung für mehr als $\frac{1}{2}$ Std. stabilisiert hatten, wurde zur partiellen Depolarisation auf eine K^+-reiche Tyrode-Lösung (19 mM K^+) für weitere 30 min umgeschaltet. Anschließend begann das eigentliche Experiment. Der Wechsel von der normalen auf die K^+-reiche Tyrode-Lösung führte regelmäßig zu einer etwa 8fachen Erhöhung der elektrischen Reizschwelle. Die während der Experimente gewählte Reizstärke entsprach jeweils der doppelten Schwellen-Spannung. In der K^+-reichen (19 mM) Tyrode-Lösung war die NaCl-Konzentration auf 140 mM reduziert, um eine normale Osmolarität beizubehalten. Alle Experimente, in denen ein Dauer-Einstich für die Zeit von etwa 2 Stunden an ein und derselben Einzelfaser nicht gelang, wurden verworfen.

Ergebnisse

Aus Abb. 1a ist im Detail zu ersehen, wie das Meerschweinchen-Myocard nach vorausgegangener partieller Depolarisation in K^+-reicher Tyrode-Lösung reagiert, wenn man die extrazelluläre Ca^{++}-Konzentration von 2 mM auf 0,4 mM, d. h. auf $\frac{1}{5}$ der Norm, senkt. Die obere Kurve (Differenzierungskurve der Ca^{++}-getragenen Aktionspotentiale) zeigt dabei die maximalen Aufstrichs-Geschwindigkeiten − als Indiz für die Geschwindigkeit des transmembranären Ca^{++}-Einstroms an. Im mittleren Bildabschnitt sind die Aktionspotentiale während eines intracellulären Dauer-Einstichs an ein und derselben Myocardfaser registriert. Darunter sind die dazugehörigen Mechanogramme des Papillarmuskels wiedergegeben. Die im Zeitabstand von 3, 6, 9 und 12 min aufgezeichneten Kurvenscharen demonstrieren die Folgen des

Ca⁺⁺-Entzug

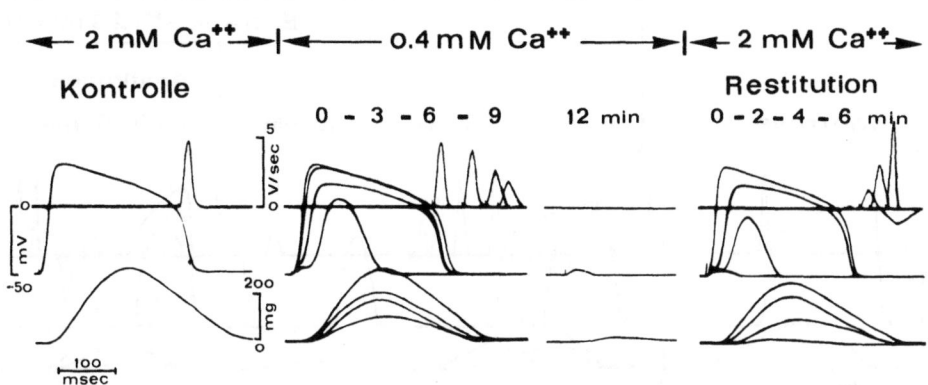

Abb. 1a–f. Abnahme der Aufstrichgeschwindigkeit ($dV/dt_{max.}$) jeweils in der oberen Zeile, der Höhe und Dauer der Ca^{++}-vermittelten Aktionspotentiale in der mittleren Zeile sowie der isometrischen Gipfelspannung in der unteren Zeile nach extracellulärem Ca^{++}-Entzug oder nach Zusatz von Ca^{++}-Antagonisten an partiell depolarisierten Meerschweinchen-Papillarmuskeln in K^+-reicher Tyrodelösung ($K_e = 19$ mM). a Senkung der extracellulären Ca^{++}-Konzentration von 2 mM auf 0,4 mM.

b Einwirkung von Nifedipin
c Einwirkung von D 600
d Einwirkung von Verapamil
e Einwirkung von Fendilin

Extracellulärer Ca^{++}-Gehalt = 2 mM

In Teilabbildung **a** erfolgt eine weitgehende Restitution der Ca^{++}-abhängigen Aktionspotentiale und der Kontraktilität nach Rückkehr in normale Tyrodelösung mit 2 mM Ca^{++}.
In den Teilabbildungen **b – e** wurde der Effekt der Ca^{++}-Antagonisten durch Zusatz von Extra-Calcium (Steigerung der extracellulären Ca^{++}-Konzentration von 2 auf 6 – 8 mM) wieder aufgehoben.
f hier erfolgt die Neutralisation von Verapamil mit Hilfe des β-adrenergen Sympathomimetikums Isoproterenol. Kontinuierliche Reizung der Papillarmuskeln mit einer Frequenz von 30/min. Versuchstemperatur 30°C

Ca^{++}-Entzugs in voller Deutlichkeit: Offensichtlich werden die elektrischen Parameter (Aufstrichsgeschwindigkeit, Overshoot, Plateaudauer und Gesamtdauer der Ca^{++}-abhängigen Aktionspotentiale) bei Ca^{++}-Mangel quantitativ und zeitlich etwa im gleichen Ausmaß reduziert wie die isometrischen Kontraktionsamplituden. Umgekehrt kommt es nach Wiederherstellung der normalen Ca^{++}-Konzentration von 2 mM zu Versuchsende innerhalb von 6 min zu einer – ebenfalls parallel laufenden – Restitution der elektrischen und mechanischen Aktivitäten bis zum Ausgangsniveau.

Ca^{++}-Antagonisten sind nun offenbar in der Lage, bei normaler Höhe der extracellulären Ca^{++}-Konzentration (2 mM) die Ca^{++}-abhängigen Aktionspotential-Parameter und die Kontraktilität partiell depolarisierter Papillarmuskeln genauso zu unterdrücken, wie dies in Abb. 1a durch eine einfache Senkung der extracellulären Ca^{++}-Konzentration auf 0,4 mM geschah. Tatsächlich produzierten die Ca^{++}-Antagonisten Verapamil, D 600, Nifedipin und Fendilin in den Abb. 1b – e praktisch die gleichen charakteristischen Kurvenverläufe wie ein extracellulärer Ca^{++}-Mangel. Lediglich die Wirkungsstärke der einzelnen Ca^{++}-Antagonisten war deutlich verschieden: Bei einer Einwirkungsdauer von 20 – 40 min erwiesen sich – beurteilt nach der Stärke der Beeinflussung der Ca^{++}-abhängigen Aktionspotential- und Kontraktilitäts-Parameter – die folgenden Konzentrationen an partiell depolari-

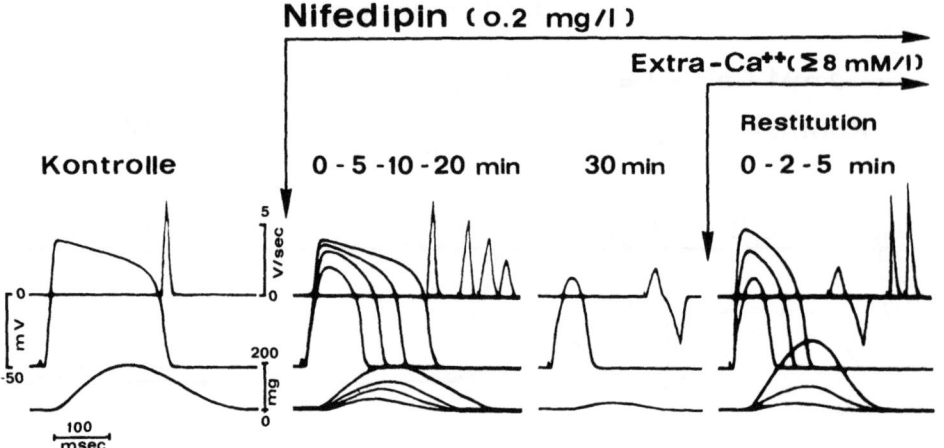

Abb. 1b

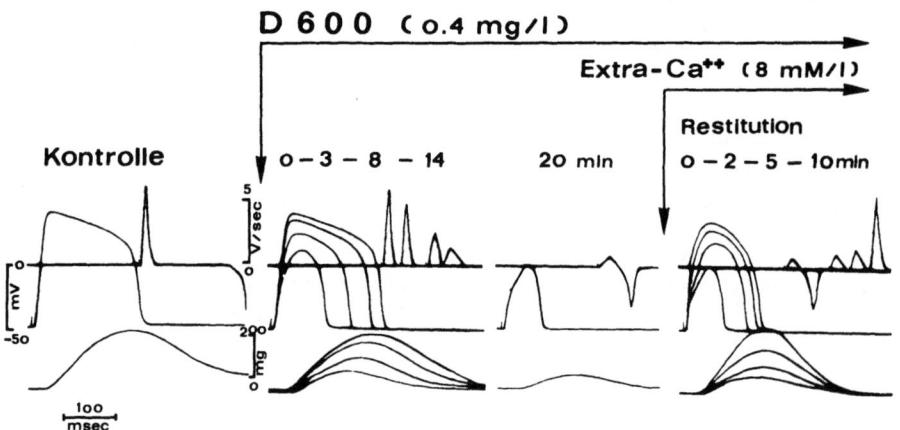

Abb. 1c

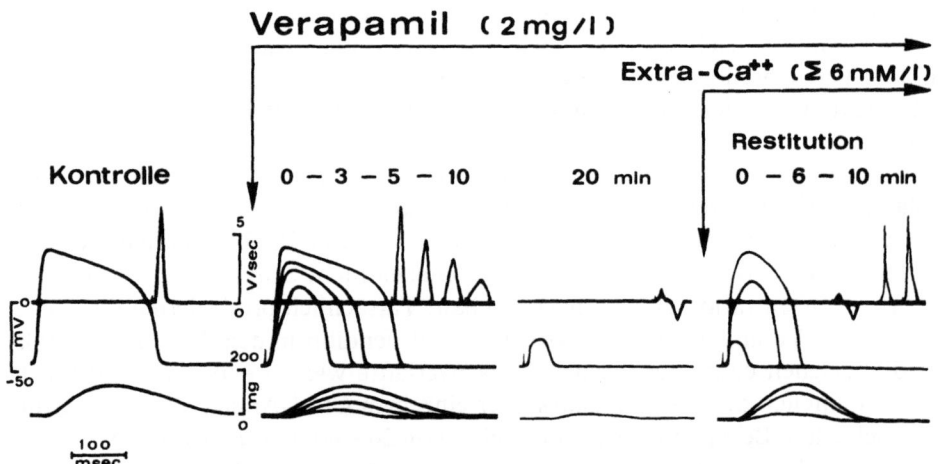

Abb. 1d

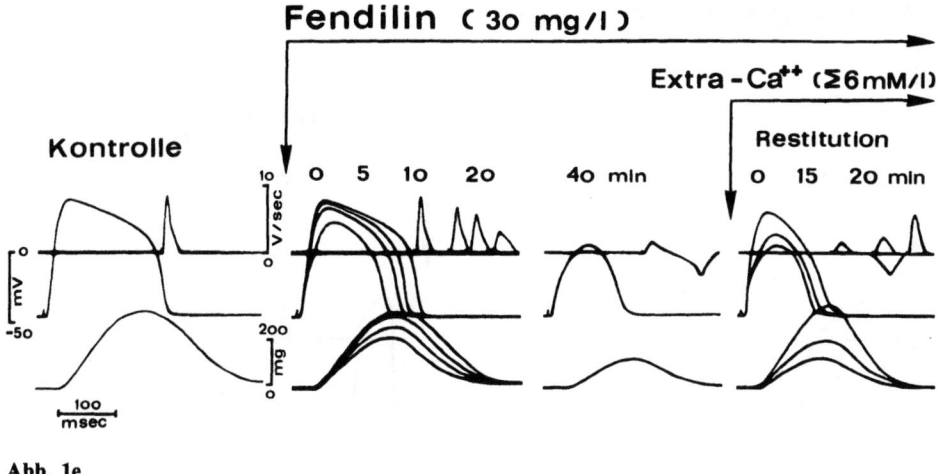

Abb. 1e

sierten Papillarmuskeln als äquipotent: Nifedipin (0,2 mg/l), D 600 (0,4 mg/l), Verapamil (2 mg/l), Diltiazem (4 mg/l), Prenylamin (25 mg/l), Fendilin (30 mg/l) und Bencyclan (30 mg/l). Durch die Gabe von Extra-Calcium (Steigerung der extracellulären Ca^{++}-Konzentration in Anwesenheit der Ca^{++}-Antagonisten von 2 auf 6 oder 8 mM) ließen sich die Effekte der Ca^{++}-Antagonisten zu Versuchsende in allen Fällen neutralisieren. Im allgemeinen kam es im Laufe von 5 bis 20 min zu einer annähernd vollen Restitution der Aufstrichsgeschwindigkeit und des Overshoot der Ca^{++}-getragenen Aktionspotentiale sowie der isometrischen Gipfelspannung. Nur die ursprüngliche Dauer der Aktionspotentiale wurde erst nach einer etwas längeren Zeit wieder erreicht. Die Wirkung von Nifedipin war nach Zusatz von Extra-Calcium am raschesten, diejenige von Fendilin am langsamsten reversibel. Außer Extra-Calcium können bekanntlich auch β-adrenerge Sympathomimetika wie z. B. Isoproterenol die Myocardeffekte der Ca^{++}-Antagonisten wieder beseitigen. β-Mimetika bringen offensichtlich den durch Ca^{++}-Antagonisten blockierten Ca^{++}-Influx wieder in Gang. Dementsprechend werden auch in dieser Situation die Ca^{++}-Aktionspotentiale jeweils im gleichen Ausmaß restituiert wie die mechanische Spannungsentwicklung. Als Beispiel ist in Abb. 1f die Neutralisation von Verapamil durch Isoproterenol wiedergegeben. Alle von uns geprüften Ca^{++}-Antagonisten lassen sich so am Herzen mit Hilfe von Extra-Calcium oder β-adrenergen Sympathomimetika überspielen.

In der folgenden Abbildungsserie 2a – e ist der Verlauf der vorausgehend wiedergegebenen Original-Experimente in Form von Diagrammen graphisch dargestellt. Die weitgehende Identität des durch Ca^{++}-Entzug verursachten Zustandes mit dem durch Ca^{++}-Antagonisten hervorgerufenen Erscheinungsbild ist bei dieser Art der Darstellung (prozentuale Veränderung der einzelnen Parameter) besonders augenfällig. Abb. 2a zeigt zunächst, daß nach Reduktion der Ca^{++}-Konzentration von 2 auf 0,4 mM die elektrischen Meßwerte (Höhe, Aufstrichsgeschwindigkeit, Plateau-Dauer und Gesamt-Dauer der Ca^{++}-Aktionspotentiale) von Minute zu Minute etwa um den gleichen Prozent-Betrag unter das Ausgangsniveau absinken wie die isometrische Spannungsentwicklung. Umgekehrt kommt es nach Normalisie-

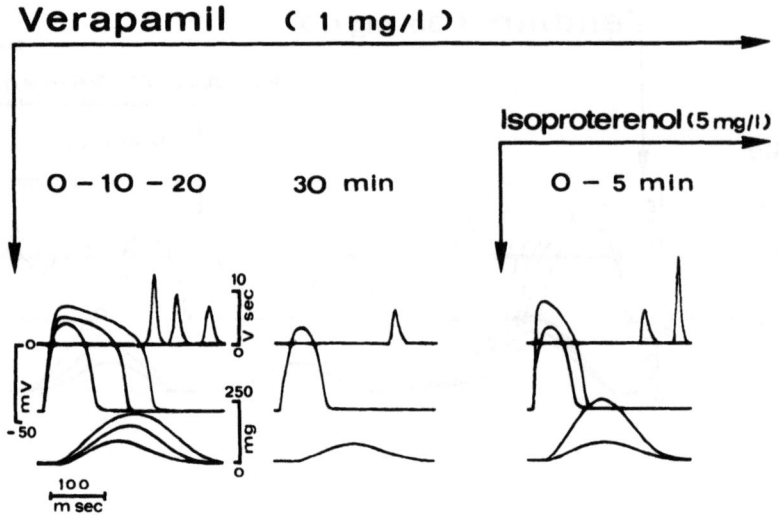

Abb. 1f

rung des extracellulären Ca^{++}-Gehaltes innerhalb von 6 min zu einer − wiederum parallel verlaufenden − Restitution der bioelektrischen und mechanischen Aktivität. Dies ist natürlich zu erwarten, da in partiell depolarisierten Myocardfasern sowohl die mechanischen Parameter der Kontraktion als auch die bioelektrischen Parameter des Aktionspotentials in gleicher Weise als eine Funktion des Ca^{++}-Einstroms durch die langsamen Kanäle zu gelten haben.

Weitgehend deckungsgleiche Kurvenverläufe ergeben sich aber auch, wenn man die prozentualen Veränderungen der Ca^{++}-Aktionspotentiale und der isometrischen Mechanogramme unter dem Einfluß der verschiedenen Ca^{++}-Antagonisten graphisch darstellt. Tatsächlich fallen an partiell depolarisierten Papillarmuskeln die bioelektrischen und mechanischen Parameter auch nach Zusatz von Nifedipin, D 600, Verapamil und Fendilin annähernd parallel zueinander ab (vgl. Abb. 2b − e). Dies gilt auch für die Beeinflussung der Ca^{++}-abhängigen Aktionspotentiale und der Kontraktilität durch die Ca^{++}-Antagonisten Diltiazem und Prenylamin. Die gleiche Kongruenz der Kurvenverläufe wird schließlich auch in der Restitutionsphase nach Zusatz von Extra-Calcium offenbar. Hierbei ergab sich eine besonders augenfällige Übereinstimmung zwischen der Regeneration des Ca^{++}-abhängigen Aktionspotential-Aufstrichs − als Ausdruck der Geschwindigkeit des transmembranären Ca^{++}-Einstroms − und der Rückkehr der kontraktilen Funktion.

Eine dritte Serie von Diagrammen ist in den Abb. 3a − c wiedergegeben. Bei dieser Art der Auswertung tritt die Existenz einer quantitativen Korrelation zwischen den einzelnen Parametern der Ca^{++}-Aktionspotentiale und der isometrischen Spannungsentwicklung sicherlich am deutlichsten zutage. So ist z. B., wie die Diagramme in Abb. 3a erkennen lassen, die Beziehung zwischen der jeweiligen Höhe der isometrischen Spannungsentwicklung (auf der Ordinate) und der *Aufstrichsteilheit der* Ca^{++}-*Aktionspotentiale* ($dV/dt_{max.}$ auf der Abszisse) eindeutig linear, unabhängig davon, welcher Ca^{++}-Antagonist zur Anwendung kommt und in welcher Konzentration er auf die partiell depolarisierten Papillarmuskeln einwirkt. Anders ausge-

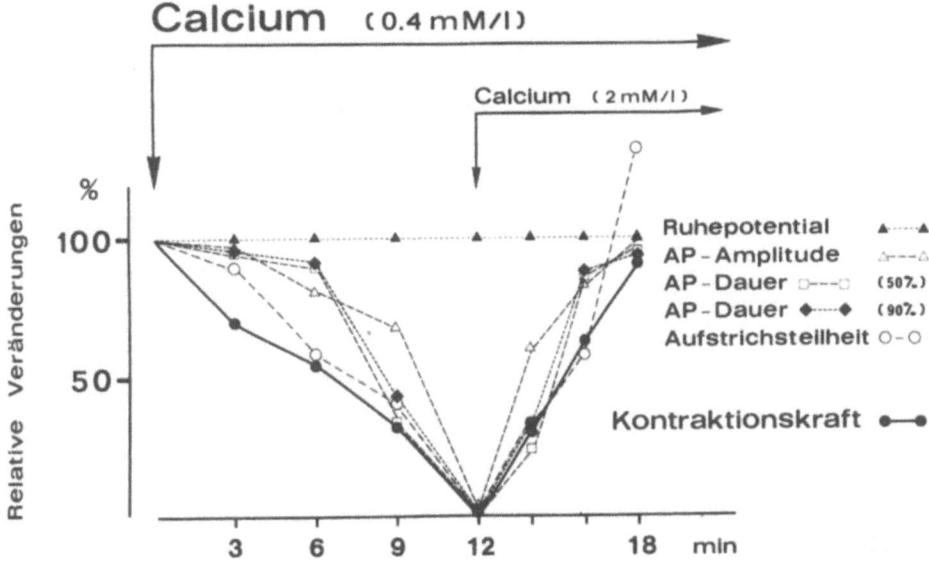

Abb. 2a – e. Parallele Beeinflussung der Ca^{++}-abhängigen Aktionspotential-Parameter (AP-Aufstrichsteilheit = $dV/dt_{max.}$; AP-Amplitude und AP-Dauer bei 50% und 90% Repolarisation gemessen) und der Kontraktionskraft (isometrische Gipfelspannung) bei partiell depolarisierten Meerschweinchen-Papillarmuskeln in K^+-reicher Tyrodelösung (19 mM K^+) nach extracellulärem Ca^{++}-Entzug (Teilabbildung **a**) oder nach Zusatz von Ca^{++}-Antagonisten (Teilabbildungen **b – e**). Graphische Darstellung der vorausgehend in Abb. 1a – f wiedergegebenen Originalkurven. Die nach Ca^{++}-Entzug bzw. Zusatz von Ca^{++}-Antagonisten ermittelten Meßdaten sind jeweils relativ in Prozent der Ausgangswerte (= 100%) angegeben. In der Restitutionsphase besteht offensichtlich eine besonders enge zeitliche Korrelation zwischen der Zunahme der Aufstrichsteilheit der Ca^{++}-abhängigen Aktionspotentiale (als Ausdruck der Intensität des elektrogenen Ca^{++}-Influx durch die langsamen Kanäle) und der Rückkehr der isometrischen Kontraktionsamplituden zu den Ausgangswerten

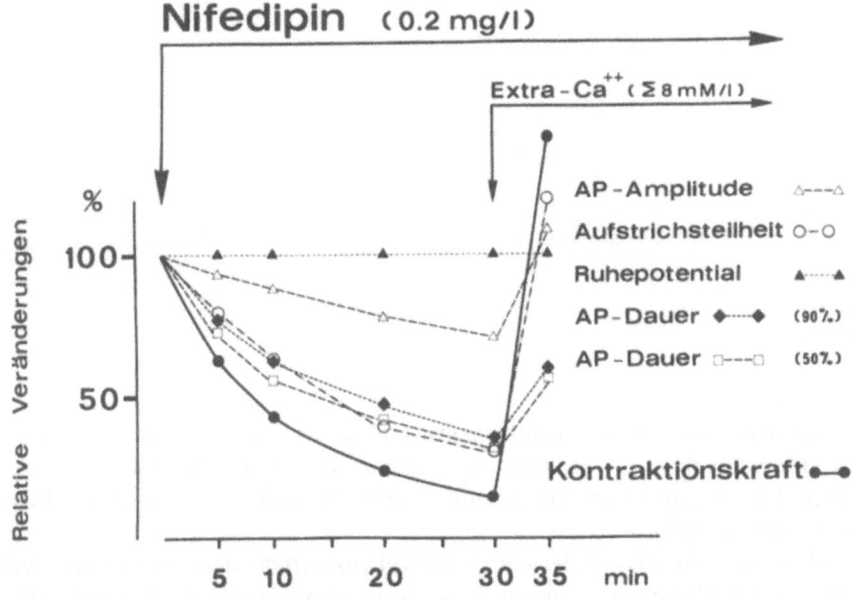

Abb. 2b

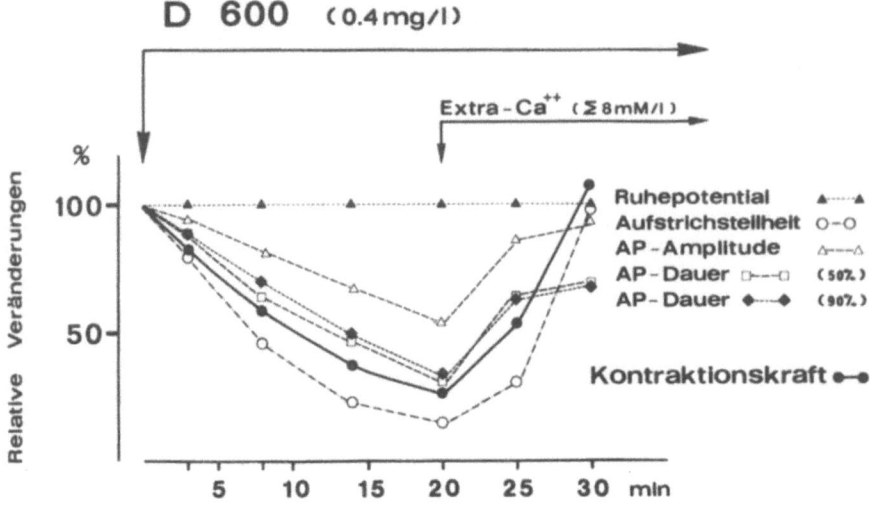

Abb. 2c

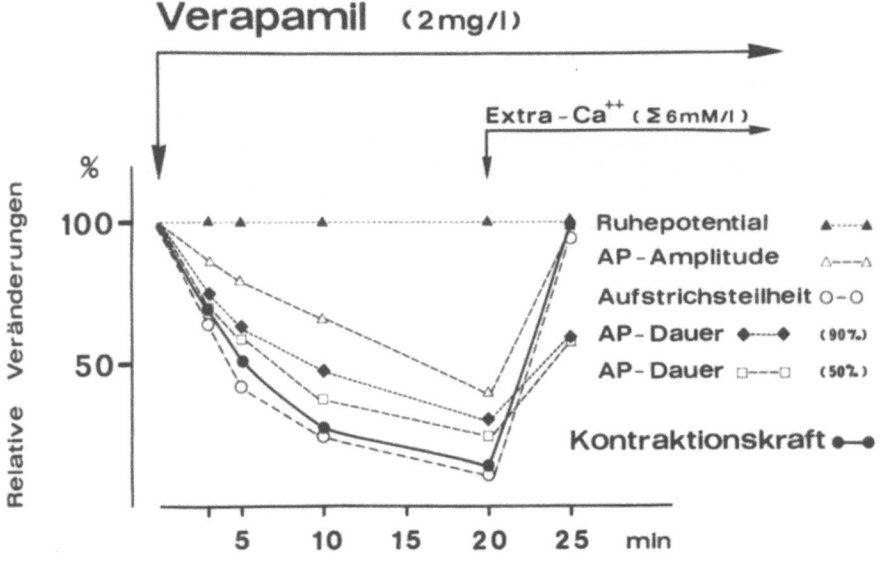

Abb. 2d

drückt wird also die Kontraktionskraft jeweils im gleichen Umfang reduziert, wie die Intensität des Ca^{++}-Einstroms – gemessen an der Abnahme von $dV/dt_{max.}$ – unter dem Einfluß von Verapamil, D 600, Nifedipin, Prenylamin, Fendilin oder Bencyclan absinkt.

Aber auch die *Dauer der Ca^{++}-Aktionspotentiale* steht in linearer Beziehung zu der Absolut-Höhe der isometrischen Kontraktionsamplituden, gleichgültig, ob man

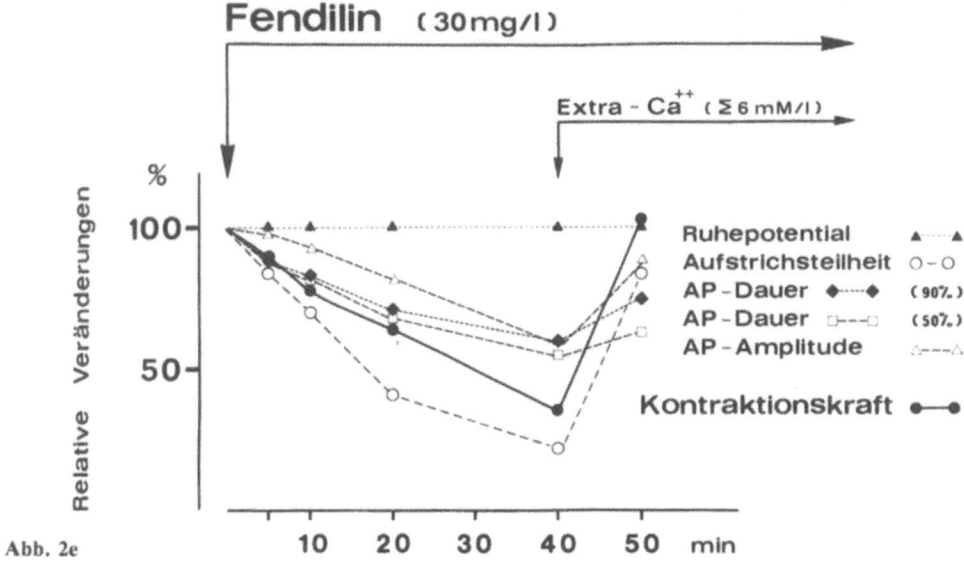

Abb. 2e

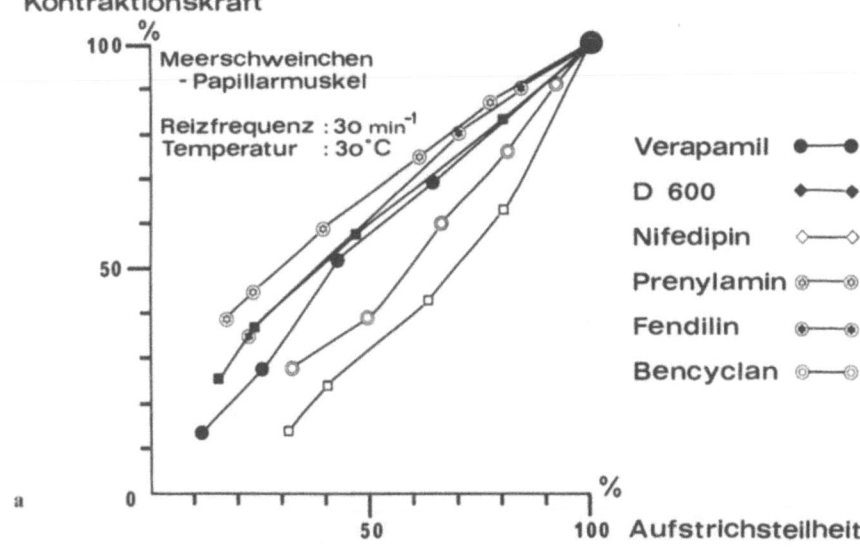

Abb. 3a – c. Lineare Beziehung zwischen dem Abfall der – durch den transmembranären Ca^{++}-Einstrom bedingten – elektrischen Aktionspotential-Parameter und dem Rückgang der dabei entwickelten isometrischen Gipfelspannung (Kontraktionskraft) unter dem Einfluß verschiedener Ca^{++}-Antagonisten. Versuche an partiell depolarisierten Meerschweinchen-Papillarmuskeln in K^+-reicher Tyrodelösung (19 mM K^+). Aufstrichsgeschwindigkeit ($dV/dt_{max.}$), Aktionspotential und Mechanogramm wurden in den einzelnen Versuchen im Abstand von 5 – 10 min nach Zusatz der Ca^{++}-Antagonisten auf einem Speicher-Oszillographen für die spätere Auswertung registriert. Die elektrischen Meßwerte wurden in den einzelnen Versuchen jeweils während eines Dauereinstichs an ein und derselben Myocardfaser gewonnen. Verwendete Konzentrationen: Verapamil (1 – 3 mg/l); D 600 (0,4 – 2 mg/l); Nifedipin (0,2 – 0,4 mg/l); Prenylamin (20 – 30 mg/l); Fendilin (20 – 30 mg/l); Bencyclan (20 – 30 mg/l). **a** Proportionalität zwischen der Abnahme der Aufstrichssteilheit ($dV/dt_{max.}$) der Ca^{++}Aktionspotentiale und dem Rückgang der Kontraktionskraft jeweils bezogen auf die Ausgangswerte vor Zusatz der Ca^{++}-Antagonisten (= 100%). **b** Proportionalität zwischen der Abnahme der Dauer der Ca^{++}-Aktionspotentiale und dem Rückgang der Kontraktionskraft. **c** Proportionalität zwischen der Abnahme der von den Ca^{++}-Aktionspotentialen umschriebenen Areale und der Verkleinerung der Mechanogramm-Flächen

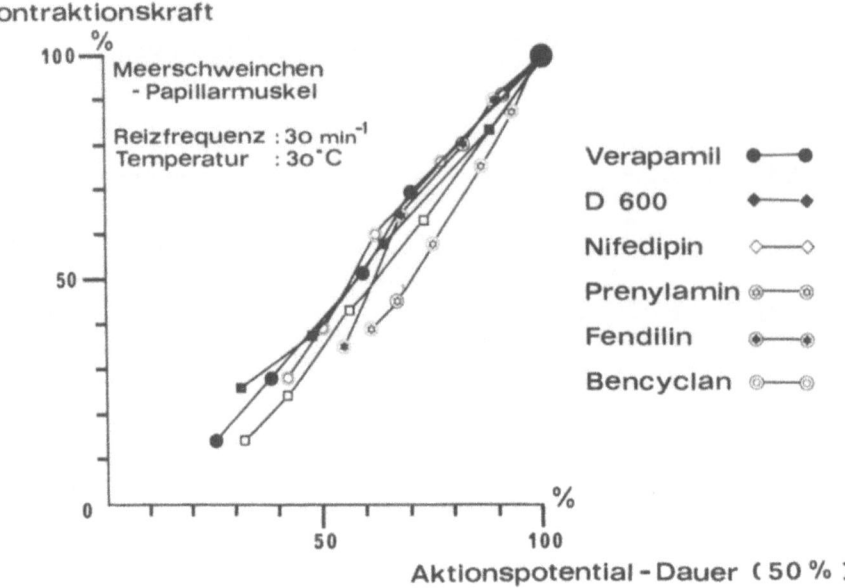

Abb. 3b

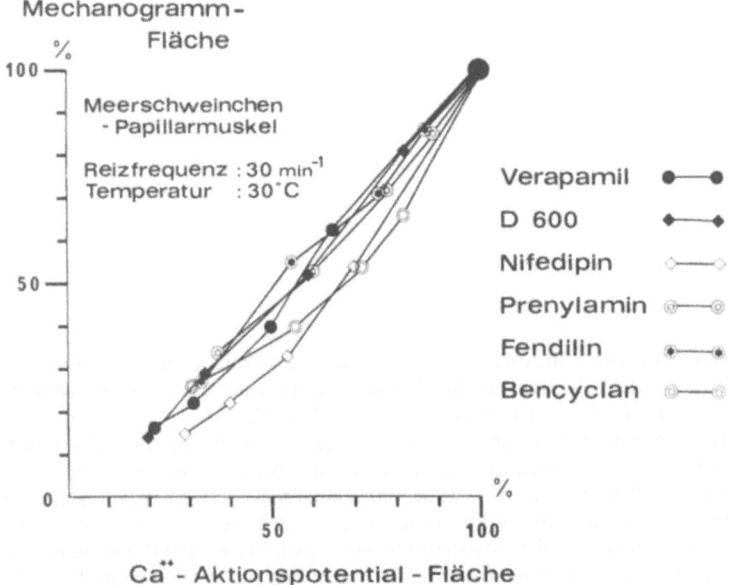

Abb. 3c

– wie in den Diagrammen in Abb. 3b – die Aktionspotential-Dauer auf dem Niveau von 50% oder bei 90%iger Repolarisation mißt. Offensichtlich bestimmt also auch die Dauer der Ca^{++}-Aktionspotentiale – als ein Maß für die Dauer des transmembranären Ca^{++}-Einstroms – die Höhe der isometrischen Spannungsentwicklung.

Eine perfekte Linearität ergibt sich schließlich auch, wenn man in Abb. 3c die Ca^{++}-Aktionspotentiale mit den Arealen der isometrischen Mechanogramme korreliert. Offensichtlich verkleinern sich also auch die von den Ca^{++}-Aktionspotentialen umschriebenen Flächen jeweils proportional zu den Arealen der isometrischen Kontraktionskurven.

Besprechung

In dem vorausgegangenen Referat ist von Fleckenstein darauf hingewiesen worden, daß sämtliche Herzwirkungen von Ca^{++}-Antagonisten (Herabsetzung von ATP-Spaltung, Kontraktionskraft und O_2-Verbrauch; Dämpfung nomotoper und ektoper Automatie-Zentren; Schutz vor Myocardnekrosen) dadurch erklärt werden können, daß diese Pharmaka den transmembranären Einstrom von Ca^{++}-Ionen ins Innere der Herzmuskelfasern und Schrittmacherzellen zu hemmen vermögen. Der prinzipielle Nachweis dieser Membranwirkung gelang zunächst am Myocard in situ mit Hilfe von radioaktiv markiertem Calcium [6] und später an isolierten Papillarmuskeln unter Verwendung einer speziellen Voltage-clamp-Technik, die eine getrennte Messung des transmembranären Na^+- und Ca^{++}-Influx gestattete [7]. Dagegen ließ sich in den Untersuchungen verschiedener Laboratorien keinerlei Hinweis auf eventuelle Angriffspunkte der Ca^{++}-Antagonisten an intracellulären Strukturen (Mitochondrien, sarkoplasmatisches Reticulum, Myofibrillen) gewinnen.

Durch unsere jetzt vorgelegten Ergebnisse wird die Hemmung des transmembranären Ca^{++}-Einstroms – als entscheidender Wirkungsmechanismus aller bisher von uns geprüften Ca^{++}-Antagonisten – noch weiter erhärtet; denn die Versuche zeigen, daß die mechanische Spannungsentwicklung der depolarisierten Myocardpräparate jeweils um denselben Betrag abnimmt, wie die Intensität und Dauer des – am Ca^{++}-Aktionspotential ablesbaren – Ca^{++}-Influx unter dem Einfluß eines Ca^{++}-Antagonisten reduziert wird. Ca^{++}-Antagonisten hemmen, Extracalcium und β-Mimetika fördern den transmembranären Ca^{++}-Einstrom und beeinflussen damit das physiologische Steuerungssystem der Myocardkontraktion an der Sarkolemm-Membran diametral entgegengesetzt. Spezifische Wirkungsunterschiede zwischen einzelnen Ca^{++}-Antagonisten sind dabei nicht zutage getreten. Hierdurch wird auch der spekulativen Annahme der Boden entzogen, der eine oder andere Ca^{++}-Antagonist übe möglicherweise noch zusätzliche Effekte auf den Ca^{++}-Stoffwechsel intracellulärer Organellen aus; denn in diesem Falle würde die – für die geprüften Ca^{++}-Antagonisten einheitlich gültige – lineare Funktion zwischen der Abnahme des Ca^{++}-Influx und der Dämpfung der Myocard-Kontraktilität durchbrochen.

Zusammenfassung

Partielle Depolarisation von Myocardfasern in einer K^+-reichen Tyrodelösung (19 mM K^+) führt zu einer Inaktivierung des schnellen Na^+-Kanals in der Sarkolemm-Membran, während der langsame Carrier-Mechanismus für Ca^{++}-Ionen seine Funktion beibehält. Partiell depolarisierte Myocardfasern sind weiterhin zur Bildung fortgeleiteter Aktionspotentiale befähigt; die Aufstrichsgeschwindigkeit sowie die Höhe und Dauer des Aktionspotentials werden jedoch in diesem Fall durch den transmembranären Einstrom von Ca^{++}-Ionen vermittelt. Ca^{++}-Antagonisten (Nifedipin, Verapamil, D 600, Diltiazem, Prenylamin, Fendilin, Bencyclan, Perhexilin) können daher an partiell depolarisierten Meerschweinchen-Papillarmuskeln — ähnlich wie ein einfacher Ca^{++}-Entzug — nicht nur die Ca^{++}-abhängige Kontraktilität hemmen, sondern auch die Ca^{++}-abhängige bioelektrische Membran-Aktivität unterdrücken. Die normalerweise Na^+-abhängigen Aktionspotentiale nicht-depolarisierter Papillarmuskeln werden hingegen durch Ca^{++}-Antagonisten kaum verändert. Die vorliegende Studie zeigt, daß die durch Ca^{++}-Antagonisten bewirkte Abnahme der mechanischen Spannungsentwicklung in K^+-reicher Tyrodelösung quantitativ und zeitlich der Hemmung des transmembranären Ca^{++}-Influx überraschend eng parallel geht, wie die strikte Korrelation zwischen den Ca^{++}-abhängigen bioelektrischen und mechanischen Parametern beweist. Extra-Calcium oder β-adrenerge Catecholamine restituieren die Ca^{++}-vermittelten Aktionspotentiale ebenso wie die kontraktilen Reaktionen selbst in Anwesenheit der Ca^{++}-antagonistischen Inhibitoren. Der gemeinsame Wirkungsmechanismus der Ca^{++}-Antagonisten beruht offensichtlich auf einer Hemmung des transmembranären Ca^{++}-Influx durch den langsamen Kanal, während intracelluläre Strukturen (Mitochondrien, Myofibrillen, sarkoplasmatisches Reticulum) nicht direkt betroffen werden.

Summary

Partial depolarization of myocardial fibres caused by Tyrode solution with high potassium (19 mM K) leads to inactivation of the fast transmembrane Na channel, whereas the slow carrier mechanism for Ca continues to operate. Partially depolarized myocardium is still capable of conducting propagated action potentials. But in this case upstroke velocity, height, and duration of action potential depend on the slow inward current of Ca. Hence in partially depolarized guinea pig papillary muscles, apart from Ca-withdrawal, Ca-antagonistic compounds such as nifedipine, verapamil, D 600, diltiazem, prenylamine, fendiline, bencyclan, and perhexiline not only suppress Ca-dependent contractility but also abolish the Ca-dependent bioelectric membrane responses, whereas normal Na-mediated action potentials remain almost unchanged. The present study demonstrates that the drug-induced decrease in contractile tension development at 19 mM K strikingly parallels quantitatively and temporally the drug-induced suppression of transmembrane Ca influx as evidenced by a strict correlation between the Ca-dependent bioelectric and mechanical parameters. Additional Ca or β-adrenergic catecholamines rapidly restore both Ca-mediated action potentials and contractile responses even in presence of the inhibitors. The common mechanism of action of the above-mentioned Ca-antagonists obviously consists of restricting Ca influx through the slow channel, whereas other structures (mitochondria, sarcoplasmic reticulum, myofibrils) are not directly involved.

Literatur

1. Reuter H, Beeler GW (1969) Calcium current and activation of contraction in ventricular myocardial fibers. Science 162:399 – 401
2. Mascher D, Peper K (1969) Two components of inward current in myocardial muscle fibres. Pfluegers Arch 307:190 – 203
3. Mascher D (1970) Electrical and mechanical responses from ventricular muscle fibres after inactivation of the sodium carrying system. Pfluegers Arch 317:359 – 372
4. Tritthart H, Volkmann R, Weiss R, Fleckenstein A (1973) Calcium-mediated action potentials in mammalian myocardium: Alteration of membrane response as induced by changes of Ca or by promoters and inhibitors of transmembrane Ca inflow. Naunyn Schmiedebergs Arch Pharmacol 280:239 – 252
5. Kohlhardt M, Fleckenstein A (1977) Inhibition of the slow inward current by nifedipine in mammalian ventricular myocardium. Naunyn Schmiedebergs Arch Pharmacol 298:267 – 272
6. Fleckenstein A (1968) Myokardstoffwechsel und Nekrose. Referat anläßlich des VI. Symposiums der Dtsch. Ges. f. Fortschritte auf dem Gebiet der Inneren Medizin, Freiburg, 8. – 9. Nov. 1968. In: Heilmeyer L, Holtmeier HJ (Hrsg) Herzinfarkt und Schock. Thieme, Stuttgart, S. 94 – 109
7. Kohlhardt M, Bauer B, Krause H, Fleckenstein A (1972) Differentiation of the transmembrane Na and Ca channels in mammalian cardiac fibres by the use of specific inhibitors. Pfluegers Arch 335:309 – 322

The Effect of Calcium-Antagonists on Atrioventricular Conduction

N. Taira, S. Motomura, A. Narimatsu, K. Satoh, and T. Yanagisawa

Experiments were carried out exclusively on the isolated, blood-perfused atrioventricular (AV) node preparation of dogs. The preparation was composed essentially of the right atrium and the ventricular septum. The preparation was perfused through the cannulated right coronary, posterior septal (PSA), and anterior septal (ASA) arteries with blood from a donor dog. Donors were anaesthetized with pentobarbitone and given heparin. The PSA supplies the atrial margin and upper part of the AV node where major AV conduction delay occurs. The ASA supplies the lower part of the AV node, His bundle, right bundle branch, Purkinje fibres and the myocardium of the ventricular septum. It has been claimed that the slow calcium channel prevails in cells in the atrial margin and upper part of the AV node, whereas the fast sodium channel prevails in cells in the more distal conduction system.

Nifedipine, verapamil, and diltiazem, that is, the drugs shown to be rather pure inhibitors of the slow channel or described as calcium antagonists in ventricular muscle, increased AV conduction time and in high doses produced complete AV block when these drugs were injected into the PSA. By contrast when these drugs were injected into the ASA, none of them impaired AV conduction. AV conduction impaired by these drugs was restored by injection of calcium chloride into the PSA, although calcium chloride scarcely modified or rather slightly suppressed AV conduction when given into the PSA under the control condition. The results suggest that the calcium-antagonistic drugs impair AV conduction by inhibition of the slow calcium channel in cells in the atrial margin and upper part of the AV node. Or conversely, the results can be taken to indicate that the slow calcium channel plays an important role in excitation of these cells.

An increase in potassium ion concentration in blood flowing through the PSA also impaired AV conduction. The impairment was also overcome by injection of calcium chloride into the same artery.

Tetrodotoxin (TTX), the relatively pure inhibitor of the fast sodium channel, when injected into the PSA, also impaired AV conduction. Similar results were obtained with quinidine and local anaesthetics like procaine and lidocaine, all of which are capable of inhibiting the fast sodium channel. Unlike impairment of AV conduction that was produced by calcium antagonists, the depressed AV conduction by TTX was not overcome by calcium chloride. The results suggest that the fast sodium channel, which is sensitive to blockade by sustained depolarization or tetrodotoxin, may also be operative in excitation of AV nodal cells that are properly nourished by arterial blood. The antagonism by exogenous calcium of the depressant action of raising extracellular potassium ion concentrations can be interpreted in such a way that the membrane will not easily be depolarized in the high extracellular calcium ion concentrations.

The three calcium antagonists injected into the PSA increased blood flow through the artery. The ratio of the dose that doubled blood flow, $ED_{100\%}$, to the dose that increased AV conduction time by 15% of control, $ED_{15\%}$, gave an estimate of the selectivity of the drug for the coronary vasculature versus the AV node. The values were about 9 for nifedipine and about 1 for verapamil and diltiazem. In other words nifedipine was about nine times as selective for the coronary vasculature as for the AV node, whereas verapamil and diltiazem were equally active on the coronary vasculature and the AV node. This is important from the therapeutic point of view. Nifedipine will not impair AV conduction in doses about nine times as much as the dose increasing coronary blood flow sufficiently, whereas verapamil and diltiazem may impair AV conduction in the same dose range that increase coronary blood flow.

Effekte antidysrhythmischer Pharmaka auf die Na$^+$- und Ca^{2+}-Permeabilität der Myokardmembran

H. A. Tritthart

Summary

Rhythmic as well as dysrhythmic cardiac activity is governed by transmembrane currents. The measurement of these currents is difficult in vitro and impossible in vivo. Antidysrhythmic compounds influence the membrane permeability and thereby modify the excitatory processes in the cardiac cell under normal and pathological conditions. The main transmembrane currents consist a) of a fast Na$^+$-influx, b) of a subsequent slow Ca^{2+} inward movement and c) of an outflow of K ions. All these currents exhibit specific susceptibilities to certain antidysrhythmic agents. In addition to the traditional Na$^+$-antagonistic compounds quinidine, lidocaine and procainamide, nowadays Ca^{2+}-antagonists, especially verapamil, are also clinically used with convincing success in the treatment of dysrhythmias. Apparently the slow Ca^{2+}-inward current, which is the prevailing current in functionally altered cardiac tissue and in pacemaker cells with a low membrane potential, plays an important role in various forms of dysrhythmias. Factors inducing membrane instability can lead to triggered or persistant automaticity and destruction of the hierarchic organization of function in the conduction system of the heart. Ca^{2+}-antagonists can inhibit these effects and block slow Ca^{2+}-dependent conduction in the myocardium making reentry less likely. Ca^{2+}-antagonistic compounds also inhibit primitive functional states of electrical activity present in cardiac cells that are damaged in a specific or nonspecific way. However the interrelationship between membrane currents (e.g. Ca^{2+}- and K$^+$-current) and the different effects on current activation and repriming processes complicates the quantitative evaluation of the individual Na- or Ca-antagonistic membrane actions of antidysrhythmic drugs. For instance the degree of inhibition of the fast Na$^+$-inflow may depend on stimulation frequency as well as on the dosis applied. Lidocaine, for instance, produces little if any Na$^+$-antagonistic inhibition of excitability at a low rate of stimulation, but will effectively suppress frequent or early incidental excitations (frequency limitation). On the other hand, procainamide reduces the maximum rate of the Na$^+$-dependent rise of the action potential only in function of the dose applied irrespective of the rates of stimulation. In therapeutic doses most antidysrhythmic compounds exhibit predominantly Na$^+$-antagonistic effects. However, inhibitory side effects on the Ca^{2+}- and K$^+$-currents may lead to a concomitant negative inotropic action or to slowing of repolarization. In contrast, verapamil and D 600 can inhibit tension development and the slow Ca^{2+}-inward current nearly completely before Na$^+$-antagonistic effects appear. Hence Ca^{2+}-antagonistic compounds, acting as selective blockers of the transmembrane Ca^{2+}-current are valuable tools for the further elucidation of the involvement of Ca ions in the pathogenesis of dysrhythmias.

Der normale Herzzyklus basiert bekanntlich auf einer zeitlich und räumlich geordneten Änderung des Potentials an den Membranen der Myokardzellen. Die zeitliche und, etwas weniger gut, die räumliche Verteilung dieser Potentialänderung erfassen wir mit dem EKG. An der einzelnen Zelle können wir in vitro den genauen Verlauf von De- und Repolarisation mit der Mikroelektrode als Aktionspotential messen (Abb. 1). Die Ursache jeder Potentialänderung ist eine Ladungsverschiebung, also ein Membranstrom; nur bei einem konstanten Membranpotential ist der Nettomembranstrom Null. Als Ladungsträger des Membranstroms kommen für die Herzmuskelzellmembran hauptsächlich die Kationen Na^+, Ca^{2+} und K^+ in Frage. Die unterschiedlichen Ionenkonzentrationen an der Innen- und Außenseite der Membran bestimmen die Richtung der wahrscheinlichen Ionenbewegungen. Solche Ionenströme bewirken, wie das Schema der Abb. 2 zeigt, entweder eine Depolarisation oder eine Re- bzw. Hyperpolarisation der Membran.

Alle elektrischen Aktivitäten im Myokard, rhythmische wie dysrhythmische, werden bestimmt durch Ionenströme, die sich in ihrer Qualität, Quantität und in der zeitlichen und räumlichen Verteilung unterscheiden können. Unter einigen vereinfachenden Annahmen ist der Membranstrom in folgender Weise zu definieren:

$$I_m = \frac{1}{R_m} V + C_m \cdot \frac{dV}{dt}; \quad I_m = \frac{d^2V}{dx^2} \cdot \frac{1}{Ri}$$

Wird z. B. in Spannungsklemmversuchen das Potential trotz Stromfluß konstant gehalten, so wird der rechte Teil der ersten Gleichung zu Null und der Membranstrom das Produkt aus Potential und Leitfähigkeit der Membran, bzw. deren Kehrwert, dem Membranwiderstand (Abb. 3). Die Messung der Membranströme bei normaler und dysrhythmischer Aktivität des Myokards und unter dem Einfluß von Antiarrhythmika steht erst ganz am Anfang. Es fehlt das ideale Einzelfaser-

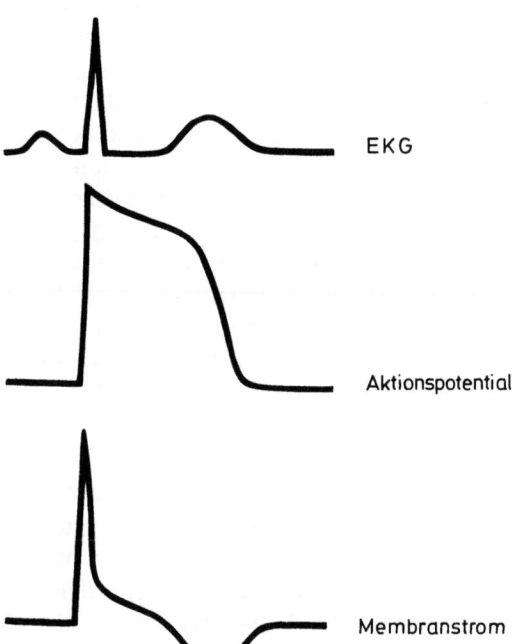

Abb. 1. Schematische Darstellung von Elektrokardiogramm (EKG), transmembranären Aktionspotential und Membranstrom

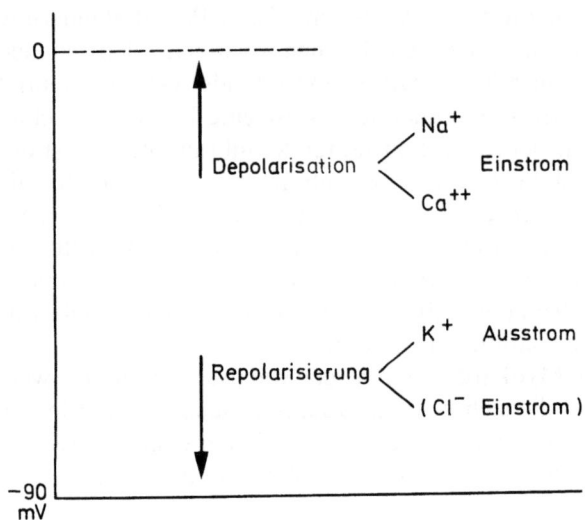

Abb. 2. Der Einfluß der transmembranären Ionen-Ströme auf das Membranpotential der Herzmuskelzellen

Präparat vom Herzmuskel, und Ergebnisse von Strommessungen sind nur mit erheblichen Vorbehalten zu interpretieren, wenn pathophysiologische Veränderungen der Membranfunktionen vorliegen, die zu dysrhythmischer Aktivität führen. Es ist deshalb noch ein weiter Weg bis zu einer speziellen Elektropathologie des Myokards und zu einer exakten Kenntnis der Membranwirkung der gebräuchlichen Antiarrhythmica.

Veränderungen der Stromstärke zeigen sich aber als Veränderung der Ladegeschwindigkeit der Membrankapazität, also durch eine Änderung der maximalen Geschwindigkeit der Depolarisation bei Einstrom bzw. der Repolarisation bei Ausstrom. In dieser Weise lassen sich die Wirkungen der Antiarrhythmika auf die transmembranären Ionenströme anhand der Veränderung des Aktionspotentials qualitativ charakterisieren und ein Einteilungsschema, wie z. B. jenes von Vaughan Williams [1] oder von Dreifuß u. Mitarb. [2], erstellen. Gerade die Einführung der Ca^{2+}-Antagonisten, Fleckenstein [3], hat ja diese richtige Betrachtungsweise entscheidend gefördert, ja z. T. erst ermöglicht; denn hierdurch wurde erstmals eine Stoffgruppe mit antidysrhythmischer Wirkung nach ihrem Einfluß auf die transmembranären Ionenströme benannt.

Die Wirkung von Antiarrhyhtmika auf die Membranströme dürfte auf einer Beeinflussung der Membranpermeabilität für Ionen beruhen, wobei wir andere, z. B. passive Membraneigenschaften ausklammern und annehmen, daß sich die Ionengradienten bzw. Gleichgewichtspotentiale für die einzelnen Stromkomponenten nicht ändern. Die Durchlässigkeit der Membran hängt davon ab, welche Energiebarriere die Membran für die Bewegung der hydratisierten Ionen darstellt. Diese Energiebarriere ist vermutlich nur an präformierten Stellen der Membran, den sogenannten Ionenkanälen, so niedrig, daß ein Ionendurchtritt wahrscheinlich ist. Ionenkanäle sind in Abhängigkeit vom Membranpotential und dem Milieu beiderseits der Membran weitgehend selektiv nur für eine Ionenart durchgängig. Für Öffnen

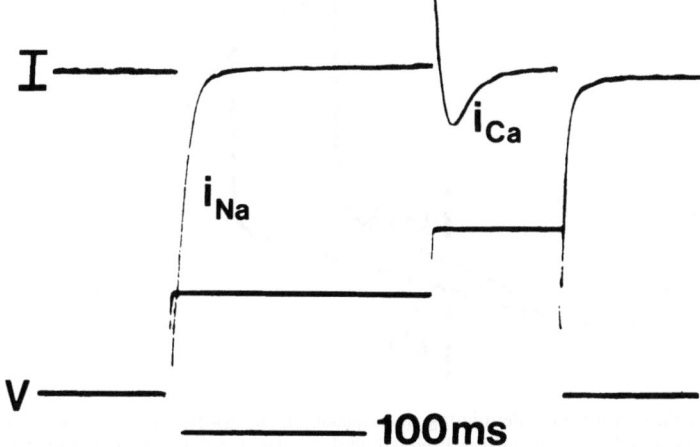

Abb. 3. Der Membranstrom (I) bei stufenweiser Änderung des Membranpotentials (V) unter Spannungsklemm-Bedingungen. Überschwellige Depolarisation bewirkt einen raschen Na^+-Einstrom (I_{Na}), nach dessen spontaner Inaktivierung ein langsamer Ca^{2+}-Einstrom (I_{Ca}) durch einen weiteren Depolarisationsschritt ausgelöst werden kann (Papillarmuskel der Katze)

und Schließen der Ionenkanäle werden 3 – 5 Reaktionsschritte postuliert. Fürs Myokard hat man die folgenden 3 Ionenkanäle wahrscheinlich gemacht: einen für den raschen *Na^+-Einstrom,* einen für den langsamen *Ca^{2+}-Einstrom,* und einen für den *K^+-Ausstrom.*

Diese Membrankanäle sind funktionell in verschiedener Weise verkettet. Jeder hat via Ionenstrom Einfluß auf das Membranpotential, welches die Funktion aller Kanäle steuert. Ca^{2+} beeinflußt den Na^+-Einstrom, und eine Mitbeteiligung von Na^+ am langsamen Ca^{2+}-Einstrom wird vermutet (welcher deshalb oft als Na^+-Ca^{2+}-Einstrom bezeichnet wird). Ca^{2+} hat an der Innenseite der Membran Einfluß auf die Leitfähigkeit der Membran für Kalium-Ionen. So ist z. B. eine Abflachung der langsamen diastolischen Depolarisation in aktuellen und latenten Schrittmachern bei einer Minderung des depolarisierenden Ca^{2+}-Einstroms ebenso zu erwarten wie bei einer Steigerung des repolarisierenden K^+-Ausstroms (Abb. 4). Wird der Ca^{2+}-Einstrom in der Diastole durch Gabe eines Ca^{2+}-Antagonisten reduziert, so tritt diese Abflachung des Potentialverlaufs ein (vgl. Abb. 5). Aber auch die Ca^{2+}-Aktivität an der Membraninnenseite dürfte hierbei absinken und so auch die Leitfähigkeit im K^+-Kanal abfallen, mit gegensinniger Membranwirkung.

Auch die qualitative und quantitative Ausstattung der Myokardmembran mit Ionenkanälen ist keine konstante Größe. Sie ist abhängig von der Zelldifferenzierung und möglicherweise auch von langfristigen Einflüssen. Die einzelne embryonale Myokardzelle (Huhn) in der Gewebekultur kann einen Einstrom nur mit Hilfe des langsamen Ca^{2+}-Kanals bilden (Abb. 5). Der Depolarisationsvorgang ist sehr langsam. Wie die Abb. 5 zeigt, werden Automatie und Erregung durch Ca^{2+}-Antagonisten prompt blockiert. Im adulten Myokard ist die Depolarisation wesentlich rascher und unempfindlich geworden gegen Ca^{2+}-Antagonisten. Die Depolarisationsgeschwindigkeit ist, wie die Differenzierung zeigt, auch dann noch unverändert, wenn der Ca^{2+}-Einstrom während des Plateaus und damit die mechanische

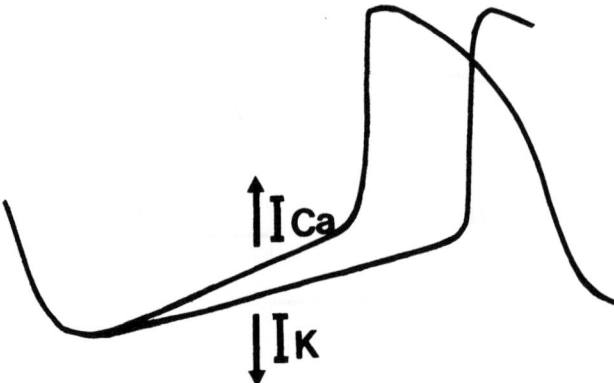

Abb. 4. Eine Beschleunigung der langsamen diastolischen Depolarisation einer Schrittmacherzelle des Herzens kann sowohl durch eine Zunahme der depolarisierenden Einströme (I_{Ca}), wie durch eine Abschwächung des repolarisierenden Ausstroms (I_K) verursacht werden

Spannungsentwicklung inhibiert ist (vgl. Abb. 5). Der Depolarisationsvorgang des adulten Arbeitsmyokards wird nur noch vom raschen Na^+-Einstrom bestimmt.

Bekanntlich besitzen wir im adulten Herzen unterschiedlich ausdifferenzierte Myokardzellen; ausgehend von den primitivsten Zellen im Sinusknoten und AV-Knoten steigt über das Reizleitungssystem zu den Zellen des Arbeitsmyokards das Ruhepotential und die Dominanz der raschen Na^+-Kanäle für die Erregbarkeit. Zahlreiche spezifische und unspezifische Schädigungen können zu einer funktionellen Rückentwicklung des Arbeitsmyokards führen; experimentell verursachen z. B. K^+-Mangel, ein Membranleck, Glykosidvergiftung oder Vergiftung mit Ba^{++} einen sogenannten Funktionswandel. Die Abb. 6 zeigt den Funktionswandel von Arbeitsmyokard zu Schrittmachergewebe durch Barium-Vergiftung (10 mM). Das Vorstadium oder das erste Anzeichen von Automatieneigung ist eine aktivitätsabhängige Automatie, sog. triggered automaticity [4]. Die Abb. 7 zeigt dieses Stadium aktivierbarer Automatie im Arbeitsmyokard nach Gabe von 5 mM $BaCl_2$. Unter Ba^{2+}-Einwirkung lösten hier 2−3 elektrische Erregungen Automatie aus. Bereits durch wenige elektrisch ausgelöste Schläge wird hierbei die Membran labilisiert, und einzelne oder mehrere spontane Schläge oder Salven von automatischer Entladung folgen. Diese Experimente zeigen in Übereinstimmung mit anderen Autoren [5, 6], daß, ebenso wie die volle Automatie im Papillarmuskel, bereits dieses Vorstadium durch Ca^{2+}-Antagonisten blockiert wird. Bereits 0,1 µg/ml D 600 heben diese Automatieneigung völlig auf; auch durch minutenlange Reizung ist keine Automatie, nicht einmal ein Doppelschlag auszulösen (Abb. 7). Ein ähnlicher Versuch bei Registrierung der mechanischen Aktivität zeigt, daß selbst 30 µg/ml Chinidin diese Automatieneigung im Papillarmuskel nicht völlig unterdrücken können (Abb. 8).

Das Membranpotential kann auch bei extrazellulärem K^+-Anstieg so vermindert sein, daß der rasche Na^+-Einstrom nicht mehr aktivierbar ist und Ca^{2+}-Aktionspotentiale gebildet werden. Hierbei ist die K^+-Leitfähigkeit aber hoch und Automatie deswegen sehr unwahrscheinlich (Abb. 9). Die Inaktivierung der raschen Na^+-Kanäle ist offensichtlich; bei einem Membranpotential um − 50 mV hat die Depolarisationsgeschwindigkeit und die Leitungsgeschwindigkeit um etwa 90% abgenommen. In diesem Stadium ist die Depolarisationsgeschwindigkeit − anders als

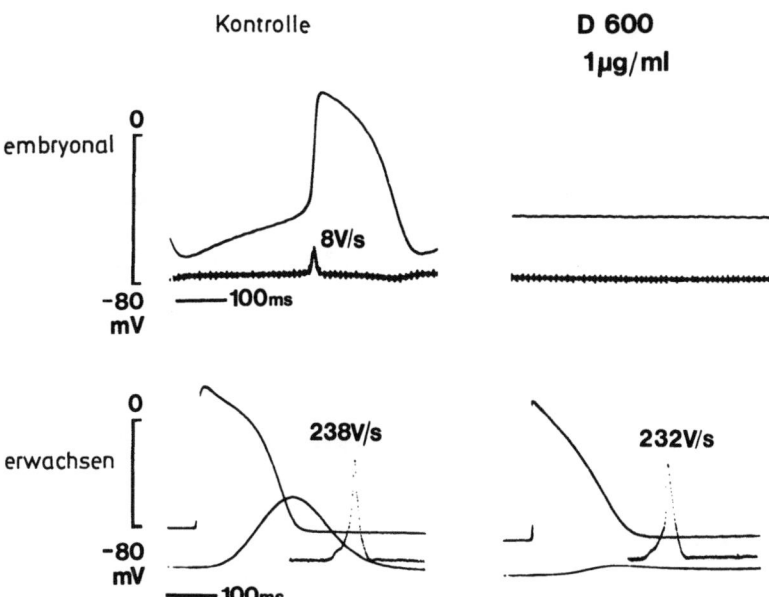

Abb. 5. Die funktionelle Differenzierung des Ventrikelmyokards (Huhn). Am Ende des ersten Drittels der Embryonalentwicklung zeigen die Ventrikelzellen Schrittmachereigenschaft und eine sehr geringe Anstiegsgeschwindigkeit des Aktionspotentials von 8 V/s. Das adulte Myokard zeigt bekanntlich ein stabiles Membranpotential und einen raschen Anstieg des Aktionspotentials (238 V/s). Blockade des Ca^{2+}-Einstroms durch D 600 hemmt die Automatie und die Erregbarkeit im embryonalen Myokard, läßt aber den raschen und Na^+-abhängigen Anstieg des Aktionspotentials von adultem Myokard praktisch unbeeinflußt. Nur das Plateau des Aktionspotentials wird abgeflacht und die Kontraktionskraft fast vollständig aufgehoben (unten rechts)

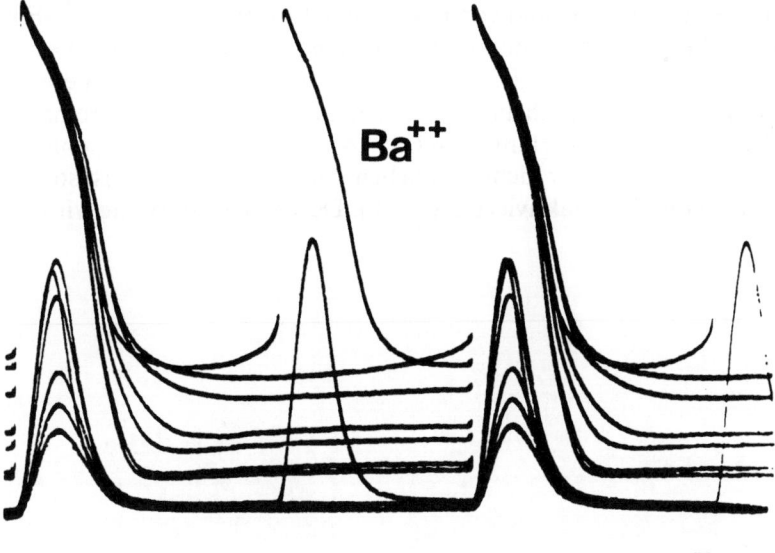

78 7 13

Abb. 6. Der Funktionswandel von Ventrikelmyokard (Papillarmuskel des Meerschweinchens) zu Schrittmachergewebe durch Barium-Vergiftung (10 mM). Wie die übereinander registrierten Aktionspotentiale unter Barium-Einwirkung zeigen, kommt es zur Reduktion des Ruhepotentials und zu so weitgehender Labilisierung der Membran, daß schließlich spontane Erregungsbildung eintritt

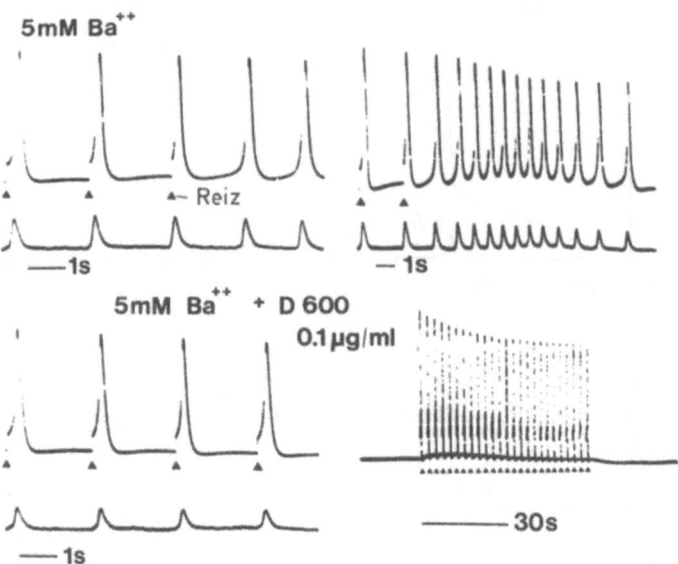

Abb. 7. Die Induktion aktivierbarer Automatie im Ventrikelmyokard (Papillarmuskel des Meerschweinchens, 5 mM BaCl$_2$). Nach Barium-Gabe läßt sich eine Salve spontaner Entladungen durch einige normale elektrische Reize im Papillarmuskel auslösen. Diese aktivierbare Automatie (triggered automaticity) ist durch Gabe des Ca^{2+}-Antagonisten D 600 vollständig zu unterdrücken (unten), selbst minutenlange Reizung kann die Membran nicht mehr zu Spontanentladungen anstoßen (vgl. unten rechts)

bei aktivierbarem Na$^+$-Strom – unmittelbar vom Ca^{2+}-Strom, der extrazellulären Ca^{2+}-Konzentration und von Faktoren mit Einfluß auf den Ca^{2+}-Einstrom abhängig (vgl. Abb. 9). Ca^{2+}-Antagonisten hemmen in sehr selektiver Weise die Bildung und Leitung dieser Ca^{2+}-Aktionspotentiale (oft als slow response bezeichnet). Die bereits normalerweise kritisch langsame Erholung des Ca^{2+}-Einstroms nach Aktivierung wird unter der Einwirkung von Ca^{2+}-Antagonisten so träge, daß selbst Ruhepausen von 1 min und länger nicht ausreichen. Der Ca^{2+}-Einstrom ist so für alle Frequenzen in vivo komplett inaktiviert (Abb. 10). Durch diese Wirkung wird auch die stark ver-

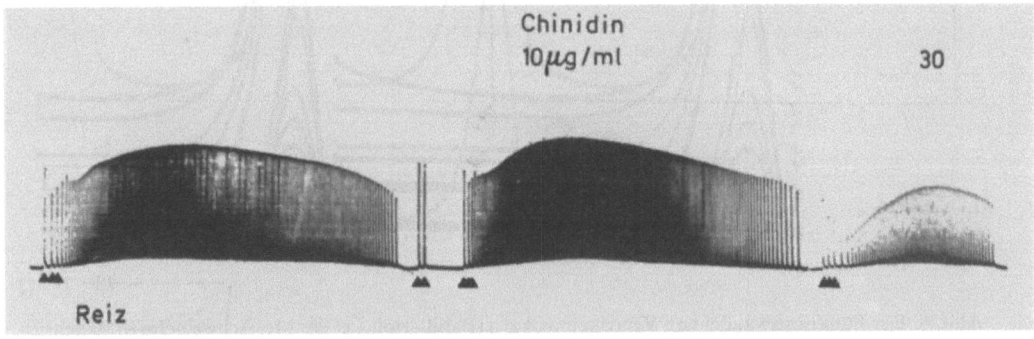

Abb. 8. Die fehlende Hemmwirkung von 10 µg/ml Chinidin auf die aktivierbare Automatie im Ventrikelmyokard (vgl. Abb. 7, Registrierung der mechanischen Aktivität, Papillarmuskel vom Meerschweinchen)

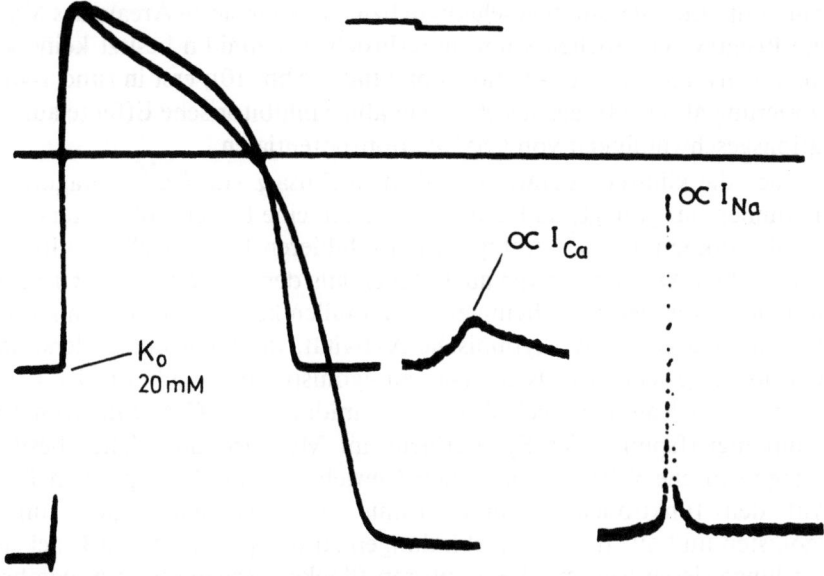

Abb. 9. Partielle Membrandepolarisation durch Erhöhung der K^+-Konzentration von 4 auf 20 mM führt zu Ausfall des raschen Na^+-Einstroms. Die Ca^{2+}-Aktionspotentiale in K^+-reichem Milieu zeigen eine sehr geringe Anstiegsgeschwindigkeit (vgl. Differenzierung des Potentials, rechts) und Ausbreitungsgeschwindigkeit und entsprechend ihrer andersartigen Genese (Ca^{2+}-Einstrom) eine völlig andere Beeinflußbarkeit durch Antiarrhythmica (vgl. Abb. 10)

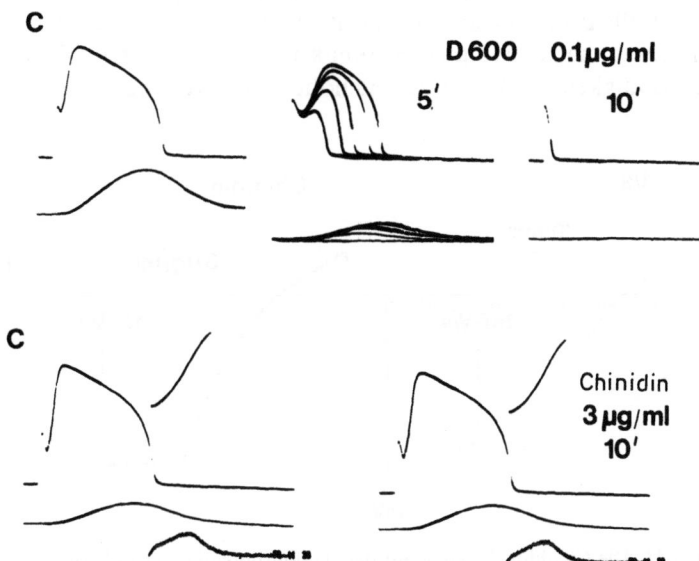

Abb. 10. An Ca^{2+}-Aktionspotentialen in K^+-reichem Milieu führt Hemmung des langsamen Ca^{2+}-Einstroms durch den Ca^{2+}-Antagonisten D 600 zum Erlöschen der Erregbarkeit. Chinidin (3 µg/ml) hat hier keine Hemmwirkung auf Erregungsablauf und Kontraktionskraft

langsamte Leitung durch geschädigte bzw. depolarisierte Areale des Myokards, welche Reentry verursachen kann, unterbrochen. Chinidin besitzt keine vergleichbare Hemmwirkung auf Ca^{2+}-Aktionspotentiale (Abb. 10); erst in rund 100fach höherer Dosierung als D 600 zeigen sich regelmäßige inhibitorische Effekte auf die Depolarisationsgeschwindigkeit von Ca^{2+}-Aktionspotentialen.

Auch die klinische Erfahrung mit dem Einsatz von Ca^{2+}-Antagonisten bei Dysrhythmien hat gezeigt, daß dem Ca^{2+}-Strom eine bisher wohl unterschätzte Schlüsselrolle zukommt. Ca^{2+}-Antagonisten inhibieren funktionell primitive Stadien der elektrischen Aktivität, in die auch Zellen aus dem Arbeitsmyokard bei spezifischen und unspezifischen Schädigungen zurückfallen können. Sie bieten so eine neuartige Absicherung gegen dysrhythmische Aktivität, die nicht nur anders, sondern auch wesentlich gezielter ist als die Na^+-antagonistische Reduktion der Erregbarkeit in Vorhof und Kammer nach Art des Chinidins. Der Ca^{2+}-Einstrom ist weiter ein Hauptangriffspunkt des Sympathicus im Myokard und daher besitzt die Ca^{2+}-antagonistische Wirkung zusätzlich Gewicht bei der Therapie von Dysrhythmien. Auf den funktionellen Antagonismus zwischen Sympathicus und Ca^{2+}-Antagonisten und auf die Querverbindungen zu den β-Rezeptoren-Blockern kann hier nur hingewiesen werden. β-Rezeptoren-Blocker besitzen häufig membranstabilisierende, chinidinartige Wirkungen.

Die Hemmwirkung von Chinidin und zahlreichen anderen Stoffen mit chinidinartiger Wirkung auf den Na^+-Einstrom vermindert bekanntlich die Depolarisationsgeschwindigkeit des normalen Aktionspotentials in Vorhof und Kammer. Die Reduktion der maximalen Aufstrichsgeschwindigkeit und proportional dazu der Erregbarkeit und der Ausbreitungsgeschwindigkeit der Erregung ist nicht nur, wie die Abb. 11 zeigt, dosisabhängig. In vielen Fällen hängt diese Hemmwirkung sehr stark von der Erregungsfrequenz ab, wie die Abb. 12 zeigt. Offensichtlich hemmen einige Stoffe, wie z. B. Procainamid, die Aktivierung des Na^+-Stroms und diese Wirkung ist für alle Frequenzen gleich groß. Andere hemmen zusätzlich oder überwiegend die Erholung nach erfolgter Stromaktivierung und reduzieren so die Aufstrichsgeschwindigkeit um so stärker, je höher die Erregungsfrequenz ist. Diese unterschied-

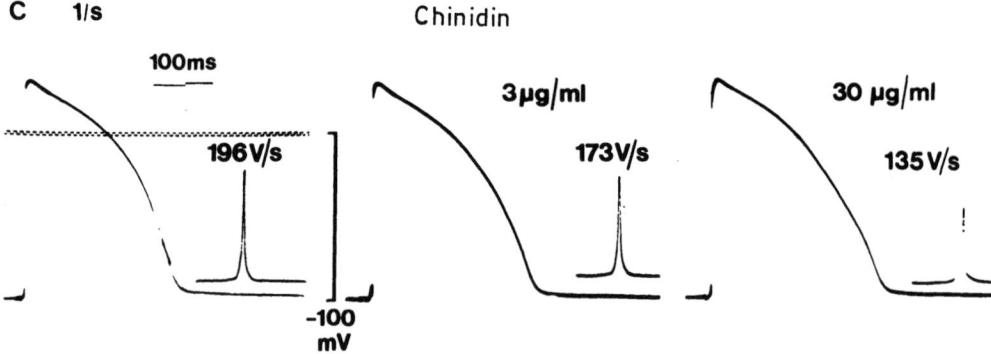

Abb. 11. Die Chinidin-Wirkung auf das Aktionspotential der isolierten elektrisch gereizten (1/s) Papillarmuskel des Meerschweinchens (K_0^+, 4 mM). Die maximale Anstiegsgeschwindigkeit (vgl. Differenzierungskurve rechts) des Aktionspotentials wird als Ausdruck der erregungshemmenden Reduktion des raschen Na^+-Einstroms vermindert. Das Plateau des Aktionspotentials wird in hoher Dosierung geringfügig abgeflacht und die Dauer des Aktionspotentials wird verlängert

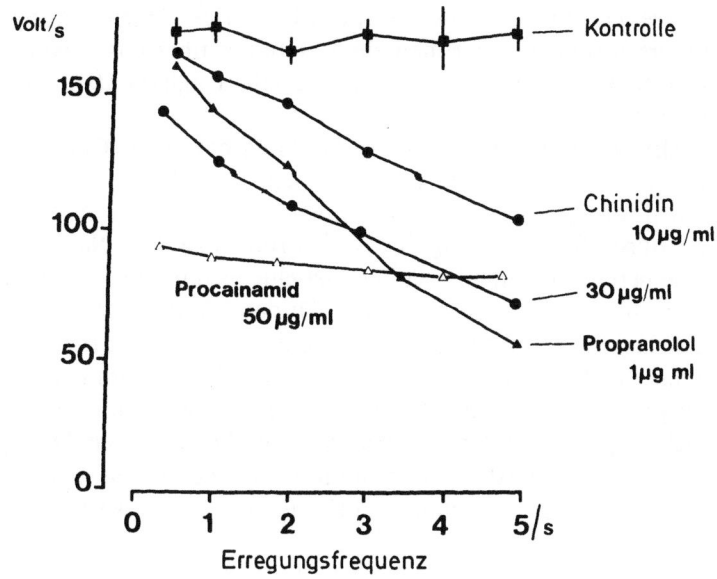

Abb. 12. Der Einfluß der Erregungsfrequenz auf die Reduktion der maximalen Anstiegsgeschwindigkeit des Aktionspotentials (gemessen in Volt/s) durch Antiarrhythmica. Bei einigen Antiarrhythmica hat neben der Dosis auch die Erregungsfrequenz einen entscheidenden Einfluß auf das Ausmaß der erregungshemmenden Reduktion des raschen Na^+-Einstroms während des Anstiegs des Aktionspotentials

lichen Effekte machen einen einfachen Dosis- bzw. Wirkungsvergleich der Antiarrhythmica schwierig. Antiarrhythmica, die bei niedrigen Frequenzen mäßige Hemmwirkung auf den Na^+-Einstrom ausüben, können dennoch die Leitung frequenter Erregung gezielt unterdrücken, also nach Art eines Frequenzfilters rhythmisierend wirken [7]. Die Wirkung einiger Antiarrhythmica und β-Rezeptoren-Blocker mit Na^+-antagonistischen, membranstabilisierenden Effekten ist in Tabelle 1 nach dem Ausmaß der Frequenzabhängigkeit im Bereich therapeutischer Dosen gruppiert. Unter dem Begriff der chinidinartigen Membran-stabilisierenden Wirkung von Antiarrhythmica werden also unterschiedliche Hemmeffekte auf den Na^+-Einstrom zusammengefaßt. Zugleich sagt dieser Begriff wenig darüber aus, in welch spezifischer Weise ein Antiarrhythmicum nur den Na^+-Strom während der Erregung erschwert. Negativ inotrope Effekte, die auf eine Reduktion des Ca^{2+}-Einstroms

Tabelle 1. Abhängigkeit der Hemmung der Anstiegsgeschwindigkeit des Aktionspotentials von der Erregungsfrequenz

+++	++	0+
Lidocaine	Quinidine	Procainamide
Prenylamine		Ajmaline
Pronethalol		Sparteine[a]
Propranolol		
Pindolol		

[a] Senges J, Ehe L (1973) Naunyn Schmiedebergs Arch Pharmacol 280:3,253

hinweisen könnten, sind bekanntlich häufige Nebenwirkungen. Doch es liegen sehr unterschiedliche experimentelle Ergebnisse über das Ausmaß dieser negativ inotropen Nebenwirkungen vor und ihre Übertragbarkeit in die klinische Situation ist fraglich.

Die klassische chinidinartige Wirkung hat nichts Gemeinsames mit den Effekten von Ca^{2+}-Antagonisten und es spricht alles dafür, daß eine klare Trennlinie zwischen solchen erregungshemmenden Wirkungen von Antiarrhythmica zu ziehen ist, die durch Beeinflussung des Ca^{2+}-Stroms bzw. des Na^+-Stroms zustande kommen. Wie bereits einleitend erläutert, ist eine exakte Quantifizierung dieser Antiarrhythmica-Wirkung erst auszuführen. Für den Kliniker hat das neue Therapie-Prinzip des Calcium-Antagonismus eine rasche Erweiterung der therapeutischen Möglichkeiten gebracht. Die Kenntnis pathophysiologischer Zusammenhänge und die differential diagnostischen Möglichkeiten der Klinik haben mit dieser raschen Entwicklung nicht angemessen Schritt gehalten. Von diesem neuen Therapie-Prinzip einer selektiv Ca^{2+}-antagonistischen Inhibition darf aber wegen seiner stimulierenden Wirkung auf Grundlagenforschung und Klinik noch viel erwartet werden.

Literatur

1. Vaughan Williams EM (1975) Classification of antidysrhythmic drugs. Pharmacol Ther [B] 1:115
2. Dreifus LS, de Azevedo I, Katz MR (1975) New antiarrhythmic drugs. In: Donoso E (ed) Current cardiovascular topics. Thieme, Stuttgart (Drugs in cardiology, part I, p 106)
3. Fleckenstein A (1977) Specific pharmacology of calcium in myocardium, cardiac pacemakers, and vascular smooth muscle. Annu Rev Pharmacol Toxicol 17:149
4. Cranefield PF (1977) Action potentials, after potentials and arrhythmias. Circ Res 41:4,415
5. Wit AL, Cranefield PF (1977) Triggered and automatic activity in the canine coronary sinus. Circ Res 41:4,435
6. Ferrier GR, Moe GK (1973) Effect of calcium on acetylstrophanthidin-induced transient depolarizations in canine Purkinje tissue. Circ Res 33:508
7. Tritthart H, Fleckenstein B, Fleckenstein A (1971) Some fundamental actions of antiarrhythmic drugs on the excitability and the contractility of single myocardial fibers. Naunyn Schmiedebergs Arch Pharmakol 269:212

The Role of Calcium-Ion Antagonists in Cardiac Arrhythmias [1]

D. M. Krikler and E. Rowland

The antiarrhythmic effects of verapamil noted clinically [1, 2] were postulated on experimental grounds [3, 4] to reflect a previously unrecognized therapeutic mechanism, selective inhibition of the transmembrane passage of calcium ions. Singh and Vaughan Williams [4] indicated that verapamil differed in its mode of action from substances that slowed the upstroke of the action potential (their class I, the paradigm of which is quinidine) as well as from beta-adrenergic blockers, with their antisympathetic action; however, part of the action of beta-blockers, predominantly in the class II of Singh and Vaughan Williams [4], was also shown to be due to an effect on calcium handling by the myocardial cell. "Calcium-antagonism", perhaps more precisely expressed as inhibition of the slow inward channel of the cell membrane (SIC-inhibition), has both practical and theoretical importance as regards the generation and treatment of cardiac arrhythmias. A new class of agents is thus available for the treatment of arrhythmias, but its role must be defined; and the relationship of such activity to the mechanisms, whereby certain arrhythmias arise; for example if the slow (rather than the fast) inward channel becomes responsible for depolarization [6]. Nevertheless, the caution expressed by Coumel [7] is wise: extrapolation from observed behaviour does not necessarily provide firm rules for therapeutic action and precise classifications depending on them can be premature. Therapeutic responses, positive and negative, noted in response to calcium-antagonists, reveal that this action is not necessarily synonymous with antiarrhythmic activity.

The slow inward channel is physiologically of prime importance in the sinoatrial and atrioventricular nodes, where the lowest resting potential during repolarization does not fall to the levels needed to activate the fast sodium-dependent inward channel (FIC) [8]. We have compared the effects of the sodium-antagonist (Class I agent) ajmaline with the calcium-antagonist verapamil in patients with paroxysmal reciprocating atrioventricular tachycardia (PRAVT) due to overt or concealed pre-excitation or AV junctional reentry. The drugs were administered by rapid intravenous injection in appropriate doses per kg body weight (ajmaline 0.75 mg, verapamil 0.15 mg, nifedipine 7.5 mcg). At this stage only the results with verapamil will be considered, those with nifedipine being mentioned later; comparison with ajmaline appears in the contribution by Rowland and Krikler (this volume). The indices explored were termination of tachycardia within 3 min and, thereafter, the ability to reinitiate PRAVT by means of programmed electric stimulation [9]. Separately, cases of PRAVT seen clinically and needing termination of episodes were given verapamil in the same dose and manner.

At electrophysiological study, verapamil terminated tachycardia in 48 of 57 cases [10]; the experience of Wellens et al. [11], with termination in nine of ten cases, is in

1 These studies are supported by the British Heart Foundation

accord with this. Our previous clinical experience showed almost universal success [2], and our current accumulated figures show termination in 195 of 199 cases [10]. The somewhat lower but still impressive responses during induced PRAVT studied electrophysiologically probably reflect the powerful reflex changes seen early in such episodes [12]: these tend to abate once the tachycardia is stable, and presumably the autonomic factors that would tend to counteract the antiarrhythmic agent no longer apply. This would explain the higher success rate in the clinical context, as the patients present during this later phase. The advantages of a specific calcium-antagonist over the beta-adrenergic antagonists are considerable: 19 of 20 cases responded to the former as compared with 8 of 20 to the latter [13]. Electrocardiographically, termination is usually abrupt (Fig. 1), though sometimes followed (as with vagotonic measures) by ventricular extrasystoles. If the terminal cycle lengths of the tachycardia show alternation this is presumptive evidence of the presence of a perhaps unsuspected accessory pathway [14], so-called concealed pre-excitation [15]. The fact that the calcium-antagonist stops the tachycardia by interrupting conduction in the AV node and not in the accessory pathway in the Wolff-Parkinson-White syndrome can be confirmed by electrophysiological study (Fig. 2).

After intravenous administration the effects of verapamil on AV nodal conduction (and on the ability to restart a tachycardia and for it to maintain itself) decline steadily. A tachycardia that could be initiated at a specific coupling interval for the extrastimulus prior to the calcium antagonist (Fig. 3) will show no response 5 min after its administration (Fig. 4) and only brief, poorly-sustained PRAVT at 10 min (Fig. 5). In most cases the effects are no longer evident or substantial 20 min after the administration of intravenous verapamil. Therapeutically verapamil slows

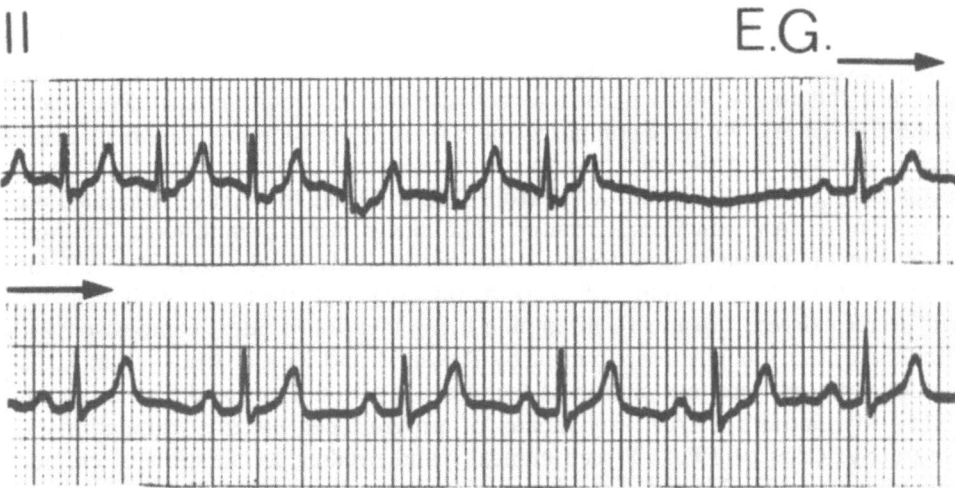

Fig. 1. ECG (lead 2) from a patient with paroxysmal reciprocating atrioventricular tachycardia. The upper panel shows the change from tachycardia (first six complexes) to sinus rhythm 30 s after intravenous verapamil (10 mg injected over 30 s). The interval between the cessation of tachycardia and the resumption of sinus rhythm is 1.2 s

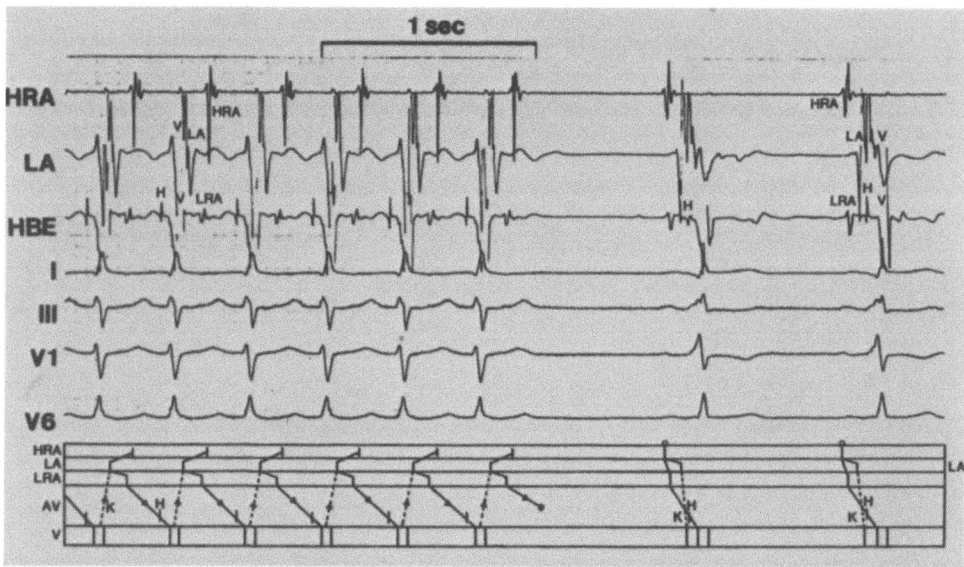

Fig. 2. Simultaneous surface and intracardiac ECG recordings taken during paroxysmal reciprocating atrioventricular tachycardia in a patient with the Wolff-Parkinson-White syndrome. HRA = high right atrial electrogram; LA = left atrial electrogram (recorded from the coronary sinus); HBE = His bundle electrogram. The first six complexes were recorded during the tachycardia, and after the sixth, the tachycardia (which showed narrow QRS complexes) is seen to terminate after atrial depolarization, i.e., anterogradely within the AV node. During tachycardia retrograde conduction to the atria was via a left-sided accessory pathway, as is shown by the fact that the first retrograde atrial depolarization was recorded in that lead. The subsequent two complexes are of sinus origin, and show the normal direction of atrioventricular conduction from proximal to distal. The QRS complexes are widened and deformed by initial delta waves, and the upright R in Vl indicates the Wolff-Parkinson-White syndrome, type A, in keeping with the fact that a left-sided pathway was used in tachycardia and now contributes, by virtue of parallel AV nodal and accessory conduction, to ventricular depolarization. The ventricular pre-excitation is confirmed because depolarization occurs simultaneously with activation of the bundle of His, thus indicating that it could not have been used by the first part of the impulse reaching the ventricles. In contrast, during tachycardia, the H-V interval is normal, reflecting anterograde AV nodal conduction. Paper speed in this and subsequent slides = 100 mm/s

the circuit conduction time so that reentry can no longer be maintained [10] and our present studies indicate that it inhibits reciprocation within the potential circuit; it does not act by preventing the occurrence of spontaneous extrasystoles, as appears to be more common with class I agents. This implies that, if adequate blood levels could be maintained, such calcium-antagonists could act prophylactically if given orally. Technical difficulties of estimation at present render precise correlations difficult [16, 17]. Isolated favourable responses to oral prophylaxis have been noted [10, 11] and we are currently investigating this by a double-blind trial.

Reciprocating sinoatrial tachycardia has also been shown to respond to verapamil, both as regards termination and prevention of acute reinitiation [18]. Slowing of AV nodal conduction reduces the ventricular rate in atrial fibrillation and flutter: uncommonly these disorders revert to sinus rhythm [19], the conversion rate being higher with flutter than fibrillation. While on theoretical grounds some ventricular tachycardias that are believed to arise because of activation of the slow

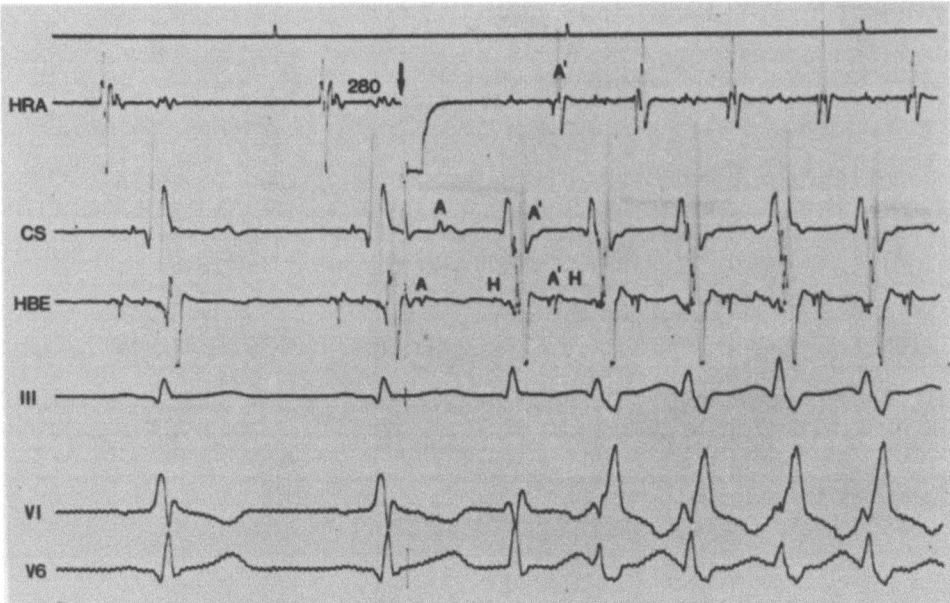

Fig. 3. Simultaneous intracardiac and surface ECGs. Conventions as in previous figure save that CS = coronary sinus, reflecting left atrial potentials. The first two complexes are sinus in origin and show pre-excitation (WPW syndrome type A, left lateral bypass). An extrastimulus 280 ms after the second sinus complex initiates reciprocating atrioventricular tachycardia using the accessory pathway retrogradely (note earliest A' in CS lead); anterograde conduction is via the AV node, with a normal HV interval but right bundle branch aberration has now appeared

inward channel [6] should be terminated by calcium-antagonists, therapeutic response is uncertain, and we are exploring this further; in about 50% of patients with ventricular extrasystoles these were suppressed by intravenous verapamil [19].

While other SIC-inhibitors have been investigated, only RO 11-1781 appears to have antiarrhythmic properties comparable to those of verapamil [20]. Indeed, nifedipine, a powerful "calcium-antagonist" now widely used for angina pectoris, was not shown to lengthen the AV conduction time in 21 patients when given alone or in combination with a beta-blocker [21]. We have studied its effects when given intravenously in ten patients; in none (all of whom responded to verapamil) did it stop paroxysmal supraventricular tachycardia, nor did it slow AV nodal conduction (Rowland et al., [22]). Whether one speculates that there may be different responses of slow inward channels in specialised tissue and working myocardium, or indeed different channels, the practical consequences suggest that it may be safe to administer beta-blockers together with nifedipine, though it is hazardous to combine them with verapamil [2, 5]. Another specific difference worth recalling is the fact that a calcium-antagonist may possess additional unrelated properties; prolongation of the QT interval is seen with prenylamine, which is prone to induce ventricular arrhythmias on this account [23].

Calcium-antagonists thus vary in efficacy (perhaps target specificity is different with different tissues), do not all have antiarrhythmic properties, and may have

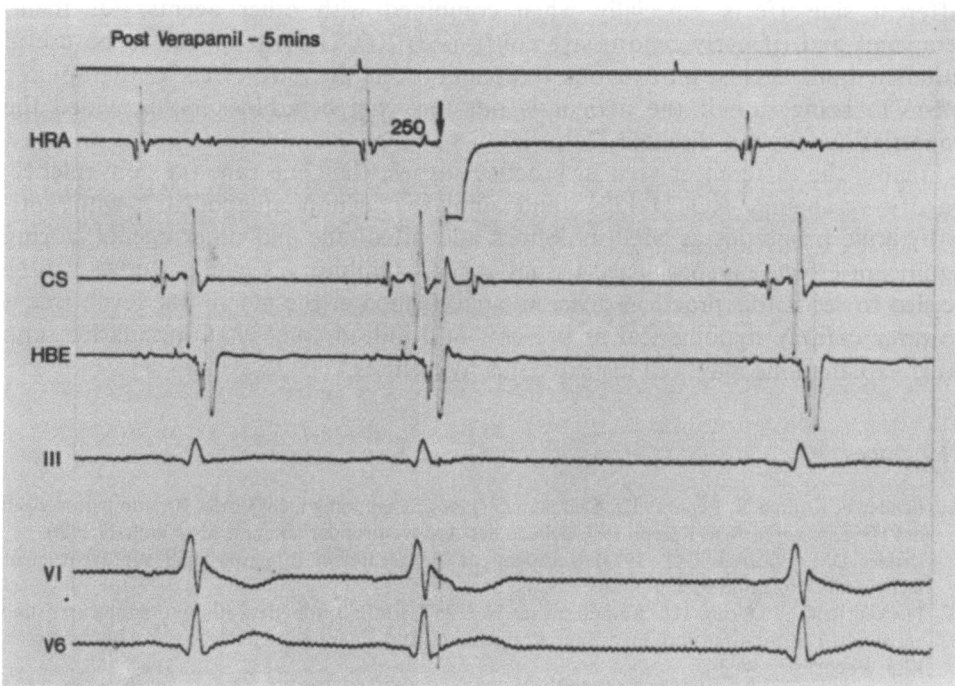

Fig. 4. Same patient as in Fig. 3, (5 min after verapamil): the tachycardia having stopped after verapamil, atrial extrastimuli over the whole cycle failed to reinitiate the arrhythmia, and at 250 ms found the atria refractory

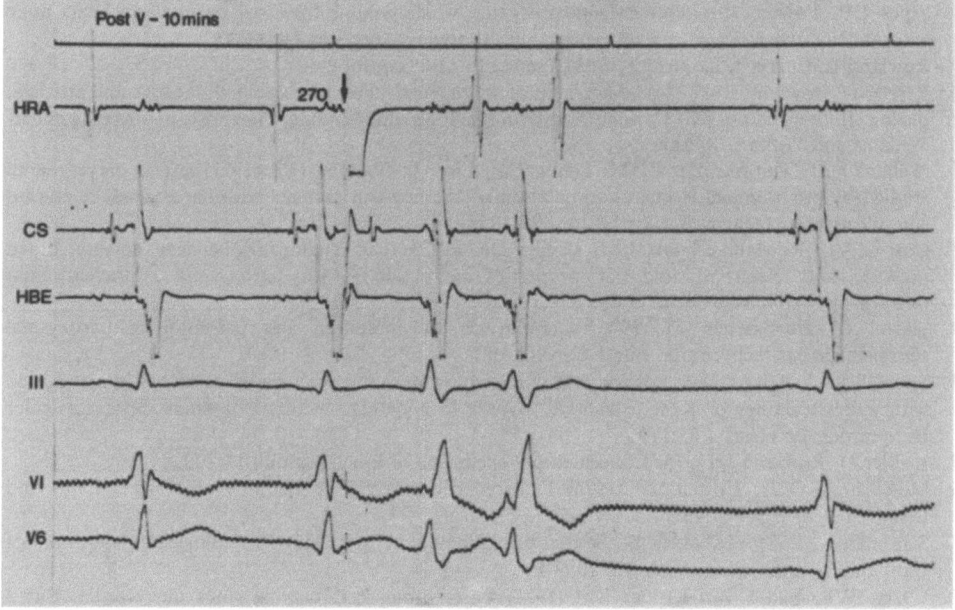

Fig. 5. Same patient 10 min after verapamil. An atrial extrastimulus 270 ms after the second sinus complex initiates atrioventricular reentry with features similar to those seen in Fig. 3, but this was sustained for only two such complexes, with immediate return to sinus rhythm

different side-effects especially when combined with other agents. Of them, verapamil and (if early reports are confirmed) RO 11-1781 appear to be useful antiarrhythmic agents: intravenous verapamil offers the most effective therapy for PRAVT, being safe if the patient is not receiving beta-blockers, provided the sinoatrial node is not diseased [24].

Finally, the differences seen in practice suggest that one can, for convenience, classify verapamil, RO 11-1781, and similar "calcium antagonists" with anti-arrhythmic properties as SIC^1-inhibitors and nifedipine and other agents lacking significant effects on specialized tissues as SIC^2-inhibitors. Cellular studies will be needed to see if this practical division is confirmed at the membrane level; this is however entirely hypothetical at present, and indeed somewhat speculative, and other explanations may well disprove this hypothesis.

References

1. Bender F, Kojima N, Reploh HD, Oelmann G (1966) Behandlung tachykarder Rhythmusstörungen des Herzens durch Beta-Rezeptorenblockade des Atrioventrikulargewebes. Med Welt 17:1120
2. Krikler DM, Spurrell RAJ (1974) Verapamil in the treatment of paroxysmal supraventricular tachycardia. Postgrad Med J 50:447
3. Fleckenstein A, Döring HJ, Kammermeier H (1968) Einfluß von Beta-Receptorenblockern und verwandten Substanzen auf Erregung, Kontraktion und Energiestoffwechsel der Myokardfaser. Klin Wochenschr 46:343
4. Singh BN, Vaughan Williams EM (1972) A fourth class of anti-dysrhythmic action? Effect of verapamil on ouabain toxicity, on atrial and ventricular intracellular potentials, and on other features of cardiac function. Cardiovasc Res 6:109
5. Nayler WG, Krikler D (1974) Verapamil and the myocardium. Postgrad Med J 50:441
6. Cranefield PF, Aronson RS, Wit AL (1974) Effect of verapamil on the normal action potential and on a calcium-dependent slow response of canine caridac Purkinje fibers. Circ Res 34:204
7. Coumel P (1978) Le choix logique d'un anti-arythmique: réalité ou gageure? Arch Mal Cœur 71:717
8. Zipes DP, Fischer JS (1974) Effects of agents which inhibit the slow channel on sinus node automaticity and atrioventricular conduction in the dog. Circ Res 34:184
9. Rowland E, Curry P, Krikler D (1978) Trans Eur Soc Cardiol 1:66
10. Krikler D, Rowland E (1979) Management of supraventricular tachycardia with drugs and artificial pacing. In: Narula OS (ed) Cardiac Arrhythmias: Electrophysiology, Diagnosis and Management. Willams and Wilkins, Baltimore, p 382
11. Wellens HJJ, Tan SL, Bar FWH, Düren DR, Lie KI, Dohmen HM (1977) Effect of verapamil studied by programmed electrical stimulation of the heart in patients with paroxysmal re-entrant supraventricular tachycardia. Br Heart J 39:1058
12. Curry PVL, Rowland E, Fox KM, Krikler DM (1978) The relationship between posture, blood pressure and electrophysiological properties in patients with paroxysmal supraventricular tachycardia. Arch Mal Cœur 71:293
13. Härtel G, Hartikainen M (1976) Comparison of verapamil and practolol in paroxysmal supraventricular tachycardia. Eur J Cardiol 4:87
14. Spurrell RAJ, Krikler DM, Sowton E (1973) Two or more intra AV nodal pathways in association with either a James or Kent extranodal bypass in 3 patients with paroxysmal supraventricular tachycardia. Br Heart J 35:113
15. Krikler D, Rowland E (1978) Concealed pre-excitation. J Electrocardiol 11:209
16. McAllister RG Jr, Howell SM (1976) Fluorometric essay of verapamil in biological fluids and tissues. J Pharm Sci 65:431
17. Schomerus M, Spiegelhalder B, Stieren B, Eichelbaum M (1976) Physiological disposition of verapamil in man. Cardiovasc Res 10:605
18. Curry PVL, Evans TR, Krikler DM (1977) Paroxysmal reciprocating sinus tachycardia. Eur J Cardiol 6:199
19. Schamroth L, Krikler DM, Garrett C (1972) Immediate effects of intravenous verapamil in cardiac arrhythmias. Br. Med J I:660

20. Gmeiner R, Ng CK, Simma H, Gstottner M (1979) The effect of a new clacium antagonist (Ro 11-1781) on the cardiac conduction system in man. Eur J Cardiol 9:77
21. Ekelund LG, Orö L (1976) Antianginal efficiency of Adalat with and without a beta-blocker. A subacute study with exercise tests. In: Jatene A, Lichtlen PR (eds) Third International Adalat Symposium: New therapy of ischemic heart disease. Excerpta Medica, Amsterdam, p 218
22. Rowland E, Evans T, Krikler D (1979) Effects of nifedipine on atrioventricular conduction as compared with verapamil. Intracardiac electrophysiological study. Br Heart J 42:124
23. Bens JL, Duboisset M, Quiret JC, Lesbre JP, Bernasconi T (1973) Syncopes par torsades de pointes induites ou favorisées par la prénylamine. Arch Mal Cœur 66:1427
24. Krikler D, Coumel P, Curry P, Oakley C (1977) Wolff-Parkinson-White syndrome type A obscured by left bundle branch block. Eur J Cardiol 5:49

Differential Responses to Sodium and Calcium Antagonists in Reciprocating Atrioventricular Tachycardia (WPW Syndrome)

E. Rowland and D. M. Krikler

Introduction

In paroxysmal reciprocating atrioventricular tachycardia (PRAVT), it is well established that anti-arrhythmic drugs may have an effect on one or more components of the re-entry circuit. These components depend for their depolarisation on fluxes of sodium or calcium ions [1], and agents that can specifically antagonise the transmembrane passage of these ions will have actions at specific sites. We have administered the sodium antagonist ajmaline and the calcium antagonist verapamil during intracardiac electrophysiological study. We have observed the ability of the drugs to terminate induced PRAVT, and then we examined the time-dependent changes in electrophysiological properties of the atrioventricular (AV) pathways, the accessory pathway (AP) on the one hand and the AV node on the other, in response to the drugs. As a result of these changes it is possible to comment on the effect on the mechanism of the tachycardia and more specifically on the ease of initiation.

These results provide guidelines for the use of these agents when used orally for long-term prophylaxis. Adverse effects may be observed which would mitigate against successful treatment irrespective of any beneficial action on the mechanism of the tachycardia. Further long-term follow-up studies are required to validate the predictions following intravenous administration.

Methods

Fourty-two patients, who were shown to have PRAVT associated with the Wolff-Parkinson-White (WPW) syndrome, underwent full electrophysiological investigation. Half of these patients received both ajmaline (0.75 mg/kg) and verapamil (0.15 mg/kg) during the study, while the other half received only one of the two drugs.

Electrophysiological testing during the control period included measurement of the sinus node recovery time, effective and functional refractory periods (ERP and FRP) of the AV node and accessory pathway in both anterograde and retrograde directions (where possible), atrial and ventricular myocardial effective refractory period and the cycle length of induced PRAVT [2]. In addition the highest 1:1 conduction rates sustained via the AV pathways in both anterograde and retrograde direction were recorded from various atrial pacing sites, and the width of the zone over which single atrial premature beats could initiate tachycardia was measured.

Each drug was given during induced PRAVT and the ability to terminate the tachycardia observed. The electrophysiological studies were repeated 5, 10 and 15 min after drug administration. If a second drug was to be given, it was done when the electrophysiological parameters had returned to the control values.

In selected patients a catheter (No. 6F) was inserted via the femoral artery and positioned in the descending thoracic aorta to record arterial pressure during the study.

Results

Table 1 and 2 illustrate the ability of ajmaline and verapamil, respectively, to terminate PRAVT following intravenous bolus administration. Five min were allowed to elapse before recording that the drug had failed to terminate the tachycardia.

Twenty-four patients received ajmaline and PRAVT was terminated in 12 of these patients (Table 1). Alongside each table the numbers in brackets refer to the response of those patients in each group who received verapamil as well (the upper table are those in whom PRAVT was terminated following verapamil and the lower figure those who did not respond). Thus the response to verapamil was equally good irrespective of whether ajmaline succeeded or failed.

Table 2 similarly illustrates the response to verapamil; 39 patients were given the drug during PRAVT and only 8 failed to terminate. The figures in brackets indicate the response to ajmaline of those who received both drugs and again there was a similar result irrespective of the response to verapamil.

The effects of the two drugs on the ability to initiate tachycardia was variable. An example of a narrowing of the initiation zone is shown in Figs. 1, 2, 3, 4. In the resting state tachycardia is induced with a premature atrial extrastimulus at a coupling interval of 280 ms (Fig. 1). Following the administration of verapamil, repeated extrastimulus testing at 5 min could not induce tachycardia (Fig. 2) because the initiation zone from the high right atrium has been abolished. At 10 min it was possible to induce tachycardia with a premature beat at 270 ms (Fig. 3), but after two cycles this was terminated spontaneously by a block in the AV node. Following a premature beat of 260 ms (Fig. 4) both AP and AV node were refractory. Thus the initiation zone at 10 min was smaller compared to the resting state and any induced tachycardia terminated spontaneously.

Table 1. The response of those patients who received ajmaline (0.75 mg/kg) during PRAVT. (+, termination; −, no termination within 5 min). Twelve responded and an equal number failed to respond. The figures in brackets refer to the response in each group of those patients who received verapamil in addition (e.g. of the 12 patients in whom PRAVT was terminated by ajmaline 10 also received verapamil, which successfully terminated in 7 and failed in 3 cases)

	+	−
WPW	$12\left(\frac{7}{3}\right)$	$12\left(\frac{8}{3}\right)$

Table 2. In a similar fashion to Fig. 1 the response to verapamil (0.15 mg/kg) of 39 patients with PRAVT associated with the WPW syndrome is shown. The figures in brackets indicate the response of those patients who received ajmaline as well (e.g. 8 patients failed to terminate with verapamil − 6 of these also received ajmaline and it succeeded in 3 and failed in 3

	+	−
WPW	$31\left(\frac{7}{8}\right)$	$8\left(\frac{3}{3}\right)$

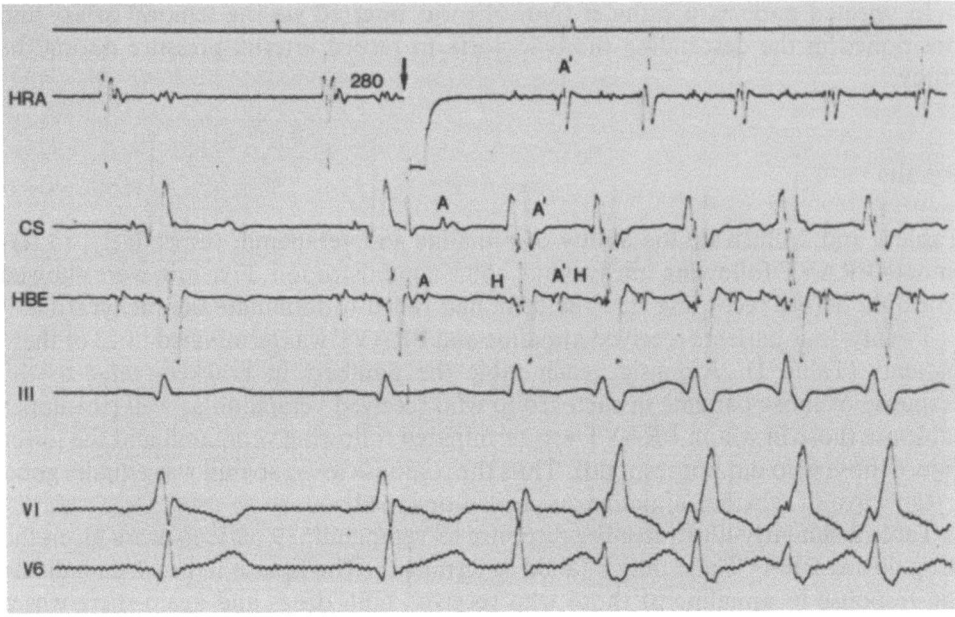

Fig. 1. The initiation of PRAVT in a patient with WPW Type A. An atrial premature beat delivered in the high right atrium (HRA) at a coupling interval of 280 ms initiates tachycardia with RBBB. Early retrograde left atrial depolarisation confirms the left-sided accessory pathway (CS, coronary sinus; HBE, His bundle electrogram; standard ECG leads III, VI and V6)

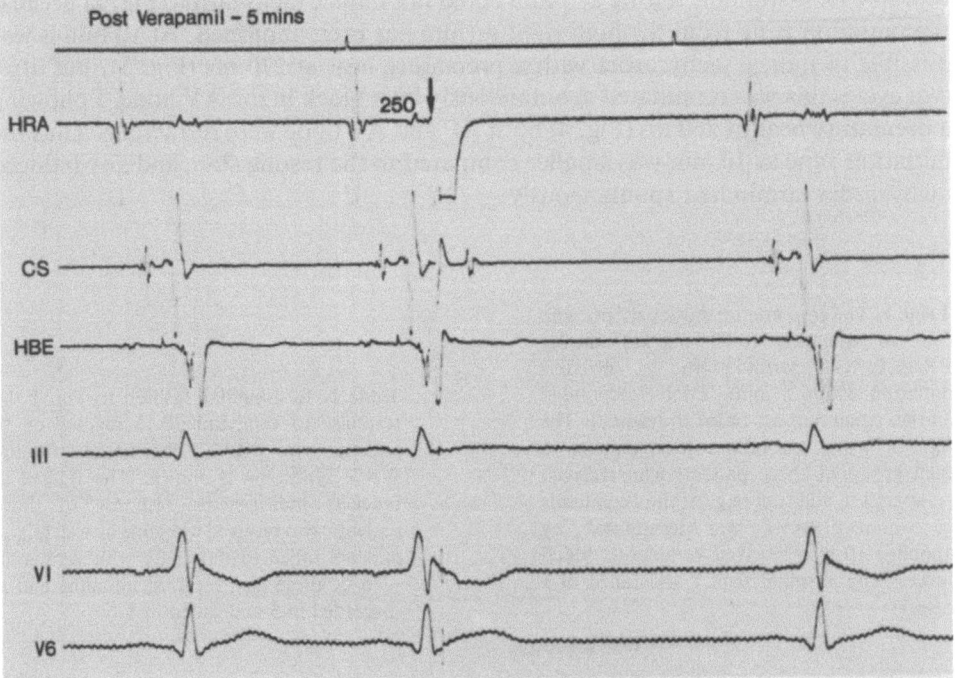

Fig. 2. In the same patient as in Fig. 3 it was not possible to induce PRAVT 5 min after the administration of verapamil. At a coupling interval of 250 ms an atrial premature beat finds the accessory pathway refractory. The AV node is also refractory indicating the abolition of an initiation zone for tachycardia

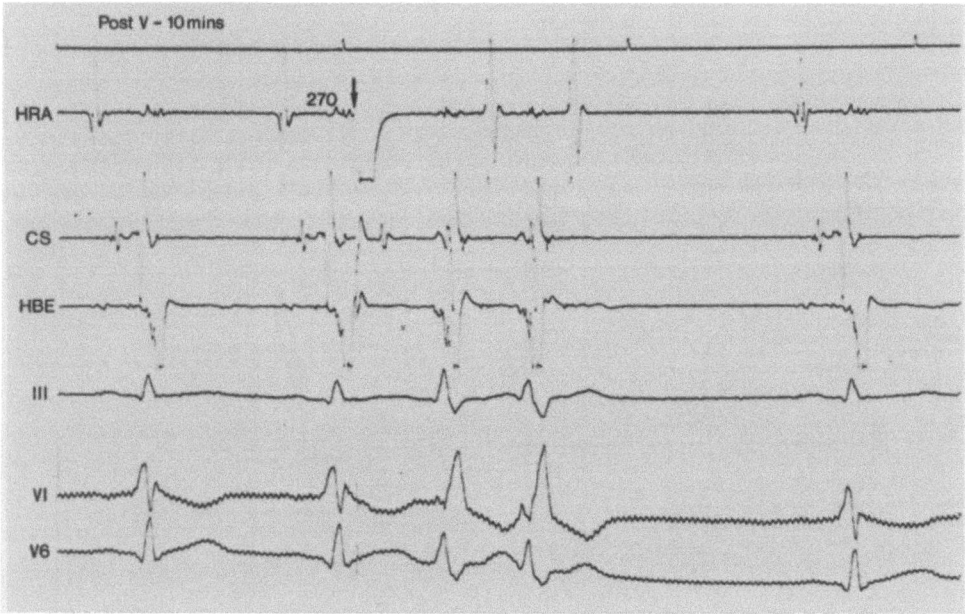

Fig. 3. The same patient as in Figs. 3 and 4, 10 min after verapamil. Following an atrial premature beat of 270 ms the accessory pathway is refractory and as AV nodal refractoriness has recovered tachycardia is initiated. However, it spontaneously terminates after two beats because of block in the AV node

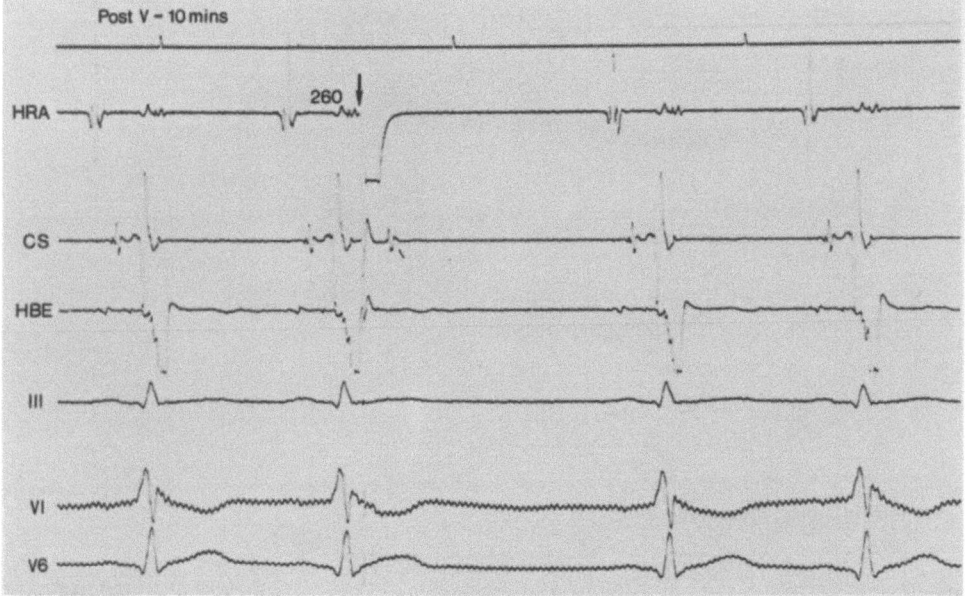

Fig. 4. An atrial premature beat at 260 ms finds both AV pathways refractory, which indicates a narrowing of the zone of initiation for PRAVT as compared to the control values

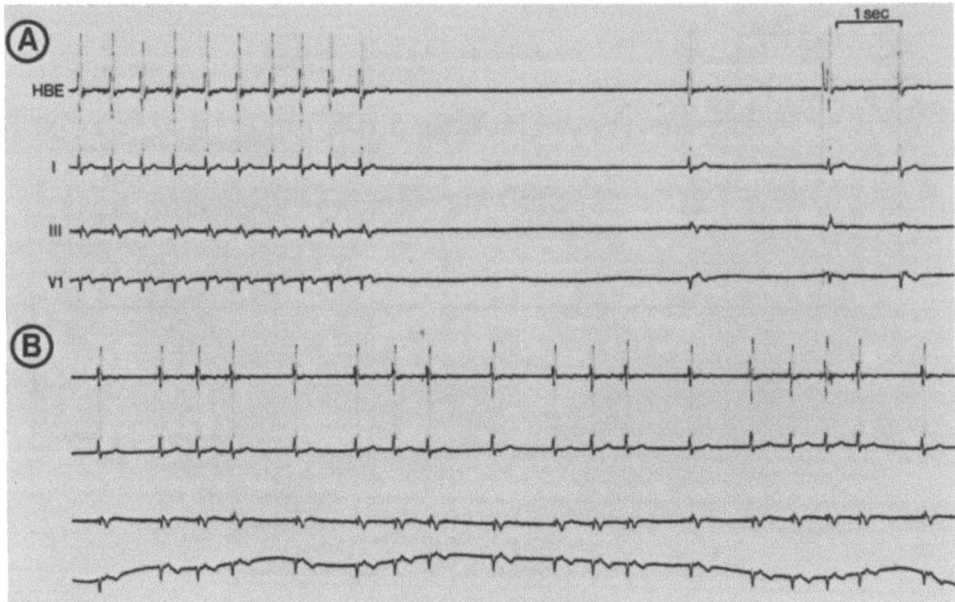

Fig. 5. Two recordings from a patients with PRAVT associated with a concealed left-sided accessory pathway – His bundle electrogram and standard leads I, III and V1 are shown. The upper trace A shows the termination of PRAVT following intravenous verapamil; 5 s elapse before a slow junctional rhythm ensues. In the lower trace B, recorded some minutes later, the junctional rhythm continuously reinitiates short paroxysms of tachycardia

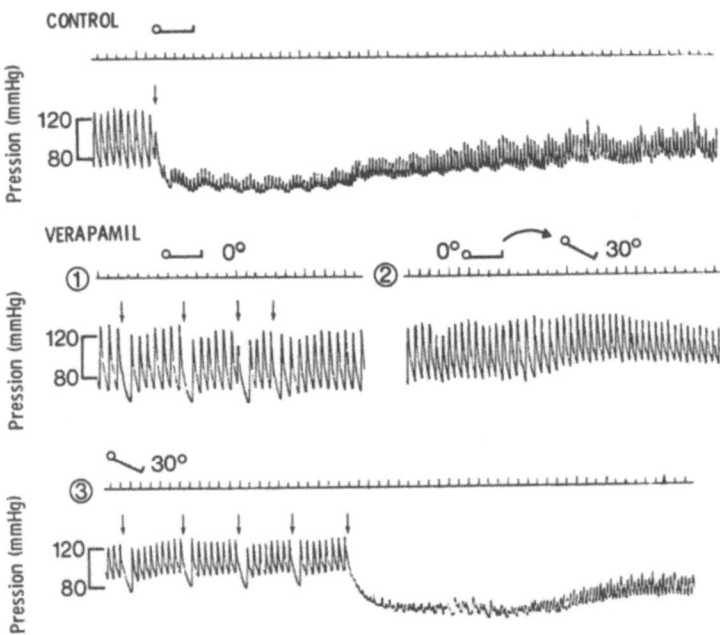

Fig. 6. Arterial blood pressure (mm Hg) recorded in a patient with PRAVT. In the upper trace tachycardia is initiated while the patient is in the horizontal position. In the middle trace atrial premature beats (↓), in the presence of verapamil, fail to induce tachycardia (1). The patient is moved from the horizontal to a position of head-up tilt (2). In the bottom trace (3), with the patient at 30° head-up tilt, an atrial premature beat can induce tachycardia. Note also how much further the blood pressure falls at the onset of tachycardia under the combined influences of verapamil and a partly upright posture

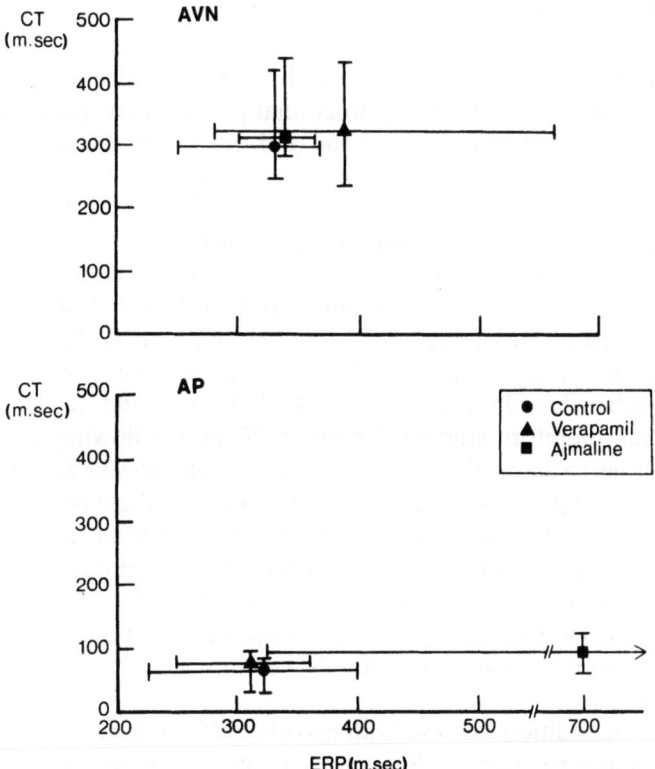

Fig. 7. The influence of verapamil and ajmaline on AV pathways. In the upper graph the effect on AV nodes (AVN) is shown. In each patient the effective refractory period (ERP) for the pathway is measured, as is the conduction time (CT) for the last conducted beat prior to the ERP, before and after drugs. The average of all the values is plotted as the central point (●, control; ▲, after verapamil; ■, after ajmaline) and the range is indicated by the bars. The lower graph shows the changes in electrophysiological properties of accessory pathways (AP) with the two drugs

Other electrophysiological effects were sometimes seen which could adversely affect a beneficial action on the re-entrant mechanism. Sinus node depression was seen in a patient in whom verapamil successfully terminated PRAVT (Fig. 5). Junctional recovery time was also prolonged and the subsequent junctional rhythm acted to continuously initiate short paroxysms of tachycardia [3].

Alterations in autonomic balance may counteract the action of verapamil [4]. The predominance of sympathetic tone that accompanies upright posture may, by reducing the depressant action of verapamil on the AV node, allow tachycardia to be initiated when this was not possible in the supine position (Fig. 6).

The specificity of ajmaline and verapamil on the AP and AV node, respectively, is not complete. Figure 7 illustrates the action of both drugs on the two groups of AV pathways. The ERP and the conduction time at the last conducted beat (CT) are measured in each patient. On each graph the central point indicates the average of these values for the group and also marked are the range of values. Verapamil prolongs both the ERP and the CT in AV nodes while having no apparent effect in APs. Ajmaline on the other hand depresses conduction and refractoriness in both types of pathways although in APs more than AV nodes.

Discussion

The PRAVT associated with the WPW syndrome is established and maintained because of the differing functional properties of parallel conducting AV pathways, the AV node on the one hand and the AP on the other [5]. The properties of each reflect the dependence for depolarisation on specific ionic fluxes. Drugs that specifically antagonise calcium or sodium ions possess specific anti-arrhythmic properties on the re-entrant mechanisms.

Given intravenously to terminate PRAVT, verapamil appears to be more effective than ajmaline [6]. It does not appear to be true that if a patient fails to respond to verapamil, ajmaline will succeed in terminating PRAVT. The serum levels of the drug immediately following intravenous bolus administration are considerably higher than during chronic oral administration [7]. The ability to reinitiate PRAVT was therefore studied for up to 20 min following intravenous administration in order to assess the time course for the changes in electrophysiological properties of the components of the re-entrant circuit. In these patients coupled atrial extrastimuli were used to assess the feasibility of reinitiating tachycardia.

An anti-arrhythmic agent may be of prophylactic benefit by abolishing atrial extrasystoles irrespective of its action on the re-entry circuit. In these patients the effect of the two drugs on the components of the circuit was variable. While in some the initiation zone was abolished, in others it was wider than during the control period.

In addition to these findings other effects were sometimes seen which would act in an adverse manner. Sinus node depression was seen with both drugs although more commonly with verapamil. The subsequent junctional rhythm was often able to reinitiate tachycardia over a wide zone.

Increase in sympathetic tone improves conduction through the AV node and shortens refractoriness. The depressant action of verapamil on the AV node will be counteracted by increasing sympathetic tone, and likewise enhanced by increasing parasympathetic tone.

The presence of other arrhythmias, such as rapidly conducted atrial fibrillation, complicating the WPW syndrome may also need to be taken into consideration when considering oral therapy. Verapamil, like other AV nodal depressing drugs, may be capable of increasing the mean ventricular rate during the arrhythmia [8].

References

1. Nayler WG (1975) The cellular basis for anti-arrhythmic therapy. In: Krikler DM, Goodwin JF (eds) Cardiac arrhythmias: The modern electrophysiological approach. Saunders, London, pp 208-222
2. Curry PVL (1975) Fundamentals of arrhythmias: modern methods of investigation. In: Krikler DM, Goodwin JF (eds) Cardiac arrhythmias: The modern electrophysiological approach. Saunders, London, pp 46-81
3. Coumel Ph, Attnel P, Slama R, Curry P, Krikler D (1976) Incessant tachycardias in Wolff-Parkinson-White syndrome. II. Role of atypical cycle length dependency and nodal-his escape beats in initiating reciprocating tachycardias. Br Heart J 38:897-905
4. Curry PVL, Rowland E, Fox KM, Krikler DM (1978) The relationship between posture, blood pressure and electrophysiological properties in patients with paroxysmal supraventricular tachycardia. Arch Mal Coeur 71:293-299

5. Coumel (1975) Supraventricular tachycardias. In: Krikler DM, Goodwin JF (eds) Cardiac arrhythmias: The modern electrophysiological approach. Saunders, London, pp 125 – 139
6. Krikler DM, Spurrell RAJ (1974) Verapamil in the treatment of paroxysmal supraventricular tachycardia. Postgrad Med J 50:447 – 453
7. Margiardi LM, Hariman RJ, McAllister RG, Bhargava V, Surawicz P, Shabetai R (1978) Electrophysiologic and hemodynamic effects of verapamil. Correlation with plasma drug concentrations. Circulation 57:366 – 372
8. Wellens HJ, Durrer D (1973) Effect of digitalis on atrioventricular conduction and circus-movement tachycardias in patients with the Wolff-Parkinson-White syndrome. Circulation 47:1229 – 1233

Calcium Currents Mediating Inotropic and Chronotropic Effects in Mammalian Cardiac Muscle

E. M. Vaughan Williams

Over a certain range of calcium concentrations, from about half to twice the normal concentration, there is a linear relation between the logarithm of the external calcium concentration and the force of cardiac contractions. Furthermore, there is very little hysteresis, so that when the calcium concentration is returned to normal for a second time the force of contraction is similar to what it was originally. This effect can, therefore, be used as a simple and convenient preliminary screening test for new drugs, to see whether they have calcium-antagonist activity (Fig. 1).

Many calcium-antagonist drugs, such as verapamil and perhexiline, are effective antiarrhythmic agents, and the question arises whether the calcium currents mediating the inotropic action passes through the same channels as are responsible for arrhythmogenesis.

Sydney Ringer discovered nearly a century ago [1] that calcium ions were necessary for cardiac contractions. When electrical recording became available with external surface electrodes, it was found that action potentials were not abolished by solutions deficient in calcium, but were almost indistinguishable from normal action potentials. The discovery that calcium currents were concerned in cardiac action potentials had to await more sophisticated recording methods, and techniques to

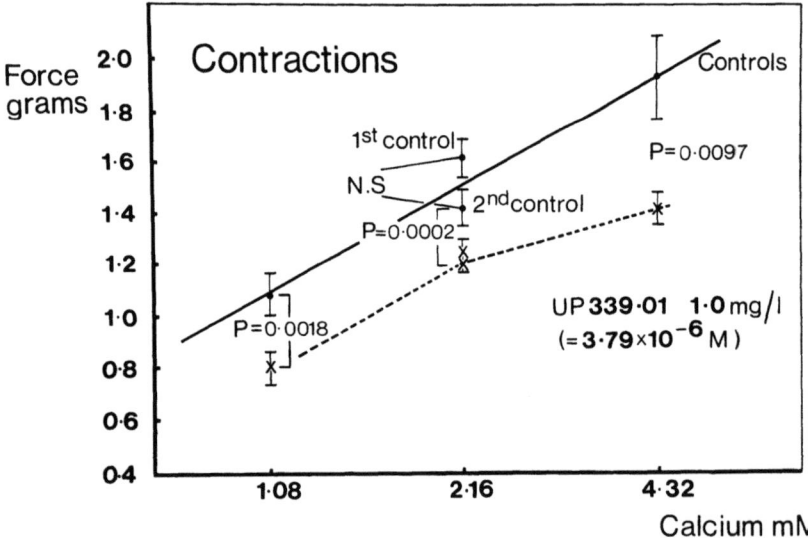

Fig. 1. Positive inotropic effects of calcium as a screening test for calcium antagonism. Over a fourfold range there is a linear relation between force of contraction and the log of the calcium concentration. There is no hysteresis, and a new compound, UP 339.01, is shown to shift the relation to the right. (Preparation: isolated rabbit atria)

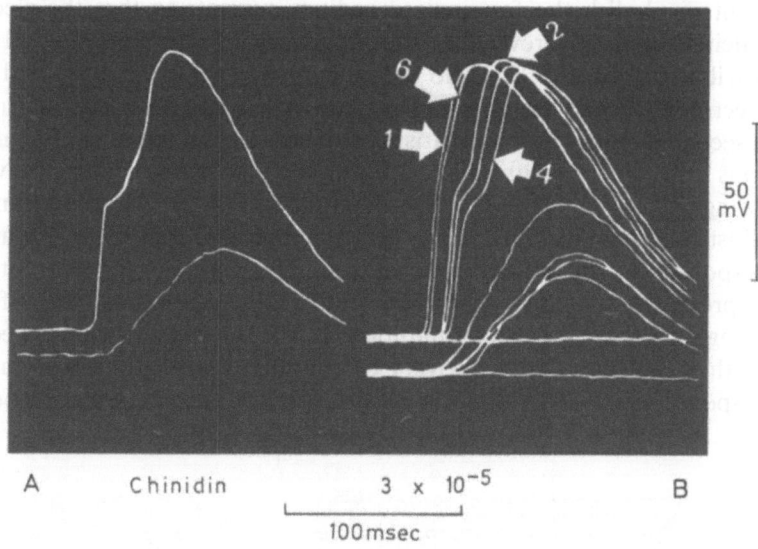

A   Chinidin 3×10^{-5} B

|—————— 100 msec ——————|

Fig. 2. Evidence for distinction between fast and slow inward current. *On the right,* responses (intracellular potentials and contractions) to six stimuli are shown. Fast inward current is progressively depressed, until the response to the fifth fails altogether. The response to the sixth stimulus, after a double interval, is again faster, illustrating the frequency-dependence of the depression by quinidine of fast inward current. The height and duration of the slow current is little affected, but the contraction after the double interval is larger. Thus the membrane current and excitation-contraction coupling current are distinguishable

Table 1. Summary of calcium movements in cardiac muscle

A. *Into cell* (Down concentration gradient)

    1. Slow inward current   Depolarising membrane current (M).
                                              Time and Voltage dependent.

    2. Excitation-contraction[a] coupling (E)   Triggered by Depolarisation.
                                                Derived from Storage Site.
                                              Combines with Troponin C.
                                              Activates Myosin ATPase.

    3. Adrenergically activated   Involves cAMP.
                                                Depolarising *and* Contraction Coupling.
                    (WHICH COMPONENT TRIGGERS OUTWARD K^+?)

B. *From Sarcoplasm* (Against concentration gradient).

    1. Uptake into Sarcoplasmic Reticulum.

    2. Uptake into Mitochondria.

    3. Extrusion into Extracellular Space.   { Na/Ca exchange
                                                         { Active pump

Associated with Relaxation of Contraction.

---

[a] *N.B.* If the storage site is intracellular, calcium released for E.C. coupling must be electrically "invisible", because calcium ions appearing in free solution must leave behind negative charges by which they had been sequestered. Consequently the net charge across the cell surface would remain unchanged

limit or abolish the fast inward sodium current, so that the electrical activity of calcium could be revealed. The discovery of the slow inward current is often attributed to Reuter [2], who used choline to replace sodium, and employed micro-electrodes for recording from Purkinje fibres, and for passing current. Evidence for a second slow inward depolarising current in contracting cardiac muscle, carried by ions other than sodium, had, in fact, been presented 9 years previously, quinidine being used to limit the fast inward current (Fig. 2). The right hand panel of Fig. 2 illustrates another difference between the fast and slow inward currents. The responses to six stimuli are shown. The fast inward current is progressively depressed by successive stimuli, until the response to the fifth stimulus fails altogether ("Wenckebach inhibition"). The double interval between the fourth and sixth stimuli permitted recovery of channels carrying the fast current, so that the response to the sixth stimulus was similar to that of the first. The contraction was

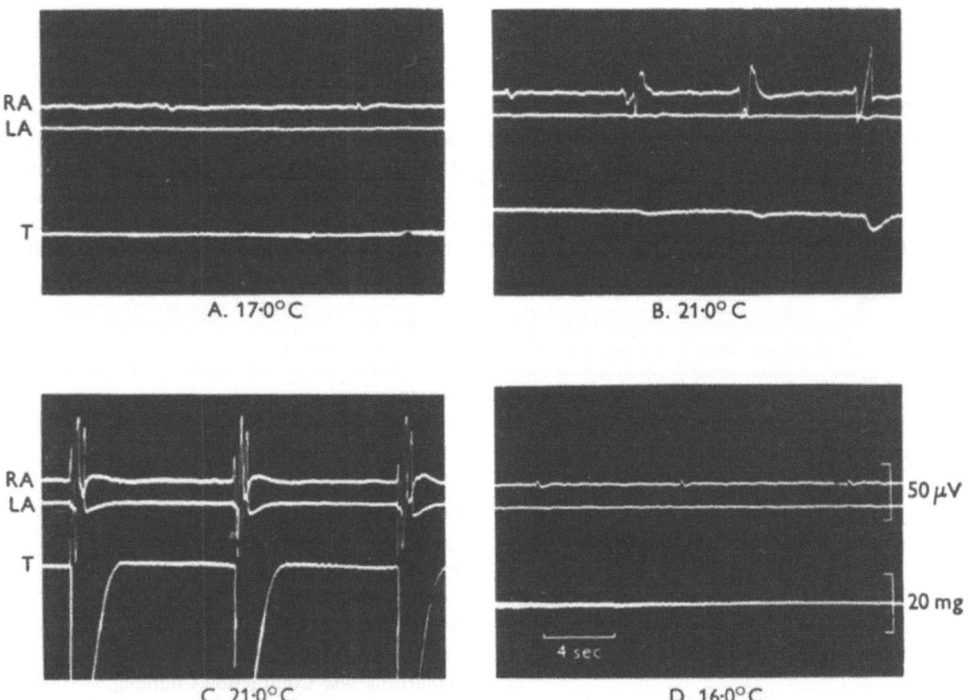

Fig. 3. Effect of low temperature on S.A. node and contracting myocardium. At 17 °C contractions were absent, but the S.A. node continued to produce potentials at a regular rate. At 21 °C, coupling between the S.A. node and contracting fibres was re-established.
(Preparation: isolated rabbit atria).
R.A. Surface recording from right atrium in the vicinity of the S.A. node.
L.A. Record from electrode on the left atrium.
T.   Tension record.
Top, Right At 21 °C potentials invaded the right atrium from the S.A. node and contractions began to appear.
Bottom, Left Potentials have now spread to the left atrium, and the contraction record goes off the screen.
Bottom, Right On recooling potentials disappear from L.A. and R.A. but pacemaker potentials persist

also larger after the double interval, implying that a larger amount of excitation-contraction coupling calcium had accumulated in the store, ready to be released by the next action potential. The height and duration of slow inward current, however, was little affected. Depression of fast inward current by quinidine is, therefore, frequency-dependent, but the slow inward current is not. A distinction must be made, also, between the slow inward current depolarising the membrane (M) and calcium current concerned in contraction coupling (E) (Table 1).

Calcium currents are important in depolarising the sinoatrial (S.A.) and atrioventricular (A.V.) nodes. The nodes, however, do not contract. If a rabbit atrium is cooled to about 17 °C, contractions cease, but the S.A. node continues to produce potentials at a regular frequency, (Fig. 3). No tension development is detectable, even though the apparatus used is sufficiently sensitive to record less than a milligram [3]. As soon as the tissue is warmed to 21 °C, conduction from the S.A. node to the atrium is re-established, and contractions return.

In the light of evidence obtained from sucrose-gap preparations containing cells from near the sinus region of the heart of the American bull frog, Brown et al. [4]

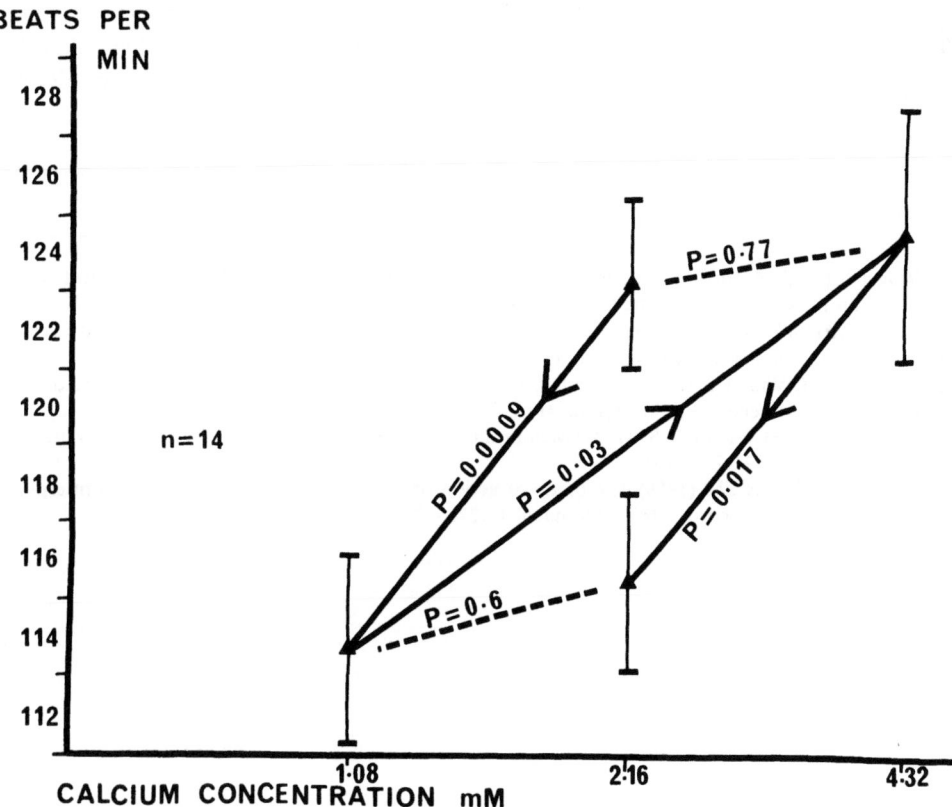

Fig. 4. Effect of calcium concentration on the S.A. node. In contrast to the relation between contractions and calcium concentration, the relation between frequency and calcium concentration exhibits considerable hysteresis. Thus the frequency in 4.32 mM calcium is not significantly different from that during the first exposure to the normal calcium concentration (2.16 mM), and the frequency in 1.08 mM calcium is not different from that during the second exposure to normal calcium

stated: "The finding that in primary pacemaker (i.e. spontaneous, tetrodotoxine-insensitive) preparations from frog sinus *only one* depolarising current is present, and that this is sensitive to Mn^{2+} ions, indicates strongly that the current involved is the slow inward current, I_{Si}, of other cardiac tissues." The chronotropic responses to changes in calcium concentration of the mammalian sinus node, however, differ from the inotropic responses of the muscle, in that they exhibit considerable hysteresis (Fig. 4).

The problem arises, therefore, whether the currents restricted by "calcium antagonist" drugs in their antiarrhythmic action are the same as those restricted in their negative inotropic action. Calcium movements into and out of cardiac cells are complex (Table 1).

The membrane capacity can be depolarised by a charge that is very much less than that which is necessary to activate contraction. Thus the small slow inward current depolarising the membrane (M) may trigger the release from a store of a much larger amount of calcium (E), sufficient to raise the intracellular calcium concentration from less than 10^{-7} M to as much as 10^{-6} M. The calcium is then actively removed by accumulation into sarcoplasmic reticulum and mitochondria, and is probably also pumped out of the cell in addition to being expelled in exchange for sodium. How it is recycled from the S.R. back to the contraction-coupling storage site, ready for release by subsequent action potentials, is not clear. Thus it is at least possible that the generic term "calcium antagonist" might be expanded to include selective antagonism by different drugs at distinct sites.

References

1. Ringer S (1882) A further contribution regarding the influence of the different constituents of the blood on the contraction of the heart. J Physiol (Lond.) 4:28 – 43
2. Reuter H (1967) The dependence of slow inward current in Purkinje fibres on the extracellular calcium concentration. J Physiol (Lond.) 192:479 – 492
3. Marshall JM, Vaughan Williams EM (1956) Pacemaker potentials. The excitation of isolated rabbit auricles by acetylcholine at low temperatures. J Physiol (Lond.) 131:186 – 199
4. Brown HF, Giles W, Noble SJ (1977) Membrane currents underlying activity in frog sinus venosus. J Physiol (Lond.) 271:783 – 816
5. Vaughan Williams EM (1958) The mode of action of quinidine in isolated rabbit atria interpreted from intracellular records. Br J Pharmacol 13:276 – 287

Verapamil Effects in the Setting of Acute Experimental Myocardial Ischemia

T. Peter, H. Hamamoto, A. McCullen, I. Yamaguchi, and W. J. Mandel

Summary

Effect of Verapamil (V) on impulse conduction in the acutely ischemic myocardium was tested in ten dogs (5 control and 5 treated) after ligation of left anterior descending artery (LAD). In the treated group V was given 0.15 mg/kg IV bolus at a rate of 2 mg/min immediately after LAD occlusion and was followed by an IV infusion at a dose of 7.5 µg/kg/min. In each dog, LAD was ligated below the second diagonal initially and 30 min later below the first diagonal. From multiple needle electrodes, endocardial bipolar (0.5 mm apart) electrograms (40–500 Hz 10 mm = 0.5 mV) were recorded prior to ligation and at 5, 15, and 30 min after each LAD occlusion. Constant rate atrial pacing (200/min.) was performed and premature stimuli were delivered at fixed coupling (50%) intervals. Conduction times (defined as the interval from premature pacing stimulus to the earliest high frequency deflection in the endocardial electrograms) were measured within the ischemic zone and within normal zone in both groups of dogs. Results showed that (1) prior to LAD ligation, the conduction within the normal myocardium was similar between the control and V treated groups of dogs; (2) following LAD ligation, conduction within the ischemic zone slowed significantly in the control group of dogs; (3) in the V treated dogs, conduction within the ischemic zone did not alter from the pretreatment values and was significantly different to the corresponding values in the control group. We conclude that post occlusion intravenous verapamil prevents deterioration of impulse conduction that normally occurs as a result of acute ischemia. This observation suggests a possible new mechanism of antiarrhythmic action of verapamil in acute ischemia and that a racemic mixture of verapamil may possess more than simple calcium antagonistic properties.

Zusammenfassung

Wir prüften die Wirkung von Verapamil (V) auf die Reizleitungszeit innerhalb des akut ischämischen Myokards bei 10 Hunden (5 Kontrollgruppe, 5 behandelt mit V) nach Unterbindung des RIVA. Verapamil wurde in einer Dosis von 0,15 mg/kg intravenös als Bolus, unmittelbar nach Koronarverschluß bei 5 Hunden verabreicht; anschließend wurde eine Dosis von 7,5 µg/kg/Min infundiert. Die Unterbindung des RIVA erfolgte in zwei Stufen: in einer ersten Phase distal vom 2. R. diagonalis und in einer zweiten Stufe 30 Min später distal vom 1. R. diagonalis. Endokardiale bipolare Elektrokardiogramme wurden mittels mehrerer Nadelelektroden vor sowie 5, 15 und 30 Min nach jeder Unterbindung aufgezeichnet. Die Untersuchung wurde bei konstanter Vorhofstimulation (200/Min) und vorzeitigen Stimuli mit einem Kopplungsintervall von 50% durchgeführt. Die Reizleitungszeit (definiert als der Zeitintervall zwischen der vorzeitigen Schrittmacherstimulation und der ersten hochfrequenten Schwingung im endokardialen EKG) wurde im ischämischen sowie normalen Muskelareal beider Untersuchungsgruppen gemessen. *Ergebnis:* (1) Vor Koronarverschluß war die Reizleitungszeit innerhalb des normalen Myokardiums bei beiden Untersuchungsgruppen gleich. (2) Nach Verschluß des RIVA verzögerte sich die Reizleitungszeit signifikant innerhalb des ischämischen Areals bei der Kontrollgruppe. (3) In der mit Verapamil behandelten Gruppe unterschied sich die Reizleitungszeit innerhalb des ischämischen Myokards nicht signifikant von Werten vor dem Koronarverschluß. Dies war signifikant unterschiedlich von Werten in der Vergleichsgruppe.

Folgerung: Nach Koronarverschluß verhindert die intravenöse Gabe von Verapamil die Verzögerung der Impulsfortleitung im ischämischen Areal. Dies läßt auf einen zusätzlichen Mechanismus der antiarrhythmischen Wirkung von Verapamil bei der akuten Ischämie schließen; möglicherweise besitzt die racemische Form von Verapamil Eigenschaften, die über seine bloße calcium-antagonistische Wirkung hinausreichen.

Introduction

Coronary Care Units have made significant contributions to our understanding of the pathophysiology of the acutely ischemic myocardium, and there is general agreement that mortality due to pump failure remains a largely unresolved problem. Controversy exists, however, regarding the role of antiarrhythmic therapy in preventing death, in spite of the fact that several new drugs have been added to the therapeutic armamentarium. A relatively new concept has been slow channel blocking agents, the prototype drug being verapamil [1]. Though there is considerable evidence in the literature that verapamil is a highly effective agent intravenously for the acute termination of reciprocating junctional tachycardias [2], its effect on ventricular arrhythmias associated with acute myocardial ischemia is less well documented and its probable effects on the electrical characteristics of the ischemic myocardium less well investigated. The purpose of the present study was to examine the effect of intravenous verapamil on the conduction of an impulse in the normal as well as in the ischemic myocardium.

Method

Preparation of the Model. Male mongrel dogs (25 – 30 kg) were premedicated with morphine sulphate intramuscularly (1.5 mg/kg) and thirty min later general anesthesia was obtained by sodium pentobarbital 5 mg/kg and 50 cc of 20% ethyl carbamate intravenously. The animal was intubated and connected to a Harvard respirator and ventilated with room air. An esophageal temperature probe was positioned and temperature was maintained within the normal range by a thermal blanket.

A right femoral venous cutdown was done and an intravenous line established for the administration of anesthesia and drugs. A No. 7 French catheter was introduced through a femoral arterial cutdown and advanced into the left ventricle (LV) and was then withdrawn to the aorta. Central aortic pressure was monitored throughout the period of the study. The left femoral vein was also exposed and a No. 7 French bipolar electrode catheter was advanced into the right ventricle (RV) by intracardiac electrogram monitoring without the aid of fluoroscopy. The signals were then filtered through 40 – 500 Hz and the catheter was positioned across the tricuspid valve to obtain a His bundle electrogram. The chest was opened via a left lateral thoracotomy through the fifth intercostal space with careful hemostasis. The lungs were gently retracted, the parietal pericardium was slit open vertically from the root of the pulmonary artery to the apex of the left ventricle and the heart was suspended in a pericardial cradle. The left anterior descending artery (LAD) was dissected at two sites: below the first diagonal branch and below the second diagonal branch and looped for subsequent ligation. Epicardial plaque electrodes were sutured on to the left atrium for atrial pacing and on to the right ventricle for obtaining a QRS signal for subsequent R-wave-triggered, premature stimuli. Multiple small intramyocardial needles were then inserted into the myocardium. These needles were constructed in our laboratory (Fig. 1) and contained three bipolar pairs of electrodes. Each bipole consisted of two silver electrodes, 1 mm long, 0.5 mm wide and 0.5 mm apart. The distance between two bipoles was 0.5 mm. The middle pair was positioned in the midwall and the remaining pairs were located each in the endocardium as well as in the epicardium. Five such needles were positioned in relation to the left anterior descending ligatures (see Fig. 2); two were positioned, one each at the level of a ligature (needles #2 and #4). The LAD was occluded transiently for 5 s at both sites, one after another, so that the myocardium was cyanotic with a clearly demarcated border and the corresponding needle was inserted precisely at this border line. The remaining three needles were positioned, one above the level of the higher ligature (needle #1), one below the level of the lower ligature (needle #5), and one in between the two ligatures (needle #3). Each needle was positioned 1 – 2 cm away from the left anterior descending artery and the intraventricular septum in the left ventricular myocardium.

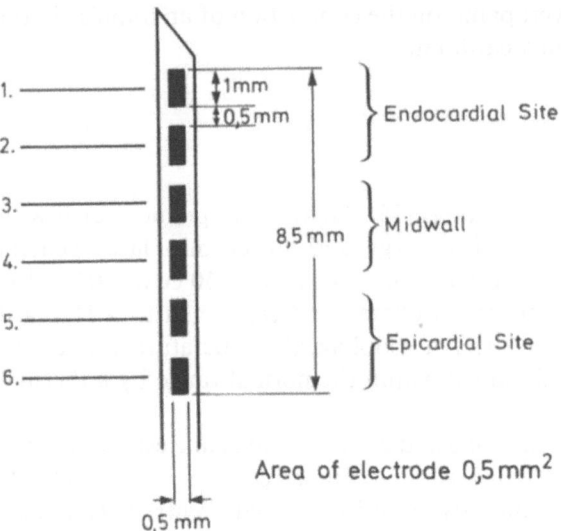

Fig. 1. Diagram of the needle electrode

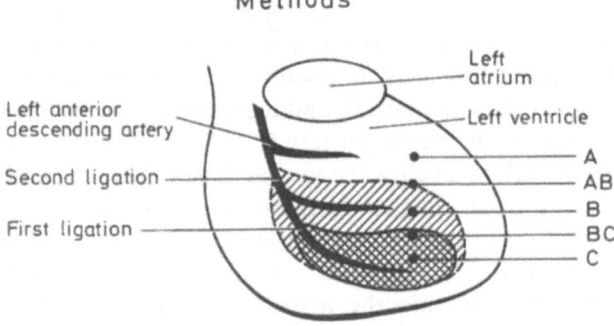

Fig. 2. Diagram of the heart with LAD and needle positions. Hatched areas represent small and large areas of ischemia. See text for details

Protocol

After control measurements, the LAD was ligated below the second diagonal branch and 30 min later below the first diagonal branch. Measurements were taken at 5, 15, and 30 min after the first and second ligation (Fig. 3). Thus, the following five myocardial areas were obtained: A = normal zone, B = normal zone during first ligation and ischemic zone during second ligation (pretreated ischemic segment), C = ischemic zone both during the first as well as the second ligation

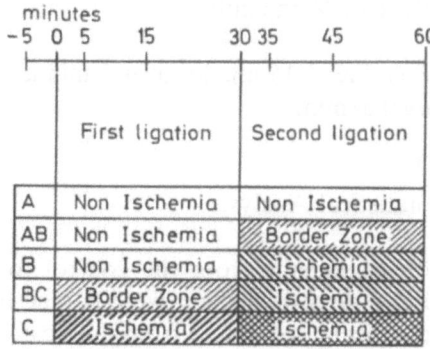

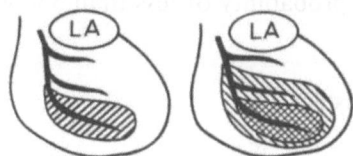

Fig. 3. Protocol of the study. First ligation indicate the 30 min period following LAD ligation at 0 hour and second ligation indicate the 30 min period following LAD ligation at 30 min. Corresponding ischemic zones are shown by hatched areas

(post-treated ischemic segment), AB = normal zone during first ligation and border zone between normal ischemic myocardium during second ligation, BC = border zone between normal and ischemic myocardium during first ligation and border zone between pretreated and posttreated ischemic segments during second ligation.

At each measurement period, atrial pacing was commenced at 200 per min and sensing from the QRS of the right ventricle epicardial electrogram, a premature stimulus at fixed coupling interval of 50% of the cycle length was delivered at the midwall at each needle site in series. Recordings were obtained with an Electronics for Medicine DR 16 recorder at a paper speed of 200 mm/s.

Definitions

Local myocardial conduction was measured as the interval between the premature pacing stimulus to the earliest high frequency deflection in the endocardial electrograms at each needle site.

Control anterograde conduction was defined as the conduction between needles 1 to 5 prior to the first LAD ligation in each group (see Fig. 2).

Conduction in the normal or nonischemic myocardium was defined as conduction between needles 1 to 4 during first ligation and between needles 1 and 2 during second ligation (see Fig. 2).

Conduction within the ischemic myocardium was divided into two subdivisions: (a) within the pretreated segment and (b) within the posttreated segment.

Pretreated segment was defined as the second zone of ischemia, i.e., area B in Fig. 3. Conduction within this area was defined as conduction between needles 2 to 4 during second ligation (30 – 60 mins.)

Posttreated segment was defined as the first zone of ischemia, i.e., area C in Fig. 3. Conduction within this area was defined as conduction between needles 4 and 5 during both ligations (0 – 60 mins.).

Dose of Verapamil

Loading: 0.15 mg/kg over 5 min after first ligation. Maintenance: IV infusion 7.5 μg/kg/min.

Statistical Analysis

Measurements from the control (or preligation), normal (or nonischemic), and ischemic myocardium were pooled in the control group of dogs and compared to identical pooled data from the treated group of dogs using unpaired Student's t test. A probability of less than 5% was considered to be significant.

Results

Following LAD ligation, the myocardium became cyanotic within 10 s in each animal with clearly demarcated borders. Needle #4 was confirmed to be precisely on the border of the cyanotic zone following the first ligation and needle #2 was confirmed to be precisely on the border of the cyanotic zone following the second ligation in each animal.

The design of the study was such that the same animal provided a normal myocardial zone, a posttreated ischemic zone and a pretreated ischemic zone. These zones will be considered separately.

The preligation values of conduction were similar between the two groups of dogs (23.03 ± 1.05 vs 20.02 ± 1.14 msec). In the normal nonischemic myocardium, the verapamil treated group and the control group of dogs had similar conduction characteristics throughout the period of the study. Thus, mean conduction in the normal zone ranged from $16.5 - 23.27$ msec in the control group and from $18.08 - 22.0$ msec in the treated group (see Table 1).

Conduction within the posttreated ischemic segment: Within C zone, ischemia depressed conduction steadily from 0 to 60 min (see Table 1) in both groups of dogs. In the control group, the depression of conduction tended to be more than the treated group at each time period, however, this difference did not reach statistical significance at any time.

Conduction within the pretreated ischemic segment: Within B zone, ischemia depressed conduction only in the control group of dogs and not in the treated group. Thus, conduction within this zone was significantly more at 35, 45, and 60 min in the treated group in contrast to the treated group in which conduction remained within the normal range.

Conduction from the pretreated to the posttreated ischemic segment: The model provided a unique opportunity to study conduction between a pretreated and a post-treated segment compared to identical segments in the control group. Verapamil protected the myocardium from the effects of ischemia so that conduction was not depressed in the treated animals. Thus, conduction was significantly more delayed at each time period in the control group compared to the treated group (see Table 1).

The conduction values from the various segments were pooled at the various time periods (Fig. 4). Following LAD ligation, verapamil did not affect the conduction in

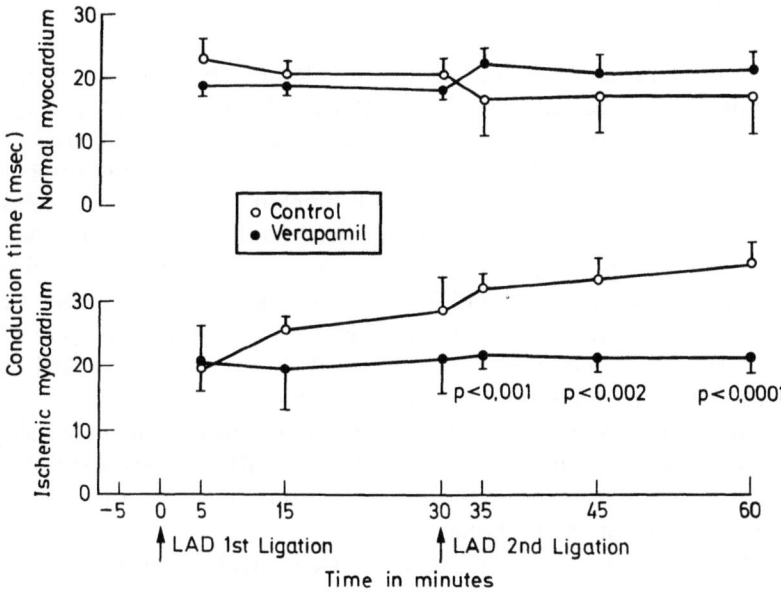

Fig. 4. Effect of verpamil on conduction. Ischemic myocardium in the verapamil group represent pooled data from both pretreated as well as posttreated ischemic segments

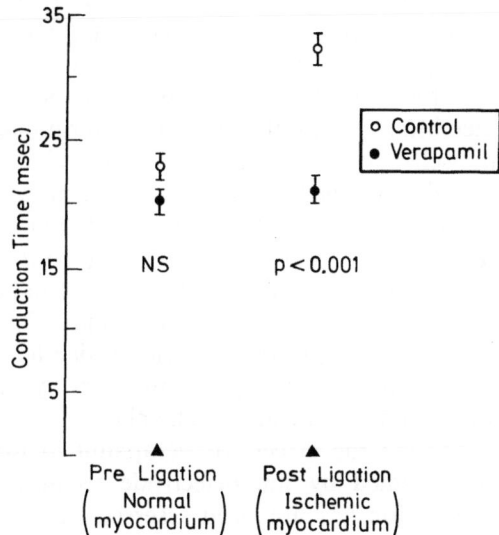

Fig. 5. Effect of verapamil on conduction within the ischemic myocardium

the normal myocardium and prevented deterioration of conduction in the ischemic zone.

The values for conduction in various ischemic segments at all time periods were pooled and compared between the control and treated group (Fig. 5). It can be noted that, compared to the preligation values, conduction was significantly depressed within the ischemic segment of the control animals. In the verapamil treated animals, however, conduction was preserved.

Discussion

Though verapamil was initially investigated for its vasoactive properties [3, 4], later studies were directed towards its antiarrhythmic properties [4 – 6] speculated to be due to β adrenoceptor blockade. The effects of verapamil were not altered, however, by the prior administration of β adergenic blocking drugs, confirming that its actions were not explained by β-blocking properties [7] (Naylor 1968). Subsequently, Fleckenstein et al. [8] reported on the mechanism of action of verapamil by selective inhibition of transmembrane conductance of calcium in different excitable tissues. Singh and Vaughan Williams [9] found that verapamil did not interfere with depolarization, was not an antisympathetic agent and did not delay repolarization and, therefore, proposed that verapamil exerted its antiarrhythmic action by its calcium antagonistic properties.

With the recent interest in the role of the calcium-mediated slow current in the genesis of arrhythmias in ischemic and/or infarcted myocardium [10], verapamil, thus provided a unique opportunity to study the effect of interruption of this current on ischemic arrhythmias.

When a myocardial cell is rendered ischemic, the transmembrane action potential is lowered by several factors including a leak of potassium ions within the cell and accumulation of lactic acid due to anerobic metabolism [10, 11 – 14]. Consequently, the fast inward current of sodium is inactivated [15], so that the remaining action potential is generated, mainly by a slow current mediated by calcium, and, to a lesser extent, sodium ions [16 – 25]. Thus, during ischemia, in the absence of the "fast" channel, a "slow" action potential results with decreased transmembrane resting potential and decreased rate of rise of phase 0. It has been well documented that the rate of rise of phase 0 of the action potential in relation to the resting membrane potential is the chief determinant of conduction velocity [26]. Therefore, in ischemic tissue, the slow rate of rise of the calcium-dependent current is postulated to be the cause for slow conduction velocity. If this were true, a calcium-antagonistic drug like verapamil should have slowed the conduction further. Our results do not suggest this. On the contrary, in our studies, verapamil preserved myocardial conduction in the ischemic tissue, the conduction being similar to that in the normal nonischemic myocardium. This observation suggests that whereas local anesthetic drugs exert their antiarrhythmic action by slowing the impulse conduction [27], verapamil may act by preventing depression of conduction that would otherwise follow ischemia.

Though the effects of verapamil in isolated cardiac tissue have been extensively studied by microelectrode techniques [10, 28], intraventricular segmental conduction has not been assessed by the method utilized in this study. Whereas microelectrode studies record the events in an individual cell, conduction in a group of cells across a bipole may be documented by the duration of the QRS complex in local electrograms. Utilizing plunge electrodes with small (0.5 mm) bipoles, verapamil has been shown to widen the QRS duration and, therefore, presumably depress conduction within the ischemic zone [29]. The present study analyzed conduction in segments of myocardium (0.5 – 6 cms) between two bipoles when the conduction was stressed not only by rapid atrial pacing but also by premature stimuli delivered at fixed coupling intervals of 50% of the atrial pacing rate. The duration of the resulting premature QRS could not be utilized to measure local conduction because of the difficulty in reproducibly measuring QRS duration in the local electrograms. The onset of the QRS complex in the five endocardial electrograms, however, was highly reproducible between independent blinded observers ($r = 0.995$). Therefore, the interval between the premature ventricular midwall stimulus and the earliest high frequency deflection of the resultant premature complex in the endocardial electrograms was considered to be an accurate representation of segmental intraventricular conduction.

Previous studies on the effect of verapamil on conduction within the ischemic myocardium have been conflicting possibly due to the variations in heart rate, dose of verapamil, recording techniques and perhaps more importantly, whether the drug was given before or after occlusion [30, 31]. Thus, when verapamil 0.2 mg/kg was given intravenously over 15 min prior to temporary (6 min) coronary occlusion, Elharrar [30] reported a significant improvement in ischemic zone epicardial conduction time and a decrease in the incidence of ventricular arrhythmias. In contrast to this, when verapamil 0.25 mg/kg was administered intravenously after coronary occlusion, Kuppersmith [31] found further depression of conduction in the ischemic epicardium. In our study, however, atrial pacing rate and coupling interval were identical in both groups of dogs, and endocardial conduction was compared in identical segments in both groups. Further, the dose of verapamil used in this study has been shown previously by us to achieve therapeutic blood levels in open chested dogs using identical anesthetic agents [29].

The design of the study provided both pretreatment as well as posttreatment ischemic segments and verapamil tended to maintain the integrity of conduction in the pretreated group and lessen the degree of ischemic damage in the posttreated group.

The possible mechanisms by which verapamil preserved myocardial conduction during acute ischemia are complex and intriguing and several factors ought to be considered. First, verapamil with its potent coronary vasodilator properties [4] could have improved myocardial blood flow to the ischemic myocardium. However, this has not been confirmed in experimental canine myocardial ischemia [32].

Secondly, verapamil has been shown to decrease myocardial oxygen demand [33] and similar to B-blockers could theoretically reduce the intensity of myocardial ischemic damage as originally suggested by Sodi-Pallares. Recently, however, reports on the ability of drugs to reduce ischemic damage have been conflicting. Verapamil was reported not to affect the tissue creatine kinase depletion of the ischemic and infarcted segments compared to a control group of animals [34]. On the contrary, Reimer et al. [35] reported that pretreatment with verapamil resulted in significantly less necrosis in dogs with circumflex artery ligation, and Naylor et al. [36] reported that in the isolated perfused heart, verapamil reduced the extent of ultrastructural damage caused by hypoxic perfusion.

Another possibility that should be considered is that the slow conduction in the ischemic myocardium may not be, in the major part, dependent on calcium flux and could possibly be due to a depressed channel of sodium ions as suggested recently by El Sherif and Lazzara [40]. Following $3 - 5$ days of coronary occlusion, they treated strips of epicardial muscle from the ischemic zone of dogs with verapamil that slightly improved the phase 0 upstroke velocity of depressed ischemic cells. These authors also utilized a fast (Na^+) channel blocker (tetrodotoxin) which further depressed or abolished action potentials of ischemic cells [37].

Finally, since a racemic mixture of the drug was used in this study, the possibility should be considered that either the *d* or *l* optical isomers may possess an action on the ischemic cell membrane that tends to restore the transmembrane potential toward normal and normalize the rate of rise of phase 0 of the action potential.

In conclusion, the results of this study are provocative with regard to mechanistic concepts of arrhythmias during acute myocardial ischemia. The data from the study suggests that under certain circumstances verapamil may be beneficial in the setting of acute ischemia, and it contrasts with most of the previous studies. Whether this is entirely by inhibition of slow current remains unclear. In light of the complex nonuniform nature of effects of ischemia, however, it is possible that multiple mechanisms may be operative on the cellular events during ischemia, including alteration in slow channel ionic currents.

References

1. Krikler D (1974) Verapamil in cardiology. Eur J Cardiol 2/1:3 – 10
2. Vohra J, Peter T, Hunt D (1974) Verapamil induced premature ventricular beats before reversion of supraventricular tachycardia. Br Heart J 36:1186 – 1193
3. Haas H, Hartfelder G (1962) x-Isopropyl-x-(N-methyl-N-homoveratryl)-y-amino-propyl)-3,4-di-methoxyphenylacetonitril, eine Substanz mit coronargefäßerweiternden Eigenschaften. Arzneim Forsch 12:549
4. Melville K, Shister HE, Huq S (1964) Iproveratril: Experimental data on coronary dilation and antiarrhythmic action. Can Med Assoc J 90:761
5. Schmid JR, Hanna C (1967) A comparison of the antiarrhythmic actions of two new synthetic compounds, iproveratril and MJ 1999, with quinidine and pronethalol. J Pharmacol Exp Ther 156:331
6. Kaumann AJ, Aramendia P (1968) Prevention of ventricular fibrillation induced by coronary ligation. J Pharmacol Exp Ther 164:326
7. Nayler WG, McInnes I, Swann JB (1968) Some effects of iproveratril (isoptin) on the cardiovascular system. J Pharmacol Exp Ther 161:247
8. Fleckenstein A, Tritthart H, Fleckenstein B (1969) Eine neue Gruppe kompetitiver CA^{++}-Antagonisten (Iproveratril, D 600, Prenylamin) mit starken Hemmeffekten auf die elektromechanische Koppelung im Warmblutermyokard. Pfluegers Arch 307:25
9. Singh BN, Vaughan Williams EM (1972) A fourth class of anti-dysrhythmic action? Effect of verapamil on ouabain toxicity, on atrial and ventricular intracellular potentials, and on other features of cardiac function. Cardiovasc Res 6:109
10. Cranefield PF, Aronson RS, Wit AL (1974) Effect of verapamil on the normal action potential and on a calcium-dependent slow response of canine cardiac Purkinje fibers. Circ Res 34:204 – 213
11. Wit AL, Bigger JT (1975) The electrophysiology of lethal arrhythmias. Possible electrophysiological mechanisms for lethal arrhythmias accompanying myocardial ischemia and infarction. Circulation [Suppl III] 52:96 – 115
12. Bigger JT, Dresdale RJ, Heissenbuttel RH (1977) Ventricular arrhythmias in ischemic heart disease. Mechanism, prevalence, significance, and management. Prog Cardiovasc Dis 19:255 – 300
13. Friedman PL, Stewart JR, Ferroglio JJ (1973) Survival of subendocardial Purkinje fibers after extensive myocardial infarction in dogs. In vitro and in vivo correlation. Circ Res 33:597 – 611
14. Lazzara R, El-Sherif N, Scherlag BJ (1974) Early and late effects of coronary artery occlusion on canine Purkinje fibers. Circ Res 35:391 – 399
15. Cranefield PF, Wit AL, Hoffman BF (1973) Genesis of cardiac arrhythmias. Circulation 47:190 – 204
16. Paes de Carvalho A, Hoffman BF, Carvalho D (1969) Two components of the cardiac action potential. I. Voltage time course and the effect of acetyl choline on atrial and nodal cells of the rabbit heart. J Gen Physiol 54:607 – 635
17. Rougier O, Vassort G, Stampfli R (1968) Voltage clamp experiments on frog atrial heart muscle fibres with the sucrose gap technique. Pfluegers Arch 301:91 – 108

18. Rougier O, Vassort G, Garnier D, Existence and role of a slow inward current during the frog atrial action potential. Pfluegers Arch 308:70 – 81
19. Cranefield PF, Klein HO, Hoffman BF (1971) Conduction of the cardiac impulse: I. Delay, block, and one-way block in depressed Purkinje fibers. Circ Res 28:199 – 219
20. Cranefield PF, Wit AL, Hoffman BF (1972) Conduction of the cardiac impulse: III. Characteristics of very slow conduction. J Gen Physiol 59: 277 – 246
21. Carmeliet E, Vereecke J (1969) Adrenaline and the plateau phase of the cardiac action potential. Pfluegers Arch 313:300
22. Beeler GW, Reuter H (1970) Membrane calcium current in ventricular myocardial fibres. J Physiol (Lond) 207:191 – 209
23. Surawicz B (1974) Calcium responses (Calcium Spikes). Am J Cardiol 33:689 – 690
24. Reuter H (1967) The dependence of slow inward current in Purkinje fibres on the extracellular calcium concentration. J Physiol (Lond) 192:479 – 492
25. Shigenobu K, Sperelakis N (1972) Calcium current channels induced by catecholamines in chick embryonic hearts whose fast sodium channels are blocked by tetrodotoxin or elevated potassium. Circ Res 31:932 – 952
26. Hoffman BF (1964) Impulse transmission in the mammalian hearts. Circ Res [Suppl II] 14:202 – 209
27. Rosen MR, Hoffman BF (1973) Mechanisms of action of antiarrhythmic drugs. Circ Res 32:1 – 8
28. Yamaguchi I, Obayashi K, Mandel WJ (to be published) The electrophysiological effects of verapamil. Cardiovasc Res
29. Barrett PA, Yamaguchi I, Mandel WJ (to be published) The mechanical and electrical effects of verapamil in experimental acute myocardial ischemia. Circulation
30. Elharrar V, Gaum WE, Zipes DP (1977) Effect of drugs on conduction delay and incidence of ventricular arrhythmias induced by acute coronary occlusion in dogs. Am J Cardiol 39:544
31. Kuppersmith J, Shiang H, Litwak RS (1976) Electrophysiologic effects of verapamil in canine myocardial ischemia. Am J Cardiol 37:149
32. Smith HJ, Singh BN, Nisbet HD (1975) Effects of verapamil on infarct size following experimental coronary occlusion. Cardiovasc Res 9:569
33. Nayler WG, Szeto J (1972) Effect of verapamil on contractility, oxygen utilization, and calcium exchangeability in mammalian heart muscle. Cardiovasc Res 6:120
34. Peter CT, Heng MK, Singh BN (1977) Epicardial ST segment reduction by verapamil without change in experimental infarct size. Presented at the annual scientific session of Cardiac Society of Australia and New Zealand. Aust NZ J Med
35 Reimer KA, Lowe JE, Jennings RB (1977) Effect of the calcium antagonist verapamil on necrosis following temporary coronary artery occlusion in dogs. Circulation 55:581 – 587
36. Nayler W, Grau A, Slade A (1976) A protective effect of verapamil on hypoxic heart muscle. Cardiovasc Res 10:650 – 652
37. El-Sherif N, Lazzara R (1978) Mechanism of action of Ca blockers and role of the slow response in ischemia related reentrant ventricular arrhythmias. Circulation [Suppl II] 58:66

Effects of Calcium-Antagonists on Automaticity and Conduction in Man[1]

L. Seipel and G. Breithardt

Electrophysiologic studies have shown that Ca-antagonists like verapamil or D 600 exert their dominant action on the slow channel response [1 – 7]. These drugs depress spontaneous depolarization and conduction within the isolated sinus and A-V node [6, 8 – 16]. In contrast, they have only little effect on action potential and refractoriness of the normal myocardium and the His-Purkinje system, which becomes more pronounced only at high concentrations [1, 6, 17 – 19]. Spontaneous diastolic depolarization in His-Purkinje fibers has been observed to be depressed by verapamil [18], whereas other investigators noted a high resistance of pacemaker activity to verapamil within the Purkinje system [20]. In addition, regenerative responses in the spontaneous beating atrial muscle seem not to be influenced by Ca-antagonists [14].

In contrast to these results in isolated preparations, most studies in intact animals could not demonstrate a depressive effect of verapamil on sinus node activity [13, 21 – 23]. Only in high doses a marked sinus depression ensued in the dog [13, 24]. Only Ross [25] observed a depressant effect of verapamil in therapeutic doses on sinus node activity. With one exception [26] studies in man have shown no significant effects on the sinus node or a decrease of cycle length and sinus node recovery (SRT) after iv administration of verapamil [27 – 34]. However, when given in patients with sick sinus syndrome, verapamil or D 600 sometimes cause a marked depression of sinus node activity [35 – 37] (Fig. 1a).

Testing the effect of verapamil (0.1 mg/kg iv) systematically in patients with and without sinus node dysfunction a different response of the two groups was found [37]. In 18 patients without clinical signs of sinus node dysfunction and a normal SRT corrected for heart rate during control stimulation (CSRT [corrected sinus node recovery time] $\leq$ 472 ms), verapamil caused a slight decrease in cycle length from 750.6 ± 172.2 ms to 703.7 ± 150.3 ms ($p < 0.05$). The CSRT showed a slight, insignificant prolongation from 225.6 ± 156.1 ms to 258.3 ± 183.1 ms. In 16 patients with sinus node dysfunction and a CSRT during control stimulation >472 ms, the response to verapamil was different. The mean cycle length increased only slightly from 1016.0 ± 174.0 to 1086.3 ± 244.7 ms though some patients showed a substantial slowing of heart rate. The CSRT increased in 11 of 16 patients and reached a critical length in four cases. The mean increase of CSRT was from 1201.7 ms during control stimulation to 5297.7 ms after verapamil ($p < 0.05$, Wilcoxon test for paired data) (Fig. 2).

It is noteworthy that in many cases with sinus node dysfunction and a very marked prolongation of SNRT after verapamil the ventricle was driven by a junctional escape rhythm preventing asystole and syncope in these patients (Fig. 1). The His bundle electrogram recorded during this period showed a His spike pre-

---

1 Supported by grant of Landesamt für Forschung NRW

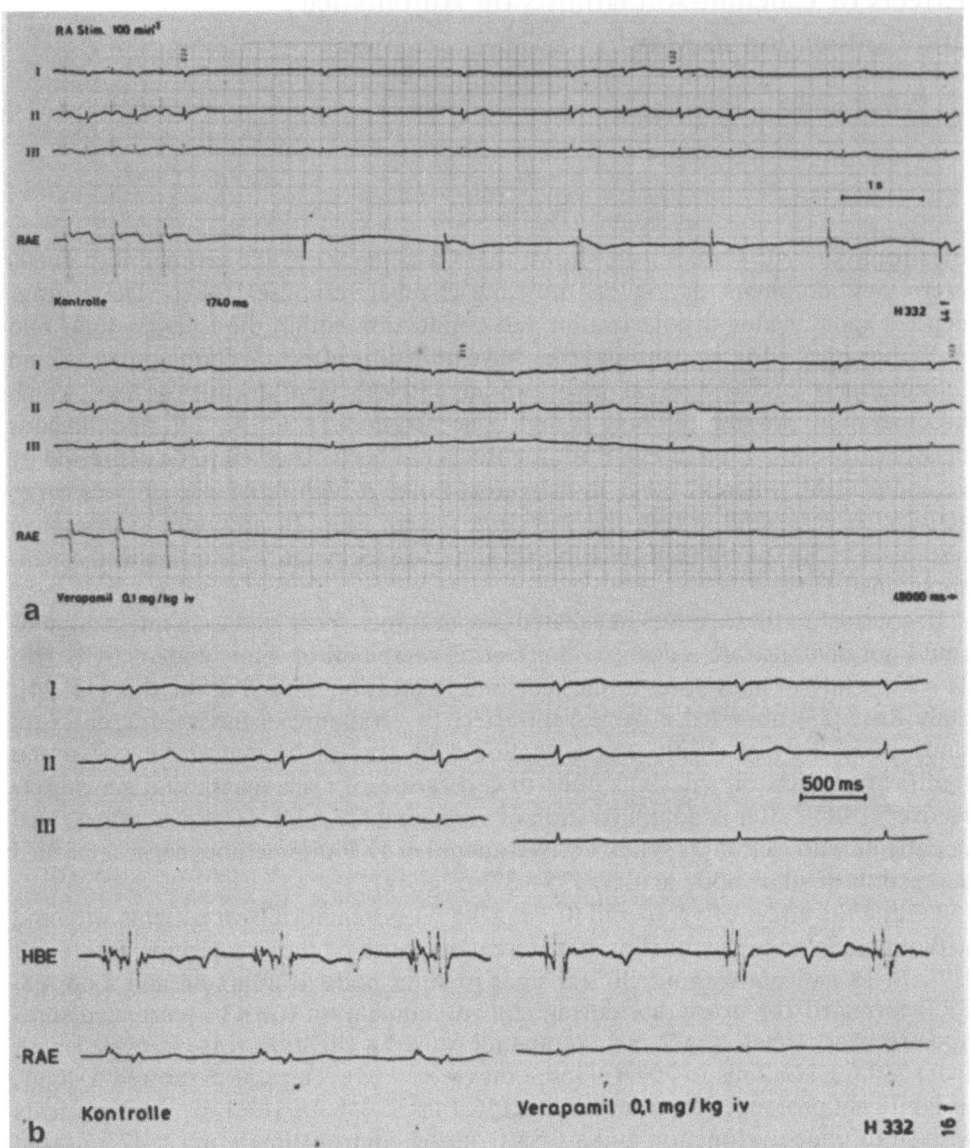

Fig. 1. a ECG (lead D I – III) and right atrial electrogram (RAE) during control stimulation (*top panel*) and after verapamil 0.1 mg/kg iv (*bottom panel*). The first three beats in each panel are paced beats. After verapamil no atrial activity is seen over a period of 49,000 ms. The ventricle is driven by a junctional escape rhythm

b His bundle electrogram (HBE) in the same patient. During control period a normal sinus rhythm is recorded (*left side*). After verapamil each ventricular complex is preceded by a His spike with a normal H-V interval. There is a retrograde block to the atrium with atrial standstil (*right side*)

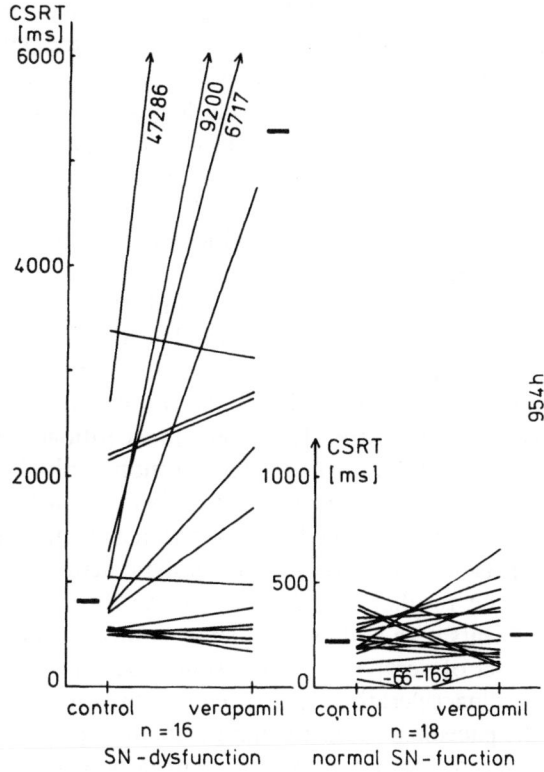

Fig. 2. Sinus node recovery time corrected for heart rate (CSRT) before and after verapamil administration (0.1 mg/kg IV) in patients with and without clinical signs of sinus node dysfunction

preceeding the V complex with a normal H-V time. The impulse from the subsidiary pacemaker was often blocked retrogradely to the atrium within the A-V node (Fig. 1b). This leads to the assumption that the pacemaker cells, which are not affected by verapamil, are located within the upper part of the His bundle. One explanation for this finding is that the A-V junction is not involved in the pathologic process that has affected the sinus node. Another possibility is that the spontaneous activity of the His bundle is not influenced by verapamil. In isolated preparations a significant increase in His bundle activity after verapamil was observed, which was explained by an catecholamine-releasing effect of this drug [38].

The calculated sinoatrial conduction time (SACT) showed an increase in the group of patients with normal sinus function from 86.4 ± 28.4 ms to 109.6 ± 53.4 ms, whereas in the patients with sinus node dysfunction a slight decrease was observed (137.8 ± 32.5 ms during control stimulation and 112.0 ± 34.1 ms after verapamil). A possible explanation for the shortening of SACT after verapamil in patients with sinus node dysfunction could be a pacemaker shift towards the border of the sinus node [37]. However, all changes were not significant.

In order to elucidate the mechanism of action of verapamil on the sinus node in man, the drug was injected before and after autonomic blockade [39, 40]. In five healthy volunteers, cycle length decreased from 1104.0 ± 111.6 ms before to 891.0 ± 67.0 ms after drug application ($p < 0.01$). During the next 15 min the cycle length increased but did not reach the control values (Fig. 3). Simultaneously, there was a significant fall in mean systemic pressure. After autonomic blockade (propranolol 0.1 mg/kg, atropine 0.02 mg/kg iv) the cycle length shortened from 961.0 ± 132.0 ms to 686.0 ± 66 ms. After additional application of verapamil a progressive increase in cycle length was observed which reached a plateau after 10 min between 690 and 712 ms. Though the changes were small, they were significant ($p < 0.01$). The fall in systemic pressure was the same as after application of verapamil alone without autonomic blockade. This increase in cycle length was not registered after autonomic blockade alone without further application of verapamil (Fig. 3).

The results show that verapamil has a dual effect on sinus node function. After autonomic blockade verapamil leads to a continuous prolongation of the cycle length, whereas without prior autonomic blockade verapamil shortens the P-P interval. Autonomic blockade is not able to prevent the verapamil-induced fall in systemic pressure. However, the cardioaccelerating effect of the fall in blood pressure is diminished after autonomic blockade and thereby the direct depressive effect of verapamil on sinus node is unmasked. In addition to these indirect reflex mechanisms induced by verapamil via the baroreceptors, a direct catecholamine-releasing effect [41] and a vagolytic action [42] of verapamil have been discussed.

The results spread light on the different effects of intravenous verapamil in patients with and without sinus node dysfunction. In normals, the direct depressive effect of verapamil on the sinus node is counteracted by the baroreceptor-induced cardioacceleration. In patients with sinus node dysfunction the responsiveness of the pacemaker cells to changes in autonomic tone is reduced [43, 44]. Therefore, the direct depressive effect of the drug prevails that can lead to dangerous bradycardia or asystole. On the other hand, iv verapamil may be useful in provoking latent

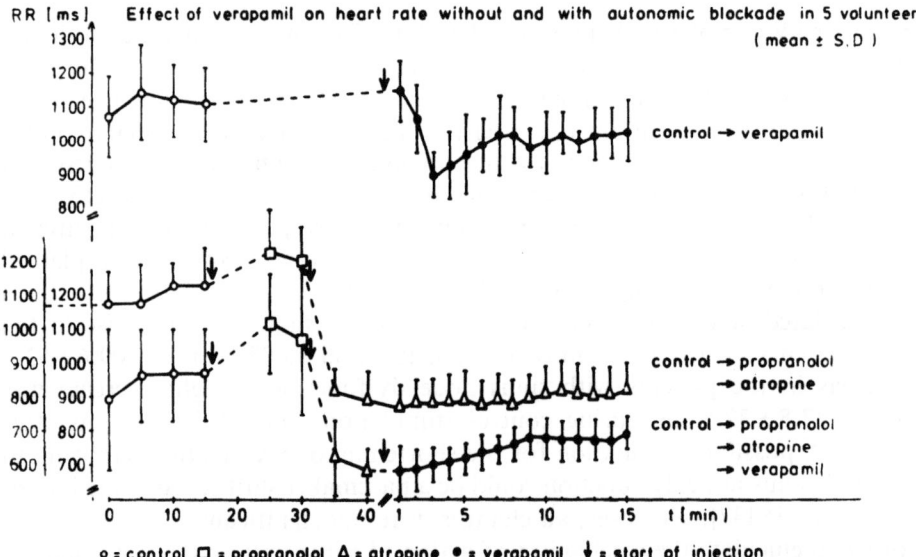

Fig. 3. Effect of verapamil 0.1 mg/kg IV on sinus cycle length in five healthy volunteers. *Top panel* represents the effect of verapamil alone, *bottom panel* the effect of verapamil after pretreatment with propranolol and atropine (autonomic blockade). The *middle panel* represents the effect of autonomic blockade alone

sinus node dysfunction. Whether the results are also applicable to oral administration remains unsettled.

As far as the A-V node is concerned, the depressive effect of verapamil prevails. In man, a significant prolongation of A-V nodal conduction time (A-H interval) as well as of the functional and effective refractory periods was found. During high rate test the Wenckebach point was lowered, i.e., the impulse was blocked within the A-V node at lower frequencies after verapamil than during control stimulation [30, 32–34, 45–48].

Comparing the effect of three different Ca-antagonists (verapamil 0.1 mg/kg, D 600, 0.03 mg/kg, Ro 11-1781 1.0 mg/kg iv) all compounds showed in principle the same depressive effect on the A-V node. However, in the dose given the effect of Ro 11-1781 was less pronounced (Table 1). Other investigators showed similar results for D 600 [35] and Ro 11-1781 [49]. However, the latter authors found a significant decrease of the Wenckebach point after Ro 11-1781 in contrast to our results. In a clinical trial a slowing of ventricular rate in patients with atrial fibrillation after application of Ro 11-1781 was seen [50]. Other Ca-antagonists do not seem to have the same electrophysiologic effects. Nifidepine, for example has only very small effects on the A-V node [51–53].

Electrophysiologic studies in man were not able to show significant effects of Ca-antagonists on atrial or ventricular conduction time and refractoriness [30, 32–34, 45, 48, 54]. In contrast, some investigators found a broading of the P waves in the surface ECG after verapamil [27, 31, 55]. In experimental studies in the dog heart in situ a change in the ratio of the monophasic action potential duration and the effective refractory period of the atrium was observed. These changes may be responsible for some antiarrhythmic effects of Ca-antagonists [22].

The electrophysiologic effects of Ca-antagonists are counteracted by atropine [30, 31, 37, 55, 56] as well as by catecholamines [27, 55]. This antagonism between Ca-antagonists and catecholamines was characterized as functional in contrast to the competitive one of the beta-blockers [57]. As a consequence, Ca-antagonists in therapeutic doses can not abolish the effect of catecholamines on sinus node activity [9, 57, 58]. Occasionally, the administration of atropine may cause a paradoxical effect. In some cases pretreated with verapamil, the additional application of atropine caused a further prolongation of the SRT (Figs. 4, 5). This "paradoxical" prolongation of SRT after atropine is perhaps due to a facilitation of sinoatrial conduction that improves sinus node sensing [56, 59, 60–62].

Table 1. Electrophysiological effects of three different Ca-antagonists on A-V node conduction and refractoriness. A-H = conduction time from the low right atrium to the His bundle (A-H interval); SR = sinus rhythm; S-S = cycle length during fixed rate pacing in ms; FRP = functional refractory period; ERP = effective refractory period; AVN = A-V node; ( ) = not significant

	A-H SR	A-H S-S 600	FRP AVN	ERP AVN	AV block S-S
verapamil 0.1 mg/kg IV	+13.2%	+15.6%	+11.0%	+24.3%	+14.0%
D 600 0.03 mg/kg IV	+14.0%	+25.0%	+12.9%	+31.2%	+13.9%
Ro 11-1781 1.0 mg/kg IV	+12.3%	(+18.1%)	(+1.9%)	(+3.0%)	(+8.9%)

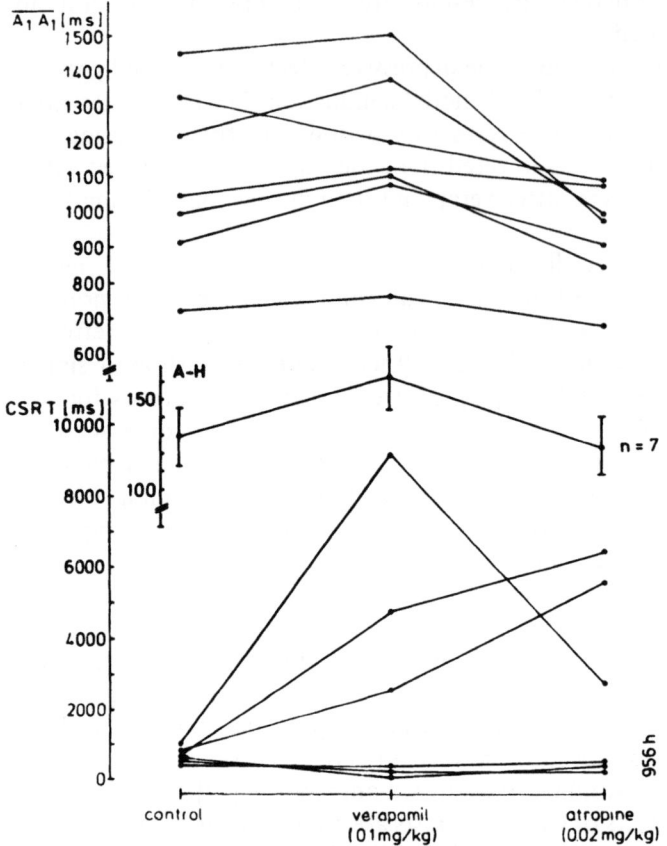

Fig. 4. Effect of atropine after pretreatment with verapamil on sinus cycle length (A-A), A-H interval, and corrected sinus node recovery time (CSRT). (In one case CSRT could not be measured after atropine). In two patients a further prolongation of CSRT after additional application of atropine occurres. The A-H interval is given as the mean value ±S.D.

From these electrophysiologic results some conclusions which are supported by clinical experience can be drawn with regard to the antiarrhythmic therapy with Ca-antagonists like verapamil. Ca-antagonists are very useful in the treatment of tachycardias in which the A-V node is involved: i.e. A-V nodal tachycardias and reentry tachycardias in patients with preexcitation. They are able to slow ventricular rate in patients with atrial tachycardias, especially atrial flutter-fibrillation, if the impulses are conducted by the normal nodal pathway. Ca-antagonists are not able to slow sinus tachycardia. (They may be effective in patients with true sinus node reentry tachycardia [63]). In spite of that, the same drugs should be used with caution in patients with sinus node dysfunction. In addition, Ca-antagonists may lead to a higher degree A-V block in patients with A-V nodal conduction disturbances. However, ventricular asystole in patients with sinus pauses or nodal block after verapamil is often prevented by junctional (His bundle?) escape rhythms, which seem not to be depressed by Ca-antagonists. Patients with intraventricular conduction defects are not at a risk to develop higher degree A-V block under treatment with Ca-antagonists.

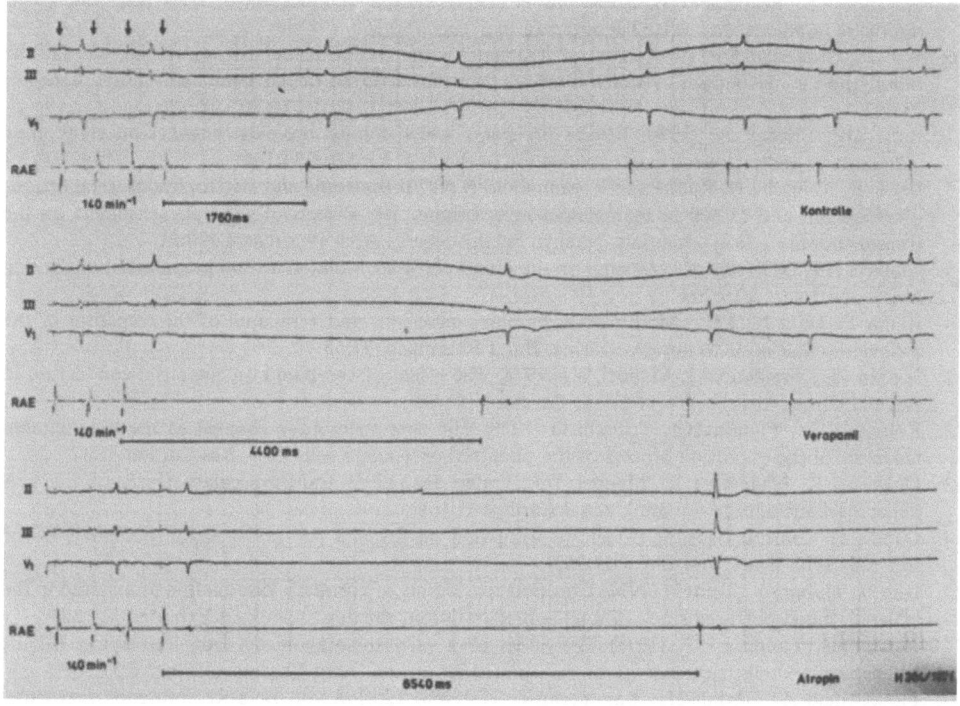

Fig. 5. ECG (lead D II, III, V1) and right atrial electrogram (RAE) during control stimulation (*top*) after application of verapamil (0.1 mg/kg IV) and after additional injection of atropine (0.02 mg/kg IV) (*bottom*). After atropine a further prolongation of the sinus node recovery time is observed

However, the results of the electrophysiologic studies in man are not able to explain the other antiarrhythmic effect of Ca-antagonists reported in the literature. There are some studies in isolated tissue that indicate that verapamil has some effects on the diseased myocardial and Purkinje fibers that may show slow channel conduction [41, 64, 65]. At the present time a gap remains between the electrophysiologic knowledge and the clinical experience. Thus, the goal of a rational antiarrhythmic therapy has not been reached today.

References

1. Cranefield PF, Aronson RS, Wit AL (1974) Effect of verapamil on the normal action potential and on a calcium depent slow response of canine cardiac purkinje fibers. Circ Res 34:204
2. Kaufmann R, Tritthart H, Rost B (1969) Trennung der Ca^{++}-antagonistischen Wirkungskomponente von den β-adrenolytischen Effekten Herz-hemmender Pharmaka an Kulturen embryonaler Herzmuskelzellen. Naunyn Schmiedebergs Arch Pharmcol 264:252
3. Kohlhardt M, Bauer B, Krause H, Fleckenstein A (1972) Differentiation of the transmembrane Na and Ca channels in the mammalian cardiac fibers by the use of specific inhibitors. Pfluegers Arch 335:309
4. Nawrath H, Ten Eick RE, McDonald TF, Trautwein W (1977) On the mechanism underlying the action of D-600 on slow inward current and tension in mammalian myocardium. Circ Res 40:408

5. Shigenobu K, Schneider JA, Sperelakis N (1974) Verapamil blockade of slow Na$^+$ and Ca^{++} responses in myocardial cells. J Pharmacol Exp Ther 190:280
6. Wit AL, Cranefield PF (1974) Effect of verapamil on the sinoatrial and atrioventricular nodes of the rabbit and the mechanism by which it arrests reentrant atrioventricular node tachycardia. Circ Res 35:413
7. Zipes DP, Fischer JC (1974) Effects of agents which inhibit the slow channel on sinus node automaticity and atrioventricular conduction in the dog. Circ Res 34:184
8. Bayer R, Kalusche D, Kaufmann R, Mannhold R (1975) Inotropic and electrophysiological actions of verapamil and D 600 in mammalian myocardium. III. Effects of the optical isomers on the transmembrane action potentials. Naunyn Schmiedebergs Arch Pharmacol 290:81
9. Chiba S (1975) Effects of verapamil on the blood-perfused, isolated atrium preparation of the dog heart. Jpn Heart J 16:709
10. Iijima T, Taira N (1976) Modification by manganese ions and verapamil of the responses of the atrioventricular node to norepinephrine. Eur J Pharmacol 37:55
11. Jordan JL, Yamaguchi I, Mandel WJ (1978) The effect of verapamil on sinoatrial conduction in isolated tissue (Abstr.). World Congr Cardiol VIII:478
12. Kohlhardt M, Figulla HR, Tripathi O (1976) The slow membrane channel as the predominant mediator of the excitation process of the sinoatrial pacemaker cell. Basic Res Cardiol 71:17
13. Obayashi K, Nagasawa K, Mandel WJ, Vyden JK (1975) Cardiovascular effects of the new antiarrhythmic agent verapamil. Am J Cardiol 35:161
14. Okada T, Konishi T (1975) Effects of verapamil on SA and AV nodal action potentials in the isolated rabbit heart. Jpn Circ J 39:913
15. Ono H, Himori N, Taira N (1977) Chronotropic effects of coronary vasodilators as assessed in the isolated, blood-perfused sino-atrial node preparation of the dog. Tohoku J Exp Med 121:383
16. Refsum H, Landmark K (1975) The effect of a calcium-antagonistic drug, nifedipine, on the mechanical and electrical activity of the isolated rat atrium. Acta Pharmacol Toxicol 37:369
17. Fleckenstein A, Döring HJ, Kammermeier H (1968) Einfluß von Beta-Rezeptorenblockern und verwandten Substanzen auf Erregung, Kontraktion und Energiestoffwechsel der Myokardfaser. Klin Wochenschr 46:343
18. Rosen MR, Ilvento JP, Gelband H, Merker C (1974) Effects of verapamil on electrophysiologic properties of canine purkinje fibers. J Pharmacol Exp Ther 189:414
19. Singh BN, Vaughan Williams EM (1972) A fourth class of anti-dysrhythmic action? Effect of verapamil on ouabain toxicity, on atrial and ventricular intracellular potentials, and on other features of cardiac function. Cardiovasc Res 6:109
20. Endoh M, Yanagisawa T, Taira N (1978) Effects of calcium-antagonistic coronary vasodilators nifedipine and verapamil, on ventricular automaticy of the dog. Naunyn Schmiedebergs Arch Pharmacol 302:235
21. Angus JA, Richmond DR, Dhumma-Upakorn P, Kobbin LB, Goodman AH (1976) Cardiovascular action of verapamil in the dog with particular reference to myocardial contractility and atrioventricular conduction. Cardiovasc Res 10:623
22. Landmark K, Amlie JP (1976) A study of the verapamil-induced changes in conductivity and refractoriness and monphasic action potentials of the dog heart in situ. Eur J Cardiol 4:419
23. Mangiardi LM, Hariman RJ, McAllister RG, Bhargava V, Surawicz B, Shabetal R (1978) Electrophysiologic and hemodynamic effects of verapamil. Circulation 57:366
24. Melville KI, Shister HE, Huq S (1964) Iproveratril: Experimental data on coronary dilatation and antiarrhythmic action. Can Med Assoc J 90:761
25. Ross G, Jorgensen CR (1967) Cardiovascular actions of verapamil. J Pharmacol Exp Ther 158:504
26. Bischoff KO, Hager W, Flohr E, Heredia D (1978) Die Beeinflussung systolischer und elektrokardiographischer Zeitintervalle herzgesunder Patienten durch den Kalziumantagonisten Ro 11-1781. Z Kardiol 67:268
27. Belz GG, Bender F (1974) Therapie der Herzrhythmusstörungen mit Verapamil. Fischer, Stuttgart
28. Grendahl H, Miller M, Sivertssen E (1975) Registration of sinus node recovery time in patients with sinus rhythm and in patients with dysrhythmias. Acta Med Scand 197:403
29. Heng MK, Singh BN, Roche AHG, Norris RM, Mercer CJ (1975) Effects of intravenous verapamil on cardiac arrhythmias and on the electrocardiogram. Am Heart J 90:487
30. Husaini MH, Kvasnicka J, Ryden L, Holmberg S (1973) Action of verapamil on sinus node, atrioventricular and intraventricular conduction. Br Heart J 35:734

31. Klempt HW, Bachour G, Reploh HD, Gradaus D, Brisse B, Bender F (1972) Untersuchungen zum Wirkungsmechanismus von Verapamil. Verh Dtsch Ges Inn Med 78:1116
32. Rizzon P, di Biase M, Calabrese P, Brindicci G, Chiddo A (1977) Electrophysiologic evaluation of intravenous verapamil in man. Eur J Cardiol 6:179
33. Seipel L, Both A, Breithardt G, Gleichmann U, Loogen F (1974) Action of antiarrhythmic drugs on his bundle electrogram and sinus node function. Acta Cardiol (Brux) [Suppl] 18:251
34. Silvertssen E, Bay G, Grendahl H (1975) The effect of propranolol and verapamil on atrial and atrioventricular refractory periods in man. Angiology 26:605
35. Beck OA, Witt E, Lehmann H-U, Hochrein H (1978) Die Wirkung von Gallopamil (D 600) auf die intrakardiale Erregungsleitung und Sinusknotenautomatie beim Menschen. Z Kardiol 67:522
36. Blömer H, Wirtzfeld A, Delius W, Sebening H (1977) Das Sinusknotensyndrom. Perimed, Erlangen p 89
37. Breithardt G, Seipel L, Wiebringhaus E, Loogen F (1978) Effects of verapamil on sinus node function in man. Eur J Cardiol 8:379
38. Cosin J, Gimero J, Baguena J (1978) Effect of antiarrhythmic drugs on the automaticity of junctional pacemaker (Abstr.). World Congr Cardiol VIII:481
39. Breithardt G, Seipel L, Wiebringhaus E (1978) Dual effect of verapamil on sinus node function in man. In: Bonke FIM (ed) The sinus node. Nijhoff The Hague, p 129
40. Breithardt G, Seipel L, Wiebringhaus E, Loogen F (1978) The role of the autonomic nervous system in the action of verapamil on the sinus node in man. Basic Res Cardiol 73:637
41. Danilo P, Hordof AJ, Delphin ES, Rosen MR (1978) Verapamil effects on blood superfused purkinje fibers: Evidence for direct and catecholamine-mediated actions (Abstr.). Am J Cardiol 41:417
42. Garvey HL (1969) The mechanism of action of verapamil on the sinus and AV nodes. Eur J Pharmacol 8:159
43. Dighton DH (1974) Sinus bradycardia. Autonomic influences and clinical assessment. Br Heart J 36:791
44. Mandel WJ, Hayakawa H, Allen HN, Danzig R, Kermaier AI (1972) Assessment of sinus node function in patients with the sick sinus syndrome. Circulation 46:761
45. Gleichmann U, Seipel L, Loogen F (1973) Der Einfluß von Antiarrhythmika auf die intrakardiale Erregungsleitung (His-Bündel Elektrographie) und Sinusknotenautomatie beim Menschen. Dtsch Med Wochenschr 98:1487
46. Neuss H, Schlepper M (1971) Der Einfluß von Verapamil auf die atrioventrikuläre Überleitung. Lokalisation des Wirkungsortes mit His-Bündel Elektrogrammen. Verh Dtsch Ges Kreislaufforsch 37:433
47. Roy PR, Spurrel RAJ, Sowton E (1974) The effect of verapamil on the cardiac conduction system in man. Postgrad Med J 50:270
48. Schlepper M, Neuss H (1974) Changes of refractory periods in the A-V conduction system induced by antiarrhythmic drugs. Acta Cardiol (Brux) [Suppl] 18:269
49. Gmeiner R, Simma H, Ng CK, Dienstl F, Knapp E (1977) Die Wirkung von Ro 11-1781, einem Kalziumantagonisten, auf die atrioventrikuläre Überleitung. Z Kardiol 66:238
50. Brisse B, Bender F, Gülker H, Niehues H (1978) Behandlung der absoluten Tachyarrhythmie bei Vorhofflimmern mit dem neuen Kalziumantagonisten Ro 11-1781. Z Kardiol 67:609
51. Narimatsu A, Taira N (1976) Effects on atrio-ventricular conduction of calcium-antagonistic coronary vasodilators, local anaesthetics and quinidine injection into the posterior and the anterior septal artery of the atrioventricular node preparation of the dog. Arch Pharmacol 294:169
52. Raschack M (1976) Differences in the cardiac actions of the calcium antagonists verapamil and nifedipine. Arzneim Forsch 26:1330
53. Resfum H, Glomstein A, Landmark K (1976) The effect of nifedipine on the isolated rat heart. Acta Pharmacol Toxicol 38:328
54. Grohmann HW, Theisen K, Jahrmärker H (1971) Einfach- und Doppelstimulation des menschlichen Vorhofs. Untersuchungen zur Refraktärzeitbestimmung. Verh Dtsch Ges Kreislaufforsch 37:460
55. Bass O, Friedman M (1971) Ein Beitrag zum antiarrhythmischen Wirkungsmechanismus von Verapamil (Isoptin). Schweiz Med Wochenschr 101:792
56. Breithardt G, Seipel L, Both A, Loogen F (1976) The effect of atropine on calculated sinoatrial conduction time in man. Eur J Cardiol 4:49
57. Görlitz BD, Wagner J, Schüren HJ (1975) Functional antagonism between calcium-antagonists and noradrenaline on isolated guinea-pig atria. Naunyn Schmiedebergs Arch Pharmacol 288:311

58. Bender F, Schmidt E, Sieger W (1968) Vergleichende Untersuchungen mit Beta-Rezeptorenblockern. Verh Dtsch Ges Inn Med 74:569
59. Bashour T, Hemb R, Wickramesekaran R (1973) An unusual effect of atropine on overdrive suppression. Circulation 48:911
60. Bisset JK, de Soyza N, Kane JJ, Schmitt NM (1976) Improved sinus node sensing after atropine. Am Heart J 91:752
61. Dhingra RC, Amat-y-Leon F, Wyndham C, Denes P, Wu D, Pouget JM, Rosen KM (1976) Electrophysiologic effects of atropine on human sinus node and atrium. Am J Cardiol 38:429
62. Reiffel JA, Bigger JT, Guardina EGV (1975) "Paradoxical" prolongation of sinus nodal recovery time after atropine in the sick sinus syndrome. Am J Cardiol 36:98
63. Curry PVL, Evans TR, Krikler DM (1977) Paroxysmal reciprocating sinus tachycardia. Eur J Cardiol 6:199
64. Hordof AJ, Edie R, Malm JR, Hoffman BF, Rosen MR (1976) Electrophysiologic properties and response to pharmacologic agents of fibers from diseased human atria. Circulation 54:774
65. Rossner KL, Sachs HS (1978) Electrophysiological study of syrian hamster hereditary cardiomyopathy. Cardiovasc Res 12:436

Effects of Altered Calcium Concentrations on AV Conduction and Interactions of Verapamil and Sodium or Calcium

Y. Watanabe

In recent years, the importance of slow inward currents in the genesis of trans-membrane action potentials of cardiac fibers has been well established as the result of various experimental observations [1-4]. Such slow inward currents are considered responsible for the maintenance of prolonged plateau characteristic of cardiac action potentials, and for the slowly rising action potentials (so-called slow responses) observed in damaged or partially depolarized myocardial fibers. In fibers of the sinoatrial (SA) and atrioventricular (AV) nodes, which physiologically show reduced membrane potentials and typical slow responses, the action potentials are said to depend predominantly on these slow inward currents [5-10]. Since it has been shown that calcium is one major charge carrier through the slow channel [1-4,6,11-15], the effects of altered calcium concentrations on AV conduction were studied in the present series of experiments using isolated hearts of the rabbit.

Material and Methods

Most of the experiments were carried out in isolated rabbit hearts. The techniques of isolation and perfusion were previously reported in detail [16]. The coronary arteries were perfused at a rate of approximately 17 ml/min with a constant flow pump (Tokyo Rika Kikai Co.). The perfusate was a modified Chenoweth's solution with the following composition in millimoles per liter: NaCl, 119.8; KCl, 4.5; $CaCl_2$, 2.4; $MgCl_2$, 2.1; $NaHCO_3$, 25.0; and dextrose, 10.0. The solution was saturated with a mixture of 95% O_2 + 5% CO_2, and its temperature maintained at $37° \pm 1°C$. The heart was positioned horizontally at the center of a metal ring 15 cm in diameter, with several silk sutures. A constant heart rate was maintained by electrically driving the right atrium through a close bipolar electrode having an interelectrode distance of 1 mm, attached near the sinoatrial node. The stimuli produced by a stimulator (Nihon Kohden Co., model MSE-49) were square pulses of 5 ms duration and twice the threshold intensity, and were isolated from the ground. A pair of unipolar surface electrodes were attached to the right ventricular apex and the left ventricular base to record a bipolar electrocardiogram. A small incision of approximately 10 mm was made in the posterolateral wall of the right atrium along the AV groove to expose the AV junctional region. A direct His bundle electrogram was recorded by attaching, on the His bundle region, a close bipolar electrode similar to the stimulating electrode. These potentials were amplified through an amplifier (Nihon Kohden Co., model RB-5) with a time constant of 0.003 s and a filter setting of 300 Hz. Transmembrane potentials of the AV junctional fibers were often recorded with a flexibly mounted microelectrode, filled with 3M KCl and having a resistance of 10-20 MΩ. The output from the microelectrode amplifier (Nihon Kohden Co., model MZ-4) was led, together with the electrocardiographic and His bundle potentials, to two dual-beam, four channel oscilloscopes (Nihon Kohden Co., model VC-7) for the purposes of monitoring and recording. Photographic records were made with a movie camera (Nihon Kohden Co., model PC-2B), usually at a paper speed of 100 mm/s.

During an initial control period lasting from 30 to 45 min, numerous records were obtained to determine the stimulus to A (St-A) interval (roughly corresponding to the intraatrial conduction time), the A-H interval (the intranodal conduction time) and the H-V interval (the His-Purkinje conduction time). Subsequently, the control perfusate was switched to various test solutions, and the recordings were repeated. The concentrations of ions and drugs in the test solutions were: (1) 0.8 mM Ca (low Ca); (2) 4.8 or 7.2 mM Ca (high Ca); (3) 7.5 mM K (high K); (4) 172 mM Na (high Na); (5) tetrodotoxin (TTX), 10 mg/l; (6) verapamil, 0,5 or 1.0 mg/l; and certain combinations thereof. When the ionic concentrations were changed, no adjustments were made to keep the osmotic pressure of the solution at a constant level.

Several additional experiments were carried out in excised right atrial preparations containing the AV junctional region and a small portion of the interventricular septum, which were superfused in a tissue bath, in order to study the changes in transmembrane action potentials and in the atrial excitation pattern produced by altered Ca concentrations. The perfusion chamber had a volume of 30 ml, the rate of flow was approximately 30 ml/min, and the perfusate was saturated with 95% O_2 + 5% CO_2 both in the reservoir and the chamber.

Results

Effects of Low and High Ca Concentrations on AV Conduction Time

In a total of ten hearts, the effects of low extracellular Ca concentration were studied. During the control period, the total AV conduction time as determined by the St-V interval measured 108.2±2.87 ms. When the Ca concentration in the perfusate was lowered to 0.8 mM, there was a slight but insignificant prolongation of the total AV interval. The St-A interval was shortened from 30.5±2.44 to 27.8±2.88 ms (a decrease of 8.9%), whereas the H-V interval was prolonged from 35.9±3.11 to 38.9±4.94 ms (an increase of 8.4%). Both these changes were, however, statistically insignificant. On the other hand, the A-H interval was significantly ($P < 0.02$) prolonged from 41.8±3.55 to 49.3±2.97 ms, or by 17.9%. Thus, the threefold decrease in extracellular Ca concentration depressed intra-AV nodal conduction, without affecting intraatrial and His-Purkinje conduction.

The effects of high Ca concentration were tested in 13 hearts. The total AV conduction time during the control perfusion measured 106.4±9.21 ms. An elevation of extracellular Ca concentration to 4.8 mM caused a 28.8% prolongation of this interval to 137.7±12.93 ms ($P < 0.01$). The St-A and H-V intervals were prolonged by 22.9 and 7.9%, respectively. The former change was significant at 1% level. However, the greatest prolongation of 56.4% occurred in the A-H interval ($P < 0.05$). Hence, the twofold increase in extracellular Ca concentration depressed conductivity in the AV node to a greater extent than the low Ca perfusion. Even occasional failure of propagation within the AV node was seen in 5 of the 13 hearts at this Ca level. Further elevation of Ca concentration to 7.2 mM in three hearts invariably produced second degree intranodal block.

The depression of AV nodal conduction by low Ca concentration may readily be expected if the action potentials of AV nodal fibers are truly dependent on slow inward currents predominantly carried by Ca [7, 8], whereas the more marked depression of intranodal conduction by high Ca concentrations appears rather contradictory. After the lowering of Ca concentration, the action potential amplitude of the AN (atrionodal) and N (true nodal) regions of the AV node tended to be decreased, although the change was statistically insignificant. The changes in the action potential characteristics of these fibers produced by high Ca concentrations were inconsistent. Since the intraatrial conduction also was significantly depressed by the elevation of Ca concentration, the spread of atrial excitation was studied by recording transmembrane action potentials from numerous fibers in the right atrium-AV junctional preparations superfused in the tissue bath.

Figure 1 summarizes the results of one such experiment. In this sketch of the preparation, stimulating electrode A was positioned near the ostium of coronary

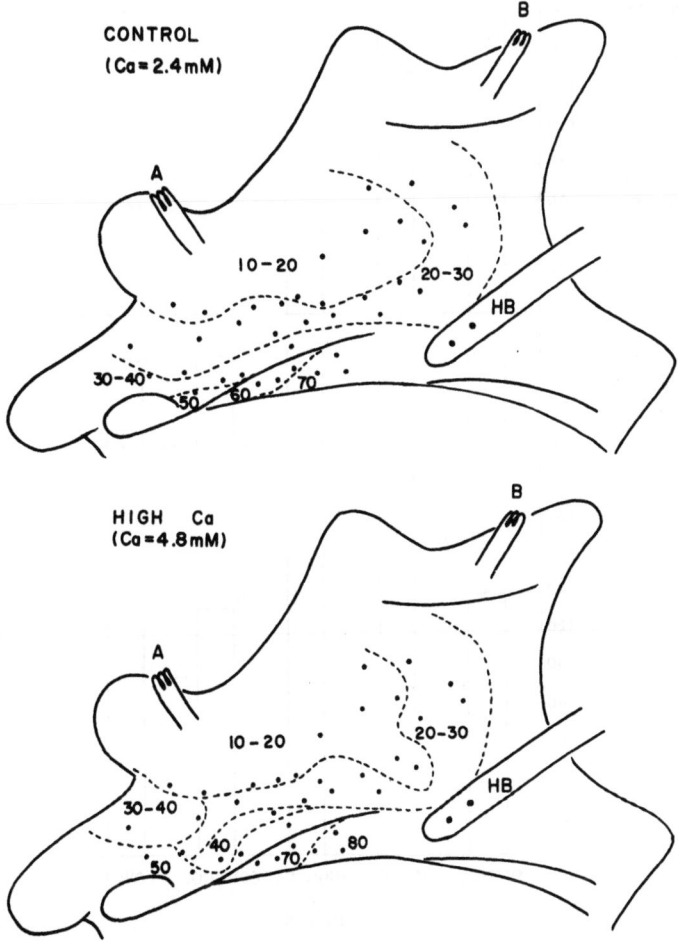

Fig. 1. Spread of atrial excitation during control (2.4 mM) and high Ca (4.8 mM) perfusion. Dots represent microelectrode recording sites. Activation times in milliseconds. HB = His bundle electrode

sinus, whereas electrode B was placed slightly anteriorly to the fossa ovalis. The preparation was electrically driven from the electrode A, and the time of activation of various fibers (*marked by dots*) were grouped at 10 ms intervals to draw the isochronus lines (*broken lines*). During the control period (*top*), atrial excitation proceeded with a relatively smooth wavefront, and depolarization of the AV nodal NH (node-His) region occurred around 70 ms after the stimulation. The timing of the A deflection on the simultaneously recorded His bundle electrogram closely corresponded to the activation time of the atrial fibers adjacent to the His electrode. Upon doubling of the Ca concentration (*bottom*), the pattern of atrial depolarization was altered, the contour of the excitation front apparently becoming more irregular. The time of activation of the NH region was delayed by approximately 10 ms. Thus, it would appear that the changes in atrial excitation played some role in depressing intranodal conduction.

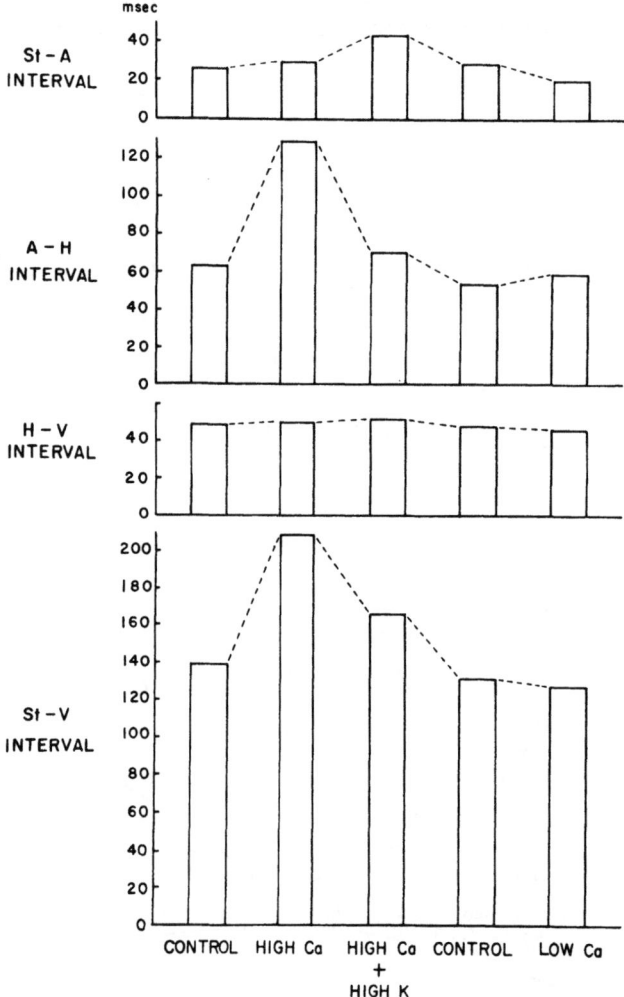

Fig. 2. Changes in various conduction times produced by alterations in Ca concentration in the perfusate. Discussion in text

Figure 2 shows the changes in the St-A, A-H, H-V and St-V (total AV) intervals by altered Ca concentrations in a representative experiment. It is evident that high Ca (4.8 mM) increased conduction times in all three portions of the AV conducting system, but the greatest prolongation was observed in the A-H interval. When the K concentration in the perfusate was elevated from 4.5 to 7.5 mM in the presence of high Ca, the St-A and H-V intervals were further prolonged, whereas the A-H interval was shortened toward the control value. After restoration of almost normal conduction times in all three portions of the AV conducting system with a fresh control perfusion, lowering of Ca concentration prolonged the A-H interval. The St-A interval was clearly shortened in this heart, causing a slight decrease in the total AV conduction time.

The interactions of Ca and K as illustrated in Fig. 2 were studied in three additional hearts. In two of these three hearts, increased extracellular K concentration in the presence of high Ca shortened the A-H interval, with a slight prolongation of the St-A and H-V intervals. In the remaining heart, a threefold increase in Ca concentration to 7.2 mM caused a second degree intranodal block with a 4:1 conduction ratio. Subsequent elevation of K to 7.5 mM restored a 1:1 conduction across the AV node, although the A-H interval remained markedly prolonged (not shown). Antagonism of high K against the depressing effects of high Ca concentrations on AV nodal conduction thus appeared to be substantiated.

Interactions of Verapamil and Various Cations on AV Conduction

Verapamil, a so-called Ca antagonist, is known to depress AV nodal conduction [7, 8]. Since it has been reported that the effects of this agent on Purkinje fiber action potentials are reversed by high Ca concentrations, interactions of verapamil and high Ca on AV conduction were tested in two hearts (Fig. 3). In the *top panel* reproduced from a representative experiment, the His bundle electrogram (HBE) and the electrocardiogram (ECG) recorded during the control period are shown. The upward arrows indicate the timing of electric stimulation applied near the SA node. Addition of verapamil to the perfusate at the concentration of 0.5 mg/l produced a second degree AV block with the Wenckebach phenomenon within 10 min, and a 2:1 block within 15 min (Fig. 3, *middle panel*). Absence of H deflection after the first and the third atrial stimuli indicates failure of conduction within the AV node. When Ca concentration in the perfusate was elevated to 7.2 mM in the presence of verapamil, 2:1 intranodal block persisted, and the A-H interval was further prolonged (*bottom panel*). Hence, high Ca concentration did not antagonize but rather exaggerated the depressing action of verapamil on AV nodal conduction.

In another experiment shown in Fig. 4, a Wenckebach type intranodal block was produced by the addition of 0.5 mg/l verapamil (*second panel*). Subsequent elevation of Na concentration in the perfusate from 144.8 to 172 mM reestablished a 1:1 AV conduction with marked shortening of the A-H interval, even though verapamil perfusion was still maintained (*bottom panel*). Such a successful reversal of verapamil-induced intranodal block by high Na concentration was observed in two other experiments.

On the other hand, it has been reported earlier that a lowering of extracellular Na concentration to 3/4 of normal (108.6 mM) significantly prolongs the conduction

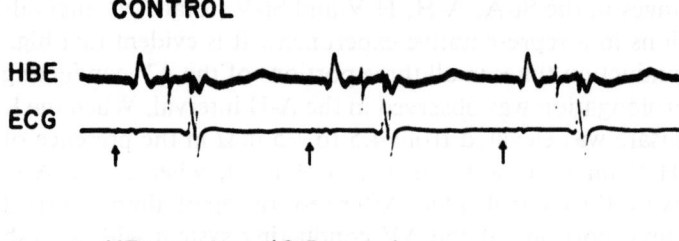

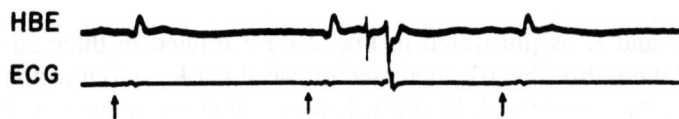

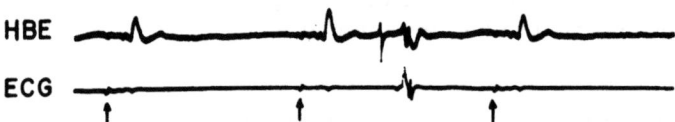

Fig. 3. Interactions of verapamil and high Ca concentration. HBE = His bundle electrogram; ECG = electrocardiogram. Arrows indicate the time of stimulation near the SA node

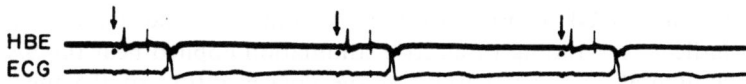

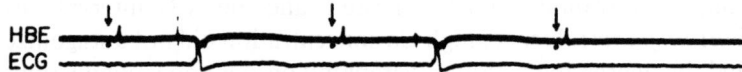

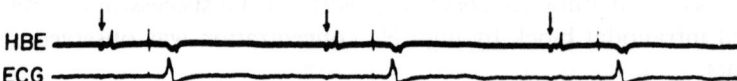

Fig. 4. Interactions of verapamil and high Na concentration. Abbreviations and arrows similar to Fig. 3

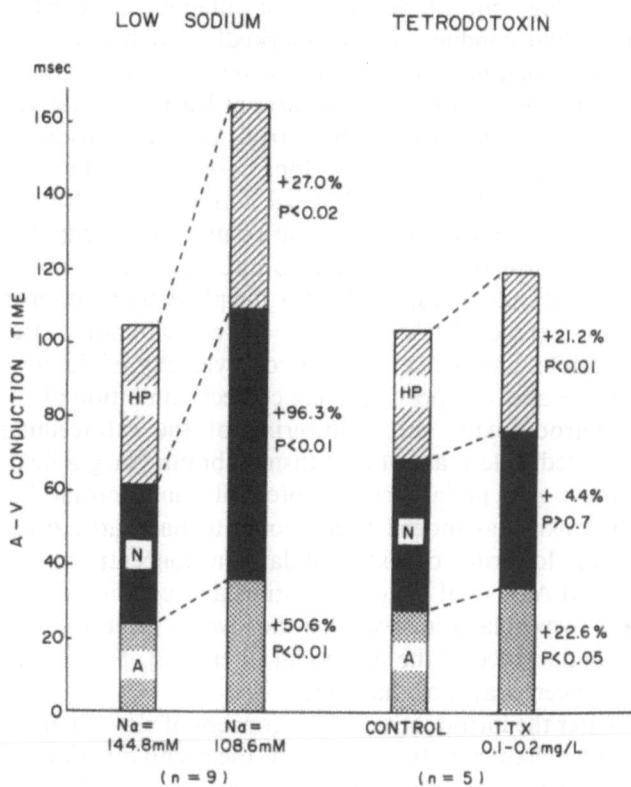

Fig. 5. Effects of low Na perfusion and tetrodotoxin (TTX) on intraatrial (A), intranodal (N) and His-Purkinje (HP) conduction times. See text for detailed discussion. (Modified from Watanabe, Y. [22])

time in all three portions of the AV transmission system, but the delay is most marked in the intranodal conduction [17], culminating in the development of second degree block within the node (Fig. 5, *left*). In contrast, TTX, which is a specific fast Na channel blocker, significantly prolonged the intraatrial as well as His-Purkinje conduction time, but failed to depress AV nodal conduction (Fig. 5, *right*), suggesting the little role played by the fast Na current in depolarizing the fibers of the AV node. These relationships were further tested in one experiment in which a second degree intranodal block with a 2:1 conduction ratio was produced by the combination of TTX (10 mg/l) and verapamil (1 mg/l). Elevation of extracellular Na concentration to 172 mM in the presence of these two agents again restored a successful 1:1 AV conduction (not shown).

Discussion

We have demonstrated earlier, in experiments using isolated, perfused rabbit hearts, that lanatoside C and low extracellular K concentration selectively depress AV nodal conduction, without significantly affecting intraatrial and His-Purkinje conduction [18 – 20]. In contrast, quinidine and high K concentration appeared to have little depressing action (and may even antagonize the effects of cardiac glycosides) on intranodal conduction, but markedly prolonged the intraatrial and His-Purkinje conduction times [19, 20]. These results indicate that the responses of AV nodal conduction to various agents are, at least quantitatively and perhaps qualitatively, different from those of the atrial and His-Purkinje conduction. A possible explanation for these observations comes from the following concept presented by Paes de Carvalho [5, 21]. Cardiac action potentials depends on two different electric events, or (1) a spike phase that results from a rapid increase (and decrease) in Na conductance of the cell membrane, and (2) a much slower and longer lasting potential change responsible for the plateau phase, probably reflecting a decrease in K conductance. In AV nodal fibers, contribution of the initial spike phase is almost negligible, and hence, the upstroke velocity of the action potential is quite low.

If the above hypothesis were correct, inhibition of the so-called Na carrier system by tetrodotoxin, and a lowering of the extracellular Na concentration, which supposedly decreases the transmembrane Na gradient, would not be expected to depress AV nodal action potentials and intranodal conduction. Although tetrodotoxin has indeed been shown to have little effect on intranodal conduction [7, 22], lowering of extracellular Na concentration invariably and markedly depressed AV nodal action potentials and conductivity (Fig. 5) [22–25]. Earlier, my tentative explanation was that the low Na perfusion might have secondarily affected K conductance of the AV nodal fibers [22]. However, no definite conclusion could have been drawn at that time.

After the introduction of the concept of slow channels and subsequent elucidation of their characteristics, genesis of the peculiar action potentials of SA and AV nodal fibers has come to be explained by a slow inward current carried mainly by Ca. The demonstration by Zipes and others that agents such as verapamil, D 600, manganese, and lanthanum, which are often called Ca-antagonists, drastically depress AV nodal conduction (and SA nodal automaticity) [7, 8, 26], appears to verify the above contention.

An earlier study by us on the effects of various cations on AV conduction revealed that both lowering and elevation of extracellular Ca concentration depressed AV conduction [17], although the reason for such diphasic action of Ca remained obscure. More recently, however, Matsuda showed that the amplitude and overshoot of the rabbit AV nodal action potential were linearly increased when the extracellular Ca concentration was increased from 0.18 to 3.6 mM [6]. This latter observation appears to be in full agreement with the above concept that slow Ca current plays an important role in the excitation of AV nodal fibers, and it was this apparent discrepancy between these two studies that prompted the present series of experiments.

As has been presented above, lowering of Ca concentration from 2.4 to 0.8 mM slightly but significantly prolonged the A-H interval. This indicates depression of AV nodal conduction by low Ca, a finding in keeping with Matsuda's report [6]. Upon elevation of Ca concentration in the perfusate to 4.8 mM (or sometimes to 7.2 mM), however, the A-H interval was again significantly and markedly prolonged (Figs. 2, 3), reconfirming our earlier experiment [17]. There are several mechanisms that may possibly explain this observation. First, since the highest level of Ca concentration studied by Matsuda was 3.6 mM, whereas the Ca level reached in the present study was much higher, the Ca ions may indeed have a diphasic action, with concentrations higher than 3.6 mM again acting to decrease the amplitude of the AV nodal action potential. Such changes in the action potential may result either from a direct modification of the transmembrane Ca current, or from a secondary change in the membrane permeability to Na and K. Indeed, an extremely high Ca concentration is considered to decrease the Na conductance (N. Toda, personal communication). Reversal of high Ca-induced AV nodal block by high K concentration (Fig. 2) may be in keeping with this concept. However, there is a report showing an increased action potential amplitude at a Ca concentration of 5 mM [25]. Second, it is possible that an altered spread of atrial excitation in the presence of high Ca perfusion (Fig. 1) decreased the efficacy of the wavefront invading the AV node and caused a more inhomogeneous intranodal conduction [27].

Third, it has been suggested recently by Toyama that the high Ca-induced depression of AV nodal conduction may be, at least in part, due to an uncoupling effect of this cation [28]. In his experiment, he measured the input resistance of the AV nodal fibers by passing a current through the microelectrode, and found a 30% increase in the resistance upon a threefold elevation of Ca concentration from 1.8 to 5.4 mM. This was associated with a 30% prolongation of the A-H interval, whereas the resting potential, action potential amplitude and the maximal rate of depolarization ($\dot{V}$max) of the AV nodal fibers were not significantly affected. From these observations, he argued that an increased intracellular accumulation of Ca, due to high extracellular Ca level, increased the resistance across the nexuses, and consequently interfered with the cell to cell propagation, without a significant depression of individual action potentials. The depression of intraatrial conduction by high Ca, with resultant inhomogeneity of wavefront secondarily affecting AV nodal conduction (Fig. 1), may also be a result of such uncoupling in the atrial tissue.

Although it cannot be determined from the present data whether only one of the above mechanisms is responsible, or all three factors are involved, these considerations clearly illustrate the fact that the phenomenon of intranodal conduction is not only dependent on the action potential characteristics of individual AV nodal fibers but also is affected by numerous other factors in a complex manner.

On the other hand, the present study demonstrated reversal of the depressing effects of verapamil on AV nodal conduction by a high Na concentration, and failure of high Ca to antagonize the action of this slow channel blocker (Figs. 3, 4). Zipes and Fischer earlier stated that neither Ca nor Na reversed the depressing effects of verapamil [7]. However, their experiment using open chest dogs probably did not permit a sufficient elevation of serum Na concentration to reveal the antagonistic action of high Na perfusion. Such a reversal of verapamil effect by Na ions is amenable to two different interpretations. First, Ruiz Ceretti and Ponce Zumino reported previously that the upstroke of AV nodal action potentials is composed of two electric events: an initial fast phase (called phase I) and a second, slower depolarization (called phase II), with an inflection point in between [25]. They suggested that the first phase is dependent on the fast Na channel, and the second phase, on slow inward currents. Shigeto and Irisawa also presented evidence for the presence of fast Na current in AV nodal fibers [29], and similar findings were reported on frog ventricular muscle [30]. If the above assumption is correct, elevation of extracellular Na concentration may enhance the initial rapid depolarization, or phase I, and improve conductivity in the AV node, even when the second, slow phase of depolarization is depressed by verapamil. However, in a heart showing second degree AV nodal block caused by a combination of tetrodotoxin and verapamil, high Na perfusion still restored a 1:1 conduction. This observation may be difficult to explain by the above concept.

Second, it has been shown by several investigators that the slow inward currents could be carried not only by Ca but also by Na ions [3, 10, 15]. Especially, Noma et al. have demonstrated that the rising phase of the spontaneous SA nodal action potential is mainly produced by Na current through the slow channel [10]. Similar ionic mechanisms may well prevail in the AV node, a tissue electrophysiologically resembling the SA node. The improvement of AV nodal conduction by high Na, after its depression by verapamil (or even combination of tetrodotoxin and verapamil), may then be explained by an enhancement of the second, slower phase of action potential upstroke dependent on the slow Na current. Marked prolongation of the AV nodal conduction time culminating in the development of second degree intranodal block by low Na concentration, and the lack of significant depressant action of tetrodotoxin (Fig. 5) [22], are also in agreement with this concept. Thus, this latter interpretation may appear more plausible, although more direct studies of ionic currents are definitely needed in the future.

In summary, the present study (1) reconfirmed the diphasic action of extracellular Ca concentrations on AV nodal conduction, with an apparent optimum Ca concentration around 2.4 mM; (2) demonstrated the reversal of verapamil-induced depression of AV nodal conduction by elevated Na concentration; and (3) suggested the role played by slow Na current in the genesis of AV nodal action potentials. Possible mechanisms for the depression of intranodal conduction by high Ca were also discussed.

References

1. Rougier O, Vassort G, Garnier D, Gargouil YM, Coraboeuf E (1969) Existence and role of a slow inward current during the frog atrial action potential. Pfluegers Arch 308:91–110
2. Beeler GW Jr, Reuter H (1970) Membrane calcium current in ventricular myocardial fibers. J Physiol 207:191–209
3. Reuter H (1973) Divalent cations as charge carriers in excitable membranes. Prog Biophys Mol Biol 26:3–43
4. Cranefield PF (1975) The conduction of the cardiac impulse. Futura, Mount Kisco NY, p 75–113
5. Paes de Carvalho A, Hoffman BF, De Paula Carvalho M (1969) Two components of the cardiac action potential. I. Voltage-time course and the effect of acetylcholine on atrial and nodal cells of the rabbit heart. J Gen Physiol 54:607–635
6. Matsuda K (1973) Function of the node of Tawara. Jpn J Clin Exp Med 50:3514–3520 (in Japanese)
7. Zipes DP, Fischer JC (1974) Effects of agents which inhibit the slow channel on sinus node automaticity and atrioventricular conduction in the dog. Circ Res 34:184–192
8. Wit AL, Cranefield PF (1974) The effects of verapamil on the sinoatrial and atrioventricular nodes of the rabbit and the mechanism by which it arrests reentrant AV nodal tachycardia. Circ Res 35:413–425
9. Noma A, Irisawa H (1976) Effects of calcium ion on the rising phase of the action potential in rabbit sinoatrial node cells. Jpn J Physiol 26:93–99
10. Noma A, Yanagihara K, Irisawa H (1977) Inward current of the rabbit sinoatrial node cell. Pfluegers Arch 372:43–51

11. Carmeliet E, Vereecke S (1969) Adrenaline and the plateau phase of the cardiac action potential: Importance of Ca^{++}, Na^+ and K^+ conductance. Pfluegers Arch 313:300–315
12. Matsubara I, Matsuda K (1969) Contribution of calcium current to the ventricular action potential of dog. Jpn J Physiol 19:814–823
13. Kohlhardt M, Bauer B, Krause H, Fleckenstein A (1972) Differentiation of the transmembrane Na and Ca channels in mammalian cardiac fibers by the use of specific inhibitors. Pfluegers Arch 335:309–322
14. Cranefield PF, Aronson RS, Wit AL (1974) Effect of verapamil on the normal action potential and on a calcium-dependent slow response of canine cardiac Purkinje fibers. Circ Res 34:204–213
15. Shigenobu K, Schneider JA, Sperelakis N (1974) Verapamil blockade of slow Na^+ and Ca^{++} responses in myocardial cells. J Pharmacol Exp Ther 190:280–288
16. Watanabe Y, Dreifus LS (1968) Sites of impulse formation within the atrioventricular junction of the rabbit. Circ Res 22:717–727
17. Watanabe Y, Dreifus LS (1968) Electrophysiological effects of major cations on atrioventricular (A-V) transmission. Proc Int Union Physiol Sci 7:460
18. Watanabe Y, Dreifus LS (1967) Electrophysiologic effects of digitalis on A-V transmission. Am J Physiol 211:1461–1466
19. Watanabe Y, Dreifus LS (1967) Interactions of quinidine and potassium on atrioventricular transmission. Circ Res 20:434–446
20. Watanabe Y, Dreifus LS (1970) Interactions of lanatoside C and potassium on atrioventricular conduction in rabbits. Circ Res 27:931–940
21. Paes de Carvalho A (1966) Excitation of the atrioventricular node during normal rhythm. Effects of acetylcholine. In: Dreifus LS, Likoff W (eds) Mechanisms and therapy of cardiac arrhythmias. Grune and Stratton, New York, p 341–352
22. Watanabe Y (1970) Effects of electrolytes and antiarrhythmic agents on atrioventricular conduction. In: Sandøe E, Flensted-Jensen E, Olesen KH (eds) Symposium on cardiac arrhythmias. Astra, Södertälje, Sweden, p 535–557
23. Kanno T, Matsuda K (1966) The effects of external sodium and potassium concentration on the membrane potential of atrioventricular fibers of the toad. J Gen Physiol 50:243–253
24. Ponce Zumino AZ, Parisii IM, Ceretti ERP (1970) Effect of ischemia and low-sodium medium on atrioventricular conduction. Am J Physiol 218:1489–1494
25. Ruiz Ceretti E, Ponce Zumino A (1976) Action potential changes under varied $[Na^+]_o$ and $[Ca^{++}]_o$ indicating the existence of two inward currents in cells of the rabbit atrioventricular node. Circ Res 39:326–336
26. Angus JA, Richmond DR, Dhumma-Upakorn P, Cobbin LB, Goodman AH (1976) Cardiovascular action of verapamil in the dog with particular reference to myocardial contractility and atrioventricular conduction. Cardiovasc Res 10:623–632
27. Watanabe Y, Dreifus LS (1965) Inhomogeneous conduction in the AV node. A model for reentry. Am Heart J 70:505–514
28. Toyama J (1978) Electrical uncoupling in the A-V node. Effects of Ca^{++} and ouabain on input resistance of A-V node cells. Presented in an International Symposium on excitation and conduction of the heart. September 20, 1978, Tokyo
29. Shigeto N, Irisawa H (1974) The effect of polarization on the action potentials of the rabbit AV nodal cells. Jpn J Physiol 24:605–616
30. Niedergerke R, Orkand RK (1966) The dual effect of calcium on the action potential of the frog's heart. J Physiol (Lond) 184:291–311

Calcium-Antagonisten in der Behandlung von supraventrikulären Tachykardien

H. Neuss, M. Schlepper, V. Mitrović und J. Thormann

Der negativ dromotrope Effekt bestimmter Calcium-Antagonisten (Verapamil, D 600) auf die Strukturen des AV-Knotens [1, 2, 3] kann als ein wesentliches therapeutisches Prinzip in der Behandlung supraventrikulärer Tachykardien angesehen werden. Auf diese Weise ist durch parenterale Gabe eines dieser Pharmaka bei chronischem Vorhofflimmern mit rascher Kammerschlagfolge meist eine zuverlässige Normalisierung der Kammerfrequenz möglich [4].

Für die orale Behandlung dieser Rhythmusstörungen liegen freilich wenig Daten über Dosis/Wirkungsbeziehungen und Wirkdauer der vorhandenen Verabreichungsformen vor. Am ehesten scheint uns hier die Analyse des Kammerfrequenzverhaltens durch Langzeit-EKG Aufzeichnungen geeignet, den therapeutischen Effekt zu objektivieren und konkrete therapeutische Empfehlungen zu erarbeiten.

So konnten wir an einem Kollektiv von 10 Patienten mit chronischem Vorhofflimmern und rascher Kammerfolge die frequenzmindernde Wirkung einer einmaligen Dosis von 100 mg D 600 über die Dauer von 8 Std − mit einem Wirkungsmaximum bei 2 Std − nachweisen. Eine vergleichende Studie über die frequenzsenkende Wirkung von Verapamil in einfacher und retardierter Form mit D 600 ist noch nicht abgeschlossen, sie scheint jedoch die Ergebnisse einer früheren Untersuchung [5] zu bestätigen, bei der durch Langzeit-Vorhofstimulation die Pharmakodynamik dieser Substanzen analysiert wurde.

Die akute Beendigung supraventrikulärer Re-entry Tachykardien durch die genannten Calcium-Antagonisten ist immer dann zu erwarten, wenn der AV-Knoten Teil der Re-entry Bahn ist. Dies gilt sowohl bei einem auf die AV-Region begrenzten Re-entry Vorgang als auch bei den typischen supraventrikulären Tachykardien des klassischen WPW-Syndroms. Während die akuten Therapieerfolge in der Literatur gut belegt sind [6], liegen keine überzeugenden Erfahrungsberichte über eine erfolgreiche Langzeitprophylaxe dieser Rhythmusstörungen vor.

Die Objektivierung eines Therapieerfolges bei diesen Patienten ist aus methodischen Gründen recht schwierig, dennoch scheint nach eigenen Erfahrungen an einem Kollektiv von 35 Patienten mit paroxysmalen Knotentachykardien die chronische Applikation von Verapamil in Tagesdosen von 240 bis 320 mg keinen zuverlässigen Schutz vor diesen Anfällen zu gewähren.

Neben pharmakokinetischen Problemen könnten hierfür elektrophysiologische Konstellationen verantwortlich sein, die für den Mechanismus dieser Tachykardien wichtig sind. Wir haben daher an 10 Patienten mit supraventrikulären Tachykardien durch AV-Knoten Re-entry die Beeinflussung der Auslöse- und Terminationsbedingungen der Paroxysmen sowie die Änderung der Refraktärparameter des AV-Knotens durch Calcium-Antagonisten im Rahmen einer His-Bündel Elektrographie untersucht.

An der Studie nahmen 10 Patienten (4 Männer, 6 Frauen) im Alter zwischen 22 und 51 Jahren teil. Nach Ermittlung der Kontrollwerte wurde eine Tachykardie ausgelöst und deren Beeinflussung durch Injektion von 4 mg D 600 (n = 7), bzw. 10 mg Verapamil (n = 3) registriert. Über 20 bis 30 min Dauer wurden dann erneut die Leitungseigenschaften des AV-Knotens, d. h. die Refraktärparameter und Leitungskapazität (Auftreten eines AV-Blocks II^0 bei Frequenzbelastung) bestimmt, die Echozone definiert und auch das Verhalten der VA-Leitung analysiert.

Die Injektion der Substanzen führte bei 9 Patienten zu einer spontanen Beendigung der Paroxysmen. Dieser Termination lag stets eine Blockierung im antegraden Schenkel des Re-entry Kreises zugrunde (Abb. 1), d. h. einem retrograden Vorhofpotential folgte kein His-Potential. Der Termination ging stets eine erhebliche Verlangsamung der Tachykardiefrequenz (im Mittel: 191/min auf 138/min − d. h. auf 72% des Ausgangswertes) vorauf. Bei einer Patientin war diese Frequenzabnahme sogar so ausgeprägt, daß die schnelleren Sinuserregungen die Tachykardie einholten und sie beendeten.

Die Zunahme der Cyclusdauer der supraventrikulären Tachykardie ging ausnahmslos auf das Konto einer Verlängerung der Laufzeit zwischen kaudalem Vorhof und Hisschem Bündel (A'-H), d. h. sie wurde durch eine Leitungsverzögerung im antegraden Schenkel des Re-entry Weges hervorgerufen. Entsprechend war die Leitungskapazität des AV-Knotens 5 min nach der Injektion deutlich vermindert. Während AV-Blockierungen II^0 in der Kontrollperiode im Mittel bei einer Frequenz von 213/min auftraten, wurden sie nach den Calcium-Antagonisten bereits bei einer mittleren Stimulationsfrequenz von 129/min beobachtet. Induzierte atriale Extrasystolen führten bei gleichem Kopplungsintervall zu ausgeprägteren Verlängerungen des A_2H_2-Intervalls, so daß bei Sinusrhythmus eine Zunahme der funktionellen Refraktärperiode des AV-Knotens von im Mittel 379±42 ms auf 470±58 ms (10 min nach der Injektion) − also einer Verlängerung um 24% entsprechend − resultierte. Auch die effektive Refraktärzeit des AV-Knotens − bei Sinusrhythmus in der Kon-

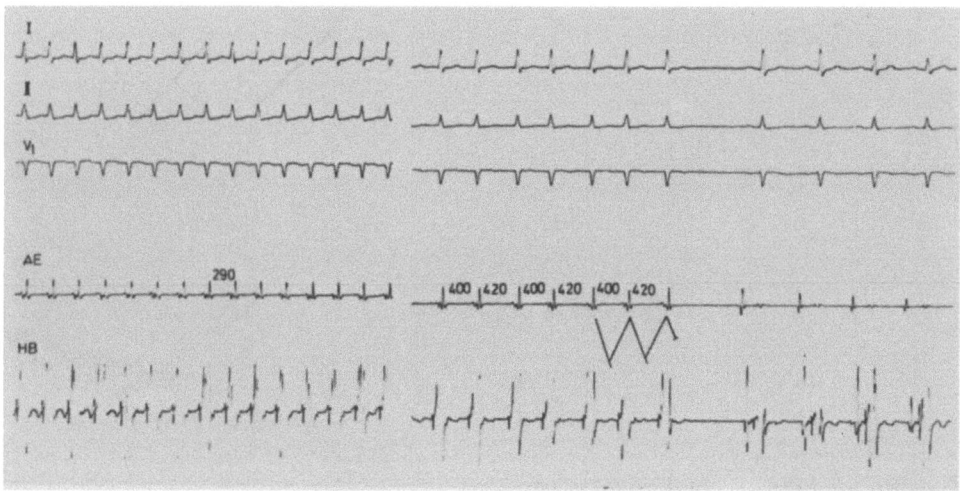

Abb. 1. Originalregistrierung einer Knotentachykardie mit EKG-Ableitungen I, II und V_1, sowie einer intraatrialen Ableitung (AE) und einer His-Bündel Ableitung (HB). Auf der linken Bildhälfte supraventrikuläre Tachykardie vor Injektion von 4 mg D 600 mit einer Zyklusdauer von 290 ms. Links Verlangsamung der Tachykardiefrequenz (Zyklusdauer 400−420 ms) und spontanes Ende durch Block zwischen A' und H unmittelbar nach Injektion des Calcium-Antagonisten

trollperiode mit einer Ausnahme durch die effektive Refraktärzeit des Vorhofs bestimmt – verlängerte sich deutlich von 250 ± 22 ms auf 327 ± 49 ms ($+31\%$).

Bei zwei Patienten wurde eine mäßige und bei zwei weiteren Patienten eine deutliche Minderung der VA-Leitungskapazität beobachtet – die retrograde Leitfähigkeit blieb also bei den meisten Patienten unbeeinträchtigt. Die AV-Leitungskapazität erholte sich rasch, und 20 min nach der Injektion konnten AV-Blockierungen II^0 erst bei einer mittleren Stimulationsfrequenz von 163/min ausgelöst werden (76% des Ausgangswertes).

Die ausgeprägte Verlängerung des A_2H_2-Intervalls nach Injektion der Calcium-Antagonisten erleichterte sogar die Auslösung von Echophänomenen. So waren bei einer Patientin supraventrikuläre Tachykardien bei Sinusrhythmus und einer stimulierten Grundfrequenz von 100/min unter Kontrollbedingungen nicht auszulösen. Erst die Applikation von Doppelstimuli führte zu einer ausreichenden A-H Verlängerung, um eine Tachykardie in Gang kommen zu lassen (Abb. 2). Nach Injektion von 4 mg D 600 war bei Sinusrhythmus bereits bei einem A_1A_2-Intervall von 400 ms die kritische Verlängerung von A_2H_2 gegeben (Abb. 3). Die Echozone erstreckte sich über 90 ms, bis bei einem A_1A_2-Intervall von 310 ms die effektive Refraktärzeit des Vorhofs erreicht war (Abb. 4). Bei einem weiteren Patienten verlängerte sich die Echozone bei Sinusrhythmus von 40 auf 120 ms, auch hier wurde sie jetzt begrenzt durch die effektive Refraktärzeit des AV-Knotens.

Insgesamt ließ sich bei 4 Patienten eine Verbreiterung der Echozone nach Gabe des Calcium-Antagonisten nachweisen. Bei 4 weiteren Patienten wurde das frühere Auftreten der Echophänomene (also bei längeren A_1A_2-Intervallen) neutralisiert durch eine Einengung auf der linken Seite der Kurve (d. h. durch eine deutliche Verlängerung der effektiven Refraktärzeit des AV-Knotens) (Abb. 5).

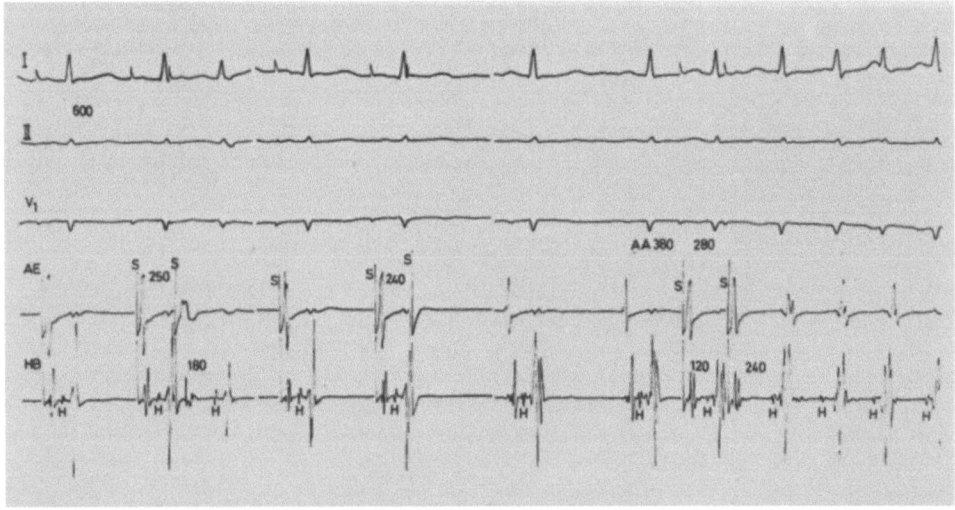

Abb. 2. Originalregistrierung von EKG (Abl. I, II und V_1), einer Ableitung aus dem hohen rechten Vorhof (AE) sowie einer His-Bündel Ableitung. Unter Kontrollbedingungen können Paroxysmen einer supraventrikulären Tachykardie bei einer stimulierten Grundfrequenz von 100/min (SS: 600 ms) nicht ausgelöst werden (links). Die effektive Refraktärzeit der AV-Leitung wird bestimmt durch die effektive Refraktärzeit des AV-Knotens (Mitte). Ein Auslösen wird erst möglich, wenn durch atriale Doppelstimuli eine AH-Verlängerung von mehr als 230 ms herbeigeführt wird (rechts)

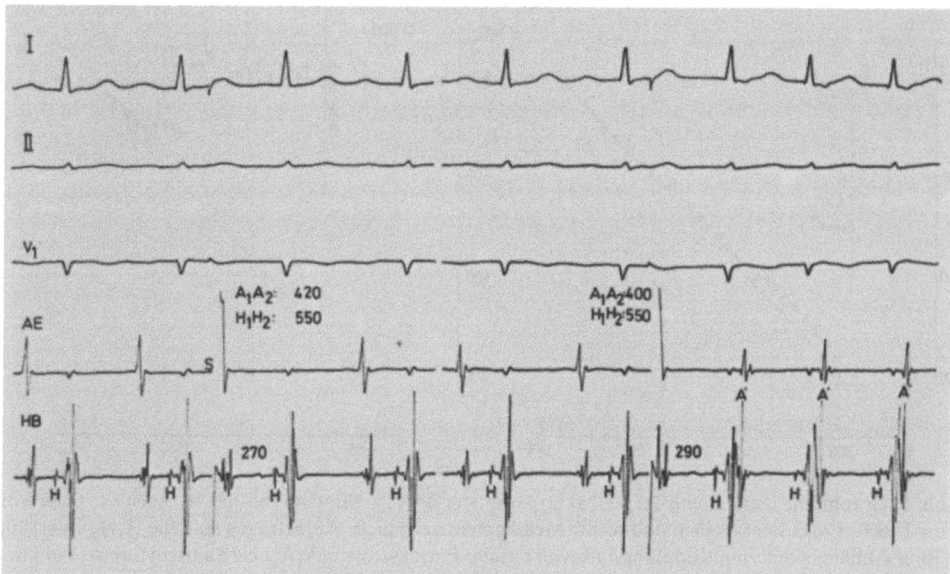

Abb. 3. Originalregistrierung von EKG (Abl. I, II, V_1), einer Ableitung aus dem hohen rechten Vorhof (AE) und einer His-Bündel Ableitung (HB) bei der gleichen Patientin wie in Abb. 2 10′ nach Gabe von 4 mg D 600. Bei Sinusrhythmus führt eine atriale Extrasystole mit einem Kopplungsintervall von 420 ms zu einer Verlängerung von A_2H_2 auf 270 ms. Eine Tachykardie wird nicht induziert (links). Die Verkürzung des Kopplungsintervalls auf 400 ms verlängert das A_2H_2-Intervall auf 290 ms und erlaubt jetzt das Ingangkommen einer Tachykardie

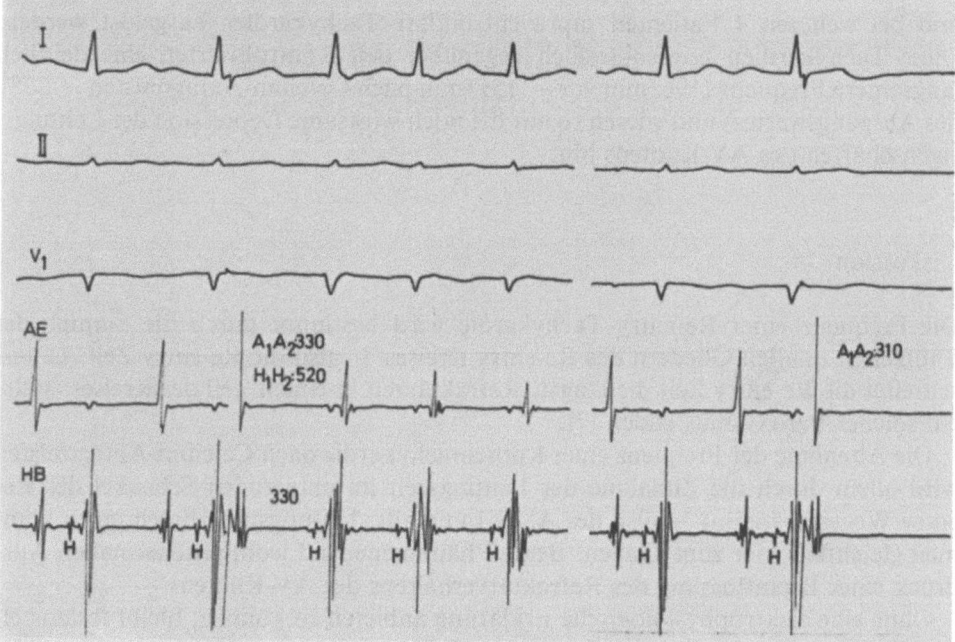

Abb. 4. Gleiche Patientin wie in Abb. 2 und 3. Nach Gabe von D 600 wird das Ende der Echozone bestimmt durch das Erreichen der effektiven Refraktärzeit des AV-Knotens, eine atriale Extrasystole mit einem Kopplungsintervall von 310 ms wird nicht zum Hisschen Bündel weitergeleitet

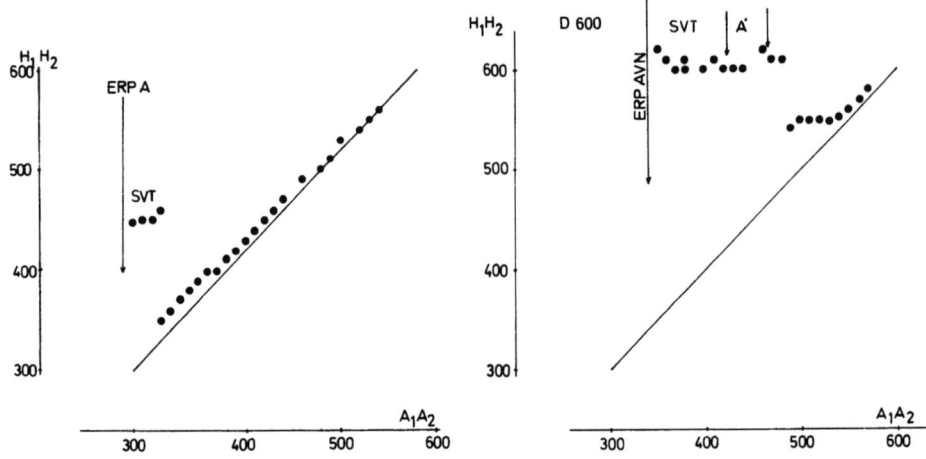

Abb. 5. Graphische Darstellung der Refraktärparameter des AV-Knotens vor und 10′ nach i.v. Gabe von 4 mg D 600. Links Leerversuch und rechts Medikamentenversuch. Aufgetragen sind die H_1H_2-Intervalle in ihrer Abhängigkeit vom Kopplungsintervall atrialer Extrasystolen (A_1A_2) bei Sinusrhythmus. Funktionelle Refraktärzeit des AV-Knotens (kürzestes H_1H_2-Intervall) im Leerversuch bei 350 ms, nach D 600: 540 ms. Die effektive Refraktärzeit der AV-Leitung wird im Leerversuch bestimmt durch die effektive Refraktärzeit des Vorhofs (ERP A = 290 ms), nach D 600 durch die effektive Refraktärzeit des AV-Knotens (ERP AVN = 340 ms). Die Echozone reicht im Leerversuch von einem A_1A_2-Intervall von 330 bis 290 ms, nach D 600 von einem A_1-A_2-Intervall von 460 ms bis zu 340 ms. SVT = supraventrikuläre Tachykardien, A′ = Vorhofechosystolen

Am Ende der Beobachtungsperiode konnten bei 4 Patienten atriale Echosystolen und bei weiteren 4 Patienten supraventrikuläre Tachykardien ausgelöst werden. Diese Tachykardien zeigten freilich gegenüber den Kontrollwerten eine deutlich langsamere Frequenz (196/min vor − 151/min nach Calcium-Antagonisten − 77% des Ausgangswertes) und wiesen so auf die noch wirksame Depression der Leitungseigenschaften des AV-Knotens hin.

Diskussion

Die Frequenz einer Re-entry Tachykardie wird bestimmt durch die Summe der Laufzeiten in allen Gliedern des Re-entry Kreises − also die Re-entry Zeit. Unterschreitet die Re-entry Zeit die längste Refraktärzeit in einem Teil des Kreises, sollte ein solcher Paroxysmus enden [7].

Die Abnahme der Frequenz einer Knotentachykardie nach Calcium-Antagonisten wird allein durch die Zunahme der Leitungszeit im antegraden Schenkel des Re-entry Weges bestimmt − also des A′-H Intervalls. Leitungsunterbrechungen kommen gleichfalls hier zum Tragen. Beide Phänomene sind wohl gleichermaßen Ausdruck einer Beeinflussung des Refraktärverhaltens des AV-Knotens.

Ohne eine elektrophysiologische Erklärung anbieten zu können, bleibt festzustellen, daß bei der Hälfte der Patienten trotz ausgeprägter Minderung der AV-Leitungskapazität die Verlängerung der antegraden Leitungszeit so ausgeprägt sein kann, daß bei der verlangsamten Tachykardiefrequenz eine stabile Re-entry Tachykardie möglich ist. Die Verlängerung der nodalen Leitungszeit neutralisiert hier die Minderung der Leitungskapazität.

Dies mag ein Problem der Dosis sein. Es scheint jedoch, daß bei Patienten mit guter Leitfähigkeit des AV-Knotens — bei Patienten mit Knotentachykardien wohl als Normalverhalten anzusehen — durch orale Gabe selbst hoher Dosen nur eine kurzfristige Senkung der AV-Leitungskapazität in einen Bereich erzielt werden kann, in dem zuverlässig nicht mehr mit dem Ingangkommen von Paroxysmen zu rechnen ist [5].

Literatur

1. Husaini MH, Kurasnicki J, Ryden I, Holmberg S (1973) Action of verapamil on sinus node, atrioventricular and intraventricular conduction. Br Heart J 35:734
2. Neuss H, Schlepper M (1971) Der Einfluß von Verapamil auf die atrioventrikuläre Überleitung. Lokalisation des Wirkungsortes mit His-Bündel Elektrogrammen. Verh Dtsch Ges Kreislaufforsch 37:433
3. Rizzon P, Di Biase M, Calabrese P, Brindicci G, Chiddo A (1977) Electrophysiologic evaluation of intravenous verapamil in man. Eur J Cardiol 6:179
4. Schamroth L (1971) Immediate effects of intravenous verapamil on atrial fibrillation. Cardiovasc Res 5:419
5. Schlepper M, Thormann J, Schwarz F (1975) The pharmacodynamics of orally taken verapamil and verapamil retard as judged by negative dromotropic effects. Arzneim Forsch 25:1452
6. Krikler D, Spurrel R (1974) Verapamil in the treatment of paroxysmal supraventricular tachycardia. Postgrad Med J 50:446
7. Antoni H (1971) Electrophysiological mechanisms underlying pharmacological models of cardiac fibrillation. Naunyn Schmiedebergs Arch Pharmacol 269:1977

Behandlung von Herzrhythmusstörungen und Hypertonien mit Calciumantagonisten

F. Bender, G. Bachour und D. Gradaus[1]

In der Absicht, eine Herzrhythmusstörung zu bessern, wurde ein Calciumantagonist erstmalig 1965 angewandt, als bei einem 36jährigen Patienten mit Zustand nach Operation eines Kammerseptumdefektes wegen eines Vorhofflatterns mit 2:1 Überleitung und Kammerfrequenz von 150/min die Injektion von 5 mg Verapamil intravenös zur höhergradigen AV-Blockierung führte. Während der folgenden Wochen und Monate wurde die blockierende Wirkung dieses Calciumantagonisten auf die AV-Leitung systematisch überprüft und dabei bestätigt, ferner die Unwirksamkeit oder nur geringe Wirksamkeit bei der durch Isoproterenol induzierten Sinustachykardie, so daß die nach Angaben in der Literatur anfänglich diskutierte Wirkungsvermittlung über eine Blockade der Beta-Rezeptoren des Herzens ausgeschlossen werden konnte. Bei Gesunden führte Verapamil regelmäßig zur Zunahme der Sinusfrequenz, wahrscheinlich reflektorisch infolge leichter Senkung des Aortendrucks.

An 6 freiwilligen Probanden wurde die Wirkung von 15 mg Verapamil i.v. auf die Zeitwerte von P, PQ, QRS und QT des EKG überprüft. Mit Maximaländerungen um 2 – 5 min nach der Injektion traten signifikante Verbreiterungen der P-Welle um 18%, signifikante Verlängerungen von PQ um 38% und Verkürzungen der QT-Dauer um 12% jeweils im Mittel auf, während die QRS-Breite unverändert blieb. Der Veränderung der QT-Dauer erwies sich bei Frequenzkorrektur als harmonisch. Durch Orciprenalin, jeweils 0,25 mg i.v. etwa 6 min nach Verapamilapplikation ließen sich die Veränderungen von P und PQ den Ausgangswerten wieder annähern, auch der zu erwartende synergestische Effekt auf die QT-Dauer wurde ermittelt [6]. Die Feststellung einer Verbreiterung der P-Welle durch Verapamil, die bereits vorher von Bass u. Friedemann [7] festgestellt worden war, kann mit der zwar seltenen, von uns aber in engem zeitlichen Zusammenhang mit der Verapamilinjektion bei tachykardem Vorhofflattern in 6 Fällen gemachten Beobachtung der Entstehung von Vorhofflimmern in Einklang gebracht werden. Die Flatterfrequenz der Vorhöfe wurde in 7 kontrollierten Fällen durch 2,5 – 10 mg Verapamil i.v. trotz Erzielung der normalen Kammerfrequenz nicht oder nur unwesentlich verringert.

Bei bisher 71 Patienten mit tachykardem *Vorhofflattern* führte die i.v. Injektion von 2,5 – 10 mg Verapamil zur prompten Reduzierung der Kammerfrequenz von 140/min (± 7) auf 82/min (± 5) im Mittel. Die Calciumantagonisten *D 600* (Fa. Knoll/Ludwigshafen) und *Ro 11-1781* (Fa. Hoffmann-La Roche/Basel) [8] sowie Verapamil wurden in ihrer Frequenzwirkung bei *Vorhofflimmern* überprüft: In 10 Fällen erfolgte nach je 2 mg D 600 i.v. eine Abnahme der Kammerfrequenz von 140 (± 12) auf 91 (± 6) pro Minute, in 9 Fällen nach je 60 – 70 mg Ro 11-1781 i.v. von 96

---

1 Neben anderen Autoren waren besonders erfolgreich Fleckenstein [1, 2] und seine Schule an der Aufklärung der Wirkungsmechanismen der Calciumantagonismen beteiligt. Haas und Härtfelder [3], Knoch u. Mitarb. [4] sowie Melville u. Mitarb. [5] wiesen auf Einzelkomponenten der Verapamileffekte am Herzen hin, die den Gedanken an eine therapeutisch am Menschen ausnutzbare antiarrhythmische Wirkung aufkommen ließen

($\pm$ 8) auf 74 ($\pm$ 5) pro Minute und in 564 Fällen nach 5 – 15 mg Verapamil i.v. von 142 ($\pm$ 6) auf 95 ($\pm$ 4) pro Minute. Im Hinblick auf den frequenzmindernden Effekt scheint bei den von uns angewandten Dosierungen kein wesentlicher Unterschied zwischen diesen Calciumantagonisten zu bestehen. Während das Wirkungsmaximum nach Verapamil und D 600 in 2 – 5 min zu registrieren ist, wird der niedrigste Kammerfrequenzwert nach Ro 11-1781 im Mittel erst nach 15 min erreicht. Bei diesen Calciumantagonisten ist nach i.v. Injektion eine vergleichsweise längere Wirksamkeit als bei Verapamil und D 600 zu erwarten.

Von Seipel [9] und anderen Autoren, auch von uns [10], wurde mit Hilfe der Frequenzbelastung im *His-Bündel-Elektrogramm* am Menschen festgestellt, daß Verapamil isoliert die AH-Zeit der AV-Überleitung verlängerte, während die HV-Zeit völlig normal blieb. Ein identisches Verhalten dieser Zeitintervalle wurde von Gmeiner u. Mitarb. [11] auch für Ro 11-1781 nachgewiesen. Die therapeutische Wirkung von Verapamil auf die *paroxysmale supraventrikuläre Tachykardie,* die heute allgemein mit Wiedereintrittsmechanismen der Erregung unter Benutzung von Bahnen des AV-Knotens erklärt werden, wurde 1966 bereits von uns beschrieben und seitdem von vielen anderen Autoren bestätigt [12].

Nach Verapamil i.v. bei *arterieller Hypertonie* des Systemkreislaufs kann während fortlaufender Registrierung bereits während der ersten Minute – also schon während der Injektion – der Beginn der Blutdrucksenkung erkannt werden, die 2 min nach Injektion das Maximum erreicht. Klinische Indikationen bestehen für Verapamil bei Blutdruckkrisen [13], z. B. auch bei Haemodialysen, ferner bei frischem Infarkt mit Hypertonie und Rhythmusstörungen, schließlich bei der oralen Dauerbehandlung der Patienten mit chronischer Hypertonie. Da das Herzzeitvolumen (Indikatormethode) nach Verapamil i.v. regelmäßig zunimmt und auch die Unterschenkeldurchblutung bei plethysmographischer Bestimmung erheblich ansteigt [6], ist eine Dilatation der Widerstandsgefäße als entscheidender Wirkungsmechanismus anzunehmen (vgl. auch [14]). Besonders von Fleckenstein-Grün [15] wurde auf die Rolle des ionisierten Calciums und der Calciumantagonisten in ausgedehnten experimentellen Studien bei der reversiblen Engstellung der peripheren Arterien in verschiedenen Gefäßprovinzen aufmerksam gemacht. Eigene Untersuchungen an 16 Patienten mit renaler Hypertonie ergaben signifikant nach je 5 mg Verapamil i.v. eine Blutdrucksenkung von 195/125 mm Hg auf 149/102 mm Hg im Mittel, wobei gleichzeitig eine Zunahme der plethysmographisch erfaßten Unterschenkeldurchblutung von 3,24 auf 4,22 ml/100 ml Gewebe/min im Mittel erfolgte. Ähnliche Werte wurden bei 9 Fällen mit nichtrenaler Hypertonie ermittelt, bei denen signifikant die Blutdrucksenkung von 179/116 mm Hg auf 145/100 mm Hg im Mittel erfolgte, während die periphere Durchblutung bei gleicher Methode von 1,97 auf 4,46 ml/100 ml Gewebe/min anstieg. Von Bachour u. Mitarb. [16] wurden telemetrisch Messungen des Blutdruckverhaltens in der perkutan sondierten Brachialarterie vorgenommen, die unter standardisierten Belastungsbedingungen bei Gesunden sowie Hypertonikern mit und ohne Vorbehandlung durch Reserpin und/oder Clonidin signifikante Minderungen des Belastungshochdrucks nach Verapamil i.v. ergaben. Auch 30 min nach oraler Einnahme von je 160 mg Verapamil konnte durch blutige, fortlaufende Messung des Brachialarteriendrucks bei Normotonikern (n = 24), Hypertonikern (n = 25) und behandelten Hypertonikern (n = 7) ein signifikant blutdrucksenkender Effekt während der standardisiert überprüften Belastungsreaktion festgestellt werden, der im Stehversuch nicht eine verstärkte orthostatische

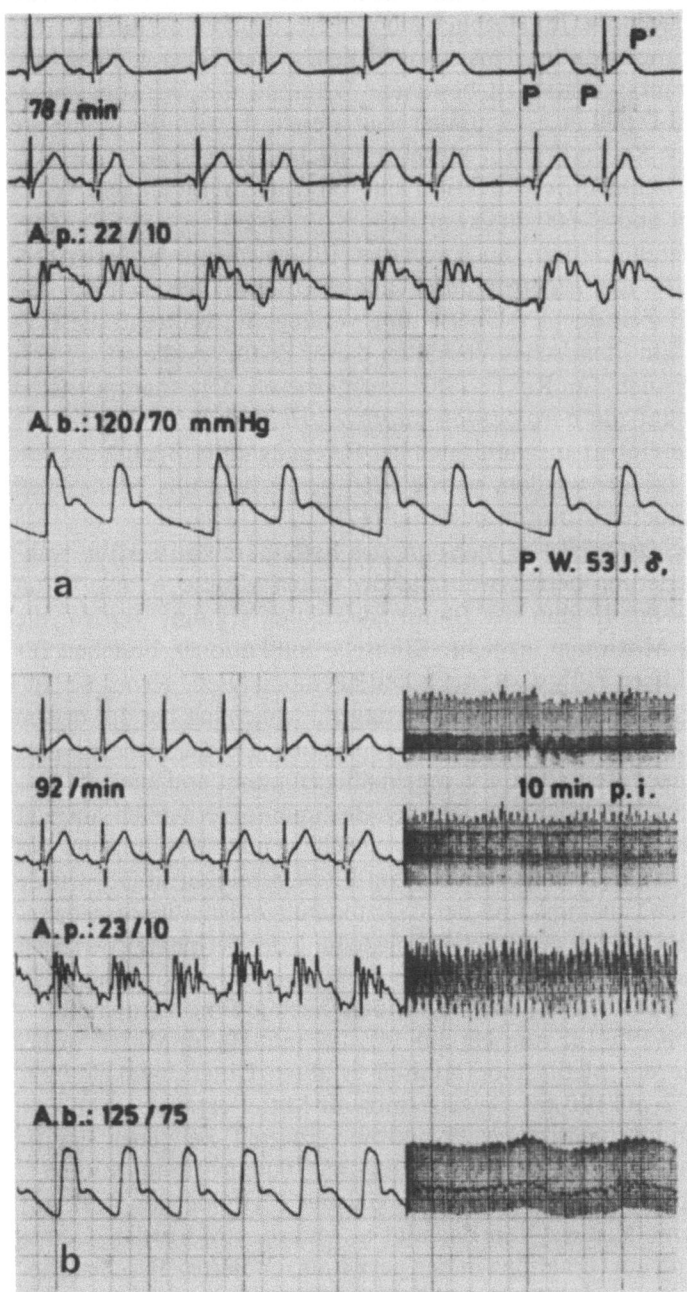

Abb. 1. a Änderungen der Hämodynamik nach 5 mg Verapamil i.v. bei 53jährigem Mann mit Vorhofbi-
geminie infolge akuten Myokardinfarkts. Beseitigung der Rhythmusstörung (unten), **b** Derselbe Fall. Be-
rechnung und graphische Darstellung hämodynamischer Parameter: Nach Verapamil (Pfeil) Abnahme
des Brachialarteriendrucks, der eine Zunahme des Schlagvolumenindex folgt. Kein Anstieg des PC-
Drucks oder rechten Vorhofdrucks

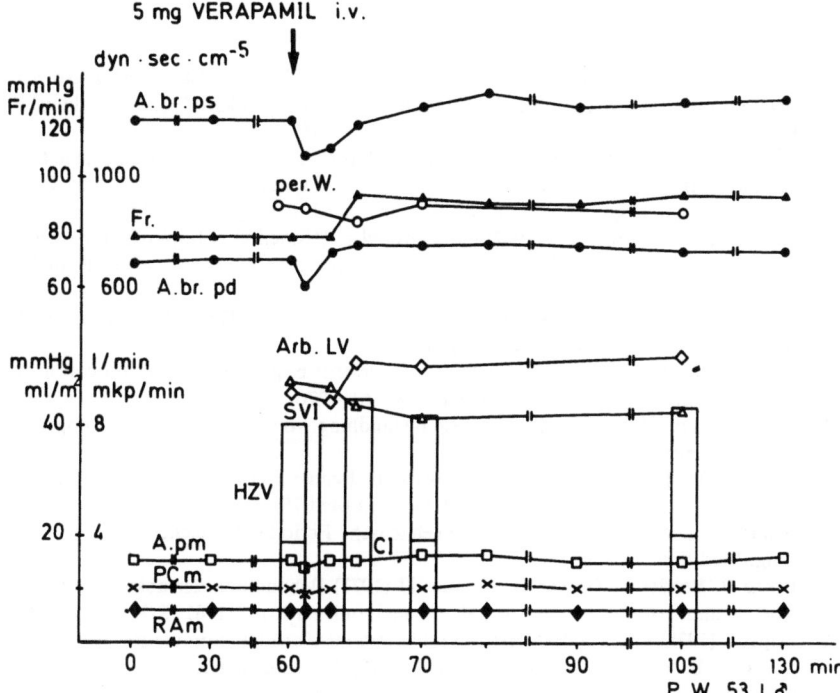

Abb. 1b

P. W. 53 J. ♂.

Druckabnahme erkennen ließ. Von Brittinger u. Mitarb. [7] wurde die Beobachtung der therapeutisch ausnutzbaren Blutdrucksenkung des Verapamil bestätigt und durch ausgedehnte Studien ergänzt.

In orientierenden Untersuchungen wurde festgestellt, daß der Calciumantagonist D 600 ebenfalls eine starke Blutdrucksenkung bei Hypertonikern bewirken kann. Die Dosisrelation zu Verapamil entspricht etwa der bei der Therapie von Rhythmusstörungen. Ob die Substanz Ro 11-1781 ähnlich eingesetzt werden kann, ist noch nicht hinreichend geklärt.

Bei *akutem Herzinfarkt* können Calciumantagonisten wegen der Wirkung auf den peripheren Gefäßwiderstand nicht nur wegen einer Hypertonie indiziert sein, sondern ähnlich wie Nitroprussidnatrium auch bei Normotomie zur Sauerstoffverbrauchsminderung des Myocards führen. Die frühere Auffassung, der Calciumantagonist Verapamil sei bei frischem Herzinfarkt grundsätzlich kontraindiziert, wird von uns also nicht unterstützt. Von Bachour u. Mitarb. [18] wurden die hämodynamischen Veränderungen durch direkte Blutdruckregistrierungen in den Pulmonal- und Brachialarterien sowie Bestimmungen des Herzzeitvolumens bei 14 Patienten mit akutem transmuralem Herzinfarkt und Tachyarrhythmien kontrolliert, wobei keine kardiodepressiven Effekte ermittelt wurden. Wolf u. Mitarb. [19] beschrieben einen günstigen Verlauf des akuten Infarktstadiums nach Anwendung dieses Calciumantagonisten. Außer Einzelinjektionen von 5 mg i.v. kamen auf der Intensivstation unserer Klinik auch i.v. Dauerinfusionen mit Tagesdosen bis 50 mg zur Anwendung. In Abb. 1a u. b ist ein Beispiel der hämodynamischen Veränderungen nach Verapamil wiedergegeben. Damit soll der negativ inotrope Effekt des Calciumantagonisten aber nicht bezweifelt oder für Fälle mit primär muskulärer Herzinsuffizienz verharmlost werden.

Literatur

1. Fleckenstein A, Kammermeier H, Döring HJ, Freund HJ (1967) Zum Wirkungsmechanismus neuartiger Koronardilatoren mit gleichzeitig Sauerstoff einsparenden Myokardeffekten, Prenylamin und Iproveratril. Z Kreislaufforsch 56:716 – 744, 839 – 858
2. Fleckenstein A, Tritthart H, Fleckenstein B, Herbst A, Grün G (1969) Eine neue Gruppe kompetitiver Ca^{++}-Antagonisten (Iproveratril, D 600, Prenylamin) mit starken Hemmeffekten auf die elektromechanische Koppelung im Warmblütermyokard. Pfluegers Arch 307:25
3. Haas H, Härtfelder G (1962) a-Isopropyl-a-((N-methyl-N-homoveratryl)-y-aminopropyl)-3,4-dimethoxyphenylacetonitril, eine Substanz mit coronargefäßerweiternden Eigenschaften. Arzneimforsch 12:549 – 558
4. Knoch G, Schlepper GM, Witzleb E (1963) Untersuchung an Gesunden und koronarkranken Patienten mit Isoptin. Med Klin 58:1485 – 1489
5. Melville KI, Shister HE, Huq S (1964) Iproveratril: Experimental data on coronary dilatation and antiarrhythmic action. Can Med Assoc J 90:761 – 770
5 Bender F (1968) Die medikamentöse Behandlung von Herzrhythmusstörungen. Therapiewoche 18:1803 – 1808
6. Klempt HW, Bachour G, Gradaus D, Brisse B, Bender F (1972) Untersuchungen zum Wirkungsmechanismus von Verapamil. Verh Dtsch Ges Inn Med 78:1116
7. Bender F, Zimmerhof K (1967) Wenckebachsche Periode als Zeichen einer Arzneimittelüberdosierung. Med Welt 18:1585
8. Brisse B, Bender F, Gülker H, Niehues H (1977) Behandlung der absoluten Tachyarrhythmie bei Vorhofflimmern mit dem neuen Calciumantagonisten Ro 11-1781. Z Kardiol 67:609 – 611
9. Seipel L (1978) His-Bündel-Elektrographie und intrakardiale Stimulation. Thieme, Stuttgart
10. Belz GG, Bender F (1974) Therapie der Herzrhythmusstörungen mit Verapamil. Fischer, Stuttgart
11. Gmeiner R, Simma CK, Ng K, Dienst F, Knapp E (1977) Z Kardiol 66:238
12. Bender F, Kojima N, Reploh HD, Oelmann G (1966) Behandlung tachykarder Rhythmusstörungen des Herzens durch Beta-Rezeptorenblockade des Atrioventrikulargewebes. Med Welt 17:1120 – 1123
13. Bender F (1970) Die Behandlung der tachykarden Arrhythmien und der arteriellen Hypertonie mit Isoptin. Arzneim Forsch 20:1310 – 1316
14. Roskamm H, Fröhlich GJ, Reindell H (1966) Die Wirkung verschiedener Coronardilatatoren auf den Sauerstoffverbrauch, die Herzfrequenz und den Blutdruck bei standardisierter Belastung auf dem Ergometer. Arzneim Forsch 16:835 – 841
15. Fleckenstein-Grün G, Fleckenstein A (1971) Ca^{++}-Antagonismus – ein neu erkanntes Prinzip der Vasodilatation. Naunyn Schmiedebergs Arch Pharmacol [Suppl] 270:48
16. Bachour G, Bender F, Wessels F, Losse H (1976) Orale Hypertoniebehandlung mit dem Calciumantagonisten Verapamil. Verh Dtsch Ges Inn Med 82:1334
17. Brittinger DW, Schwarzbeck A, Wittenmeier KW, Twittenhoff WD, Stegaru B, Huber W, Ewald RW, von Henning GE, Fabricius M, Strauch M (1970) Klinisch-experimentelle Untersuchungen über die blutdrucksenkende Wirkung von Verapamil. Dtsch Med Wochenschr 95:1871 – 1877
18. Bachour G, Bender F, Hochrein H (1977) Antiarrhythmische Wirkungen und hämodynamische Reaktionen unter Verapamil bei akutem Herzinfarkt. Herz Kreislauf 2:89 – 95
19. Wolf R, Nötges A, Witt E, Habel F, Everling F, Hochrein A (1975) Der Einfluß von Verapamil (Isoptin®) auf die Hämodynamik und Ausdehnung des acuten Myokardinfarktes. Z Kardiol [Suppl II] 62

Cardioprotective Actions of Calcium-Antagonists in Myocardial Anoxia and Ischaemia[1]

W. G. Nayler, F. Ferrari, and A. Slade

Summary

When cardiac muscle becomes hypoxic or ischaemic the cells become oedematous and the fine ultrastructure of the mitochondria is altered. Developed tension declines and resting tension increases. The cellular stores of ATP and CP are depleted and the mitochondria exhibit an altered respiration, characterized by a reduced state III respiration and a lowered respiratory control index. The calcium accumulating activity of the mitochondria is enhanced. During reperfusion the calcium content of the mitochondria increases and total tissue calcium rises. Using these changes in function as indices of the severity of the damage caused by hypoxia, ischaemia, and reperfusion we have investigated whether pretreatment with the slow channel Ca^{2+} antagonists verapamil and nifedipine provides protection.

Adult male New Zealand White rabbits were injected twice daily with either saline, verapamil, or nifedipine for $2-3$ days before starting the experiments. The drugs were given subcutaneously or intraperitoneally and the last injection was given 2 h before killing the animals. The hearts were isolated, Langendorff perfused and then made ischaemic. Ischaemia was induced by occluding the coronary perfusion line. If hypoxic conditions were required they were established by substituting 95% N_2 and 5% CO_2 for 95% $O_2 + 5\%$ CO_2 in the gas mixture.

Pretreatment with either verapamil or nifedipine protected the mitochondria against the ischaemic- and hypoxic-induced changes in mitochondrial function. This pretreatment also prevented the mitochondria from accumulating excessive amounts of calcium; it resulted in the preservation of the fine ultrastructure of the myocardium and in the maintenance of its high energy phosphate (ATP and CP) reserves: a similar protective effect was observed when the drugs were added directly to the coronary perfusion circuit.

During the past decade more intensive efforts have been expended in the search for a universally successful form of treatment for ischaemic heart disease than in any other area of adult cardiology. Most of the early forms of treatment were based on clinical empiricisms and consequently were limited by a lack of understanding of the various regulatory control mechanisms governing oxygen availability and utilization in the ischaemic myocardium. Recently the tenuous nature of the balance between oxygen supply and utilization has been recognised, and knowing that the oxygen requirements of the heart are critically dependent upon several haemodynamic parameters, including heart rate, contractility, wall tension, and afterload, new approaches have been devised for the clinical treatment of patients with coronary

1 These investigations were supported by grants from The Wellcome Foundation and the Medical Research Council

artery disease, myocardial infarction, and angina pectoris. In general, therapies that have been designed to protect the ischaemic heart either improve energy production through changes in metabolic pathways (e.g. the glucose-potassium-insulin treatment) or they limit the heart's requirement for oxygen — as in the case of the slow channel Ca^{2+}-antagonist drugs, the β-adrenoceptor antagonists, and the peripheral vasodilators. Agents that act in other ways have also been used, for example, hyaluronidase, which probably increases extracellular diffusion and capillary permeability in the ischaemic tissue, and steroids, including methylprednisolone, which may stabilize membrane structure and hence retard the release the Iysosomal enzymes. In general, however, the drugs that reduce the oxygen requirements of the heart seem to have the greatest potential value for use in the treatment of ischaemic heart disease.

It was the introduction in the early 1960's of the β-adrenoceptor blocking drugs that, by stimulating the search for other compounds for use in the treatment of ischaemic heart disease, resulted in the development of the drugs now commonly referred to as "calcium-antagonist" [1]. Drugs belonging to this group include prenylamine, verapamil, nifedipine, and diltiazem. These drugs share certain pharmacological properties. They all depress the contractile activity of cardiac and smooth muscle. Like nitroglycerin they are potent coronary vasodilators, and like nitroprusside they reduce peripheral vascular resistance. They all reduce myocardial oxygen uptake [2] and they lack β-adrenoceptor blocking activity [3]. Their use in the treatment of ischaemic heart diseases apparently depends upon their ability to act at the level of the cell membrane to suppress the slow inward calcium current which flows during the plateau phase of the action potential (Fig. 1). Strictly speaking, of course, these drugs should be called "inhibitors of the slow calcium current" and not "calcium-antagonists", their effect on calcium transport being

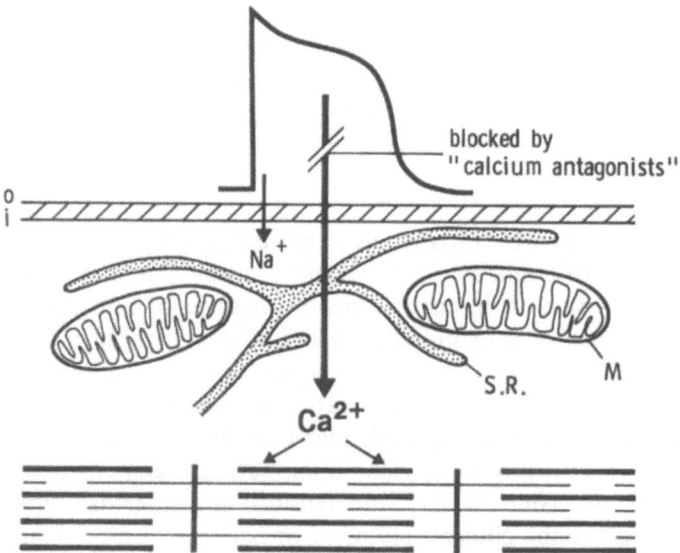

Fig. 1. Schematic representation of the mode of action of the "calcium-antagonist" drugs S.R., sarcoplasmic reticulum; M, mitochondrion

specific for the transport of those calcium ions that act as charge carries and that are displaced inwards during the plateau phase of the action potential. Drugs such as verapamil and nifedipine have no effect on the bulk movement of calcium into cardiac and smooth muscle cells nor do they have any effect on the calcium sodium exchange system.

To establish whether the calcium antagonist drugs have a potentially useful protective effect on heart muscle that is inadequately oxygenated – either because of an inadequate coronary blood flow or arterial desaturation – we have performed a series of experiments using hearts excised from animals that have been pretreated with either verapamil or nifedipine. The excised hearts were made either hypoxic or ischaemic and the effects of these procedures monitored in a variety of ways, including enzyme release, ultrastructural, and mitochondrial function studies. In some studies the mechanical performance of the heart was followed and in others the hearts were assayed for energy-rich phosphates. Our results show that pretreatment with either verapamil or nifedipine does protect heart muscle against the deleterious effects of hypoxia and ischaemia.

Methods

Perfusion

Hearts excised from adult male albino rabbits (New Zealand strain) were perfused at 37 °C by the Langendorff technique [4]. The perfusate was Krebs-Henseleit buffer solution gassed with 95% O_2 + 5% CO_2, delivered to the aortic cannula (Fig. 2) via a two-way stopcock, at a mean pressure of 60 mmHg. The hearts were electrically paced to beat at a constant rate of 180/min.

After 30 min equilibration at 37 °C and under the perfusion conditions described above, the hearts were randomly divided into three groups. In one group the

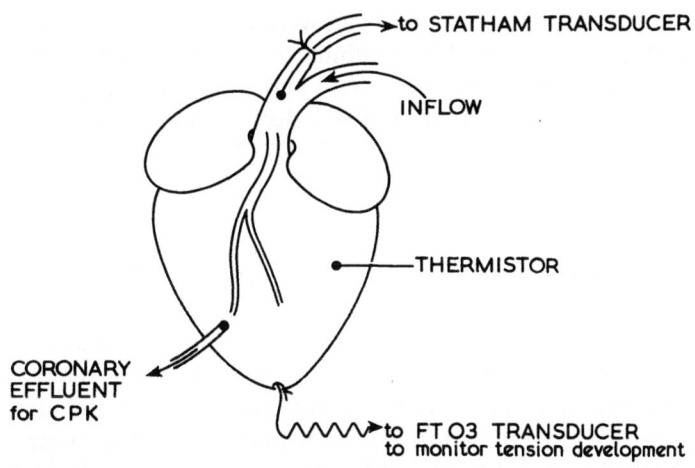

Fig. 2. Diagramatic representation of the isolated heart used in these studies

perfusate was gassed continuously with 95% O_2 + 5% CO_2 — referred to as *aerobic perfusion*. In the second group the perfusate was gassed with 95% N_2 + 5% CO_2, to provide *hypoxic conditions*. In the third group the perfusate was continuously gassed with 95% O_2 + 5% CO_2 but coronary flow was stopped. Hearts in this group were therefore *totally ischaemic*. Other hearts were made partially ischaemic by reducing the coronary flow. A Grass FT O3 transducer was attached via a fine nylon ligature to the ventricular apex and used to monitor peak developed and resting tension.

CPK Activity of Coronary Effluent

Coronary flow was measured by timed collection, and samples of coronary effluent collected into chilled glass vials were analysed on the same day for CPK activity. CPK activity was assayed spectrophotometrically using a Gilford 300 N spectrometer.

Tissue ATP and CP

Some of the hearts were used for ATP and CP determination. The perfusion of these hearts was terminated by freezing the hearts between large stainless steel tongs precooled in liquid nitrogen [5]. The frozen tissue was assayed for ATP and CP as previously described [6].

Electronmicroscopy

Other hearts were used for ultrastructural studies. After the required period of perfusion under either aerobic, hypoxic, or ischaemic conditions these hearts were perfusion-fixed for electron microscopy, as follows: the Krebs-Henseleit buffer solution in the perfusion system was replaced with 4% glutaraldehyde prepared in 0.2 mol/l sodium cacodylate buffer, pH 7.3. Ten min later papillary muscle or biopsies of left ventricular wall were cut into 1 mm^3 cubes, fixed in glutaraldehyde and post-fixed in 1% osmium tetroxide, prepared in cacodylate buffer. The specimens were then dehydrated and embedded in epoxy resin. Silver sections were cut and examined in an AEI 901 electron microscope.

Mitochondrial Studies

Respiratory Function and Ca^{2+}-Accumulating Activity

The remaining hearts were used for mitochondrial studies. After the required period of aerobic, hypoxic, or ischaemic perfusion, left ventricular muscle was excised, gently homogenized, and then differentially centrifugated to provide a pellet that consisted predominantly of mitochondria [6]. The composition of the pellets was checked enzymatically and by electronmicroscopy. Oxidative phosphorylation was monitored polarigraphically at 25 °C, using a Clark O_2 electrode. The incubation medium contained 125.0 mmol/l KCl; 1.25 mmol/l Tris-HEPES (N-2-hydro-xyethylpiperazine, N'-2-hydroxyethylpiperazine, N'-2-ethanesulphoric acid) buffer, pH 7.2; 3 mmol/l Tris pyruvate or glutamate as substrate, 3.0 mM K_2HPO_4; 0.5 mmol/l EDTA-2% dextran, 0.75 mg mitochondrial protein/ml and 0.25 mmol/l ADP. The following indices of mitochondrial function were used:

a) P/O ratio (nmol ADP used per n atoms O_2 consumed);

b) Oxygen uptake (QO_2; state III) (n atoms O_2 uptake in response to the addition of 0.25 mmol/l ADP;

c) RCl: respiratory control index: ratio of O_2 consumed in the presence of ADP to that taken up after phosphorylation to ATP) and

d) Ca^{2+}-accumulating activity (nmol Ca^{2+}-accumulated per mg protein per min). This was measured by dual beam spectrometry as described by Scarpa and Graziotti [7].

Ca^{2+} Content

The mitochondria that were assayed for Ca^{2+} content were isolated, as described by Peng et al. [8], to ensure that they neither gained nor lost Ca^{2+} during their extraction. When isolated, HNO_3 digests were analysed by atomic absorption spectrometry for Ca^{2+} content.

Drug Administration

The rabbits were either pretreated with the drugs (1.0–2.0 mg/kg given either intraperitoneally or subcutaneously twice daily for 3–5 days before the start of each experiment) or the drugs were added directly to the coronary perfusion circuit. If the rabbits were pretreated the last dose of the drug was given 2 h before the start of the experiment.

Statistical Analysis

The significance of the results was analysed by Student's t, taking $p = 0.05$ as the limit of significance.

Results

Control Studies

Preliminary control studies showed that 90 min of aerobic perfusion failed to cause any significant change in either the mechanical performance, fine ultrastructure, or metabolism of isolated rabbit hearts irrespective of whether the donor rabbits had been pretreated with either verapamil or nifedipine. Resting and peak-developed tension remained relatively constant and the tissue stores of ATP and CP (Tables 1 and 2) were well maintained. There was no evidence of intracellular oedema, the

Table 1. Effect of Ischaemia on Myocardial Stores of ATP (ATP µmoles/gm dry weight)

Experiment	Untreated	Verapamil	Nifedipine
90 min aerobic perfusion	18.4 ± 1.2	19.1 ± 1.8	18.9 ± 1.1
90 min ischaemia	4.6 ± 0.8	14.8 ± 0.9[a]	14.3 ± 1.0[a]
90 min ischaemia + reperfusion	4.2 ± 0.3	15.6 ± 1.2[a]	15.9 ± 0.8[a]

[a] $p < 0.001$.

Each result mean $\pm$ S.E. of 6 experiments.

Tests of significance relate to the difference from the untreated series.

Table 2. Effect of Ischaemia on Myocardial Stores of CP — CP (µ moles/gm dry weight)

Experiment	Untreated	Verapamil	Nifedipine
90 min aerobic perfusion	34.6 ± 3.2	35.1 ± 2.9	34.9 ± 3.2
90 min ischaemia	2.1 ± 0.2	19.8 ± 1.4[a]	18.6 ± 2.2[a]
90 min ischaemia + reperfusion	1.8 ± 0.3	24.3 ± 1.8[a]	26.2 ± 1.3[a]

[a] $p < 0.001$.

Each result is mean $\pm$ S.E. of 6 experiments.

Test of significance relate to the difference from the untreated series.

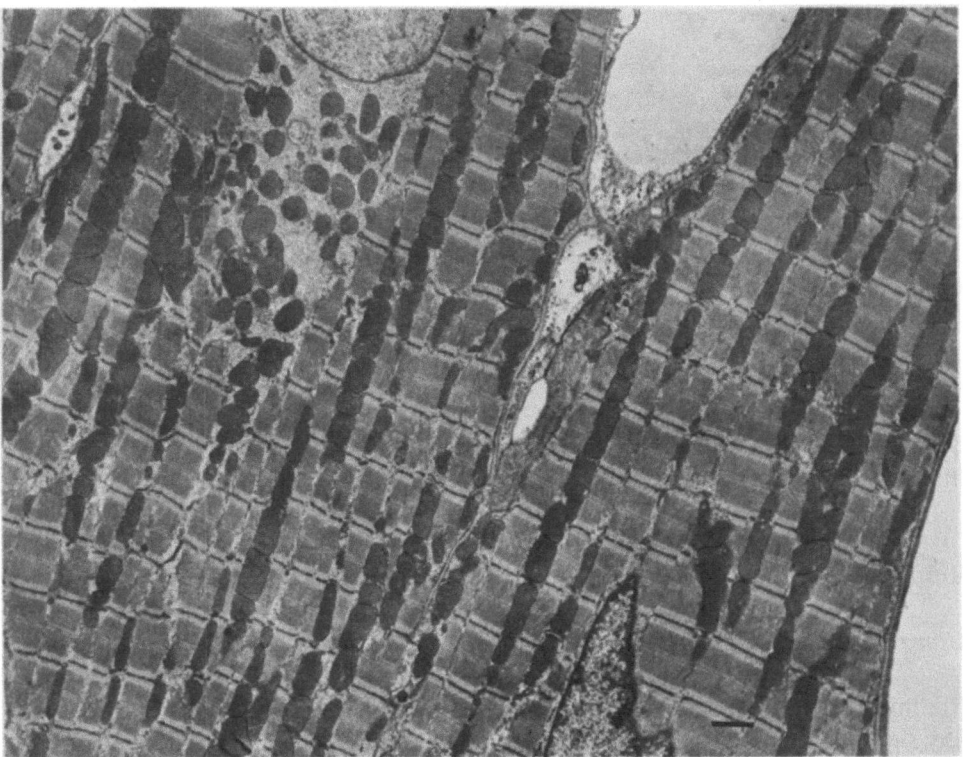

Fig. 3. Longitudinal section through the left ventricular wall of an aerobically perfused heart. Note that the myofibrils are in array and the mitochondria are packed with cristae. There is no oedema and the cytosol contains glycogen. Mag: 7,000

Table 3. Effect of Propranolol, Verapamil, and Nifedipine Treatment

Experiment	Heart Rate (Beats/Minute)	Developed Tension (GM)
Untreated	142 ± 13 (37)	8.3 ± 2.5 (37)
Propranolol	130 ± 25 (14)	7.3 ± 1.7 (10)
Verapamil	108 ± 50 (20)	4.2 ± 2.7 (17)
Nifedipine	122 ± 20 (14)	5.3 ± 1.3 (14)

Numbers in parenthesis are the number of separate experiments performed.
Results are mean ± S.D.

myofibrils remained in array and the mitochondria (Fig. 3) were densely packed with cristae. When isolated the mitochondria exhibited normal respiratory activity and they contained between 15 and 17 nmoles Ca^{2+} per mg protein.

Hearts isolated from rabbits that had been pretreated with either verapamil or nifedipine exhibited a slowed spontaneous heart rate and developed less tension (Table 3) during contraction than saline treated controls.

Effect of Ischaemia and Reperfusion

Total Ischaemia

The total cessation of coronary flow in the hearts taken from untreated rabbits resulted in a decline in the tissue stores of ATP and CP (Tables 1 and 2). At the same time (Table 4) resting tension increased and there were marked changes in the fine ultrastructure of the myocardium. These changes in the fine ultrastructure included clumping of the chromatin material in the nucleus (Fig. 4a), intracellular oedema (Fig. 4a & b), disruption of the myofibrils (Fig. 4b), the appearance of lipid droplets (Fig. 4b), the disappearance of glycogen from the cytosol, and (Fig. 4c) the appearance of electron dense bars in the mitochondria (Fig. 4c).

Mitochondria that were isolated from these hearts after they had been ischaemic for 90 min exhibited a reduced RCl (Fig. 5) and QO_2 (Fig. 6) and they contained large amounts of calcium (Fig. 7).

Table 4. Effect of Ischaemia and Reperfusion on Resting Tension. Change in Resting Tension (GM)

Perfusion		90 min Aerobic	90 min Ischaemia	After 30 min Reperfusion
Untreated	(17)	0	1.7 ± 0.3	6.6 ± 0.7
Propranolol	(10)	0	1.1 ± 0.2^a	3.5 ± 0.5^a
Verapamil	(10)	0	0.8 ± 0.2^b	1.8 ± 0.2^b
Nifedipine	(14)	0	1.2 ± 0.3^a	1.3 ± 0.1^b

[a] $p < 0.01$.
[b] $p < 0.001$.
Tests of significance calculated with respect to difference from the untreated preparations.

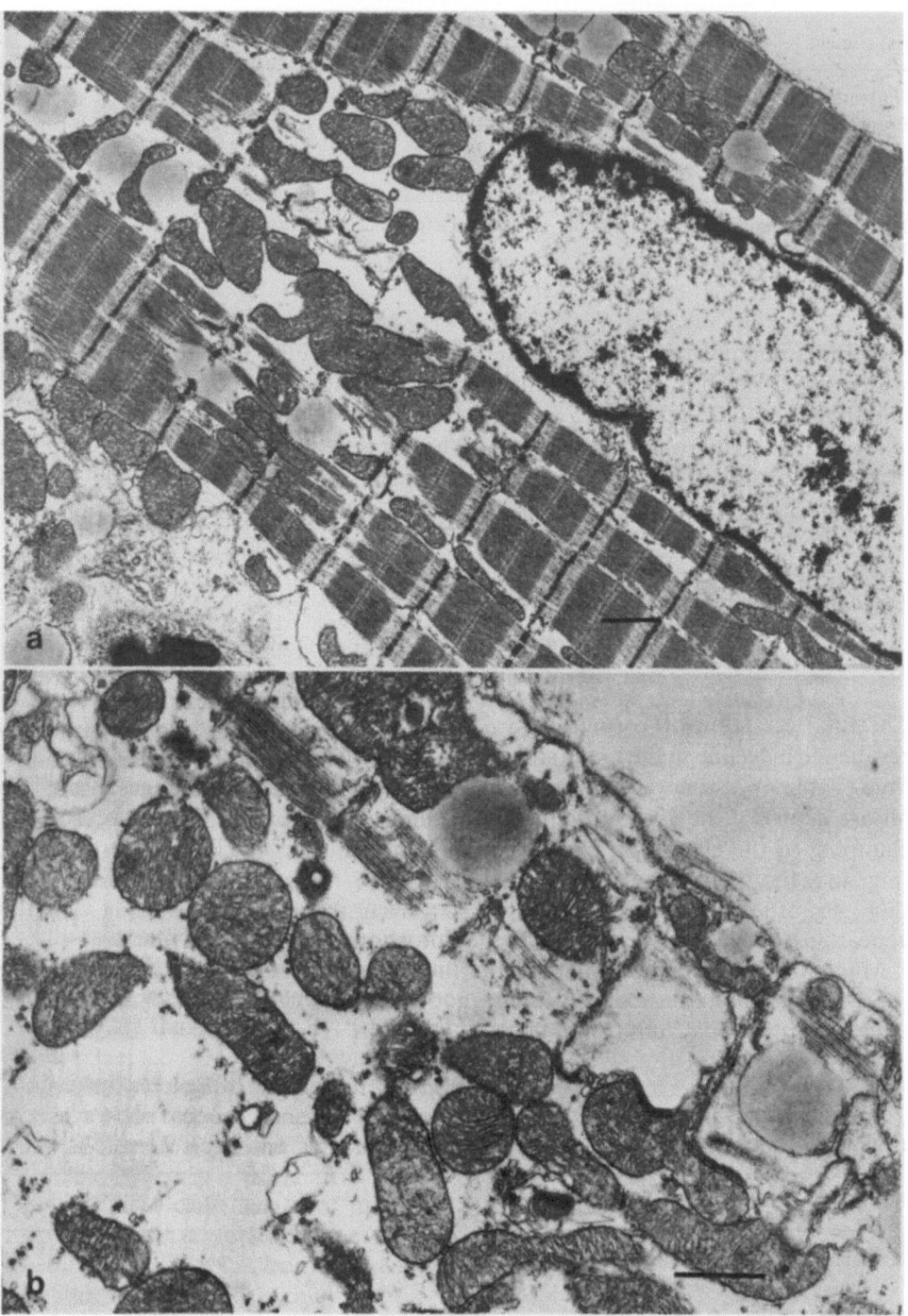

Fig. 4a – c. Longitudinal sections of left ventricular wall muscle perfusion-fixed after 90 min ischaemia. Note the presence of oedema, the absence of glycogen, the presence of lipid droplets and the presence of electron dense bars in the mitochondria. In some cells (Fig. 4b) the myofibrils are lysed. Mag: **a**, 13,000; **b**, 20,000; **c**, 35,000

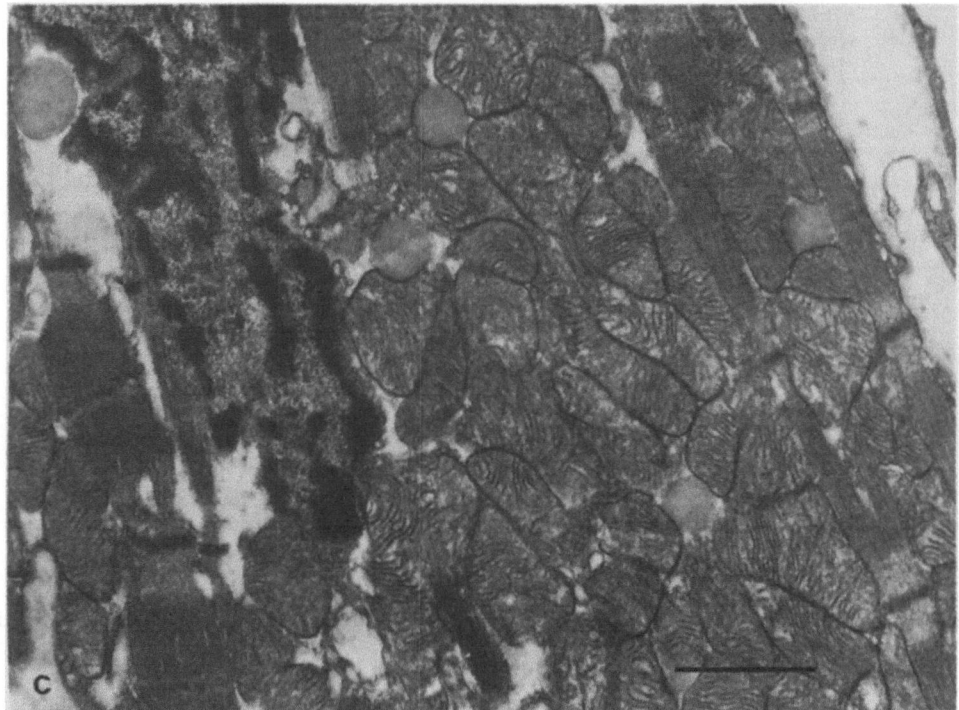

Fig. 4c

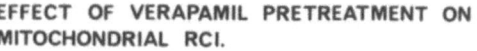

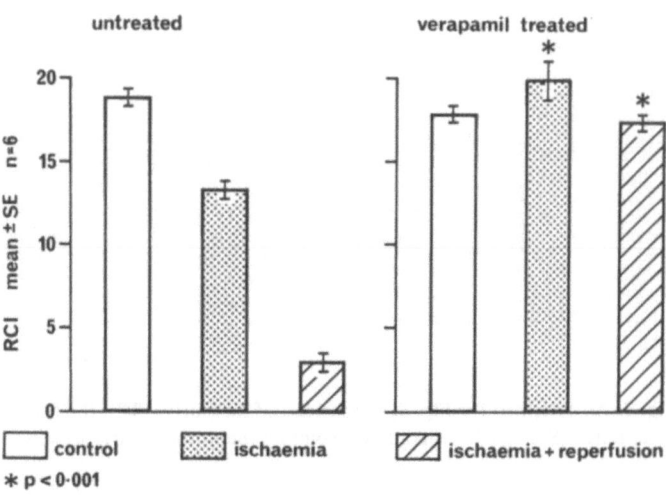

Fig. 5. Respiratory control values of mitochondria isolated from the hearts of untreated and verapamil treated rabbits. The hearts were either perfused under aerobic conditions for 90 min (control) or they were made ischaemic for 90 min (ischaemia) or they were reperfused

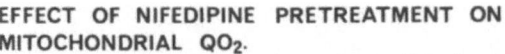

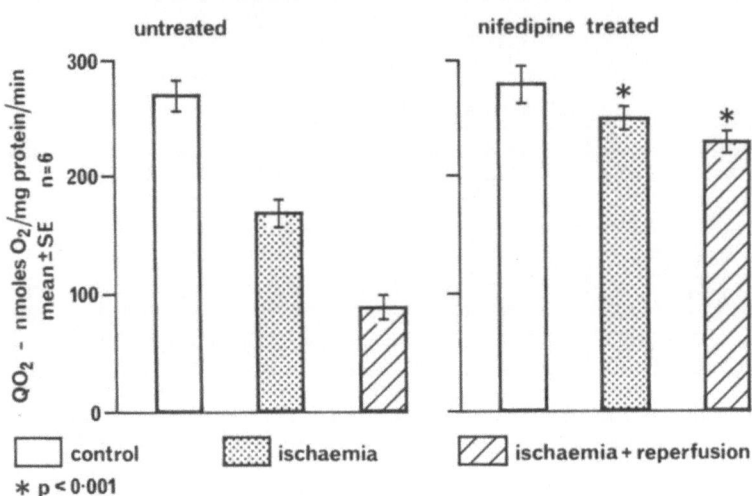

Fig. 6. Experiments performed as described for Fig. 5, but the state III respiration (QO_2) of the isolated mitochondria was measured

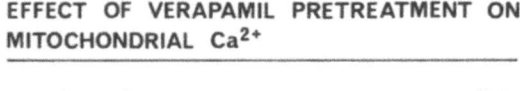

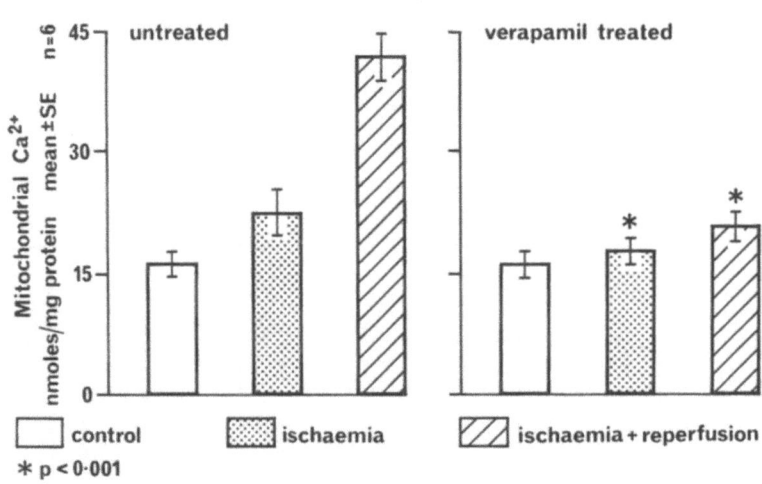

Fig. 7. As described for Fig. 5, but instead of measuring RCl, the Ca^{2+} content of the mitochondria was determined (See text for method of isolating the mitochondria for Ca^{2+} determination)

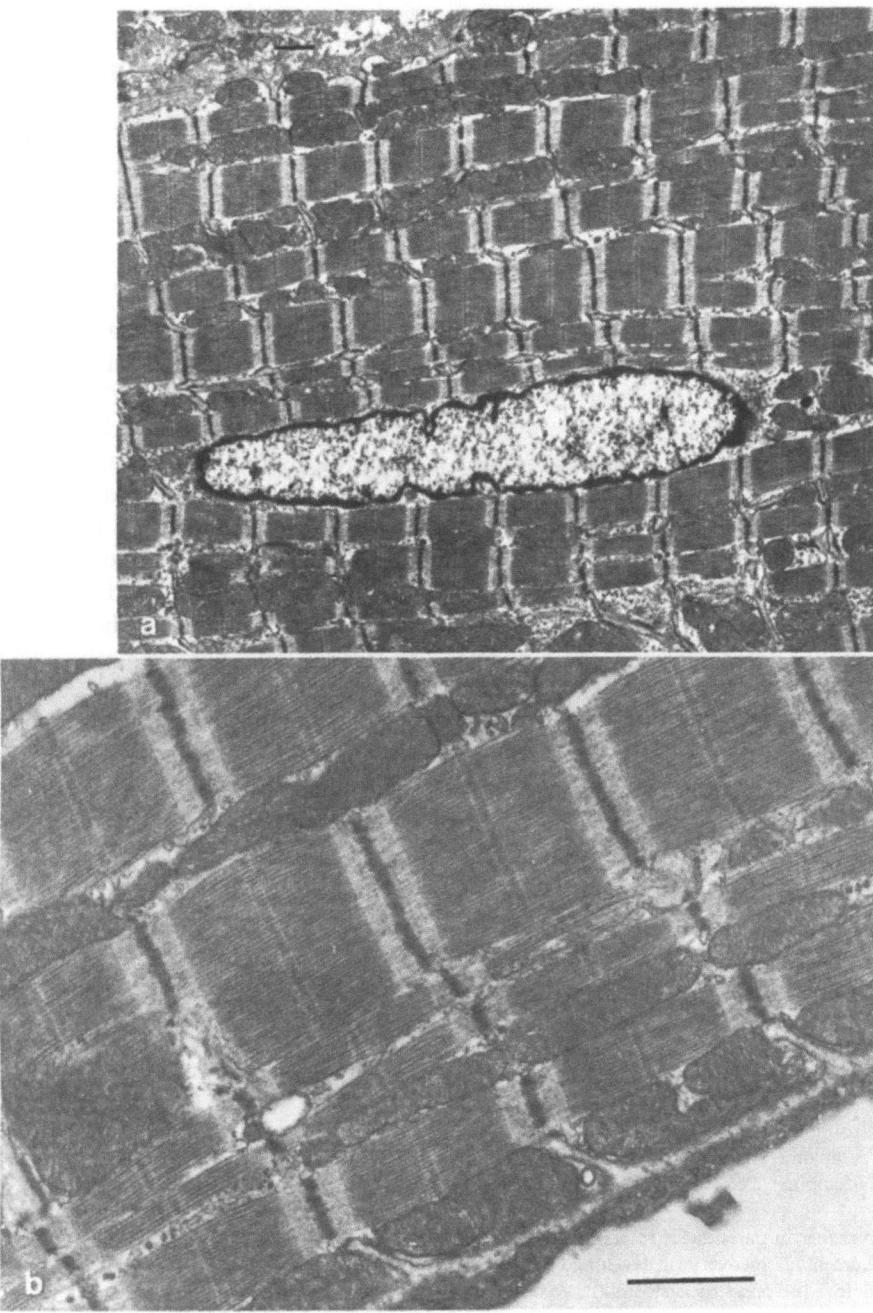

Fig. 8a,b. Electronmicrographs of longitudinal sections of left ventricular free wall of rabbits that had been pretreated with verapamil prior to making the hearts ischaemic for 90 min. Note the myofibrils are in array, and there is little oedema. Mag: **a**, 8,000; **b**, 28,000

Reperfusion

Reperfusing hearts that previously had been made ischaemic (for 90 min) resulted in an exacerbation of the ischaemic-induced damage. Thus (Table 4) there was a further rise in resting tension ($p < 0.001$) and additional deterioration in mitochondrial function — assayed in terms of RCl (Fig. 5), QO_2 (Fig. 6) and Ca^{2+} content (Fig. 7).

Effect of Pretreatment with Verapamil on the Ischaemic
and Reperfusion-Induced Damage

The data shown in Tables 1, 2, and 4 and in Fig. 5 – 7 show that pretreating the rabbits with verapamil provided some protection against the deleterious effects of total ischaemia and reperfusion. Thus the cardiac stores of ATP (Table 1) and CP (Table 2) were better maintained, relative to the untreated series, there was a significant reduction in the amount by which resting tension increased during either the ischaemic period or during reperfusion (Table 4) and the respiratory activity (Figs. 5 and 6) and calcium content of the mitochondria (Fig. 7) remained within normal limits. Examination of the fine ultrastructure of the muscle revealed further evidence of the protection that resulted from pretreatment with verapamil, the myofibrils remaining in array (Fig. 8a) and oedema (Fig. 8a & b) being absent. The mitochondria retained their normal appearance and were densely packed with cristae.

When electrically paced hearts from untreated rabbits were made ischaemic for 90 min and then reperfused they developed only 24% of the tension they had developed prior to the onset of the ischaemic episode (Table 5). This contrasts with the results obtained for hearts excised from rabbits that had been pretreated with verapamil, where the tension developed during contraction was 72% of that (Table 5) developed prior to their being made ischaemic and then reperfused.

Table 5. Percentage Recovery of Developed Tension During Reperfusion After 90 min Ischaemia

Experiment	% Recovery of Developed Tension
Untreated	24 (11)
Propranolol	56 (10)
Verapamil	72 (7)
Nifedipine	74 (14)

Number in parenthesis refers to number of experiments performed.
Percentage recovery of developed tension calculated with respect to the tension developed immediately before the onset of ischaemia.

Effect of Adding Verapamil to the Coronary Perfusion Buffer in Hearts Made
Partially Ischaemic by Reducing the Coronary Flow from 25 to < 2 ml/min

In the experiments described so far the hearts were made totally ischaemic by abolishing coronary flow, and under these conditions the hearts of rabbits that had been pretreated with verapamil were found to be protected against the deleterious effects of ischaemia.

Because partial obstruction of the coronary flow, rather than total obliteration, may be more like the situation that occurs clinically, some additional experiments were performed reducing the coronary flow from 25 to < 2 ml/min and simultaneously adding verapamil to the coronary perfusion line. The results of these experiments are summarized in Fig. 9 – 12. These results show that adding verapamil to provide a final concentration of 0.1 mg/l in the coronary perfusion buffer resulted in less CPK (Fig. 9) being released ($p < 0.001$) during the "ischaemic" episode. At the same time rise in resting tension (Fig. 10) was reduced ($p < 0.001$), and the tissues stores of ATP and CP (Fig. 11) were better preserved. Mitochondria that were isolated from hearts made partially ischaemic in the presence of verapamil exhibited a higher state III respiration (Fig. 12) than mitochondria from the untreated partially ischaemic preparations and (Fig. 13) they accumulated calcium at a relatively normal rate.

In general, therefore, experiments in which verapamil either has been added directly to the perfusion line or the animals have been pretreated prior to the onset of the ischaemic episode indicate that this drug can provide protection under conditions of inadequate oxygenation caused by inadequate flow.

Effect of Verapamil on Hearts Perfused Under Hypoxic Conditions

Evidence relating to the protective effect of verapamil on hearts made hypoxic by gassing the coronary perfusion circuit with 95% + 5% N_2, instead of 95% O_2 +

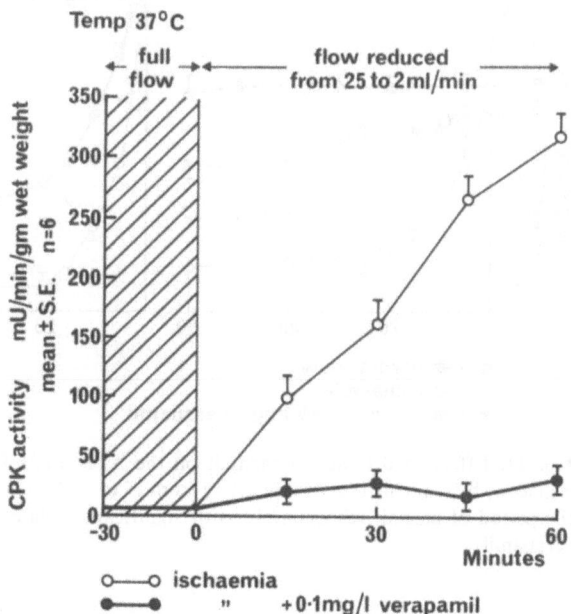

Fig. 9. Release of CPK (creatine kinase) from hearts made partially ischaemic by reducing the coronary flow from 25 to < to 2 ml/min. Note that adding verapamil to the coronary perfusion line resulted in a reduced rate of CPK leakage into the coronary effluent. Partial ischaemia was induced at zero on time scale

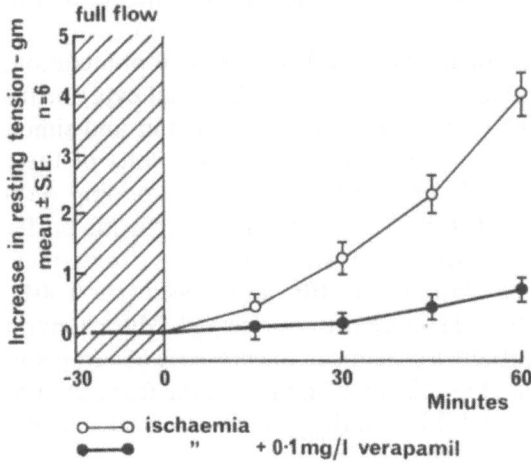

Fig. 10. Effect of partial ischaemia on resting tension exhibited by isolated electrically paced rabbit hearts. Partial ischaemia was induced at time zero, as described for Fig. 9. Verapamil was introduced into the coronary perfusion circuit co-incident with the onset of the partial ischaemia

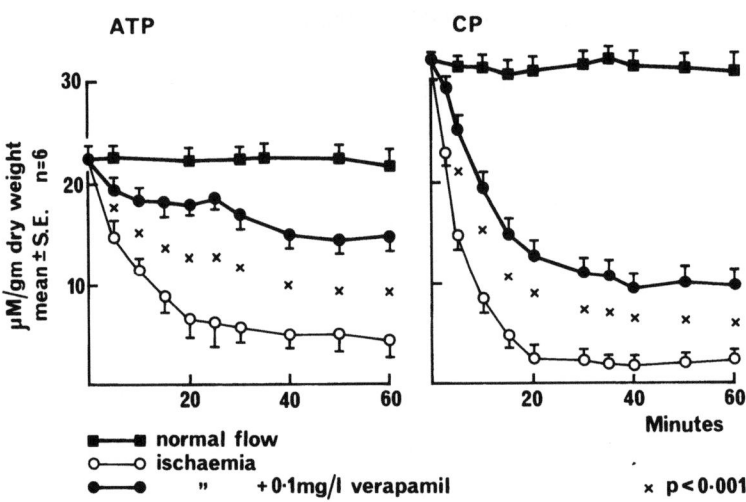

Fig. 11. Effect of 0.1 mg/l verapamil on the ATP and CP reserves of heart muscle made partially ischaemic by reducing the coronary flow from 25 to < 2 ml/min. The verapamil was added at the start of the period of partial ischaemia. Tests of significance relate to the difference made by the presence of verapamil

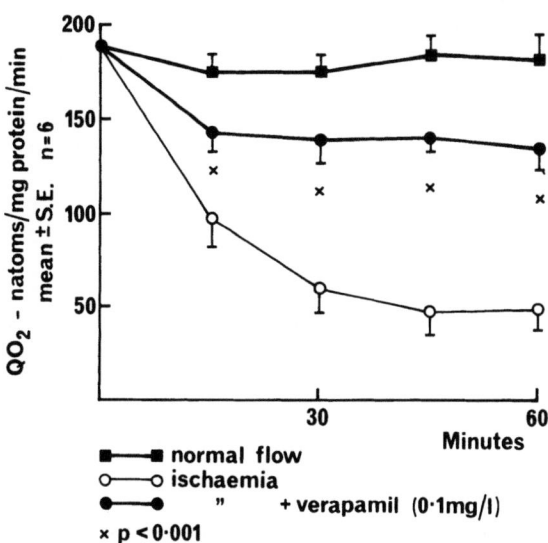

Fig. 12. Mitochondrial state III respiration in hearts made partially ischaemic as described for Figs. 10 and II, with and without verapamil in the coronary perfusion circuit. Tests of significance relate to the difference made by the presence of verapamil

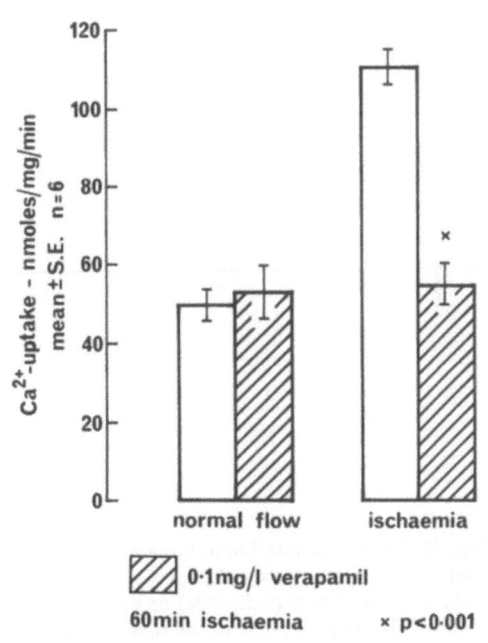

Fig. 13. Calcium uptake by mitochondria isolated from normoxic heart muscle and from heart muscle made partially ischaemic for 60 min by reducing the coronary flow from 25 to < 2 ml/min. Note that mitochondria isolated from the hearts perfused under conditions of partial ischaemia but in the presence of 0.1 mg/l verapamil accumulated calcium at a relatively slow rate

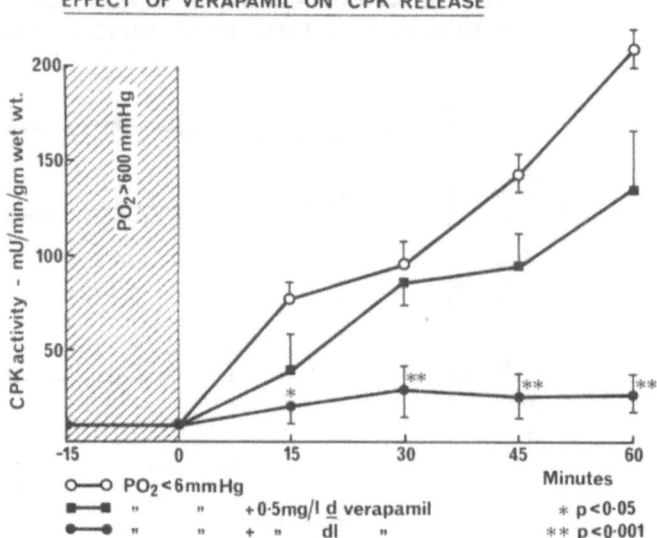

Fig. 14. Effect of *dl* and the *d* isomer of verapamil on the rate of enzyme leakage from hearts made hypoxic by gassing the perfusate with 95% N_2 + 5% CO_2 instead of 95% O_2 + 5% CO_2. Hypoxic conditions were introduced at zero on the time scale. Results are mean ± SE, 6 experiments p O_2 > 600 mm Hg refers to preliminary period of perfusion under aerobic conditions

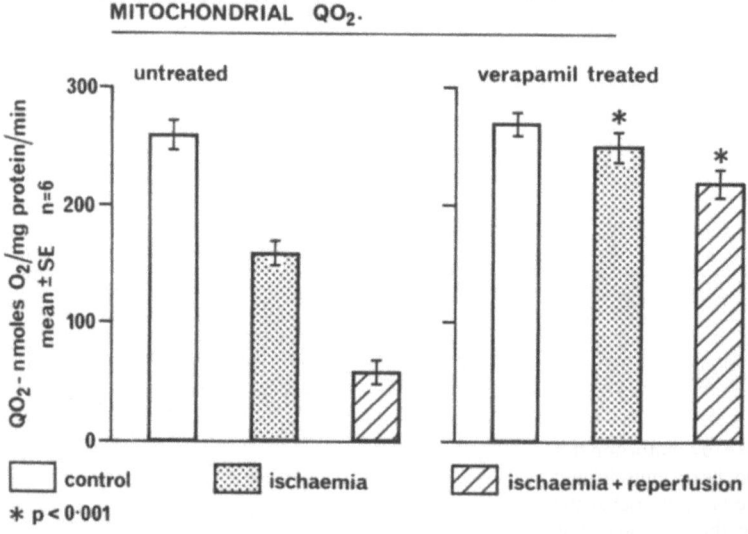

Fig. 15. State III respiration of mitochondria isolated from hearts of untreated and nifedipine — treated rabbits. The hearts were either perfused under aerobic conditions (control) or they were made totally ischaemic for 90 min (ischaemia) or they were made totally ischaemic for 90 min and then reperfused. Tests of significance relate to the significance of the difference made by the nifedipine pretreatment

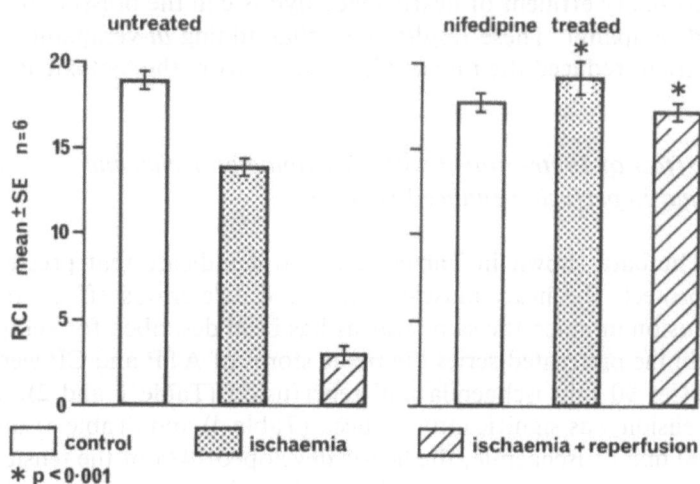

Fig. 16. As described for Fig. 15, except that instead of measuring State III respiration the respiratory control index was monitored

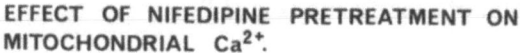
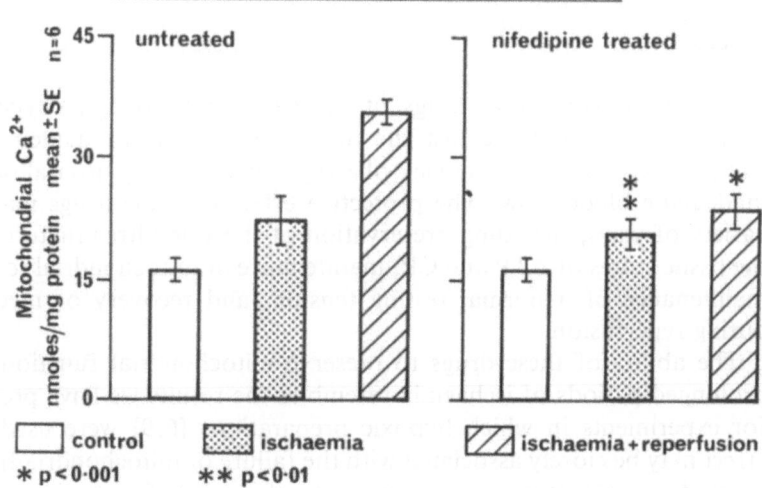

Fig. 17. As described for Fig. 15, except that the calcium content of the mitochondria was determined

5% CO_2, have already been described in detail in the literature [6,9]. Further evidence of this protection is shown in Fig. 14, which relates to CPK release into the coronary effluent of hearts made hypoxic in the pressure or absence of either *dl-* or *d*-verapamil. These results show that adding *dl*-verapamil directly to the coronary circuit reduced the rate of CPK leaked from the hypoxic muscle.

Effect of Pretreatment with Nifedipine on Ischaemic and Reperfusion-Induced Damage

The data shown in Tables 1, 2 and 4 indicate that pretreatment with nifedipine protects the heart muscle against the deleterious effects of ischaemia and reperfusion in much the same way as has been described for verapamil. Thus in the nifedipine pretreated series the tissue stores of ATP and CP were well maintained even after 90 min ischaemia and reperfusion (Table 1 and 2). The increase in resting tension was significantly reduced (Table 4) and (Table 5) during reperfusion, after 90 min of ischaemia, the hearts developed 74% of the tension they were developing prior to the introduction of the ischaemic conditions.

The mitochondrial function studies showed similar evidence of a protective effect for nifedipine. Thus the QO_2 values were well maintained despite 90 min of ischaemia with and without reperfusion (Fig. 15); the RCl values were well maintained (Fig. 16) and the Ca^{2+} content of the mitochondria was reduced, particularly after the period of reperfusion (Fig. 17).

Discussion

These results show that drugs of the verapamil-nifedipine type can be used to protect heart muscle against the deleterious effects of inadequate oxygenation, irrespective of whether the lack of oxygen is caused by arterial desaturation or an inadequate blood flow. The protective effect of these drugs manifests itself in a variety of ways, including preservation of the fine ultrastructure, maintenance of the tissue stores of ATP and CP, maintenance of mitochondrial respiratory activity, maintenance of a normal resting tension, and recovery of mechanical function during reperfusion.

The ability of these drugs to preserve mitochondrial function even after quite prolonged periods of ischaemia resembles the results we have previously described for experiments in which hypoxic preparations [6,9] were used. This protective effect may be closely associated with the failure of mitochondria from the protected hearts to accumulate excessive amounts of calcium for, in liver mitochondria, the presence of excessive amounts of calcium triggers a failure of the mitochondria to rephosphate ADP to ATP.

In general terms it seems highly likely that the ability of the drugs studied here to protect hypoxic and ischaemic muscle depends ultimately upon their ability to maintain the tissue stores of ATP and CP. This, in turn, could be due in part to the decreased contractile state of the heart. In addition it may be the result of the better maintenance of mitochondrial function. We can easily devise a scheme whereby the maintenance of the tissue stores of ATP and CP, even during phases of acute ischaemia, results in the maintenance of the fine ultrastructure of the heart and in the continued activity of its various ATP-dependent systems — including those that are responsible for regulating the cytosolic Ca^{2+}, and those which, via the Na^+K^+-ATPase enzyme, regulate the movement of Na^+ and K^+, and hence, of water, across the cell membrane.

The protection that drugs of the nifedipine-verapamil type provide to the ischaemic-hypoxic heart resembles that provided (Tables 4 and 5, and [9]) by propranolol. The advantage of the slow channel Ca^{2+}-antagonists is, of course, that they can be administered without interfering with the support provided by the sympathetic system.

As yet the factors that determine infarct size are not yet clearly defined [10], but our results together with those already reported in the literature [11 – 15] indicate that both nifedipine and verapamil should be of considerable value, provided, of course, that these drugs are given at an early stage. In addition, because of their vasodilator activity we can expect them to be useful for the treatment of variant angina.

References

1. Fleckenstein A (1971) Specific inhibitors and promoters of calcium action in the excitation-contraction coupling of heart muscle and their role in the prevention on production of myocardial lesions. In: Harris P, Opie L (eds) Calcium and the heart. Academic Press, London-New York, pp 135 – 188
2. Nayler WG, Szeto J (1972) Effect of verapamil on contractility, oxygen utilization and calcium exchangeability in mammalian heart muscle. Cardiovasc Res 6:120 – 128
3. Nayler WG, McInnes I, Swann JB, Price JM, Carson V, Race D, Lowe TE (1968) Some effects of iproveratril (Isoptin) on the cardiovascular system. J Pharmcol Exp Ther 161:247 – 260
4. Langendorf O (1895) Untersuchungen am überlebenden Säugetierherzen. Pfluegers Arch 61:291 – 332
5. Wollengerger A, Ristau O, Schoffa G (1960) Eine einfache Technik der extrem schnellen Abkühlung größerer Gewebestücke. Pfluegers Arch 270:399 – 412
6. Nayler WG, Grau A, Slade A (1976) A protective effect of verapamil on hypoxic heart muscle. Cardiovasc Res 10:650 – 662
7. Scarpa A, Graziotti P (1973) Mechanism of intracellular calcium regulation in heart. Stopped flow measurement of Ca^{2+} uptake by cardiac mitochondria. J Gen Physiol 62:756 – 772
8. Peng CF, Kane JJ, Murphy MC, Straub KD (1977) Abnormal mitochondrial oxidative phosphorylation of ischaemic myocardium reversed by Ca^{2+} chelating agents. J Mol Cell Cardiol 9:897 – 908
9. Nayler WG, Fassold E, Yepez C (1978) The pharmacological protection of mitochondrial function in hypoxic heart muscle: effect of verapamil, propranolol and methylprednisolone. Cardiovasc Res 12:151 – 161
10. Maroko PR, Kjekshus JK, Aobel BE, Watanabe T, Covell JW, Ross J Jr, Braunwald E (1971) Factors influencing infarct size following experimental coronary artery occlusion. Circulation 43:67 – 82
11. Reimer KA, Lowe JE, Jennings RB (1977) Effect of the calcium antagonist verapamil on necrosis following temporary coronary artery occlusion in dogs. Circulation 55:581 – 587
12. Robb-Nicholson C, Currie WD, Wechsler AS (1978) Effects of verapamil on myocardial tolerance to ischemic arrest: Comparison to potassium arrest. Circulation [Suppl II] 58:119 – 123
13. Shuchleib R, Borda LJ, Roberts R, Williamson JR, Sobel BE (1978) Effects of nifedipine on myocardial perfusion and ischaemic injury in dogs. Circ Res 43:372 – 380
14. Smith HJ, Goldstein RA, Griffith JM, Kent KM, Epstein SE (1976) Selective depression of ischaemic myocardium by verapamil. Circulation 54:629 – 635
15. Henry PD, Shuchleib R, Davis J, Weiss ES, Sobel BE (1977) Myocardial contracture and accumulation of mitochondrial calcium in ischemic rabbit heart. Am J Physiol 233:H677 – H684

Effect of Verapamil on Energy Consumption and Development of Contracture During the Calcium Paradox[1]

T. J. C. Ruigrok, A. B. T. J. Boink, A. N. E. Zimmerman, and F. L. Meijler

Summary

Reperfusion of calcium-deprived rat hearts with normal calcium-containing medium results in massive release of cell constituents, rapid depletion of tissue high-energy phosphate stores, and development of irreversible contracture (calcium paradox).

In an attempt to protect the heart against the calcium paradox, the slow channel calcium-antagonist drug verapamil (1 mg $\cdot$ litre^{-1}) was added to the calcium-free medium and the reperfusion medium. Cell damage was quantitated in terms of creatine kinase (CK) release into the effluent medium, depletion of tissue creatine phosphate (CP) and adenosine triphosphate (ATP) stores, and development of contracture.

Verapamil did not reduce the initial rate of CK release from the hearts upon reperfusion with calcium-containing medium, but reduced the initial rate of myocardial CP and ATP depletion, and lessened the severity of the contracture.

Introduction

Reperfusion of isolated rat hearts with calcium-containing medium, after a short period of calcium-free perfusion, results in the occurrence of the calcium paradox [2]. This phenomenon is characterized by massive release of cell constituents [2], exhaustion of tissue high-energy phosphates [3], and the rapid onset of myocardial contracture [4].

It has been postulated that during calcium-free perfusion the permeability of the sarcolemma to calcium changes in such a way that reperfusion with calcium-containing medium results in intracellular calcium overload [5]. The calcium paradox forms an extreme example of the damaging effects of an imbalance in calcium homeostasis and can also be evoked in other species [6].

In an attempt to reduce the damaging effect of sequential perfusion with a calcium-free and a calcium-containing medium, the slow channel calcium-antagonist drug verapamil [7–9] was added to the calcium-free medium and the reperfusion medium. Cell damage was quantitated in terms of enzyme leakage, depletion of high-energy phosphates, and development of myocardial contracture.

Methods

Male Wistar rats were anaesthetized with diethyl ether. The rats were heparinized and the hearts quickly removed and subsequently perfused at 37°C by the

---

1 Full text will be published elsewhere [1]

Langendorff technique at a constant pressure of 10.0 kPa (75 mmHg). The standard perfusion medium had the following composition (mmol · litre^{-1}): NaCl, 124; KCl, 4.7; CaCl$_2$, 1.3; MgCl$_2$, 1.0; NaHCO$_3$, 24.0; Na$_2$HPO$_4$, 0.5; glucose, 11.0. During calcium-free perfusion, calcium was omitted from the standard medium without correction for the small change of osmolarity. The media were equilibrated with 95% O$_2$ − 5% CO$_2$; the pH of the media was 7.40 ± 0.05. The isotonic contractions of the heart were recorded according to Meijler et al. [10].

After 15 min of perfusion with standard medium, the perfusion was changed to the calcium-free medium. After 4 min of calcium-free perfusion, the hearts were reperfused with the calcium-containing standard medium. When required, 1 mg · litre^{-1} verapamil (Knoll AG, Ludwigshafen, F.R.G.) was added to the calcium-free and the reperfusion medium.

Samples of the effluent medium were collected and analysed for creatine kinase (CK) activity. CK activity was assayed [11, 12] using a Vitatron Automatic Kinetic Enzyme System (AKES) at 25 °C. Enzyme activity was expressed in IU released · min^{-1} · g^{-1} dry heart tissue (± SEM).

For the determination of tissue creatine phosphate (CP) and adenosine triphosphate (ATP), hearts were freeze-clamped at various points in the perfusion sequence and assayed as previously described [3]. Results were analysed for significance by Student's t test, taking $p = 0.05$ as the limit of significance.

Results and Discussion

During the control perfusion period (0 − 15 min) and subsequent calcium-free period (15 − 19 min) the hearts released negligible amounts of CK. During the reperfusion phase, however, massive release of CK was observed (Table 1). When verapamil was added to the calcium-free and the reperfusion medium, the initial rate of CK release during reperfusion with calcium-containing medium was even higher than that from untreated hearts, although the difference was not significant. This difference was probably caused by the higher coronary flow in the verapamil-treated hearts. The increase in coronary flow may be due to the less pronounced contracture (Table 3) or the vasodilator action of the drug [7], thus giving rise to a more rapid removal of CK from the damaged cells.

At the end of the control perfusion period myocardial CP and ATP stores amounted to 29.6 and 18.8 μmol · g^{-1} dry wt, respectively (Table 2). Subsequent calcium-free perfusion for 4 min resulted in a slight increase of the endogenous stores of CP and ATP, irrespective of whether verapamil was present. During the first minute of reperfusion with calcium, myocardial CP fell from 35.6 to 4.6 μmol · g^{-1} dry wt in the absence of verapamil, and from 33.1 to 15.0 μmol · g^{-1} dry wt in the presence of verapamil ($p < 0.001$). In the same period myocardial ATP fell from 20.8 to 6.3 μmol · g^{-1} dry wt in the absence of verapamil, and from 20.6 to 13.2 μmol · g^{-1} dry wt in the presence of verapamil ($p < 0.001$). During the next 3 min of reperfusion, CP and ATP stores decreased gradually (Table 2).

During the control perfusion period isotonic contractions of the hearts were recorded as changes in length of the longitudinal axis of the left ventricle [4]. Omitting calcium from the medium caused rapid arrest in diastole. Verapamil had no effect on the degree of relaxation achieved during diastole. Reperfusion with

Table 1. Effect of verapamil (1 mg · litre^{-1}) on the release of CK from isolated rat hearts during successive perfusion with a calcium-free and calcium-containing medium

Perfusion period (min)	CK release (IU · min^{-1} · g^{-1} dry wt)		
	no verapamil	+ verapamil	p
Control perfusion (0 – 15)			
9 – 10	0		
Ca^{2+}-free perfusion (15 – 19)			
16 – 17	0	0.8 ± 0.1	
18 – 19	0	1 ± 0.1	
Reperfusion with Ca^{2+} (19 – 23)			
19 – 19.5	78 ± 15	78 ± 24	NS
19.5 – 20	304 ± 15	476 ± 69	NS
20 – 20.5	366 ± 70	478 ± 54	NS
20.5 – 21	393 ± 14	432 ± 36	NS
21 – 21.5	330 ± 56	407 ± 16	NS
21.5 – 22	281 ± 35	300 ± 9	NS
22 – 22.5	223 ± 17	202 ± 9	NS
22.5 – 23	167 ± 13	178 ± 9	NS

Results are expressed as mean ± SEM of 4 perfusion experiments. During the different perfusion periods the effluent medium was collected and analysed for CK activity. When verapamil was present it was added to the calcium-free and the reperfusion medium. Tests of significance relate to significance of change in CK release caused by the presence of verapamil. NS = not significant ($p > 0.05$).

Table 2. Effect of verapamil (1 mg · litre^{-1}) on the depletion of myocardial CP and ATP stores, induced by reperfusion with calcium after a calcium-free period of 4 min

Perfusion sequence	CP (µmol · g^{-1} dry wt)			ATP (µmol · g^{-1} dry wt)		
	no verapamil	+ verapamil	p	no verapamil	+ verapamil	p
plus Ca^{2+}: 15 min	29.6 ± 2.1			18.8 ± 0.8		
minus Ca^{2+}: 4 min	35.6 ± 2.9	33.1 ± 2.6	NS	20.8 ± 1.4	20.6 ± 1.5	NS
plus Ca^{2+}: 1 min	4.6 ± 3.2	15.0 ± 2.2	<0.001	6.3 ± 2.7	13.2 ± 1.2	<0.001
2 min	4.0 ± 2.3	5.6 ± 2.3	NS	4.8 ± 1.8	6.2 ± 1.6	NS
4 min	1.6 ± 1.2	1.9 ± 1.1	NS	2.9 ± 1.0	2.9 ± 0.9	NS

Values are given as mean ± SD (n = 4). When verapamil was present it was added to the calcium-free and the reperfusion medium. Tests of significance relate to the significance of the difference between CP and ATP levels in hearts perfused in the presence and absence of verapamil. NS = not significant ($p > 0.05$).

calcium resulted in the development of an irreversible contracture, expressed as shortening of the length (mm) of the longitudinal axis of the left ventricle. In the presence of verapamil contracture was significantly reduced (Table 3).

The energy sparing effect of verapamil during the first few minutes of reperfusion with calcium-containing medium (Table 2) may account for the reduction in magnitude of myocardial contracture (Table 3), because ATP depletion is a

Table 3. Effect of verapamil ($1 \text{ mg} \cdot \text{litre}^{-1}$) on the development of myocardial contracture, induced by reperfusion with calcium after a calcium-free period of 4 min

Reperfusion with Ca^{2+}	contracture (mm)		
	no verapamil	+ verapamil	p
0.5 min	0.74 ± 0.14	0.26 ± 0.14	<0.001
1.0 min	0.82 ± 0.13	0.41 ± 0.11	<0.001
1.5 min	0.79 ± 0.12	0.44 ± 0.10	<0.001
2.0 min	0.72 ± 0.10	0.41 ± 0.10	<0.001
2.5 min	0.61 ± 0.10	0.37 ± 0.10	<0.005
3.0 min	0.52 ± 0.09	0.34 ± 0.11	<0.02
3.5 min	0.45 ± 0.10	0.31 ± 0.11	NS
4.0 min	0.41 ± 0.08	0.29 ± 0.10	NS

Spontaneously beating rat hearts went into diastolic arrest as soon as calcium was omitted from the medium. Reperfusion with calcium resulted in the development of irreversible contracture. Contracture is expressed as shortening of the length (mm) of the longitudinal axis of the left ventricle. Values are given as mean ± SD (n = 4). Tests of significance relate to the significance of the difference between contracture of hearts perfused in the presence and absence of verapamil. NS = not significant ($p >$ 0.05).

determining factor in the development of irreversible myocardial contracture [13]. Ultrastructural data revealed [1] that after 30 min of reperfusion all cells contained contracted myofibrils, irrespective of whether verapamil was present. Hence, the decrease of contracture, which began within 2 min of reperfusion (Table 3), was possibly caused by loss of the normal architecture of the heart, rather than by relaxation of the myofibrils.

Our results on the energy sparing effect of verapamil show a qualitative resemblance to the data obtained by Nayler et al. [14] from hypoxic heart muscle. Verapamil reduced the rate at which myocardial CP and ATP stores were depleted, although it failed to prevent the hypoxic muscle from gaining calcium. In case of an increased permeability of the sarcolemma to calcium, brought about by hypoxia [14], ischemia [15], or calcium-free perfusion (this study), verapamil appears to have a direct effect on the intracellular high-energy phosphate metabolism.

References

1. Ruigrok TJC, Boink ABTJ, Slade A, Zimmerman ANE, Meijler FL, Nayler WG (1980) The effect of verapamil on the calcium paradox. Am J Pathol 98: in the press
2. Zimmerman ANE, Hülsmann WC (1966) Paradoxical influence of calcium ions on the permeability of the cell membranes of the isolated rat heart. Nature 211:646 – 647
3. Boink ABTJ, Ruigrok TJC, Maas AHJ, Zimmerman ANE (1976) Changes in high-energy phosphate compounds of isolated rat hearts during Ca^{2+}-free perfusion and reperfusion with Ca^{2+}. J Mol Cell Cardiol 8:973 – 979
4. Ruigrok TJC, Burgersdijk FJA, Zimmerman ANE (1975) The calcium paradox: a reaffirmation. Eur J Cardiol 3:59 – 63
5. Zimmerman ANE, Daems W, Hülsmann WC, Snijder J, Wisse E, Durrer D (1967) Morphological changes of heart muscle caused by successive perfusion with calcium-free and calcium-containing solutions (calcium paradox). Cardiovasc Res 1:201 – 209

6. Hearse DJ, Humphrey SM, Boink ABTJ, Ruigrok TJC (1978) The calcium paradox: metabolic, electrophysiological, contractile and ultrastructural characteristics in four species. Eur J Cardiol 7:241 – 256
7. Haas H, Härtfelder G (1962) α-Isopropyl-α-[(N-methyl-N-homoveratryl)-γ-aminopropyl]-3,4-dimethoxyphenylacetonitril, eine Substanz mit coronargefäßerweiternden Eigenschaften. Arzneim Forsch 12:549 – 563
8. Fleckenstein A (1971) Specific inhibitiors and promoters of calcium action in the excitation-contraction coupling of heart muscle and their role in the prevention or production of myocardial lesions. In: Harris P, Opie LH, Calcium and the heart. Academic Press, London, pp 135 – 188
9. Nayler WG, Krikler D (1974) Verapamil and the myocardium. Postgrad Med J 50:441 – 446
10. Meijler FL, Van de Bogaard F, Van der Tweel LH, Durrer D (1962) Postextrasystolic potentiation in the isolated rat heart. Am J Physiol 202:631 – 635
11. Oliver IT (1955) A spectrophotometric method for the determination of creatine phosphokinase and myokinase. Biochem J 61:116 – 122
12. Rosalki SB (1967) An improved procedure for serum creatine phosphokinase determination. J Lab Clin Med 69:696 – 705
13. Katz AM, Tada M (1972) The "stone heart": a challenge to the biochemist. Am J Cardiol 29: 578 – 580
14. Nayler WG, Grau A, Slade A (1976) A protective effect of verapamil on hypoxic heart muscle. Cardiovasc Res 10:650 – 662
15. Robb-Nicholson C, Currie WD, Wechsler AS (1978) Effects of verapamil on myocardial tolerance to ischemic arrest. Comparison to potassium arrest. Circulation [Suppl 1] 58:119 – 124

Prevention of Myocardial Degeneration in Hamsters with Hereditary Cardiomyopathy[1]

G. Jasmin and L. Proschek

The high calcium level within the heart cells at early stages of the hamster cardiomyopathy has been claimed as a major pathologic event in the development of this hereditary disease [1]. Whether this is due to a structural defect in the plasma membrane or to some abnormality in cell organelles involved in the calcium pumping system is still questionable. In searching for membrane damage in cardiomyocytes, we were struck by the inconspicuous perivascular cell infiltrate reminiscent of heart lesions induced by catecholamines [2]. Investigations carried out by Fleckenstein on the other hand have contributed in emphasizing the prominent role of calcium in the development of cardiac necroses induced by isoproterenol [3]. Interestingly, just as is the case of isoproterenol heart lesions, calcium antagonistic drugs and, to a lesser extent, β-adrenergic blockers prevent the development of hamster cardiomyopathy [4,5].

More recently Wrogemann and Nylen [6] succeeded in demonstrating calcium overloading in heart mitochondria of 49% of cardiomyopathic hamsters aged between 21 and 412 days, but could not detect any abnormality in oxidative phosphorylation of these organelles except when exposed to increased concentration of calcium in the test medium. Under such conditions, the cardiomyopathic mitochondria are more susceptible to the uncoupling effect of calcium. Using the UM-X7.1 cardiomyopathic hamster strain, we were able to demonstrate that there exists a defective oxidative phosphorylation in isolated heart mitochondria that correlates with the progression of the disease [2].

In the present paper, we will report investigations dealing with the effect of cardioprotective drugs upon oxidative phosphorylation in heart mitochondria isolated from normal and myopathic hamsters. Our studies also concern the sensitivity of isolated mitochondria from treated and untreated animals to exogenous calcium introduced in the test medium. Finally, these findings will be analyzed in relation to the abnormal rise of cholesterol in heart subfractions of cardiomyopathic hamsters, which is unaffected by Verapamil treatment.

Materials and Methods

Male and female hamsters of the UM-X7.1 myopathic line, 20 – 140 days old, were used in this study. Unrelated healthy hamsters (Lakeview strain) served as controls. All the animals were maintained under controlled housing conditions and given Purina Laboratory Chow and tap water ad libitum. Drugs were either administered as supplied in their vehicle or solubilized in physiologic saline or in a phosphate buffer (pH 7) and administered subcutaneously or intraperitoneally in a volume of

1 This work was supported by grants from the Muscular Dystrophy Association of Canada and The Medical Research Council of Canada

0.1 ml. Verapamil (Knoll AG, Ludwigshafen, FRG) was injected twice daily in doses of 5 mg/kg body wt. during the 1st week and of 12 mg/kg body wt. until the end of the experiment. Prenylamine (Hoechst, Montreal) was injected in a single dose of 50 mg/kg body wt. each day during the first 3 days and thereafter at the same dose twice daily until the end of the experiment. Propranolol (Ayerst Laboratories, Montreal) was injected in doses of 20 mg/kg body wt. twice daily via the subcutaneous and intraperitoneal routes alternatively. Compound D 600 (Knoll AG, Ludwigshafen, FRG) was injected subcutaneously twice daily in ascending doses of 0.5 – 1.0 mg/kg body wt. during the first week and at the steady dose of 1.3 mg/kg body wt. thereafter.

Mitochondria were isolated by a proteinase method basically similar to that described by Wrogemann and Blanchaer [7] (Fig. 1). Respiratory rates and oxidative phosphorylation were determined polarographically using a Gilson oxygraph

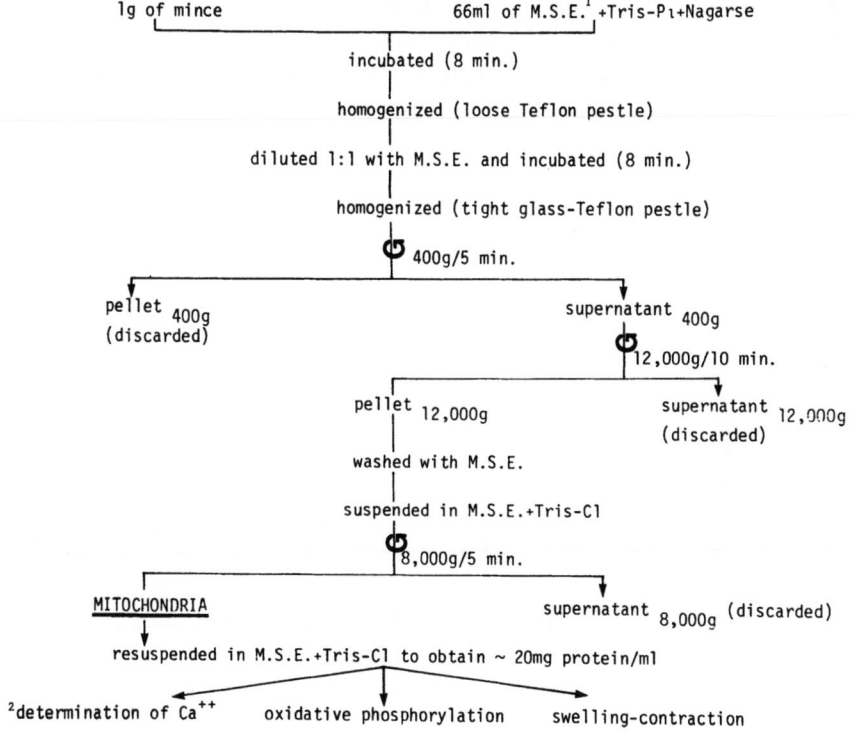

ISOLATION OF MITOCHONDRIA*

The tissue trimmed, washed, weighed and minced.

1g of mince   66ml of M.S.E.[1] +Tris-P₁+Nagarse

incubated (8 min.)

homogenized (loose Teflon pestle)

diluted 1:1 with M.S.E. and incubated (8 min.)

homogenized (tight glass-Teflon pestle)

400g/5 min.

pellet 400g   supernatant 400g
(discarded)
                     12,000g/10 min.

pellet 12,000g   supernatant 12,000g
                     (discarded)

washed with M.S.E.

suspended in M.S.E.+Tris-Cl

8,000g/5 min.

MITOCHONDRIA   supernatant 8,000g (discarded)

resuspended in M.S.E.+Tris-Cl to obtain ~ 20mg protein/ml

[2]determination of Ca++   oxidative phosphorylation   swelling-contraction

* All solutions and equipments are kept ice-cold and procedures are carried
out at cold (0-4°C).

[1] Mannitol-Sucrose-EDTA pH 7.4.

[2] 2.5μM ruthenium red added to all media.

Fig. 1. Experimental procedure

equipped with a Clarke electrode. The isolated heart mitochondria were assayed with pyruvate/malate as a substrate. To the test medium (mannitol, sucrose, EDTA, Tris-Cl and potassium phosphate, pH 7.2) saturated with air at 28 °C were added normal, myopathic, and myopathic-treated mitochondria containing approximately 1 mg of protein prior to the addition of $250-260 \, \mu M$ ADP and 5 mM pyruvate plus 1 mM L-malate. Respiratory control ratios (RCR) and ADP:0 were calculated according to the method of Chance and Williams [8]. Numbers along the curves indicate respiration rates (μM of O_2/min/gm of mitochondrial proteins) during states III and IV. All parameters were calculated after the second addition of ADP. Mitochondrial calcium content was measured with a Unicam atomic absorption spectrophotometer after extraction with 0.5 N HCl according to the method of Reynafarge and Lenninger [9]. $LaCl_3$ 1% was added to eliminate an interference by other ions.

Results

Heart and Skeletal Muscle Lesions

The severity of cardiac and skeletal muscle lesions was assessed on an arbitrary scale of $0-3$ and the means of the microscopic readings with the corresponding standard errors are given in Fig. 2. As a rule treatments were initiated in 30-day-old hamsters

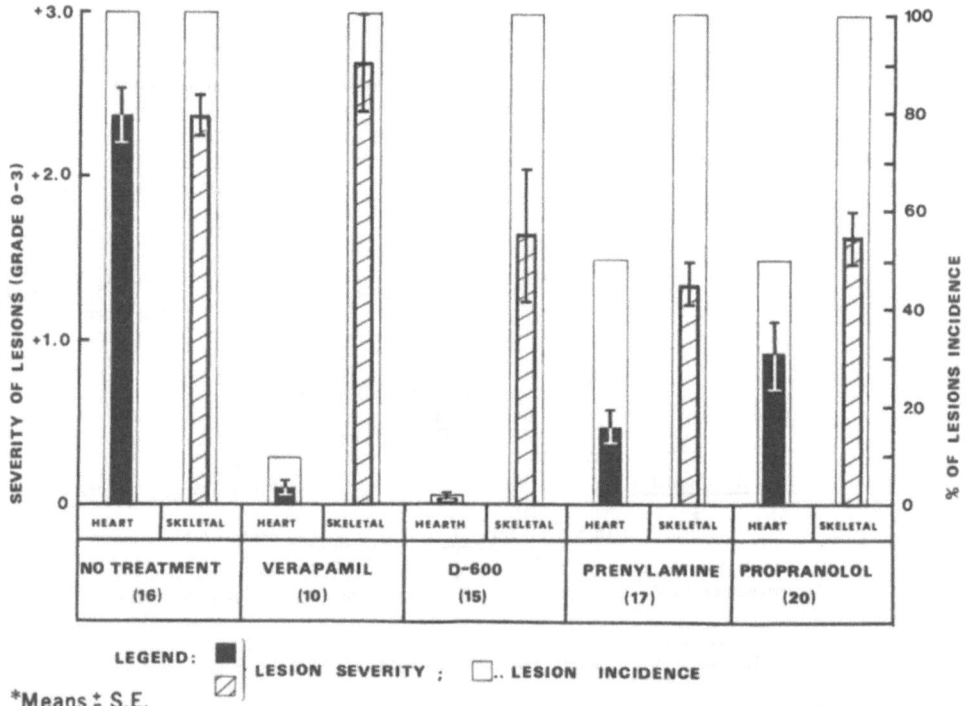

Fig. 2. Effect of calcium-antagonists and of a β-blocker on the development of pathologic changes in heart and skeletal muscles of polymyopathic hamsters UM-X7.1

when lesions are not histologically demonstrable and the experiment lasted 28 days. At autopsy, the heart necrotic changes were already severe in the untreated group and almost entirely prevented by Verapamil and Compound D 600; the lesions were significantly reduced in groups treated with Prenylamine and Propanolol. Regarding the skeletal muscle changes, our results are less conclusive. Treatment with Compound D 600, Prenylamine, and the β-blocker afforded some protection but only in terms of severity.

Mitochondrial Respiratory Patterns

The next graph (Fig. 3) represents the polarographic records of 5 mitochondrial preparations from healthy controls, nontreated and treated myopathic hamsters, all groups averaging 48 days of age, using pyruvate/malate as a substrate. The curves and values show that oxidative phosphorylation after the second cycle of state III and state IV in cardiomyopathic hamsters is so-called "loosely coupled". The respiratory control ratio was significantly depressed (30%) as well as the ATP formation (20% – 25%); the latter values are not shown in the graph. There was a slight reduction in the rate of oxygen consumption in state III (15% – 20%) and, on the contrary, a rise in state IV (5% – 10%) as indicated by the figures in brackets. Interestingly this "loose coupling" phenomenon was almost totally prevented by all cardioprotective drugs. The ADP:0 ratio, on the other hand, remained somewhat unaltered in all groups.

In Vitro Exposure of Mitochondria to Calcium

The dose effect of calcium on respiratory control ratio is illustrated in Fig. 4. As expected, there is a diminution of the respiratory control ratio with increasing

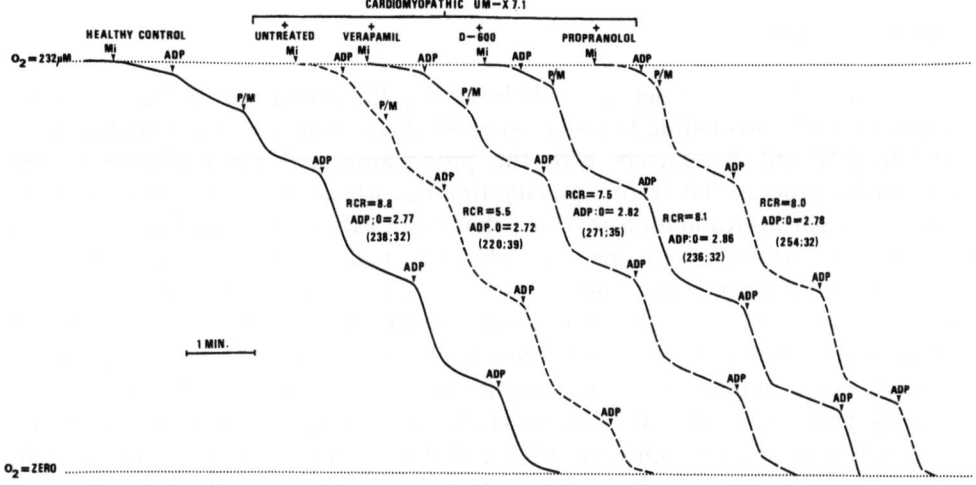

Fig. 3. Polarographic records of mitochondrial respiratory function

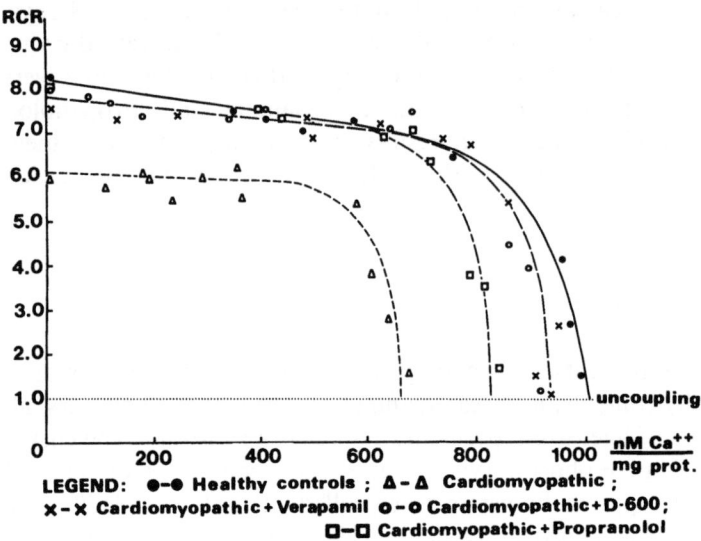

Fig. 4. Dose effect of exogenous Ca^{++} on oxidative phosphorylation of heart mitochondria from treated and untreated cardiomyopathic hamsters

concentrations of calcium, but the fact that cardiomyopathic organelles were sensitive to lower doses of calcium (600 – 700 nM/mg protein) would indicate that a proportion of mitochondria are already loaded with the cation or that they are in a loose state of coupling.

Mitochondria from Verapamil and Compound D 600-treated hamsters on the other hand were more resistant to the calcium uncoupling effect that occurred within the same dose range of calcium (950 M/mg proteins) as exhibited by the healthy-control group. The action of Propranolol was less evident with uncoupling at about 800 nM Ca/mg proteins.

Correlative Studies

Knowing that there is a progressive diminution in the severity of the heart necrotic changes in cardiomyopathic hamsters after 80 days of age, we then attempted to correlate different parameters with the progression and the evolution of the degenerative process. These preliminary findings which arise from groups of six animals at each determination revealed that there exists a remarkable parallelism between the severity of the necrotic changes, their calcium content, and the depression in the respiratory control ratio (Fig. 5). These results further illustrate the importance of relating the progression of the disease process to the age of animals when studying the pathomechanism of this hereditary cardiomyopathy.

Finally, with reference to a possible defect in heart membranes of the cardiomyopathic hamsters, let us mention that investigations carried out in 50-day-old healthy and diseased animals indicate that the amount of free cholesterol in cardiac microsomal mitochondrial and soluble supernatant fractions was significantly higher than control values. Verapamil on the other hand did not affect

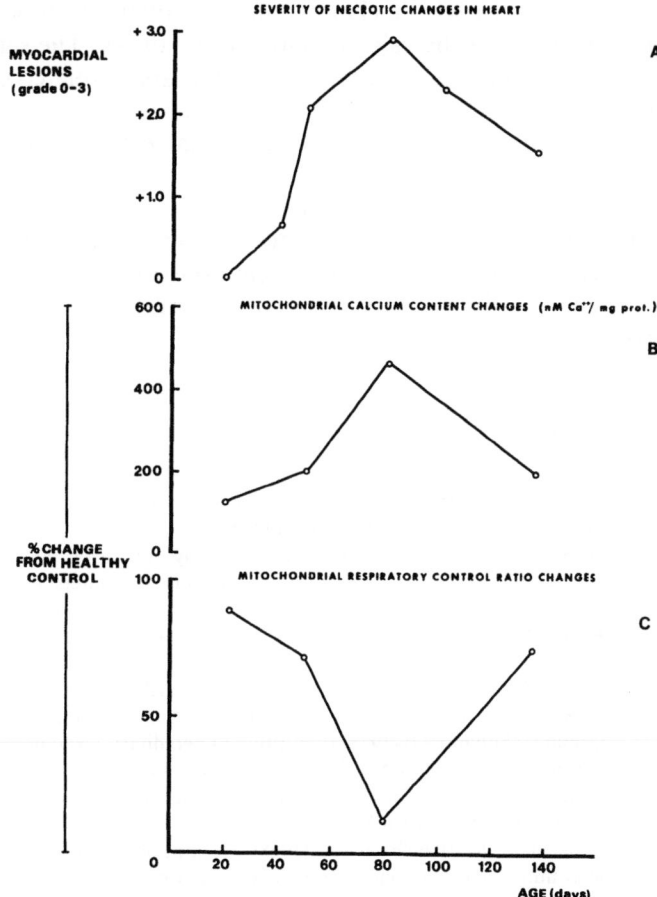

Fig. 5. Time course of cardiac necrotization, mitochondrial calcium overload, and loss of mitochondrial respiratory control in cardiomyopathic hamsters

the elevation of cholesterol in cardiac membrane even in absence of any demonstrable histopathologic changes [10].

Conclusion

The above described experiments have enabled us to demonstrate that the development of heart lesions in hamsters with hereditary cardiomyopathy is completely prevented by calcium antagonistic drugs and to a lesser degree by an adrenergic β-blocker. The most efficient cardioprotective agent is Compound D 600, being well tolerated in our experimental animals to the extent that the cardiomyopathy does not develop as long as animals remain under treatment (studies to be reported elsewhere).

We further observed a depression of mitochondrial respiratory control ratio in cardiomyopathic hamsters. This phenomenon, which coincides with the development of heart necrotic changes and concomitant mitochondrial calcium overloading, is prevented by calcium antagonistic drugs. The same drugs afford protection against the uncoupling effect of calcium upon isolated cardiomyopathic mitochondria.

It is thus inferred that the beneficial effect of the drugs consists mainly in restricting transmembrane calcium influx in cardiocytes without modifying the cholesterol content of membranes, which was found abnormally high in cardiomyopathic hamsters. These findings provide additional support to the concept that hamster hereditary cardiomyopathy is primarily a membrane disease and that calcium transmembrane abnormal flux plays a prominent role in its pathogenesis.

References

1. Bajusz E, Lossnitzer K (1968) A new disease model of chronic congestive heart failure: studies on its pathogenesis. Trans NY Acad Sci 30:939
2. Jasmin G, Eu HY (1979) The cardiomyopathy in hamster dystrophy. Ann NY Acad Sci 317:46
3. Fleckenstein A (1971) Specific inhibitors and promoters of calcium action in the excitation-contraction coupling of heart muscle and their role in the prevention or production of myocardial lesions. In: Harris P, Opie LH (eds) Calcium and the heart. Academic Press, London New York, p 135
4. Jasmin G, Bajusz E (1973) Polymyopathie et cardiomyopathie héréditaire chez le hamster de Syrie. Inhibition sélective des lésions du myocarde. Ann Anat Pathol (Paris) 18 (1):49
5. Jasmin G, Solymoss B (1975) Prevention of hereditary cardiomyopathy in the hamster by Verapamil and other agents. Proc Soc Exp Biol Med 149:193
6. Wrogemann K, Nylen EG (1978) Mitochondrial calcium overloading in cardiomyopathic hamsters. J Mol Cell Cardiol 10:185
7. Wrogemann K, Blanchaer MC (1968) Respiration and oxidative phosphorylation by muscle and heart mitochondria of hamsters with hereditary myocardiopathy and polymyopathy. Can J Biochem 46:323
8. Chance B, Williams GR (1956) The respiratory chain and oxidative phosphorylation. Adv Enzymol 17:65
9. Reynafarge B, Lenninger AL (1969) High affinity and low affinity binding of calcium by rat liver mitochondria. J Biochem Chemistry 244:584
10. Jasmin G, Solymoss B, Proschek L (1979) Therapeutic trials in hamster dystrophy. Ann NY Acad Sci 317:338

Kardioprotektion durch Kalziumantagonisten bei erblich kardiomyopathischen Hamstern

K. Lossnitzer, A. Konrad und M. Jakob

Einleitung

Die klinischen, morphologischen, hämodynamischen und gewisse biochemische Charakteristika der Kardiomyopathie des syrischen Goldhamsters wurden 1968 [1] sowie 1975 [2] zusammenfassend beschrieben. Es wurde gezeigt, daß sich das autosomal rezessiv vererbte Herzleiden histologisch anfänglich in multifokalen Myokardnekrosen zusammen mit dem Auftreten von hauptsächlich verkalkenden Riesenzellen ausdrückt, wobei diese Veränderungen sich aber erst um den 40. Lebenstag manifestieren [3]. Sowohl chemische, cytophotometrische und Gewichtsuntersuchungen [4] als auch elektrokardiographische [5] Beobachtungen beim Stamm BIO 8262 erbrachten keinen eindeutigen Hinweis auf die Ausbildung einer Herzmuskelhypertrophie während der verschiedenen Phasen der Erkrankung, so daß diese unter dem Aspekt der sie begleitenden Skelettmuskeldystrophie als dystrophische Kardiomyopathie bezeichnet werden kann. Im Gegensatz dazu konnte durch elektronenoptische Untersuchungen beim Stamm BIO 14.6 jedoch eine eindeutige Tendenz zur Herzmuskelhypertrophie im linken Ventrikel festgestellt werden [6]. Wie aus früheren Untersuchungen hervorgeht, bewirkt eine einmalige Gabe des von Fleckenstein als „Kalziumpromotor" [7] bezeichneten β-Rezeptorenstimulators Isoproterenol bei den kardiomyopathischen Hamstern sowohl eine akute Steigerung der myokardialen Radiokalziumaufnahme, als auch eine deutliche Zunahme des myokardialen Gesamt-Kalziumgehaltes [8]. Diese Phänomene treten bei den kardiomyopathischen Tieren deutlicher hervor als bei den erbgesunden Kontrollen, weshalb eine latente Störung des myokardialen Kalziumstoffwechsels bei den erbkranken Hamstern schon in der pränekrotischen Phase ihrer Erkrankung angenommen wird [9].

Durch die Verknüpfung biochemischer mit morphologischen Untersuchungen hat sich herausgestellt, daß dem Herzleiden der gestörte myokardiale Kalziumstoffwechsel wohl als entscheidender pathogenetischer Schritt zugrunde liegt, und eine synchron mit der Myokarddegeneration spontan auftretende myokardiale Kalziumakkumulation als biochemisch meßbares Äquivalent der Manifestation des Herzleidens aufgefaßt werden kann [9, 10, 11].

Da am pharmakologischen Isoproterenolmodell der Ratte von Fleckenstein und seiner Arbeitsgruppe ein kardioprotektiver Effekt von Substanzen nachgewiesen wurde, die entweder die transmembranäre Kalziumkonduktivität des Sarkolemms [7, 12 – 15] oder die intrazellulären Bindungsstellen von Kalziumionen in Herzmuskelzellen blockieren [16], lag es nahe zu prüfen, ob sich nicht auch am erblichen Krankheitsmodell des kardiomyopathischen Goldhamsters eine Wirksamkeit dieser Substanzen nachweisen läßt. Damit wäre der Brückenschlag zwischen der am pharmakologischen Experiment beobachteten Wirksamkeit solcher kalziumantagonistischer Pharmaka gegenüber der Entwicklung von Myokardnekrosen und ihrer klinischen Bedeutung bei der Behandlung von spontanen Kardiomyopathien angebahnt.

Material und Methoden

Für die Untersuchungen wurden 29 – 31tägige kardiomyopathische Hamster des In-
zuchtstammes BIO 8262 beiderlei Geschlechts herangezogen, welche in diesem Lebensalter noch keine histologisch feststellbaren Myokardveränderungen aufweisen
[3]. Ihr Körpergewicht betrug anfänglich zwischen 36 und 49 g. Die Tiere wurden in
vollklimatisierten Räumen bei einer Temperatur von 21 °C und einem 12 Std Hell-
Dunkel-Rhythmus bei künstlichem Licht gehalten. Sie erhielten Ssniff-H-Hamster-
futter in gepreßten Klötzchen und Leitungswasser ad libitum.
    Nach akuter bzw. chronischer Applikation der nachfolgend aufgeführten Sub-
stanzen wurden die Hamster unter Äthernarkose thorakotomiert und das Herz per
Scherenschlag exzidiert. Nachfolgend wurden dann die Vorhöfe von den Ventrikeln
sowie der rechte Ventrikel vom restlichen Myokard abgetrennt. Der verbleibende
linke Ventrikel samt Septum wurde mit einem sauberen Gazetupfer von Blutresten
gesäubert und bis zur Gewichtskonstanz bei 95 °C getrocknet. Nach anschließender
Feuchtveraschung mit konzentrierter Salpetersäure und Perchlorsäure in Teflonbe-
chern bei ca. 100 °C auf einem Sandbad erfolgte die Bestimmung des myokardialen
Kalziumgehaltes mittels Atomabsorptionsspektralphotometrie [17].

Akute Experimente

Für jede geprüfte Substanz wurde grundsätzlich folgendes Versuchsprogramm
durchgeführt:
    Aus verschiedenen Würfen wurde eine Anzahl von Hamstern als unbehandelte,
eine zweite Anzahl von Tieren als Isoproterenol-behandelte und eine dritte Anzahl
von Tieren als Isoproterenol- und Testsubstanz-behandelte Gruppe aufgestellt.

*Einfluß des Kalziumantagonisten Verapamil auf die Isoproterenol-bewirkte
myokardiale Kalziumakkumulation*

Eine Kontrollgruppe von 13 Tieren blieb unbehandelt, einer weiteren Gruppe von 10
Tieren wurde 1 mg/kg Körpergewicht (KG) Isoproterenol subcutan unter die
Nackenhautfalte injiziert, und 33 Hamstern, unterteilt in 4 Gruppen zu 7, 7, 11 bzw.
8 Tieren, wurden jeweils gleichzeitig zu Isoproterenol 10, 5, 3 bzw. 1 mg/kg KG
Verapamil subcutan unter die Oberschenkelhaut injiziert. Nach einer Expositions-
zeit von 6 Std wurden die Tiere getötet.

*Einfluß des Kalziumantagonisten Fendilin auf die Isoproterenol-bewirkte
myokardiale Kalziumakkumulation*

Eine Kontrollgruppe von 7 Tieren blieb unbehandelt, einer weiteren Gruppe von 7
Tieren wurde 1 mg/kg KG Isoproterenol subcutan unter die Nackenhautfalte injiziert und 39 Hamstern unterteilt in 7 Gruppen zu 6, 5, 7, 7, 7 bzw. 7 Tieren wurden
jeweils gleichzeitig zu Isoproterenol 0,06, 0,1, 0,2, 0,6, 2,0 und 6,0 mg/kg KG Fendilin unter die Oberschenkelhaut injiziert. Die Expositionszeit betrug hier ebenfalls
6 Std.

Einfluß des β-Rezeptorenblockers Propranolol auf die Isoproterenol-bewirkte myokardiale Kalziumakkumulation

Eine Kontrollgruppe von 10 Tieren blieb unbehandelt, einer weiteren Gruppe von 10 Tieren wurde 1 mg/kg KG Isoproterenol subcutan unter die Nackenhautfalte injiziert und 31 Hamstern, unterteilt in 6 Gruppen zu 6, 9, 8 und 8 Tieren, wurden 0,3, 1,0, 3,0 und 10,0 mg/kg KG Propranolol gleichzeitig mit Isoproterenol subcutan unter die Oberschenkelhaut injiziert. Die Expositionszeit betrug ebenfalls 6 Std.

Einfluß des β-Rezeptorenblockers Atenolol auf die Isoproterenol-bewirkte myokardiale Kalziumakkumulation

Eine Kontrollgruppe von 10 Tieren blieb unbehandelt, einer weiteren Gruppe von 10 Hamstern wurde 1 mg/kg KG Isoproterenol subcutan unter die Nackenhautfalte injiziert und 29 Hamstern, unterteilt in 3 Gruppen zu 10, 9 bzw. 10 Tieren, wurden jeweils gleichzeitig zu Isoproterenol 10, 30 und 100 mg/kg KG Atenolol subcutan unter die Oberschenkelhaut injiziert. Die Expositionszeit betrug auch hier 6 Std.

Einfluß von Magnesiumaspartathydrochlorid auf die Isoproterenol-bewirkte myokardiale Kalziumakkumulation

Eine Kontrollgruppe von 10 Tieren blieb unbehandelt, einer weiteren Gruppe von 11 Hamstern wurde 1 mg/kg KG Isoproterenol subcutan unter die Nackenhautfalte injiziert und 30 Hamstern, unterteilt in 3 Gruppen zu je 10 Tieren wurden 30 Minuten vor der subcutanen Isoproterenol-Injektion 2,3, 7,7 bzw. 23,0 mVal/kg KG Magnesiumaspartathydrochlorid über eine Schlundsonde direkt in den Magen appliziert. 6 Std nach der Isoproterenol-Injektion bzw. 6,5 Std nach der Magnesiumaspartathydrochlorid-Verabreichung wurden die Tiere getötet.

Chronische Experimente

Die chronischen Experimente erfolgten nach folgendem Versuchsprogramm:
   Aus verschiedenen Würfen wurde jeweils eine Anzahl von 30tägigen Tieren als unbehandelte Kontrollgruppe zusammengestellt und eine weitere Anzahl von Tieren, in Untergruppen unterteilt, über 30 Tage mit unterschiedlich hohen Pharmakadosen behandelt. Die Hamster wurden anfänglich und in Abständen von 7 Tagen nach Beginn des Experiments gewogen und die Injektionsmenge entsprechend dem Körpergewicht adjustiert. Der Zeitraum zwischen den zweimaligen täglichen Applikationen des Pharmakons betrug 12 ± 3 Std. Am 60. Lebenstag wurden die Tiere etwa 8 bis 9 Std nach der letzten Pharmakon-Verabreichung getötet.

Einfluß des Kalziumantagonisten Verapamil auf die spontane myokardiale Kalziumakkumulation

13 Tiere blieben unbehandelt, 37 Tieren, unterteilt in 4 Gruppen zu 5, 10, 9 bzw. 13 Tieren, wurden zweimal täglich 1,0, 3,0, 5,0 bzw. 10,0 mg/kg KG Verapamil subcutan unter die Nackenhautfalte injiziert.

Einfluß des Kalziumantagonisten Fendilin auf die spontane myokardiale Kalziumakkumulation

10 Tiere blieben unbehandelt und eine weitere Gruppe von 10 Tieren erhielt zweimal täglich 20 mg/kg KG Fendilin über eine Schlundsonde direkt in den Magen.

Einfluß des β-Rezeptorenblockers Propranolol auf die spontane myokardiale Kalziumakkumulation

15 Tiere blieben unbehandelt, 35 Tieren, unterteilt in 4 Gruppen zu 8, 9, 8 bzw. 10 Tieren, wurden zweimal täglich 1,0, 3,0, 10,0 bzw. 30,0 mg/kg KG Propranolol subcutan unter die Nackenhautfalte injiziert.

Einfluß des β-Rezeptorenblockers Atenolol auf die spontane myokardiale Kalziumakkumulation

12 Tiere blieben unbehandelt; 37 Tieren, unterteilt in 4 Gruppen mit 10, 10, 8 und 9 Tieren, wurden zweimal täglich 10, 30, 100 bzw. 300 mg/kg KG Atenolol subcutan unter die Nackenhautfalte injiziert.

Einfluß von Magnesiumaspartathydrochlorid auf die spontane myokardiale Kalziumakkumulation

11 Tiere blieben unbehandelt, 29 Tiere, unterteilt in 3 Gruppen zu 11, 11 bzw. 7 Hamstern, erhielten zweimal täglich 8,0, 23,0 bzw. 46,0 mVal/kg KG Magnesium-aspartathydrochlorid über eine Schlundsonde direkt in den Magen.

Pharmaka

Als Isoproterenol wurde 1:60 verdünnte, 1%ige Aludrin®-Lösung (Fa. C. H. Boehringer Sohn, Ingelheim) verwendet. Als Verdünnungsmittel diente Aqua bidest, das mit 1-n Salzsäure auf einen pH-Wert von 3,5 titriert worden war. Pro Hamster wurde entsprechend dem Körpergewicht ein Volumen von mindestens 0,22 ml und höchstens 0,29 ml injiziert.

Als Verapamil wurde Isoptin®-Lösung in Ampullen (5 mg in 2 ml) verwendet (Fa. Knoll, Ludwigshafen). Bei der Höchstdosis von 10 mg/kg KG wurde die Originallösung verwendet, bei den niedrigeren Dosen wurde entsprechend mit physiologischer Kochsalzlösung verdünnt, so daß das Injektionsvolumen pro Tier mindestens 0,14 ml und nicht mehr als 0,81 ml betrug.

Als Fendilin verwendeten wir eine 0,2%ige Lösung der Reinsubstanz in Aqua bidest (Fa. Dr. Thiemann, Lünen). Für die Akutuntersuchungen wurde diese Lösung mit physiologischer Kochsalzlösung entsprechend weiterverdünnt, so daß das Injektionsvolumen pro Tier mindestens 0,3 ml und nicht mehr als 0,7 ml betrug. Für die chronischen Experimente wurde die 0,2%ige Originallösung verwendet und pro Tier mindestens 0,36 ml und höchstens 0,81 ml verabreicht.

Als Propranolol wurde die Reinsubstanz in Pulverform (Fa. ICI-Pharma, Plankstadt) in physiologischer Kochsalzlösung aufgelöst, so daß das Injektionsvolumen pro Tier mindestens 0,11 ml, aber nicht mehr als 0,81 ml betrug.

Als Atenolol wurde die Reinsubstanz in Pulverform (Fa. ICI-Pharma, Plankstadt) in physiologischer Kochsalzlösung aufgelöst, so daß das Injektionsvolumen pro Tier mindestens 0,12 ml, höchstens aber 0,97 ml betrug.

Magnesiumaspartathydrochlorid (9,61% Mg) als Reinsubstanz in Pulverform (Fa. Verla-Pharm, Tutzing) wurde in Aqua bidest (1,5 bzw. 4,5 g in 10 ml) gelöst, so daß das pro Tier verabreichte Volumen mindestens 0,11 ml und nicht mehr als 0,94 ml betrug.

Ergebnisse

Akute Experimente

Einfluß des Kalziumantagonisten Verapamil auf die Isoproterenol-bewirkte myokardiale Kalziumakkumulation

In Tabelle 1 ist der myokardiale Kalziumgehalt unbehandelter wie behandelter kardiomyopathischer Hamster aufgeführt. In Abb. 1 ist die Dosis-Wirkungskurve von Verapamil auf die Isoproterenol-induzierte myokardiale Kalziumakkumulation dieser Hamster dargestellt. Der Kalziumgehalt im Myokard unbehandelter Tiere beträgt $7,9 \pm 1,84$ mVal/kg Trockengewicht (TG). 6 Std nach der subcutanen Injektion von 1 mg/kg KG Isoproterenol steigt er um ca. 37% über den Wert der unbehandelten Tiere, d. h. auf $10,8 \pm 2,02$ mVal/kg TG an. Unter dem gleichzeitigen Einfluß von Verapamil läßt sich seine dosisabhängige Senkung bis etwa auf den Ausgangswert unbehandelter Hamster erkennen. 10 mg/kg KG Verapamil können dabei die Wirkung von 1 mg/kg KG Isoproterenol kompensieren.

Tabelle 1. Myokardialer Kalziumgehalt 29- bis 31tägiger kardiomyopathischer Hamster nach subcutaner Gabe von Isoproterenol und Verapamil. Die Ergebnisse sind als Mittelwert ± Standardabweichung, die Tierzahl ist in Klammern angegeben

	myokardialer Kalziumgehalt (mVal/kg Trockengewicht)	% über unbehandelt
Unbehandelt	$7,9 \pm 1,84$ (13)	
Isoproterenol (1 mg/kg KG)	$10,8 \pm 2,02$ (10)	+ 37%
Verapamil (1 mg/kg KG) + Isoproterenol (1 mg/kg KG)	$10,3 \pm 1,36$ (7)	+ 30%
Verapamil (3 mg/kg KG) + Isoproterenol (1 mg/kg KG)	$8,9 \pm 1,17$ (7)	+ 13%
Verapamil (5 mg/kg KG) + Isoproterenol (1 mg/kg KG)	$8,3 \pm 0,65$ (11)	+ 5%
Verapamil (10 mg/kg KG) + Isoproterenol (1 mg/kg KG)	$8,0 \pm 1,11$ (8)	+ 1%

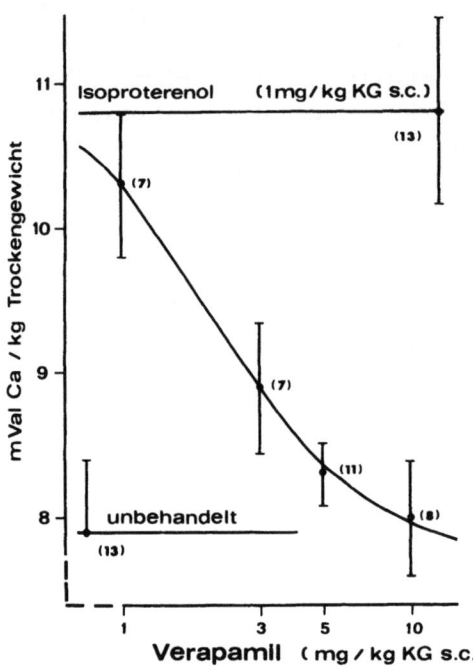

Abb. 1. Myokardialer Kalziumgehalt 29- bis 31tägiger kardiomyopathischer Hamster (Stamm BIO 8262) unter dem kombinierten Einfluß von Verapamil und Isoproterenol 6 Std nach simultaner subcutaner Pharmakongabe. Angegeben sind die Mittelwerte ± SEM. Tierzahl in Klammern

Einfluß des Kalziumantagonisten Fendilin auf die Isoproterenol-bewirkte myokardiale Kalziumakkumulation

In Tabelle 2 und Abb. 2 sind analog zur Tabelle 1 und Abb. 1 die myokardialen Kalziumgehalte unbehandelter und behandelter kardiomyopathischer Hamster sowie die Dosis-Wirkungskurve von Fendilin auf die Isoproterenol-induzierte myokardiale Kalziumakkumulation dieser Tiere aufgezeigt. Dabei beträgt diesmal der Kalziumgehalt im Myokard unbehandelter Hamster 7,7 ± 0,9 mVal/kg TG und er steigt unter Isoproterenol auf 11,8 ± 2,51 mVal/kg TG, d. h. um ca. 53% über den Ausgangswert an. Unter dem gleichzeitigen Einfluß von Fendilin zu Isoproterenol läßt

Tabelle 2. Myokardialer Kalziumgehalt 29- bis 31tägiger kardiomyopathischer Hamster nach subcutaner Gabe von Isoproterenol und Fendilin. Die Ergebnisse sind als Mittelwert ± Standardabweichung, die Tierzahl ist in Klammern angegeben

	myokardialer Kalziumgehalt (mVal/kg Trockengewicht)	% über unbehandelt
Unbehandelt	7,7 ± 0,91 (7)	
Isoproterenol (1 mg/kg KG)	11,8 ± 2,51 (7)	+ 53%
Fendilin (0,06 mg/kg KG) + Isoproterenol (1 mg/kg KG)	10,6 ± 1,83 (7)	+ 38%
Fendilin (0,10 mg/kg KG) + Isoproterenol (1 mg/kg KG)	9,7 ± 1,83 (6)	+ 26%
Fendilin (0,20 mg/kg KG) + Isoproterenol (1 mg/kg KG)	8,9 ± 0,78 (5)	+ 16%
Fendilin (0,60 mg/kg KG) + Isoproterenol (1 mg/kg KG)	8,4 ± 0,63 (7)	+ 9%
Fendilin (2,0 mg/kg KG) + Isoproterenol (1 mg/kg KG)	8,0 ± 0,66 (7)	+ 4%
Fendilin (6,0 mg/kg KG) + Isoproterenol (1 mg/kg KG)	7,6 ± 0,78 (7)	− 1%

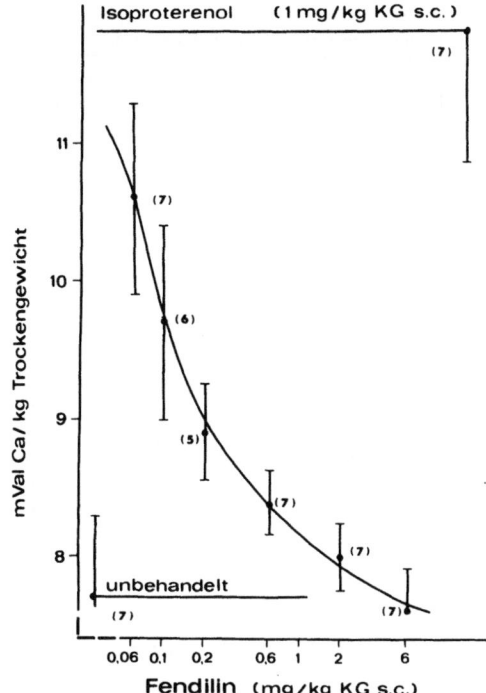

Abb. 2. Myokardialer Kalziumgehalt 29- bis 31 tägiger kardiomyopathischer Hamster (Stamm BIO 8262) unter dem kombinierten Einfluß von Fendilin und Isoproterenol 6 Std nach simultaner subcutaner Pharmakongabe. Angegeben sind die Mittelwerte ± SEM. Tierzahl in Klammern

sich die myokardiale Kalziumakkumulation ebenfalls dosisabhängig supprimieren. 6 mg/kg KG Fendilin sind dabei in der Lage die kalziumpromotorische Wirkung von 1 mg/kg KG Isoproterenol vollständig auszugleichen.

Einfluß des β-Rezeptorenblockers Propranolol auf die Isoproterenol-bewirkte myokardiale Kalziumakkumulation

Tabelle 3 und Abb. 3 geben die myokardialen Kalziumgehalte unbehandelter und behandelter Hamster sowie die Dosis-Wirkungskurve von Propranolol auf die Isoproterenol-bewirkte Kalziumakkumulation im Myokard dieser erbkranken Tiere

Tabelle 3. Myokardialer Kalziumgehalt 29- bis 31 tägiger kardiomyopathischer Hamster nach subcutaner Gabe von Isoproterenol und Propranolol. Die Ergebnisse sind als Mittelwert ± Standardabweichung, die Tierzahl ist in Klammern angegeben

	myokardialer Kalzium- gehalt (mVal/kg Trockengewicht)	% über unbehandelt
Unbehandelt	7,5 ± 0,67 (10)	
Isoproterenol (1 mg/kg KG)	11,0 ± 2,43 (10)	+ 47%
Propranolol (0,3 mg/kg KG) + Isoproterenol (1 mg/kg KG)	10,9 ± 1,02 (6)	+ 45%
Propranolol (1,0 mg/kg KG) + Isoproterenol (1 mg/kg KG)	8,9 ± 1,66 (9)	+ 19%
Propranolol (3,0 mg/kg KG) + Isoproterenol (1 mg/kg KG)	7,5 ± 0,99 (8)	± 0%
Propranolol (10,0 mg/kg KG) + Isoproterenol (1 mg/kg KG)	7,2 ± 0,86 (8)	− 4%

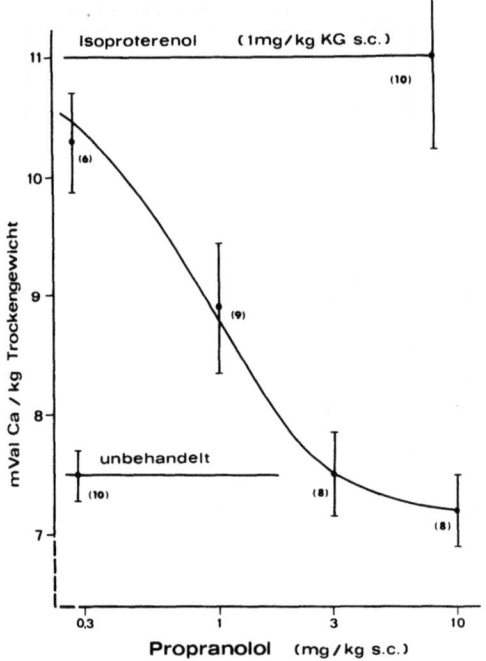

Abb. 3. Myokardialer Kalziumgehalt 29- bis 31tägiger kardiomyopathischer Hamster (Stamm BIO 8262) unter dem kombinierten Einfluß vom Propranolol und Isoproterenol 6 Std nach simultaner subcutaner Pharmakongabe. Angegeben sind die Mittelwerte ± SEM. Tierzahl in Klammern

wieder. Der Kalziumgehalt im Herzen unbehandelter Hamster beträgt hier 7,5 ± 0,67 mVal/kg TG und läßt sich unter dem Einfluß von Isoproterenol auf 11,0 ± 2,43 mVal/kg TG, d. h. um ca. 47% steigern. Unter dem Einfluß von Propranolol kommt es aber ebenfalls wie unter Verapamil oder Fendilin zu einer dosisabhängigen Unterdrückung der Isoproterenol-induzierten Kalziumakkumulation im Myokard. Dabei kompensieren 3 mg/kg KG Propranolol die Wirkung von 1 mg/kg KG Isoproterenol komplett. Die nächsthöhere Dosis von 10 mg/kg KG Propranolol senkt den myokardialen Kalziumgehalt auf ca. 7.2 ± 0.86 mVal/kg TG, d. h. unter den Ausgangswert von 7,5 ± 0,67 mVal/kg TG der unbehandelten Gruppe.

Einfluß des β-Rezeptorenblockers Atenolol auf die Isoproterenol-bewirkte myokardiale Kalziumakkumulation

Der myokardiale Kalziumgehalt behandelter und unbehandelter kardiomyopathischer Hamster sowie die Dosis-Wirkungskurve von Atenolol auf die Isoproterenol-induzierte Kalziumakkumulation dieser in der sog. pränekrotischen Phase ihres Herzleidens befindlichen Tiere sind in Tabelle 4 bzw. Abb. 4 wiedergegeben. Bei den unbehandelten Hamstern liegt der myokardiale Kalziumgehalt um 7,7 ± 1,11 mVal/ kg TG. Unter dem Einfluß von Isoproterenol steigt er um ca. 44% auf 11,1 ± 2,87 mVal/kg TG an, um unter der gleichzeitigen Gabe von Atenolol dosisabhängig bis auf 7,8 ± 1,25 mVal/kg TG, etwa auf den Basiswert unbehandelter Tiere, abzusinken.

Tabelle 4. Myokardialer Kalziumgehalt 29- bis 31tägiger kardiomyopathischer Hamster nach subcutaner Gabe von Isoproterenol und Atenolol. Die Ergebnisse sind als Mittelwert ± Standardabweichung, die Tierzahl ist in Klammern angegeben

	myokardialer Kalziumgehalt (mVal/kg Trockengewicht)	% über unbehandelt
Unbehandelt	7,7 ± 1,11 (10)	
Isoproterenol (1 mg/kg KG)	11,1 ± 2,87 (10)	+ 44%
Atenolol (10 mg/kg KG) + Isoproterenol (1 mg/kg KG)	10,8 ± 1,29 (10)	+ 40%
Atenolol (30 mg/kg KG) + Isoproterenol (1 mg/kg KG)	8,2 ± 0,93 (9)	+ 7%
Atenolol (100 mg/kg KG) + Isoproterenol (1 mg/kg KG)	7,8 ± 1,25 (10)	+ 1%

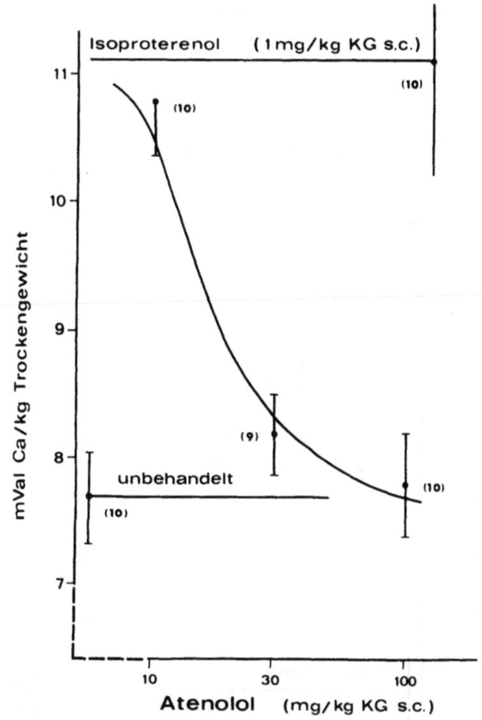

Abb. 4. Myokardialer Kalziumgehalt 29- bis 31tägiger kardiomyopathischer Hamster (Stamm BIO 8262) unter dem kombinierten Einfluß von Atenolol und Isoproterenol 6 Std nach simultaner subcutaner Pharmakongabe. Angegeben sind die Mittelwerte ± SEM. Tierzahl in Klammern

Einfluß von Magnesiumaspartathydrochlorid auf die Isoproterenol-bewirkte myokardiale Kalziumakkumulation

In Tabelle 5 bzw. Abb. 5 sind der myokardiale Kalziumgehalt unbehandelter und entsprechend behandelter kardiomyopathischer Hamster sowie die Dosis-Wirkungskurve von Magnesiumaspartathydrochlorid auf die Isoproterenol-induzierte Kalziumakkumulation im Myokard dieser Hamster dargestellt. Der 7,8 ± 0,94 mVal/kg TG betragende myokardiale Kalziumgehalt unbehandelter Tiere läßt sich unter dem Einfluß von Isoproterenol in dieser Experimentalserie auf 11,8 ± 2,66 mVal/kg TG, d.h. um ca. 51% anheben. Nach vorheriger Verabrei-

Tabelle 5. Myokardialer Kalziumgehalt 29- bis 31tägiger kardiomyopathischer Hamster nach subcutaner Gabe von Isoproterenol und oraler Gabe von Magnesiumaspartathydrochlorid. Die Ergebnisse sind als Mittelwert ± Standardabweichung, die Tierzahl ist in Klammern angegeben

	myokardialer Kalzium- gehalt (mVal/kg Trockengewicht)	% über unbehandelt
Unbehandelt	7,8 ± 0,94 (10)	
Isoproterenol (1 mg/kg KG)	11,8 ± 2,66 (11)	+ 51%
Magnesiumaspartathydrochlorid (2,3 mVal/kg KG) + Isoproterenol (1 mg/kg KG)	10,5 ± 1,07 (10)	+ 35%
Magnesiumaspartathydrochlorid (7,7 mVal/kg KG) + Isoproterenol (1 mg/kg KG)	9,1 ± 1,24 (10)	+ 17%
Magnesiumaspartathydrochlorid (23,0 mVal/kg KG) + Isoproterenol (1 mg/kg KG)	7,8 ± 0,93 (10)	± 0%

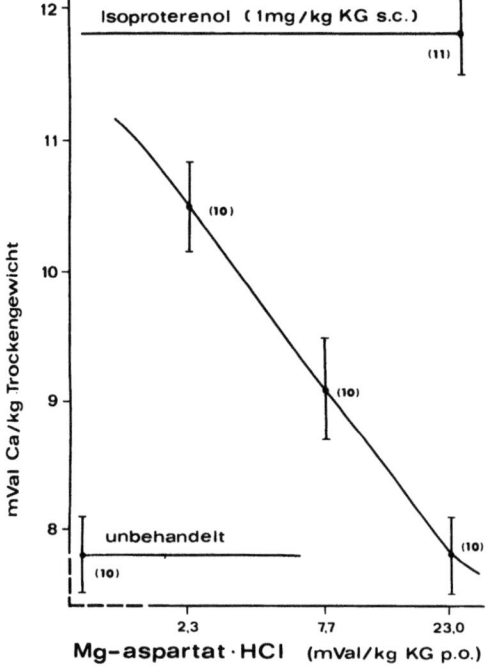

Abb. 5. Myokardialer Kalziumgehalt 29- bis 31tägiger kardiomyopathischer Hamster (Stamm BIO 8262) unter dem kombinierten Pharmakoneinfluß 6,5 bzw. 6 Std nach peroraler Gabe von Magnesiumaspartathydrochlorid bzw. subcutaner Gabe von Isoproterenol. Mittelwerte ± SEM. Tierzahl in Klammern

chung von Magnesiumaspartathydrochlorid resultiert aber eine dosisabhängige Suppression der Isoproterenol-induzierten Kalziumakkumulation im Myokard. 23 mVal/kg KG Magnesiumaspartathydrochlorid sind dabei in der Lage, die Isoproterenolwirkung völlig zu verhindern, der myokardiale Kalziumgehalt entspricht hier mit 7,8 ± 0,93 mVal/kg TG demjenigen unbehandelter Tiere von 7,8 ± 0,94 mVal/kg TG.

Chronische Experimente

Einfluß von Verapamil auf die spontane myokardiale Kalziumakkumulation

In Tabelle 6 sind die myokardialen Kalziumgehalte der unbehandelten und chronisch behandelten Hamster wiedergegeben. Abbildung 6 zeigt die Dosis-Wirkungskurve von Verapamil auf den myokardialen Kalziumgehalt der chronisch behandelten Versuchsgruppe. Der Kalziumgehalt im Myokard unbehandelter Tiere beträgt 209,1 ± 130,8 mVal/kg TG. Nach Applikation steigender Dosen Verapamil fällt er dosisabhängig bis auf 9,8 ± 2,2 mVal/kg TG ab.

Tabelle 6. Myokardialer Kalziumgehalt 60tägiger kardiomyopathischer Hamster nach chronischer subcutaner Gabe von Verapamil. Die Ergebnisse sind als Mittelwert ± Standardabweichung, die Tierzahl ist in Klammern angegeben

	myokardialer Kalziumgehalt (mVal/kg Trockengewicht)
Unbehandelt	209,1 ± 130,8 (13)
Verapamil 2 × 1 mg/kg KG	85,8 ± 136,6 (5)
Verapamil 2 × 3 mg/kg KG	37,0 ± 15,9 (10)
Verapamil 2 × 5 mg/kg KG	25,5 ± 22,1 (9)
Verapamil 2 × 10 mg/kg KG	9,8 ± 2,2 (13)

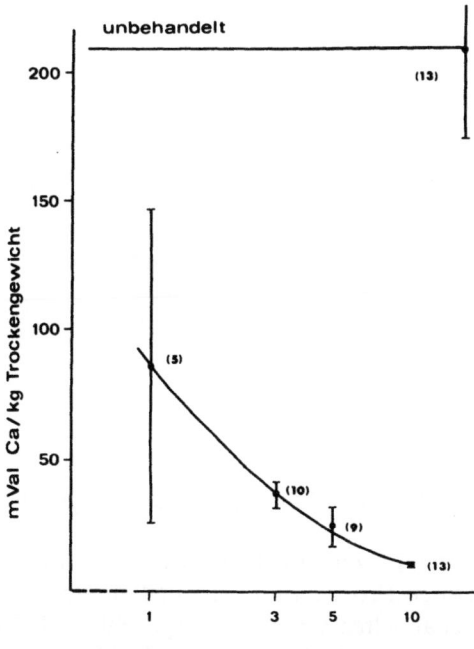

Abb. 6. Myokardialer Kalziumgehalt 60tägiger kardiomyopathischer Hamster (Stamm BIO 8262) nach chronischer subcutaner Gabe verschieden hoher Dosen von Verapamil. Angegeben sind die Mittelwerte ± SEM. Tierzahl in Klammern

Einfluß von Fendilin auf die spontane myokardiale Kalziumakkumulation

In Tabelle 7 ist der myokardiale Kalziumgehalt der unbehandelten Hamster sowie jener der chronisch mit Fendilin behandelten Tiere angegeben. Dabei zeigt sich, daß er bei den unbehandelten Hamstern $186,7 \pm 125,8$ mVal/kg TG beträgt, während er mit $16,7 \pm 0,9$ mVal/kg TG bei den behandelten Tieren über zehnmal niedriger liegt. In Abb. 7 ist dieses Verhalten graphisch dargestellt.

Tabelle 7. Myokardialer Kalziumgehalt 60tägiger kardiomyopathischer Hamster nach chronischer peroraler Gabe von Fendilin. Die Ergebnisse sind als Mittelwert ± Standardabweichung, die Tierzahl ist in Klammern angegeben

	myokardialer Kalziumgehalt (mVal/kg Trockengewicht)
Unbehandelt	$186,7 \pm 125,8$ (10)
Fendilin 2×20 mg/kg KG	$16,7 \pm 0,9$ (10)

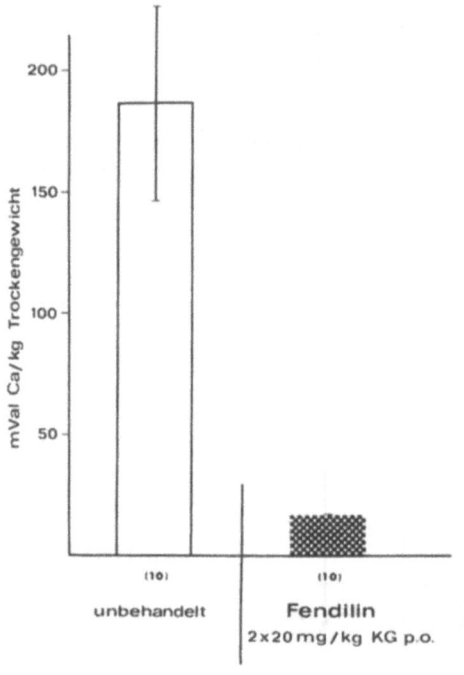

Abb. 7. Myokardialer Kalziumgehalt 60tägiger kardiomyopathischer Hamster (Stamm BIO 8262) nach chronischer peroraler Gabe von Fendilin. Angegeben ist der Mittelwert ± SEM. Tierzahl in Klammern

Einfluß von Propranolol auf die spontane myokardiale Kalziumakkumulation

Tabelle 8 zeigt die Ergebnisse der unbehandelten sowie der chronisch mit steigenden Dosen Propranolol behandelten Hamster. Der myokardiale Kalziumgehalt der unbehandelten Gruppe beträgt $169,3 \pm 162,4$ mVal/kg TG. Er fällt unter chronischer Propranololbehandlung dosisabhängig bis auf $8,4 \pm 0,8$ mVal/kg TG bei zweimal

Tabelle 8. Myokardialer Kalziumgehalt 60tägiger kardiomyopathischer Hamster nach chronischer subcutaner Gabe von Propranolol. Die Ergebnisse sind als Mittelwert ± Standardabweichung, die Tierzahl ist in Klammern angegeben

	myokardialer Kalziumgehalt (mVal/kg Trockengewicht)
Unbehandelt	169,3 ± 162,4 (15)
Propranolol 2× 1 mg/kg KG	59,4 ± 20,3 (8)
Propranolol 2× 3 mg/kg KG	29,7 ± 23,4 (9)
Propranolol 2×10 mg/kg KG	17,4 ± 8,0 (8)
Propranolol 2×30 mg/kg KG	8,4 ± 0,8 (10)

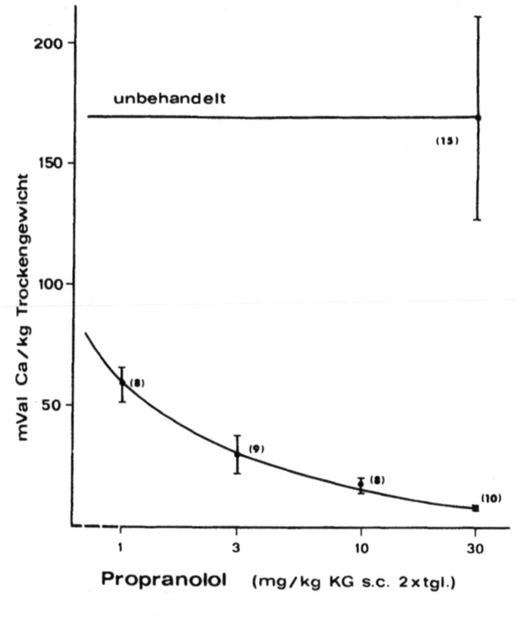

Abb. 8. Myokardialer Kalziumgehalt 60tägiger kardiomyopathischer Hamster (Stamm BIO 8262) nach chronischer subcutaner Gabe verschieden hoher Dosen von Propranolol. Angegeben sind die Mittelwerte ± SEM. Tierzahl in Klammern

tgl. 30 mg/kg KG Propranolol ab. Abbildung 8 zeigt das Dosis-Wirkungsverhalten von Propranolol auf den myokardialen Kalziumgehalt im chronischen Experiment.

Einfluß von Atenolol auf die spontane myokardiale Kalziumakkumulation

In Tabelle 9 sind die myokardialen Kalziumgehalte der unbehandelten und chronisch mit Atenolol behandelten Hamster aufgeführt. Ohne Behandlung beträgt der myokardiale Kalziumgehalt 225,2 ± 110,1 mVal/kg TG. Unter der chronischen Applikation von Atenolol läßt sich die spontane myokardiale Kalziumakkumulation nur gering supprimieren. Bei der Dosis von zweimal 300 mg/kg KG Atenolol beträgt der myokardiale Kalziumgehalt immer noch 64,3 ± 42,1 mVal/kg TG. In Abb. 9 ist die Wirkung der verschiedenen Atenololdosen auf die spontane myokardiale Kalziumakkumulation bei der Kardiomyopathie der Hamster wiedergegeben.

Tabelle 9. Myokardialer Kalziumgehalt 60tägiger kardiomyopathischer Hamster nach chronischer subcutaner Gabe von Atenolol. Die Ergebnisse sind als Mittelwert ± Standardabweichung, die Tierzahl ist in Klammern angegeben

	myokardialer Kalziumgehalt (mVal/kg Trockengewicht)
Unbehandelt	225,2 ± 110,2 (12)
Atenolol 2× 10 mg/kg KG	221,2 ± 166,6 (10)
Atenolol 2× 30 mg/kg KG	192,5 ± 179,4 (10)
Atenolol 2×100 mg/kg KG	164,9 ± 147,6 (8)
Atenolol 2×300 mg/kg KG	64,3 ± 42,1 (9)

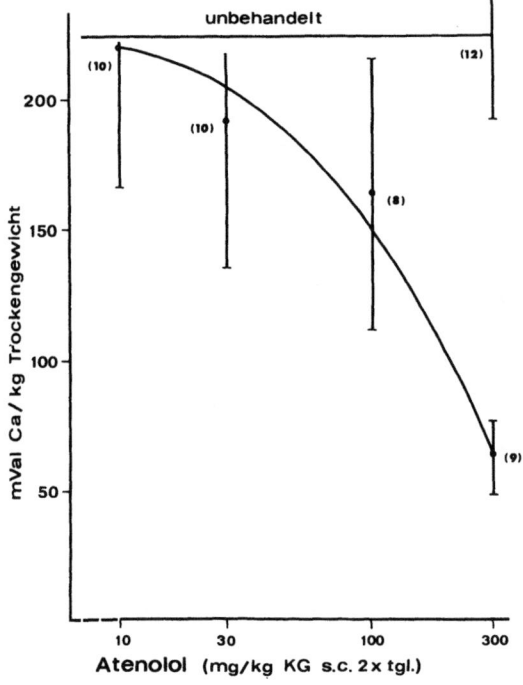

Abb. 9. Myokardialer Kalziumgehalt 60tägiger kardiomyopathischer Hamster (Stamm BIO 8262) nach chronischer subcutaner Gabe verschieden hoher Dosen von Atenolol. Angegeben sind die Mittelwerte ± SEM. Tierzahl in Klammern

Einfluß von Magnesiumaspartathydrochlorid auf die spontane myokardiale Kalziumakkumulation

Tabelle 10 zeigt den myokardialen Kalziumgehalt unbehandelter Hamster im Vergleich zu den Kalziumgehalten, die sich im Myokard unter den verschiedenen Dosen der chronisch mit Magnesiumaspartathydrochlorid behandelten Hamster ergeben. Mit ansteigenden Magnesiumaspartathydrochloriddosen sinken die myokardialen Kalziumgehalte von 245,3 ± 161,1 mVal/kg TG der unbehandelten Gruppe bis auf 13,2 ± 1,9 mVal/kg TG unter einer Dosis von zweimal 46 mVal/kg KG. In Abb. 10 ist die Dosis-Wirkungsbeziehung zwischen Magnesiumaspartathydrochlorid und Reduktion der myokardialen Kalziumakkumulation im chronischen Experiment dargestellt.

Tabelle 10. Myokardialer Kalziumgehalt 60tägiger kardiomyopathischer Hamster nach chronischer peroraler Gabe von Magnesiumaspartathydrochlorid. Die Ergebnisse sind als Mittelwert ± Standardabweichung, die Tierzahl ist in Klammern angegeben

	myokardialer Kalziumgehalt (mVal/kg Trockengewicht)
Unbehandelt	245,3 ± 161,1 (11)
Magnesiumaspartathydrochlorid 2× 8 mVal/kg KG	142,5 ± 58,6 (11)
Magnesiumaspartathydrochlorid 2×23 mVal/kg KG	41,6 ± 12,2 (11)
Magnesiumaspartathydrochlorid 2×46 mVal/kg KG	13,2 ± 1,9 (7)

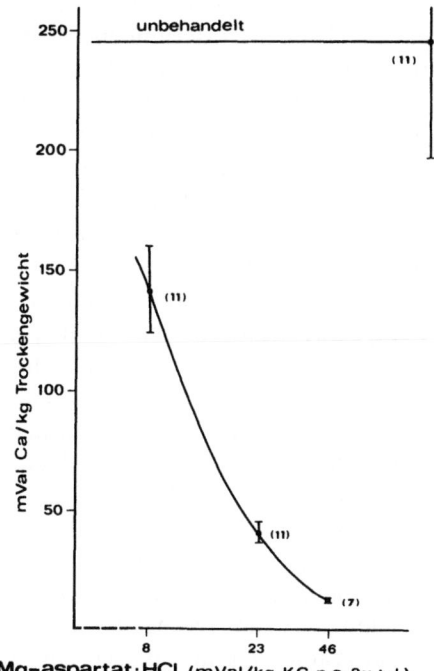

Abb. 10. Myokardialer Kalziumgehalt 60tägiger kardiomyopathischer Hamster (Stamm BIO 8262) nach chronischer peroraler Gabe verschieden hoher Dosen von Magnesiumaspartathydrochlorid. Angegeben sind die Mittelwerte ± SEM. Tierzahl in Klammern

Diskussion

Die Versuchsergebnisse zeigen in ihrer Gesamtheit, daß alle geprüften Substanzen – Kalziumantagonisten, β-Rezeptorenblocker und Magnesiumsalz – sowohl die durch Isoproterenol induzierte als auch die spontane Kalziumakkumulation im Myokard der kardiomyopathischen Hamster zu unterdrücken in der Lage sind.

Betrachtet man die Wirksamkeit der Kalziumantagonisten Verapamil und Fendilin, so läßt sich die Isoproterenol-induzierte Kalziumakkumulation im Akutversuch durch beide Substanzen vollständig unterdrücken. Bislang wurde diese Wirkung von Fendilin am Isoproterenol-Modell noch nicht direkt gezeigt, während derartige Untersuchungen mit Verapamil wohlbekannt sind [7, 9, 12 – 15, 18]. Demgegenüber konnte der nekroseverhütende Effekt sowohl von Verapamil [7, 18] als auch von

Fendilin [19] am Myokard bereits früher nachgewiesen werden. Aus unseren Untersuchungen geht außerdem hervor, daß Fendilin dosisbezogen eine etwas günstigere Wirksamkeit als Verapamil zu besitzen scheint.

Im chronischen Experiment demonstrieren unsere Ergebnisse, daß Verapamil bei subcutaner Applikation die spontane, mit Myokardnekrosen einhergehende [9,10], Kalziumakkumulation vollständig supprimieren kann; denn der in früheren Experimenten [10] ermittelte Kalziumgehalt im Myokard 61- bis 82tägiger erbgesunder syrischer Goldhamster liegt mit $8,9 \pm 1,10$ mVal/kg TG im Streubereich des Ergebnisses von $9,9 \pm 2,15$ mVal/kg TG, das jetzt unter chronischer Behandlung mit zweimal tgl. 10 mg/kg KG Verapamil bei den 60tägigen kardiomyopathischen Tieren erlangt werden konnte. Die chronische perorale Verabreichung von Fendilin weist ebenfalls einen eindeutigen kalziumsuppressorischen Effekt am Myokard auf. Dieser ist aber bei der gewählten Dosis und Applikationsform nicht vollständig. Doch darf man bei entsprechender Dosierung auch von dieser Substanz eine vollständige kardioprotektive Wirkung bei der erblichen Kardiomyopathie des Hamsters annehmen.

Bei Vergleich der akuten mit den chronischen Versuchen an mit β-Rezeptorenblockern behandelten Hamstern stellen sich unterschiedliche Ergebnisse dar. Im Akutversuch zeigen beide Pharmaka – Propranolol sowie Atenolol – dosisabhängig eine vollständige Suppression der durch den β-Rezeptorenstimulator Isoproterenol bewirkten myokardialen Kalziumakkumulation. Hierbei erweist sich, daß erst bei der Dosisrelation von 1:33 zwischen Propranolol (3 mg/kg KG) und Atenolol (100 mg/kg KG) ein identischer Effekt eintritt. Unter der Annahme, daß diese Wirkung beider Substanzen auf einer β-Rezeptorenblockade beruht, ergibt sich der Hinweis auf eine schwächere Potenz des β-Rezeptorenblockers Atenolol gegenüber Propranolol. Damit steht unser am kardiomyopathischen Hamster gewonnenes Ergebnis nicht in vollem Einklang mit demjenigen von Meesmann et al. [20] bzgl. (dp/dt) max. am infarktgeschädigten Herzen des Hundes sowie dem von Fitzgerald [21] bzgl. der atrio-ventrikulären Überleitung beim Hund. An diesen beiden Modellen hatten Propranolol und Atenolol etwa ähnliche Wirkungsstärken.

Unter der höchsten applizierten Propranololdosis (10 mg/kg KG) läßt sich außerdem eine Reduktion des myokardialen Kalziumgehaltes unter den Ausgangswert unbehandelter Hamster messen. Die Erklärung könnte darin liegen, daß infolge Äthernarkose und Operationsstreß eine zusätzliche – neben der exogen zugeführten – endogene Katecholaminwirkung durch die höchste Dosis des β-Rezeptorenblockers abgefangen wird. Für diese Annahme einer streßbedingten Katecholaminfreisetzung könnte die von Bloom u. Davis [22] beobachtete Reduktion des myokardialen Kalziumgehaltes bei mit Äther narkotisierten Ratten nach alleiniger β-Rezeptorengabe (Propranolol) gegenüber unbehandelten Tieren sprechen.

Im chronischen Versuch weisen nun Propranolol und Atenolol einen recht unterschiedlichen Einfluß auf die spontane myokardiale Kalziumakkumulation auf. Während Propranolol in einer Dosis von zweimal 30 mg/kg KG eine komplette Verhütung derselben bewirkt, ist Atenolol selbst mit der extremen Dosis von zweimal 300 mg/kg KG sowie einer wesentlich längeren Halbwertzeit als Propranolol [23,24] lediglich in der Lage, eine teilweise Suppression zu erzielen. Aller Wahrscheinlichkeit nach ist für dieses differente Verhalten der beiden β-Rezeptorenblocker die bekannte membranunspezifische Eigenwirkung von Propranolol [20, 25] bzw. ihr Fehlen oder zumindest ihre Abschwächung bei Atenolol [20] verantwortlich. Durch diese Wirkungskomponente ist wie unter dem Einfluß der Kalziumantagonisten an Myokardzellen eine direkte Blockierung transsarkolemmaler Kalziumkanäle zu erreichen. Deutliche Hinweise hierfür geben der negativ-inotrope Einfluß von Propranolol auf isolierte Meerschweinchenvorhöfe [25], sowie der stetige Abfall von (dp/dt) max. am infarktvorgeschädigten Hundeherzen [20]. Der nur mäßige Effekt selbst höchster Dosen von Atenolol auf die spontane myokardiale Kalziumakkumulation der Hamster läßt weniger das Vorliegen einer sog. adrenergen Kardiopathie mit einer Tangierung des Adenylcyclase-Systems als vielmehr einen Defekt an den Herzmuskelzellen selbst, höchstwahrscheinlich am Sarkolemm, vermuten. Der Hinweis auf eine relative Wirkungslosigkeit reiner β-Rezeptorenblockade erscheint um so wichtiger, als Angelakos et al. [26, 27] an Hamstern des kardiomyopathischen Stammes BIO 14.6 während der pränekrotischen Phase des Herzleidens eine gesteigerte Noradrenalin-Synthese sowie Noradrenalin-Aufnahme beobachten konnten und parallel mit der Entwicklung von Herzmuskelzellnekrosen eine Erhöhung des myokardialen Noradrenalingehaltes bei diesen Tieren einsetzte. Höchstwahrscheinlich steht aber die Myokardnekroseentwicklung bei dem Erbleiden eher in pathogenetischem Zusammenhang mit einer von Bester et al. [28] bei den kardiomyopathischen Hamstern beobachteten Proteinsynthesestörung, die sich nicht nur − wie vermutet − am kontraktilen Apparat, sondern auch am Sarkolemm der Herzmuskelzellen abspielen mag. Die Störung einer speziellen Barrierenfunktion dieses Zellorganells könnte daher zur pathogenetisch für die Myokardnekrotisierung entscheidenden Überladung der Zellen mit Kalziumionen führen. Die Noradrenalinstoffwechselstörung wäre somit nur von sekundärem Charakter und lediglich als Antwort auf eine Synthesestörung der kontraktilen Proteine anzusehen.

Aufgrund der Untersuchungen von Fleckenstein und seinem Arbeitskreis [7, 12−15] sind sowohl Kalium- als auch Magnesiumsalze in der Lage, eine Isoproterenol-induzierte Steigerung der myokardialen Radiokalziumaufnahme und Akkumulation von Gesamtkalzium zu unterdrücken. Dadurch ist eine Erklärung für den kardioprotektiven Effekt dieser Salze gefunden, den schon Selye [29] sowie Bajusz [30] bei verschiedenen experimentellen Herzmuskelzellnekrose-Modellen beobachten konnten. Auch in unseren akuten sowie chronischen Experimenten mit Magnesiumaspartathydrochlorid war eine vollständige bzw. nahezu vollständige Unterdrückung der Isoproterenol-induzierten bzw. spontanen myokardialen Kalziumakkumulation bei den kardiomyopathischen Hamstern möglich. Von Janke et al. [16] wird hierbei eine kompetitive Hemmung intrazellulärer Kalziumbindungsstellen durch Magnesiumionen als ein zweiter kalziumantagonistischer Mechanismus am Myokard postuliert. Damit wäre also auch über diesen Mechanismus eine Kardioprotektion bei der erblichen Kardiomyopathie der Hamster möglich.

Durch den Nachweis der Wirksamkeit kalziumantagonistischer Pharmaka bzw. von Substanzen mit kalziumantagonistischer Komponente bei einer erblichen Kardiomyopathie stellt sich eine allgemeine Gültigkeit der von Fleckenstein [7, 12−15, 18] am pharmakologischen Modell gewonnenen Erkenntnis einer myokardialen Kalziumüberladung als entscheidender, Myokardnekrosen verursachender Faktor heraus. Gleichzeitig wird aber auch dadurch die Bedeutung der kalziumantagonistisch wirksamen Pharmaka für die Klinik hervorgehoben.

Interessanterweise haben Kaltenbach et al. [31] bzgl. der subjektiven Beschwerden, aber auch vor allem des Rückgangs der Linksherzhypertrophie und des Herzvolumens eine bessere Wirksamkeit von Verapamil als von Propranolol bzw. Pindolol bei der hypertrophisch-obstruktiven Kardiomyopathie des Menschen nachgewiesen. Auch in unseren Experimenten ergibt sich eine bessere Dosis-Wirkungs-Relation bei Verapamil als bei Propranolol. Natürlich erhebt sich die Frage, welche weiteren Zusammenhänge zwischen der dystrophischen Kardiomyopathie des syrischen Goldhamsters und der hypertrophisch-obstruktiven Kardiomyopathie des Menschen bestehen. Zum einen scheint die gehäuft vorkommende Erblichkeit bei Kardiomyopathien eine gemeinsame Grundlage zu sein, wie aus der Übersichtsarbeit von Kuhn [32] hervorgeht. Zum anderen ist durch die Untersuchungen von Meerschwam u. Hootsmans [33] bei Patienten mit hypertrophisch-obstruktiver Kardiomyopathie ein kombinierter Befall von Herz- und Skelettmuskulatur deutlich geworden, ähnlich wie aufgrund der Untersuchungen von Weisenfeld u. Messinger [34], Rubin u. Buchberg [35], James [36], Perloff et al. [37], Beckmann u. Schmit [38] und Schmidt-Redemann et al. [39] bei erblicher progressiver Muskeldystrophie sowie durch die Untersuchungen von Graham [40] bei Friedreichscher Erkrankung. Der günstige Einfluß kalziumantagonistisch wirkender Pharmaka bei der dystrophischen Hamsterkardiomyopathie sowie bei der hypertrophischen Kardiomyopathie des Menschen weist geradezu darauf hin, daß evtl. beide Leiden generell unter dem Aspekt einer Systemerkrankung der quergestreiften Muskulatur mit unterschiedlicher Ausprägung zu sehen sind, denen biochemisch ein gestörter myokardialer Kalziumstoffwechsel zugrunde liegen könnte. Dadurch würde auch die durch Wrogemann u. Pena [41] in Anlehnung an die Befunde von Fleckenstein [7, 12 – 15, 18] erweiterte Hypothese einer zellulären Kalziumüberladung als genereller Mechanismus für die Ausbildung von Nekrosen bei muskulären Erkrankungen größere Bedeutung erlangen. Nicht zuletzt könnte unter gewissen Voraussetzungen ein gestörter myokardialer Kalziumstoffwechsel aber auch den Stimulus für einen myokard-hypertrophischen Prozeß abgeben. Das unterschiedliche Bild der erblichen Kardiomyopathie bei Hamstern des Stammes BIO 8262 mit alleiniger Myokarddystrophie einerseits [4] und bei Tieren des Stammes BIO 14.6 in Kombination mit Myokardhypertrophie andererseits [6], beide Stämme hängen genetisch eng zusammen [2] und weisen einen gestörten myokardialen Kalziumstoffwechsel [2, 8, 10, 17] als gemeinsames biochemisches Kennzeichen auf, verstärkt diese Vermutung. Weitere detaillierte biochemische, pharmakologische, morphologische und klinische Untersuchungen müssen jedoch in Zukunft die Richtigkeit dieser Vorstellung bestätigen.

Zusammenfassung

Vermutlich wird bei der erblichen dystrophischen Kardiomyopathie des syrischen Goldhamsters (Stamm BIO 8262) infolge einer Proteinsynthesestörung, die sich nicht nur am myofibrillären Apparat sondern auch am Sarkolemm abspielen mag, eine myokardiale Kalziumstoffwechselstörung induziert. Da von Fleckenstein und seinem Arbeitskreis eine myozelluläre Kalziumüberladung generell als entscheidender Faktor für die Auslösung von Herzmuskelnekrosen angesehen wird, erschien es von großem Interesse, der Frage nachzugehen, ob sich durch Wirksamkeitsnachweis sog. kalziumantagonistischer Substanzen bei dem spontan auftretenden Erbleiden diese am pharmakologischen Modell der Isoproterenol-behandelten Ratte entwickelte Hypothese erhärten läßt.

Bei den kardiomyopathischen Tieren wurde der Einfluß der Kalziumantagonisten Verapamil und Fendilin, des mit einer membranunspezifischen Komponenete ausgestatteten β-Rezeptorenblockers Propranolol sowie des „reinen" β-Rezeptorenblockers Atenolol und von Magnesiumaspartathydrochlorid sowohl auf die Isoproterenol-induzierte als auch auf die spontane myokardiale Kalziumakkumulation untersucht. In früheren Experimenten hatte sich nämlich herausgestellt, daß sich schon in der pränekrotischen Phase des Herzleidens durch Isoproterenol eine latente myokardiale Kalziumstoffwechselstörung manifestieren läßt, und die spontan mit der Myokardnekrotisierung einsetzende myokardiale Kalziumakkumulation als biochemisch meßbarer Ausdruck der Kardiomyopathie aufgefaßt werden kann.

Während die Kalziumantagonisten und das Magnesiumsalz sowohl die Isoproterenol-induzierte als auch die spontane Kalziumakkumulation im Myokard unterdrücken konnten, verhielten sich die β-Rezeptorenblocker Propranolol und Atenolol nicht einheitlich. Beide Pharmaka waren zwar in der Lage, die Isoproterenol-induzierte Kalziumakkumulation voll zu kompensieren, doch versagte Atenolol gegenüber der spontanen myokardialen Kalziumakkumulation. Die positive Wirkung beider Substanzen gegenüber Isoproterenol wird auf ihre gemeinsame β-rezeptorenblockierende Eigenschaft, und die günstige Wirkung von Propranolol gegenüber der spontanen Kalziumakkumulation auf seine membranunspezifische Wirkungskomponente bezogen. Letztere ist bekanntlich dem „reinen" β-Rezeptorenblocker Atenolol nicht zu eigen.

Aufgrund dieser Befunde wird das Vorliegen einer adrenergen Kardiopathie bei den kardiomyopathischen Goldhamstern mit hoher Wahrscheinlichkeit ausgeschlossen und eine Proteinsynthesestörung als wesentliches Glied in der pathogenetischen Kette dieses Leidens erachtet. Doch die Wirksamkeit der Kalziumantagonisten und des Magnesiumsalzes gegenüber der myokardialen Kalziumakkumulation bei der erblichen Kardiomyopathie der Hamster rückt die Bedeutung der myozellulären Kalziumüberladung als entscheidenden Auslöser für den Myokardnekroseprozeß mehr in den Vordergrund als die wahrscheinlich primär vorhandene myokardiale Proteinsynthesestörung. Gleichzeitig erlangt aber auch dadurch die von Fleckenstein am pharmakologischen Modell gewonnene Erkenntnis einer myokardialen Kalziumüberladung als entscheidender Myokardnekrosen verursachender Faktor allgemeinere Gültigkeit. Weiterhin wird noch die Bedeutung kalziumantagonistisch wirksamer Pharmaka für die Klinik, insbesondere bei der Behandlung von Kardiomyopathien, hervorgehoben. Die von Kaltenbach u. Mitarb. geschilderten guten therapeutischen Ansätze mit Kalziumantagonisten vor β-Rezeptorenblockern bei der hypertrophisch-obstruktiven Kardiomyopathie des Menschen sind eventuell unter dem Aspekt eines direkten myokardialen Angriffspunktes dieser Pharmaka zu sehen. Mögliche Zusammenhänge zwischen der Kardiomyopathie des syrischen Hamsters und der hypertrophisch-obstruktiven Kardiomyopathie des Menschen und die zentrale Stellung eines gestörten myokardialen Kalziumstoffwechsels dabei werden erörtert.

Literatur

1. Bajusz E, Lossnitzer K (1968) Ein neues Krankheitsmodell: Erbliche nichtvaskuläre Myokarddegeneration mit Herzinsuffizienz. Muench Med Wochenschr 31:1756–1768
2. Lossnitzer K (1975) Genetic induction of a cardiomyopathy. In: Schmier J, Eichler O (eds) Heart and circulation. Springer, Berlin Heidelberg New York (Handbuch der experimentellen Pharmakologie, vol XVI/3, pp 309–344)

3. Mohr W, Lossnitzer K (1974) Morphologische Untersuchungen an Hamstern des Stammes BIO 8262 mit erblicher Myopathie und Kardiomyopathie. Beitr Pathol 153:178 – 193

4. Mohr W, Lossnitzer K, Schwarz J (1978) The cardiomyopathy of the Syrian hamster (strain BIO 8262) – hypertrophic or dystrophic? Basic Res Cardiol 73:34 – 46

5. Lossnitzer K, Grewe N, Konrad A, Adler J (1977) Electrocardiographic changes in cardiomyopathic Syrian hamsters (strain BIO 8262). Basic Res Cardiol 72:421 – 435

6. Büchner F, Onishi S (1970) Herzhypertrophie und Herzinsuffizienz in der Sicht der Elektronenmikroskopie. Urban & Schwarzenberg, München Berlin Wien

7. Fleckenstein A (1971) Specific inhibitors and promotors of calcium action in the excitation-contraction coupling of heart muscle and their role in the prevention or production of myocardial lesions. In: Harris P, Opie L (eds) Calcium and the heart. Academic Press, London New York, pp 135 – 188

8. Lossnitzer K, Janke J, Hein P, Stauch M, Fleckenstein A (1975) Disturbed myocardial calcium metabolism: A possible pathogenetic factor in the hereditary cardiomyopathy of the Syrian hamster. In: Fleckenstein A, Rona G (eds) Recent advances in studies on cardiac structure and metabolism, vol 6. University Park Press, Baltimore, pp 207 – 217

9. Lossnitzer K, Mohr W, Konrad A, Guggenmoos R (1978) The hereditary cardiomyopathy in the Syrian golden hamster – influence of verapamil as calcium antagonist. In: Kaltenbach M, Loogen F, Olsen EGJ (eds) Cardiomyopathy and myocardial biopsy. Springer Verlag, Berlin Heidelberg New York, pp 27 – 37

10. Lossnitzer K, Steinhardt B, Grewe N, Stauch M (1975) Charakteristische Elektrolytveränderungen bei der erblichen Myopathie und Kardiomyopathie des syrischen Goldhamsters (Stamm BIO 8262). Basic Res Cardial 70:508 – 520

11. Mohr W, Hersener J, Lossnitzer K (1973) Der Nachweis von Kalzium-Phosphat in der Herzmuskulatur mittels Röntgenmikroanalyse. Virchows Arch [Pathol Anat] 358:259 – 264

12. Fleckenstein A (1975) Biochemische Veränderungen im Myokard als Ursache koronarogener und nicht-koronarogener Strukturläsionen. In: Holtmeier H-J, Siegenthaler W (eds) Koronarinsuffizienz. Thieme, Stuttgart, S 134 – 144

13. Fleckenstein A, Janke J, Döring HJ, Leder O (1971) Die intrazelluläre Überladung mit Kalzium als entscheidender Kausalfaktor bei der Entstehung nicht-coronarogener Myokard-Nekrosen. Verh Dtsch Ges Kreislaufforsch 37:345 – 353

14. Fleckenstein A, Janke J, Döring HJ, Pachinger O (1973) Ca-overload as the determinant factor in the production of catecholamine-induced myocardial lesions. In: Recent advances in studies on cardiac structure and metabolism, vol 2. In: Bajusz E, Rona G (eds) University Park Press, Baltimore, pp 455 – 466

15. Fleckenstein A, Janke J, Döring HJ, Leder O (1974) Myocardial fiber necrosis due to intracellular Ca-overload – A new principle in cardiac pathophysiology. In: Dhalla NS (ed) Recent advances in studies on cardiac structure and metabolism, vol 4. University Park Press, Baltimore, pp 563 – 580

16. Janke J, Fleckenstein A, Hein B, Leder O, Sigel H (1975) Prevention of myocardial Ca overload and necrotization by Mg and K salts or acidosis. In: Fleckenstein A, Rona G (eds) Recent advances in studies on cardiac structure and metabolism, vol 6. University Park Press, Baltimore, pp 33 – 42

17. Lossnitzer K, Bajusz E (1974) Water and electrolyte alterations during the life course of the BIO 14.6 Syrian golden hamster. A disease model of a hereditary cardiomyopathy. J Mol Cell Cardiol 6:163 – 177

18. Fleckenstein A, Janke J, Döring HJ, Leder O (1975) Key role of Ca in the production of coronarogenic myocardial necrosis. In: Fleckenstein A, Rona G (eds) Recent advances in studies on cardiac structure and metabolism, vol 6. University Park Press, Baltimore, pp 21 – 32

19. Ciplea AG, Bock PR (1976) Kardioprotektion durch perorale Anwendung des Calcium-Antagonisten Sensit. Arzneim Forsch 26:1819 – 1826

20. Meesmann W, Stephan K, Hübner H (1976) Beeinflussung der Gesamtkontraktilität des Infarktherzens durch 4 differente Beta-Sympatholytika in Abhängigkeit von ihrer "Intrinsic Activity". In: Ganten D, Dietz R, Lüth B, Gross F (Hrsg) Beta-adrenerge Blocker und Hochdruck. Thieme, Stuttgart, S 37 – 41

21. Fitzgerald JD (1975) Beta-blocking drugs as antiarrhythmic agents. Int J Clin Pharmacol Biopharm 11:235 – 256

22. Bloom S, Davis D (1974) Isoproterenol-induced myocytolysis and myocardial calcium. In: Dhalla NS (ed) Recent advances in studies on cardiac structure and metabolism, vol 4. University Park Press, Baltimore, pp 581 – 590

23. Johnsson G, Regardh CG (1976) Clinical pharmacokinetics of β-adrenoceptor blocking drugs. Clin Pharmacokinet 1:233 – 263
24. Waal-Manning HJ (1976) Hypertension: Which beta-blocker? Drugs 12:412 – 441
25. Saameli K (1972) Die pharmakologische Charakterisierung β-sympathikolytischer Substanzen. In: Dengler HJ (Hrsg) Die therapeutische Anwendung β-sympathikolytischer Stoffe. Schattauer, Stuttgart New York, S 3 – 30
26. Angelakos ET, Carballo LC, Daniels JB, King MB, Bajusz E (1972) Adrenergic neurohumors in the heart of hamsters with hereditary myopathy during cardiac hypertrophy and failure. In: Bajusz E, Rona G (eds) Recent advances in studies on cardiac structure and metabolism, vol 1. University Park Press, Baltimore, pp 262 – 278
27. Angelakos ET, King MB, Carballo LC (1973) Cardiac adrenergic innervation in hamsters with hereditary myocardiopathy: Chemical and histochemical studies. In: Bajusz E, Rona G (eds) Recent advances in studies on cardiac structure and metabolism, vol. 2. University Park Press, Baltimore, pp 519 – 531
28. Bester AJ, Gevers W, Hawtrey AO (1973) A possible defect in protein synthesis underlying inherited cardiomyopathy of Syrian hamsters. In: Recent advances in studies on cardiac structure and metabolism, vol 2. University Park Press, Baltimore, pp 533 – 541
29. Selye H (1961) The pluricausal cardiopathies. Thomas, Springfield/Ill
30. Bajusz E (1963) Conditioning factors for cardiac necroses. Karger, Basel New York
31. Kaltenbach M, Hopf R, Keller M (1976) Calciumantagonistische Therapie bei hypertrophisch-obstruktiver Kardiomyopathie. Dtsch Med Wochenschr 101:1284 – 1287
32. Kuhn E (1978) Kardiomyopathien. Fortschr Med 96:705 – 708
33. Meerschwam IS, Hootsmans WJM (1971) An electromyographic study in hypertrophic obstructive cardiomyopathy. In: Wolstenholme GEW, O'Connor M (eds) Hypertrophic obstructive cardiomyopathy (CIBA Foundation Group 37.) Churchill, London, pp 55 – 62
34. Weisenfeld S, Messinger WJ (1952) Cardiac involvement in progressive muscular dystrophy. Am Heart J 43:170 – 187
35. Rubin JL, Buchberg AS (1952) The heart in progressive muscular dystrophy. Am Heart J 43:161 – 169
36. James TN (1962) Observations on the cardiovascular involvement, including the cardiac conduction system, in progressive muscular dystrophy. Am Heart J 63:48 – 56
37. Perloff JK, Roberts WC, De Leon AC, O'Doherty D (1967) The distinctive electrocardiogram of Duchenne's progressive muscular dystrophy. Am J Med 42:179 – 188
38. Beckmann R, Schmit B (1976) Das Herz bei Muskelerkrankungen. Med Klin 71:1135 – 1145
39. Schmidt-Redemann B, Beckmann R, Schaupeter W, Schmidt-Redemann W, Vogt J (1978) Kardiomyopathie bei Duchenne'scher Muskeldystrophie. Med Klin 73:1621 – 1626
40. Graham GR (1964) Friedreich's disease. In: Wolstenholme GEW, O'Connor M (eds) Cardiomyopathies (CIBA Foundation Symposium). Churchill, London, pp 358 – 370
41. Wrogemann K, Pena SDJ (1976) Mitochondrial calcium overload: A general mechanism for cell-necrosis in muscle diseases. Lancet I:672 – 674

Klinische Ergebnisse der calciumantagonistischen Therapie bei Patienten mit hypertroph obstruktiver Kardiomyopathie

R. Hopf, R. Lemke, G. Kober und M. Kaltenbach

Der erste pathologisch-anatomische Bericht über die ätiologisch noch immer ungeklärte hypertroph obstruktive Kardiomyopathie (HOCM) stammt von Schmincke [1]. In der Folgezeit geriet das Krankheitsbild in Vergessenheit, bis sich ab 1952, beginnend mit einer Publikation von Davies [2], weitere Berichte häuften.

Mit der Einführung der Beta-Sympatholytika (Propranolol im Jahre 1964) schien eine spezifische Behandlungsmöglichkeit gefunden zu sein [3 – 5]. Verlaufskontrollen konnten jedoch zeigen, daß der gewünschte Therapieerfolg weder durch Beta-Sympatholytika noch durch die alternativ in Betracht kommende Operation [6 – 8] sicher erreicht werden konnte [9, 10].

Da die Entwicklung der Hypertrophie bei der HOCM nicht nur durch einen erhöhten Sympathikotonus hervorgerufen sein kann, da sonst die betasympatholytische Therapie erfolgreich sein müßte, galt es, Alternativen zu suchen. Wiederholt wurde die Bedeutung des Calciums bei bestimmten Formen von Kardiomyopathien und eine erfolgversprechende Behandlungsmöglichkeit mit Calcium-Antagonisten beschrieben [5, 11, 12, 13]. Es lag daher trotz der Unterschiede gegenüber anderen Kardiomyopathien nahe, die Behandlungsmöglichkeit der HOCM mit Calcium-Antagonisten zu überprüfen. Erste Ergebnisse waren ermutigend [14, 15], so daß diese Form der Therapie an einer größeren Patientenzahl über längere Zeit hinweg überprüft werden sollte.

Patienten und Methode

39 Patienten mit HOCM wurden in die Untersuchung einbezogen. Es handelte sich um 31 Männer und 8 Frauen im Alter zwischen 15 und 63, im Mittel von 43,3 Jahren. In allen Fällen war die Diagnose durch Rechts- und Linksherzkatheterismus mit selektiver Koronarangiographie sowie Kineangiographie des linken und in einigen Fällen auch zusätzlich des rechten Ventrikels gesichert. Bei 35 Patienten ließ sich ein sicherer linksventrikulärer Druckgradient zwischen 15 und 200, im Mittel von 82 mmHg, bestimmen. 13 Patienten hatten einen rechtsventrikulären Druckgradienten zwischen 5 und 15, im Mittel von 9,5 mmHg. In allen Fällen wurde die Diagnose zusätzlich echokardiographisch gesichert.

28 der 39 Patienten konnten vor Einleitung der calciumantagonistischen Therapie zwischen 1 und 100 Monaten, im Mittel über 26,4 Monate, beobachtet werden. 13 dieser Patienten waren mit Beta-Sympatholytika behandelt worden, 2 hatten Digitalispräparate erhalten. Nach Absetzen dieser Medikationen erhielten 38 Patienten als alleinige Therapie Verapamil, 1 Patientin erhielt Nifedipin. Verapamil wurde in zeitlich kurzen Schritten auf 480 mg täglich gesteigert oder sofort mit 480 mg täglich begonnen. In 4 Fällen erfolgte eine Erhöhung der täglichen Dosis auf 720 mg. Von 9 Patienten ist eine schlechte Einnahmedisziplin bekannt, zumindest vorübergehend

wurde die Tagesdosis eigenmächtig reduziert. 1 Patient weigerte sich nach 22 Monaten wegen inzwischen subjektiv guten Befindens weiterhin Verapamil einzunehmen. Das bei einer Patientin zur Behandlung eingesetzte Nifedipin wurde mit 30 mg oral täglich dosiert.

Die Behandlungsdauer beträgt inzwischen 3 bis 56, im Mittel 25,7 Monate. 11 der 39 Patienten konnten unter der calciumantagonistischen Behandlung länger als 36 Monate beobachtet werden.

Die Patienten wurden in regelmäßigen Abständen nachuntersucht, wobei neben der Zwischenanamnese und dem klinischen Befund, dem Elektrokardiogramm mit mindestens 12 Ableitungen, dem Herzvolumen und Thoraxröntgenbefund sowie dem Echokardiogramm besondere Bedeutung beigemessen wurden. Neben den üblichen Laboratoriumuntersuchungen wurden bei der letzten Kontrolle zusätzlich die Verapamil-Serumspiegel bestimmt. Hierbei wurden morgens nüchtern und damit etwa 12 bis 14 Std nach der letzten Medikamenteneinnahme der „Basisspiegel" und dann 60 min nach Einnahme der morgendlichen Dosis der „Maximalspiegel" gemessen.[1]

Ergebnisse

30 der 39 Patienten gaben unter der calciumantagonistischen Therapie eine Abnahme ihrer Beschwerden und eine Verbesserung ihrer körperlichen Leistungsfähigkeit an. Bei einem Teil dieser Fälle kam es zu völliger Beschwerdefreiheit. 8 Patienten konnten keine wesentliche Änderung ihres Befindens bemerken, bei ihnen handelte es sich vorwiegend um Kranke mit primärer Beschwerdefreiheit, oder solchen mit nur gering ausgeprägten Beschwerden. In einem Fall nahmen die Beschwerden bei unveränderten objektiven Befunden allmählich zu. Auch in den Fällen, die unter calciumantagonistischer Therapie den objektiven Parametern nach gering progredient waren, wurde meist eine subjektive Besserung angegeben.

Leichte subjektive Nebenwirkungen, wie Schwitzneigung und geringer Kopfschmerz, waren in keinem Fall sicher auf die Therapie zu beziehen und klangen in allen Fällen spontan wieder ab. Eine Patientin verweigerte nach 17 Monaten die weitere Tabletteneinnahme, weil eine schon vorbestehende Oedemneigung zugenommen habe.

Auf Grund der objektiven Kontrollbefunde war in 25 der 39 Fälle eine Besserung des Krankheitsbildes zu sichern. Unverändert blieben die Befunde von 8 Patienten. In den restlichen 6 Fällen ergaben sich Hinweise auf eine langsame Progredienz der Krankheit.

Der klinische Untersuchungsbefund änderte sich während der Behandlungszeit nicht eindeutig. Erwähnenswert ist eine bei einem Teil der Patienten zu beobachtende Abschwächung des systolischen Geräuschbefundes. Bei Hypertonikern konnte eine Erniedrigung des Blutdruckes beobachtet werden, hypotone Dysregulationen wurden unter der Langzeitbehandlung nicht beobachtet.

Meß- und auswertbare Veränderungen wiesen Elektrokardiogramm, Röntgen- und echokardiographische Befunde auf.

---

1 Die Bestimmung erfolgte durch: Zentrum der Pharmakologie, Abteilung II, Klinikum der Johann Wolfgang Goethe-Universität, Frankfurt am Main (Leiter: Prof. Dr. med. Rietbrock)

Als elektrokardiographisch bedeutsamer Parameter wurde das Verhalten der Linkshypertrophiezeichen untersucht (Abb. 1). Der Sokolow-Lyon-Index (festgelegt nach tiefster S-Zacke und höchster R-Zacke in den Brustwandableitungen) nahm in der Vorbeobachtungszeit signifikant von im Mittel 4,46 auf 4,87 mV zu ($p < 0,0005$), obwohl 12 dieser 25 Patienten betasympatholytisch behandelt wurden.

Um den Einfluß der calciumantagonistischen Therapie beurteilen zu können, wurde unter Berücksichtigung der jeweils in diesem Zeitraum nachuntersuchten Patienten die Gesamtdauer der Behandlung in 6monatige Intervalle unterteilt und für sich betrachtet. Im Verlauf der ersten 6 Monate der calciumantagonistischen Therapie kam es zu einer Abnahme des Sokolow-Index auf 3,97 mV ($p < 0,0005$). Die Abnahme des Sokolow-Index betrug durchschnittlich 0,55 mV entsprechend 11,6% und ließ sich über 42 Monate hinweg beobachten (Abb. 2 u. 3).

Die mittlere Ruhe-Herzfrequenz (Abb. 4) lag vor Einleitung der calciumantagonistischen Therapie bei 71/min. Durch die Behandlung wurde sie signifikant um 9/min, entsprechend 12,4%, gesenkt ($p < 0,0125$). Der Effekt war in den ersten 6 bis 12 Monaten am deutlichsten und bildete sich dann langsam zurück.

Die konventionellen Thorax-Röntgenbilder erbrachten weder qualitativ noch quantitativ Befundänderungen und ließen eine unter Therapie auftretende Linksherzinsuffizienz ausschließen.

Auffallend war eine Verkleinerung des röntgenologisch ermittelten Herzvolumens (Abb. 5). Während der Vorbeobachtungszeit (teilweise unter betasympatholytischer Therapie) konnte eine durchschnittliche Vergrößerung des Herzvolumens von 879 auf 939 ml/1,73 m² Körperoberfläche beobachtet werden (obere Normgrenze für Männer 790 und für Frauen 690 ml/1,73 m² Körperoberfläche). Dieser signifikanten

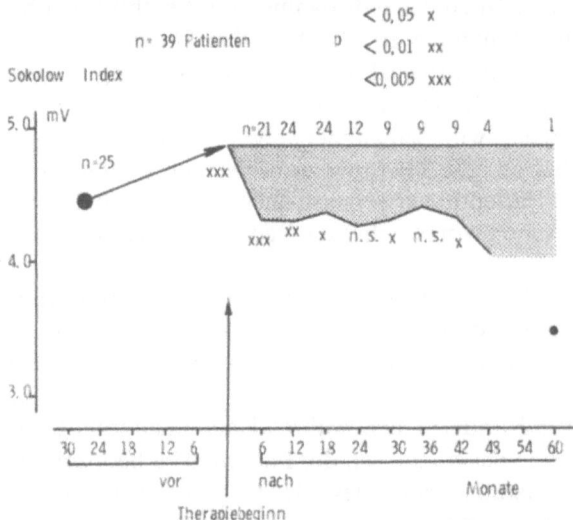

Abb. 1. Verhalten der Linkshypertrophiezeichen im EKG (Sokolow-Lyon-Index): Während einer durchschnittlich 26,4monatigen Vorperiode bei 25 der 39 Patienten mit HOCM nahm der Sokolow-Index von 4,46 auf 4,87 mV zu; 12 dieser Patienten wurden mit Beta-Sympatholytika behandelt. Unter der calciumantagonistischen Therapie nahm der Sokolow-Index durchschnittlich um 0,5 mV entsprechend 11,6% ab. Der Behandlungserfolg bleibt, mit einem Maximum nach 6 bis 12 Monaten, über 42 Monate nachweisbar

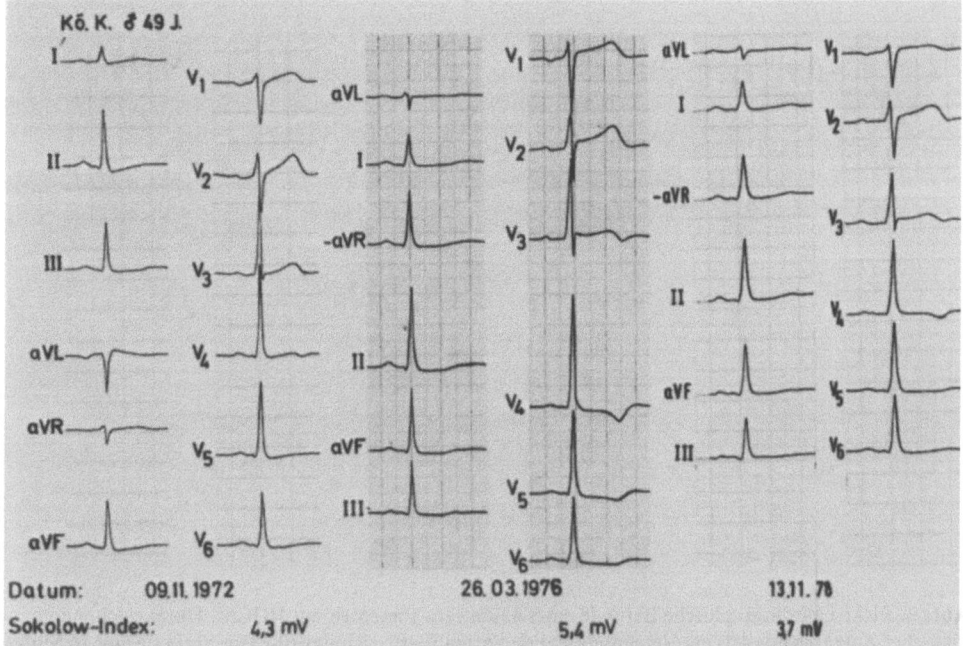

Abb. 2. Elektrokardiographische Befunde eines 49jährigen Patienten mit HOCM. Die Hypertrophiezeichen im EKG nahmen trotz betasympatholytischer Therapie vom November 1972 bis März 1976 langsam zu. Gleichzeitig vergrößerte sich das Herzvolumen von 600 auf 860 ml/1,73 m² Körperoberfläche. Unter Therapie mit 480 mg Verapamil täglich erniedrigte sich der Sokolow-Index unter gleichzeitiger Abnahme der Endteilveränderungen. (Das Herzvolumen verkleinerte sich auf 830 ml/1,73 m² Körperoberfläche)

Größenzunahme ($p < 0,0005$) folgte unter Behandlung mit Calcium-Antagonisten im Verlauf von 24 Monaten eine Verkleinerung um 110 ml entsprechend 11,9% ($p < 0,0025$). Danach nahmen die Herzvolumina in Einzelfällen wieder langsam an Größe zu.

Die Abnahme der Hypertrophiezeichen im EKG und des röntgenologischen Herzvolumens werden durch echokardiographische und angiographische Befunde in Einzelfällen bestätigt und teilweise erklärt:

Die echokardiographischen Befunde lassen zwar derzeit eine statistische Auswertung noch nicht zu, da viele Patienten nicht vom Behandlungsbeginn an sonographisch verfolgt werden konnten, es zeichnet sich jedoch folgendes Resultat ab: Alle Patienten haben kleine Ventrikel mit hoher Auswurffraktion, die sich auch unter Behandlung nicht ändern. Patienten mit großem Herzvolumen haben auffallend vergrößerte linke Vorhöfe, die sich unter calciumantagonistischer Behandlung deutlich, der Herzvolumenänderung entsprechend, verkleinern.

Einzelbefunde von solchen Patienten, die bereits vor Beginn der calciumantagonistischen Behandlung echokardiographisch untersucht werden konnten, zeigen, wie am Beispiel einer 25jährigen Patientin belegt, Abnahme von Septum- und Hinterwanddicke. Das Beispiel einer weiteren, 42jährigen Patientin, zeigt die Abnahme und das Verschwinden der systolischen Vorwärtsbewegung des vorderen Mitralsegels (SAM), klinisch verbunden mit einem letztlich nicht mehr hörbaren, zuvor lauten Mitralinsuffizienzgeräusch (Abb. 6 u. 7).

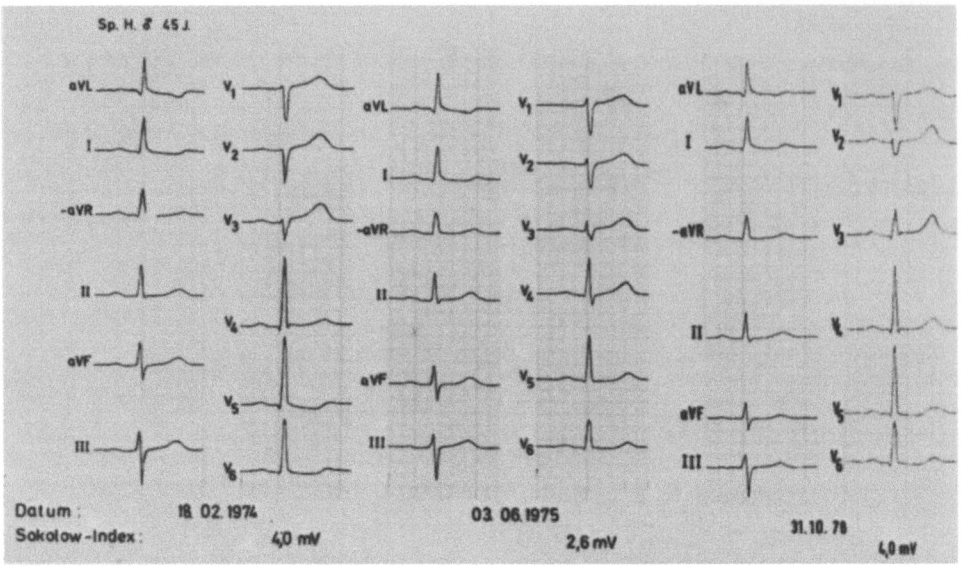

Abb. 3. Elektrokardiographische Befunde eines 45jährigen Patienten mit HOCM. Unter calciumantagonistischer Therapie mit 480 mg Verapamil täglich normalisierte sich das EKG im Verlaufe von 16 Monaten. In dieser Zeit nahm das Herzvolumen von 900 auf 775 ml/1,73 m² Körperoberfläche ab. Wegen eingetretener Beschwerdefreiheit setzte der Patient eigenmächtig die Therapie ab; in der Folgezeit nahmen die Hypertrophiezeichen wieder langsam zu. Das Herzvolumen vergrößerte sich auf 880 ml/1,73 m² Körperoberfläche

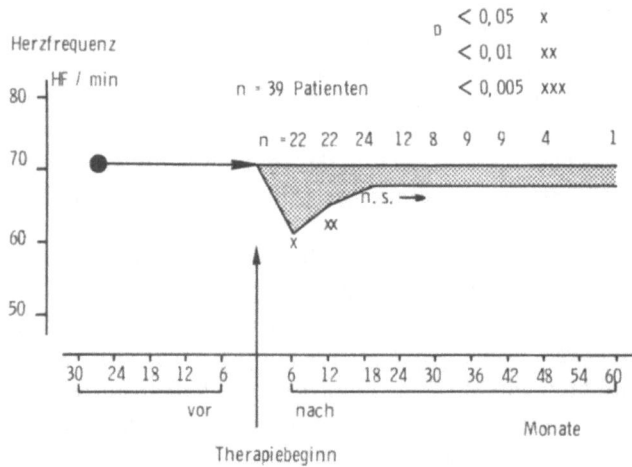

Abb. 4. Abnahme und allmähliches Wiederansteigen der Ruhefrequenz unter Verapamil-Behandlung

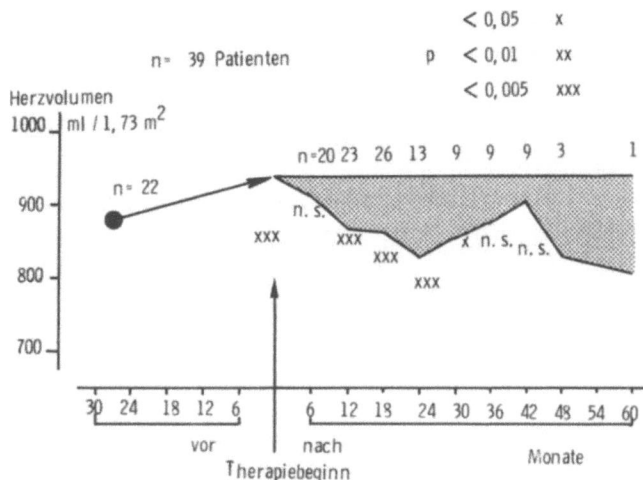

Abb. 5. Während der Vorperiode nahm das röntgenologisch bestimmte Herzvolumen von durchschnittlich 879 auf 939 ml/1,73 m² Körperoberfläche zu. Unter Verapamil-Behandlung kam es nach 24 Monaten zu einer Verkleinerung auf 811 ml/173 m². In Einzelfällen nahm danach das Herz langsam wieder an Größe zu

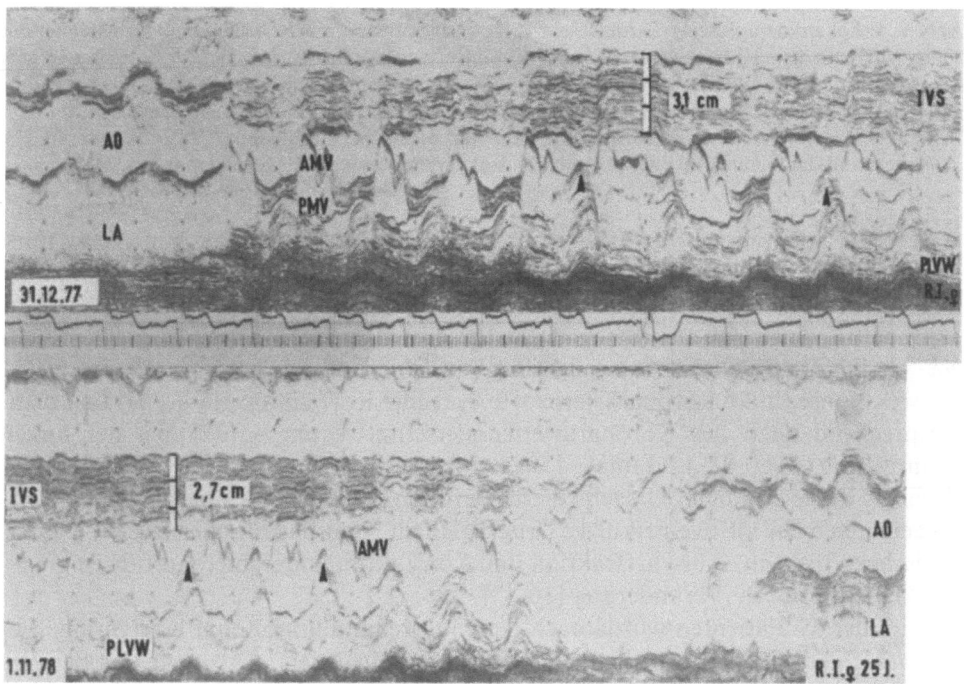

Abb. 6. Echokardiographischer Befund einer 25jährigen Patientin mit HOCM. Unter calciumantagonistischer Behandlung mit 480 mg Verapamil täglich nahmen Septum- und Hinterwanddicke ab. *Zeichenerklärung:* AO = Aorta; LA = linker Vorhof; IVS = Septum; PLVW = Hinterwand des linken Ventrikels; AMV = vordere Mitralklappe; PMV = hintere Mitralklappe; ▲ = systolische Vorwärtsbewegung der Mitralklappe (SAM)

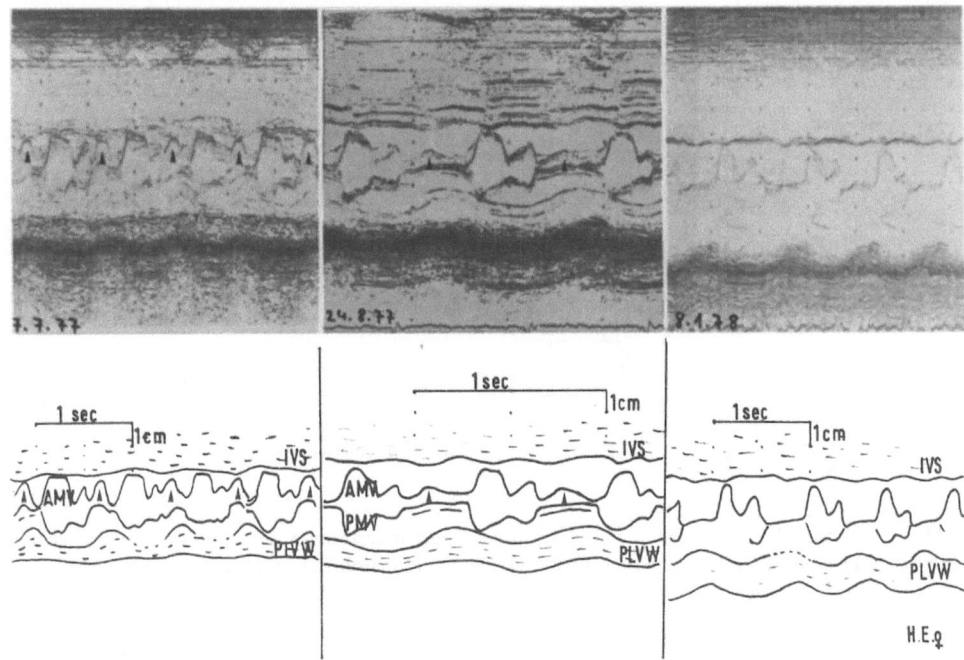

Abb. 7. Echokardiographischer Befund einer 42jährigen Patientin mit HOCM. Unter Behandlung mit 30 mg Nifedipin täglich verschwand das laute Mitralinsuffizienzgeräusch, echokardiographisch zeigt sich ein Verschwinden der systolischen Vorwärtsbewegung des vorderen Mitralsegels (SAM). Die Herzgröße nahm im Verlauf der 17monatigen Behandlung von 890 auf 760 ml/1,73 m² Körperoberfläche ab.
Zeichenerklärung: AMV = vordere Mitralklappe; PMV = hintere Mitralklappe; IVS = Septum; PLVW = Hinterwand des linken Ventrikels; systolische Vorwärtsbewegung der Mitralklappe (SAM) ▲

Bei 10 Patienten wurde nach einer durchschnittlich 19monatigen Verapamil-Behandlung im Anschluß an ein kurzes therapiefreies Intervall eine Kontrollkathe-teruntersuchung vorgenommen.

Im Mittel hatte sich bei diesen Patienten die linksventrikuläre Muskelmasse um 9% verringert, parallel damit ging eine Verkleinerung des Koronararteriendurch-messers einher (linke Koronararterie − 9%, rechte Koronararterie − 8%) und dem-entsprechend auch des Koronararterienquerschnittes um − 17% bei der linken Kranzarterie ($p < 0,01$) und um − 15% bei der rechten Kranzarterie ($p < 0,01$) [10]. Wohl als Folge und nicht Ursache dieser Befunde reduzierte sich parallel dazu über-wiegend auch der intraventrikuläre Druckgradient. Enddiastolischer Druck, enddia-stolisches Volumen, Auswurffraktion und Kontraktilitätsparameter erfuhren hinge-gen keine gerichtete Veränderung [16, 17].

Bei 7 der 39 Patienten wurde nach dem 30. Behandlungsmonat eine geringe Be-fundverschlechterung beobachtet. Hierfür könnte in 3 der 7 Fälle eine von den Pa-tienten angegebene nachlassende Disziplin in der Tabletteneinahme verantwortlich sein. In anderen Fällen könnte jedoch auch ein Gewöhnungseffekt gegenüber Calcium-Antagonisten und die bei manchen Patienten zu beobachtende deutliche Progradienz der HOCM ursächlich in Frage kommen.

Bei 4 der 39 Patienten erfolgte ein Medikamentenauslaßversuch, in einem Fall, weil der Patient keine Medikamente mehr nehmen wollte, in drei Fällen mußte die

Behandlung wegen größerer Operationen vorübergehend ausgesetzt werden. In allen Fällen kam es zu einer Zunahme der Hypertrophiezeichen im EKG und zu einer Größenzunahme des Herzens. In den drei letzteren Fällen ließ sich nach Wiederaufnahme der Therapie der Behandlungserfolg reproduzieren.

Zusammenfassung und Diskussion

Die vorgelegten Befunde zeigen, daß eine hochdosierte orale Behandlung mit Calcium-Antagonisten bei einem Großteil der Patienten mit HOCM eine erstaunliche subjektive und objektive Besserung des Krankheitsbildes erbringen kann.

Erste Messungen des Verapamil-Serumspiegels lassen eine positive Beziehung zwischen Blutspiegel und Ausmaß des Therapieerfolges vermuten.

Die Befundbesserung läßt sich objektivieren durch:

1. eine Abnahme der subjektiven Beschwerden,
2. eine Leistungsverbesserung,
3. einer Verkleinerung des Herzens,
4. eine Abnahme der Hypertrophiezeichen im EKG, wobei
5. die Verkleinerung des Herzens, quantifiziert durch das röntgenologisch ermittelte Herzvolumen, insbesondere auf eine Volumenabnahme des linken Vorhofes zurückzuführen ist. Die Abnahme der Hypertrophiezeichen im EKG, bzw. die teilweise völlige Normalisierung, entspricht einer echokardiographisch und angiographisch nachweisbaren Wanddickenabnahme des linken Ventrikels.

Über den Wirkungsmechanismus der Calcium-Antagonisten bei der Therapie der HOCM können bislang nur Vermutungen angestellt werden. Zu diskutieren sind:

1. ein direkter Angriff der Calcium-Antagonisten an der Herzmuskelzelle, der im Gegensatz steht zu der extrazellulären Beta-Blockade,
2. eine periphere Wirkung mit anhaltender Verminderung der Nachbelastung des Herzens, ohne reflektorische Frequenz- und Kontraktilitätserhöhung.

Literatur

1. Schmincke A (1970) Über linksseitige muskuläre Conusstenosen. Dtsch Med Wochenschr 33:1082
2. Davies DH (1952) A familial heart disease. Br Heart J 14:206
3. Bliss HA, Moffat JE, Gautt CL (1967) Effects of chronic oral propranolol therapy in idiopathic hypertrophic subaortic stenosis. Circulation [Suppl II] 35,36:72
4. Cherian G, Brockington IF, Shah PM, Oakly CM, Goodwin JF (1966) Beta-adrenergic blockade in hypertrophic obstructive cardiomyopathy. Br Med J I:895
5. Lossnitzer K (1975) Genetic induction of cardiomyopathy. In: Borm GVR, Eichler O, Farah A, Herken H, Welch AD (Hrsg) Springer, Berlin Heidelberg New York (Handbuch der experimentellen Pharmakologie, Bd 16/3, S 309–344)
6. Epstein SE, Morrow AG, Henry WL, Clark CE (1973) The role of operative treatment in patients with IHSS. Circulation 48:677
7. Heinrich F (1967) Die hypertrophischen Subaortenstenosen. Med Welt 18:1528,1567
8. Morrow AG (1975) Operative treatment in hypertrophic subaortic stenosis. Techniques and the results of pre- and postoperative assessments in 83 patients. Circulation 52:88–102
9. Kuhn H, Loogen F (1978) Die Anwendung von Beta-Rezeptorenblockern bei hypertrophischer obstruktiver Kardiomyopathie. Internist (Berlin) 19:527–531

10. Loogen F, Krelhaus W, Kuhn H (1976) Verlaufsbeobachtungen der hypertrophischen obstruktiven Kardiomyopathie (HOCM). Z Kardiol 65:511 – 521
11. Daniels JR, Billingham ME, Gelhart A, Bristow MR (1976) Effect of verapamil and propranolol on adriamycin-induced cardiomyopathy in rabbits. 4th Sess Am Heart Assoc Abstr 70
12. Fleckenstein A (1969) Myokardstoffwechsel und Nekrose. In: Heilmeyer L, Holtmeier HJ (Hrsg) Herzinfarkt und Schock. Thieme, Stuttgart, S 94 – 109
13. Wrogemann K, Pena SDJ (1976) Mitochondrial calcium overload. A general mechanism for cell necrosis in muscle disease. Lancet I:672
14. Hopf R, Keller M, Kaltenbach M (1976) Die Behandlung der hypertrophen obstruktiven Kardio-myopathie mit Verapamil. Verh Dtsch Ges Inn Med 82:1054 – 1057
15. Kaltenbach M, Hopf R, Keller M (1976) Calciumantagonistische Therapie bei hypertroph-obstruktiver Kardiomyopathie. Dtsch Med Wochenschr 101:1284 – 1287
16. Kaltenbach M, Hopf R, Kober G, Bussmann W-D, Keller M, Petersen Y (1978) Verapamil treatment of hypertrophic obstructive cardiomyopathy. In: Kaltenbach M, Loogen F, Olsen EGJ (eds) Cardiomyopathy and myocardial biopsy. Springer, Berlin Heidelberg New York, pp 316 – 331
17. Kaltenbach M, Hopf R, Kober G, Bussmann W-D, Keller M, Petersen Y (1979) Treatment of hypertrophic obstructive cardiomyopathy with verapamil. Br Heart J 42:35 – 42
18. Wolstenholme GEW, O'Connor M (1964) Cardiomyopathies. Ciba Found. Symp. J. a. A. Churchill, London

Protection of the Globally Ischemic Heart with Calcium-Antagonists: Improved Recovery After Cardiopulmonary Bypass

P. D. Henry, R. E. Clark, and J. R. Williamson

Calcium plays an important role in the regulation of the energy metabolism of cardiac muscle [1–4], and disturbances in the amount and distribution of intracellular calcium may be expected to affect the energetics of myocardial cells. In a number of studies, myocardial injury has been found to be associated with myocardial accumulation of calcium [5–9].

In most tissues calcium is highly compartmentalized with ionic activities across cellular and subcellular membranes differing often by a factor of 1,000 or more [10]. As cell membranes and membranes of subcellular organelles are not impermeable to calcium, the very high differences in calcium activities across membranous boundaries must be maintained by active mechanisms. Metabolic alterations interfering with such active processes may be expected to result in passive electrolyte shifts across membranes along prevailing electrochemical activity gradients [9]. It has been indeed well documented that ischemic or otherwise metabolically inhibited cells tend to lose potassium, magnesium, and phosphate, and gain sodium, calcium, and chloride, changes that may be explained on the basis of passive electrolyte shifts. In muscle cells accumulation of calcium might be particularly deleterious as it may enhance ATP hydrolysis by inappropriately activating the myofibrillar apparatus, and inhibit ATP synthesis by interfering with oxidative phosphorylation in the mitochondria [1,4]. Such a process could conceivably aggravate and perpetuate the energy crisis of the cell.

In previous studies we have demonstrated that isolated rabbit hearts perfused at low flow undergo a contracture that is associated with an accumulation of calcium in the mitochondrial fraction [9]. Administration of nifedipine during the period of low flow inhibited the development of contracture, prevented the accumulation of mitochondrial calcium, and promoted mechanical recovery during subsequent reperfusion [9]. In other experiments, nifedipine was found to increase collateral flow and minimize ischemic injury in conscious dogs subjected to acute coronary occlusion [11].

It is well known that the globally ischemic heart during cardiopulmonary bypass may undergo a contracture and that myocardial infarction may complicate open heart surgery [12]. In view of our previous experiments on global ischemia in the perfused rabbit heart and in myocardial infarction in conscious dogs, we wondered whether administration of calcium antagonists during cardiopulmonary bypass may exert a protective effect on the ischemic myocardium. Furthermore, we have performed additional experiments with isolated perfused hearts to determine mechanisms that may be operative in promoting the explosive deterioration of the ischemic heart subjected to reperfusion. Results indicate that nifedipine protects the globally ischemic heart during cardiopulmonary bypass and that mechanical factors may play an important role in determining the precipitous deterioration of the ischemic heart during reperfusion.

Materials and Methods

Isolated Perfused Heart Preparation

Rabbit hearts were isolated and perfused retrograde at 37 °C through the aorta as previously described [9]. The perfusate contrained (mM): NaCl, 118; KCl, 3.8; KH$_2$PO$_4$, 1.2; CaCl$_2$, 2.5; MgSO$_4$, 1.2; NaHCO$_3$, 25; and glucose, 5. After equilibration with a 5% CO$_2$ − 95% O$_2$ gas mixture, the pH was approximately 7.4. If not otherwise specified the rate of perfusion was maintained at 22 ml/min with a roller pump. The right atrium was opened widely, and multiple cuts were performed with microscissors in the A-V nodal area until the perfused heart went into ventricular standstill. A latex balloon mounted around a micromanometer (Konigsberg Model P 3.5) was inserted into the left ventricular cavity for measurement of left ventricular pressure and dP/dt. The balloon was connected via a short cannula to a pulse duplicator (pulsatile pump). A bipolar electrode was attached to the right ventricular free wall and the heart paced at a frequency of 180/min. The manometric system including the balloon and the pump was gradually filled with deaerated saline until end-diastolic pressure stabilized between 5 and 8 mm Hg. Thus, in this preparation, major determinants of cardiac performance including ventricular preload and afterload, cardiac frequency, coronary flow, and temperature were controlled, and left ventricular dP/dt and end-diastolic pressure were used as indexes of contractility and diastolic elastic stiffness (compliance), respectively. During electric pacing and with the pulsatile pump in "off" position, pressure events reflected the contractile activity of the heart. With the pacer in "off" position hearts went into immediate ventricular standstill. By actuating the pump it was possible to produce inside of the manometric system pulsatile pressure events that mimicked in contour and frequency those generated by ventricular contraction. In addition, a manometric servo-mechanism permitted peak pressure to be held at the same level as that observed during active beating. All hearts were equilibrated for 30 min at a coronary flow rate of 22 ml/min and a paced frequency of 180/min. In one group of hearts, perfusion under these conditions was continued for another 60 min. In another group, perfusion at low flow (.22 ml/min) was instituted and continued for 60 min under continued electric pacing. At the end of this low flow period all hearts were in ischemic ventricular standstill. In the high flow group, asystole at the end of the 60 min period was produced by switching off the pacer. Subsequently, all hearts were passively pulsed to a peak pressure of approximately 80 mm Hg at a rate of 180/min for 15 s. At the end of passive mechanical pulsing, the hearts were perfused under a hydrostatic pressure of 80 mm Hg with 1.5% gluteraldehyde and 1.25 formaldehyde for fixation for light and electron-microscopic studies [13].

Cardiopulmonary Bypass in Dogs

For studies of global ischemia, dogs were subjected to cardiopulmonary bypass [14]. In one series of experiments, conditions were designed to mimic those currently utilized clinically and included systemic hypothermia (28 °C), topical hypothermia, priming with Ringer's lactate containing glucose (30 mM), KCl (40 mM), insulin

(60 U/l), and mannitol (60 mM). After institution of hypothermia the animals were placed on total cardiopulmonary bypass for 2 h. A systemic loading dose of nifedipine, 20 µg/kg, was administered followed by continuous infusion into the aortic root of nifedipine and saline at a rate of 5 µg/kg/h. The amount of saline infused into the aorta was 2.5 ml/kg/h and was the same for treated and control animals. No drug was administered before or after bypass.

In other experiments, dogs were subjected to 1 h of cardiopulmonary bypass under normothermic conditions (37 °C). In these experiments, nifedipine in saline was administered into the aortic root at the rate of 2 µg/kg/h. The amount of saline infused into the aorta was 12 ml/kg/h in both control and treated animals. Additional control experiments were performed in which Normosol, or saline containing 25 mM KCl, or a cardioplegic solution were infused at the same rate of 12 ml/kg/h. The cardioplegic solution contained (mM): Na, 154; K, 24.3; Mg, 2.7; Cl, 115; HCO_3, 23; acetate, 23; and gluconate, 22. The solution contained also 60 mM glucose; insulin, 1.8 U/l; and lidocaine, 0.4 g/l.

Results

Isolated Heart Experiments

Figure 1 illustrates how the turning off of the pacer produced instantaneous asystole. Note that upon restarting the pacer there was an initial strong beat followed by a weak beat and a gradual, staircase-like increase in the force of the contractions, a phenomenon that was very reproducible.

Figure 2 depicts an experiment with a heart perfused at high flow for 60 min. After this interval, asystole was produced by switching the pacer off, and the heart was subsequently passively pulsed for 15 s. It can be seen that peak pressure was practically identical to that produced by the heart during electric pacing and that diastolic pressure did not change. Practically identical results were obtained in 12 hearts perfused at high flow.

Figure 3 is a representative tracing of an experiment with a heart subjected to low flow perfusion. Immediately after institution of low flow, there was a precipitous decline in developed left ventricular pressure. Mechanical standstill occurred 18 min after onset of ischemia. Subsequently, nonpulsatile ventricular pressure gradually rose and was 54 mm Hg at the end of 60 min of ischemia. In 12 hearts subjected to

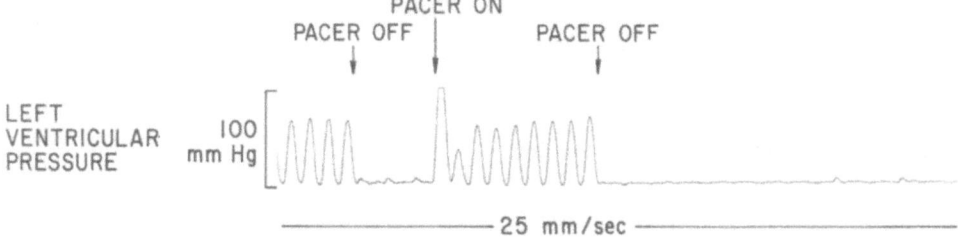

Fig. 1. Isolated perfused rabbit heart with excised A-V node

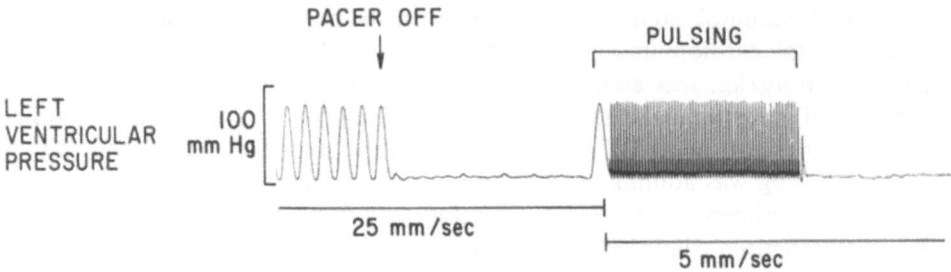

Fig. 2. Pulsing of non-ischemic heart

this protocol, ischemic standstill occurred after 17.5 ± 1.1 (SE) min, and contracture pressure at 60 min averaged 55 ± 4 mm Hg. In contrast to the high flow hearts, diastolic pressure during passive pulsing fell on average by 11 ± 1 mm Hg, a change that was significant to the 0.001 level by paired t-test. Thus, mechanical changes illustrated in this figure were highly reproducible.

Figure 4 shows representative electronmicrographs from the left ventricular free wall of hearts perfused for 60 min at high flow *(left hand side)* or low flow *(right hand side)* without subsequent passive pulsing. Note that in the high flow heart the mitochondria are present in their electron-dense configuration, whereas the low flow heart exhibits swollen mitochondria typical of myocardial ischemia. Absence of myofibrillar contracture in the ischemic heart may reflect the fact that the isovolumic preparation prevents muscle shortening. Pulsing was without effect on the ultrastructure of high flow hearts (Fig. 5), but markedly altered cellular organization in low flow hearts (Fig. 6). Disarrays as shown in Fig. 6 were never observed in ischemic hearts not subjected to passive pulsing.

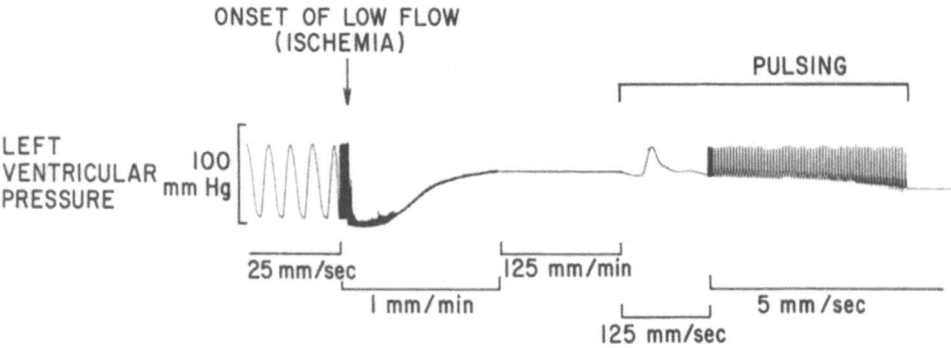

Fig. 3. Pulsing of heart after 60 min of low flow

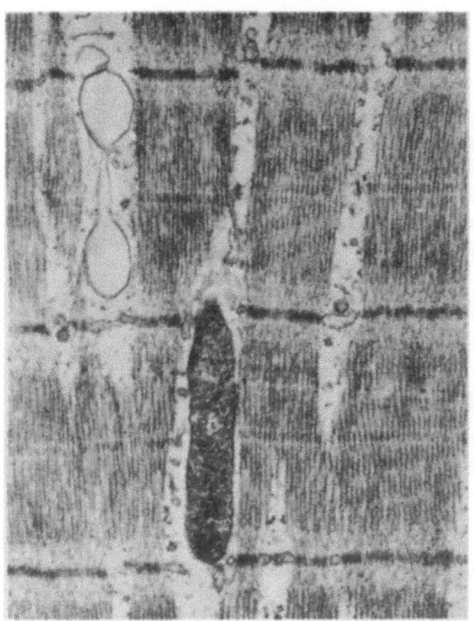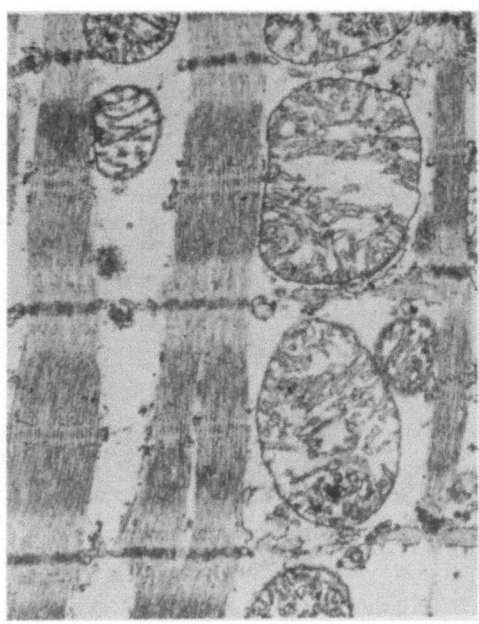

Fig. 4

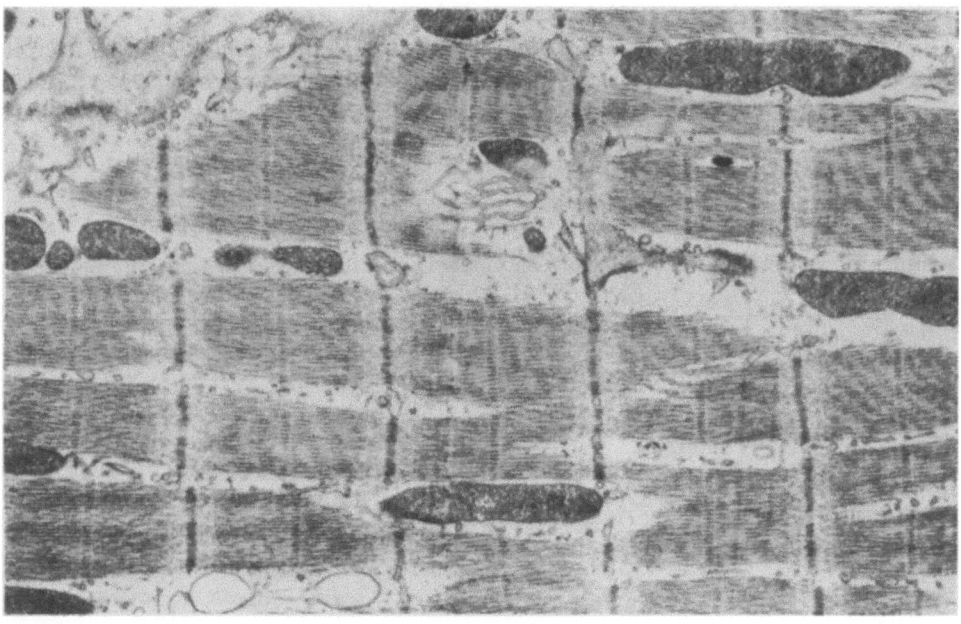

Fig. 5

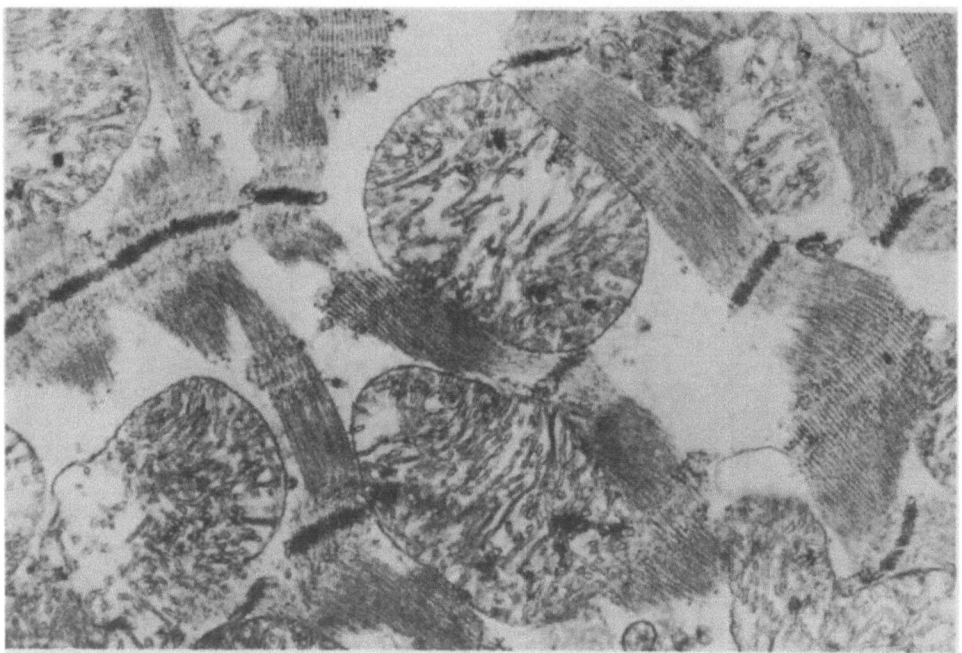

Fig. 6

Light microscopy revealed no histological differences between high flow hearts without passive pulsing and those with passive pulsing.

In summary, passive pulsing produced no appreciable changes in end-diastolic pressure and structure in nonischemic hearts. In contrast, passive pulsing produced in ischemic hearts a fall in end-diastolic pressure, an index of elastic stiffness, and a disruption of cellular architecture.

Table 1. Light microscopic frequency of cellular ruptures in low flow (ischemic) hearts with and without passive pulsing

Cell fractures in control and ischemic hearts, with and without mechanical pulsing			
	Not pulsed	Pulsed	p-Value
Non-ischemic	1.00[a] (n = 6)	1.11 ± 0.73 (n = 6)	>0.1
Ischemic	4.11 ± 0.26 (n = 6)	8.33 ± 0.58 (n = 6)	<0.05

[a] Relative units

Cardiopulmonary Bypass Experiments

Table 2 summarizes hemodynamic data of control and nifedipine-treated dogs after 2 h of hypothermic cardiopulmonary bypass. Control animals showed a severe depression in cardiac performance and attempts to wean the dogs from the bypass with various therapeutic maneuvers (variation in preload, norepinephrine, calcium

Table 2. Hemodynamics after hypothermic bypass with and without treatment with Ca^{++}-antagonist

Comparison of mean hemodynamic values before and after two hours of myocardial ischemia

Determination	Control Dogs (n = 7)			Drug-Treated Dogs (n = 6)		
	Before	After	p-Value	Before	After	p-Value
LAP (mmHg)	3.5	9.3	<0.001	5.7	10	<0.001
HR (beats/min)	157	155	NS	159	150	NS
LVP max (mmHg)	156	87	<0.001	142	140	NS
LVEDP (mmHg)	0.3	14	<0.001	1.0	7.7	<0.001
CVP (mmHg)	4.9	9.6	<0.001	4.9	7.3	NS
MAP (mmHg)	115	63.7	<0.001	81	90	NS
CO (l/min)	2,300	700	<0.001	1,820	1,320	<0.003
SV (ml/beat)	14.6	4.52	<0.001	11.5	8.8	NS
LV dP/dt (mmHg/sec)	3,981	1,853	<0.001	3,406	2,76	

Table 3. Hemodynamics after normothermic bypass with selected pharmacological regimens

	Pre-Bypass	On Hour on Bypass at 37°C Plus Two Hours Off Bypass				
		Control Groups			Treatment Groups	
	Pre-Bypass	Normal Saline	Normal Saline + 25 mEq/L KCl	Normosol R pH 7.4	Clinical Cardio-plegic Solution	Nifedipine in Saline
Stroke Work Index (g · m/m²) (SWI)	22.4 ± 1.0	7.1 ± 0.6	11.4 ± 1.7	10.6 ± 0.5	16.9 ± 2.9	21.7 ± 5.8
% Change from Preischemic Value	–	– 68	– 49	– 53	– 25	– 3
LVdP/dt (mmHg sec.)	3500 ± 188	2525 ± 340	2350 ± 210	2300 ± 264	2566 ± 550	3290 ± 452
% Change from Preischemic Value	–	– 28	– 33	– 34	– 27	– 6
LVEDP (mmHg)	8.3 ± 0.9	18.3 ± 2.9	17.8 ± 3.3	15.3 ± 5.5	15.7 ± 0.9	11.4 ± 2.8
% Change from Preischemic Value	–	+ 120	+ 113	+ 84	+ 88	+ 37
Number of Dogs	21	4[a]	4[a]	3	3	5

[a] One additional dog in each group, not included in these data failed to come off bypass

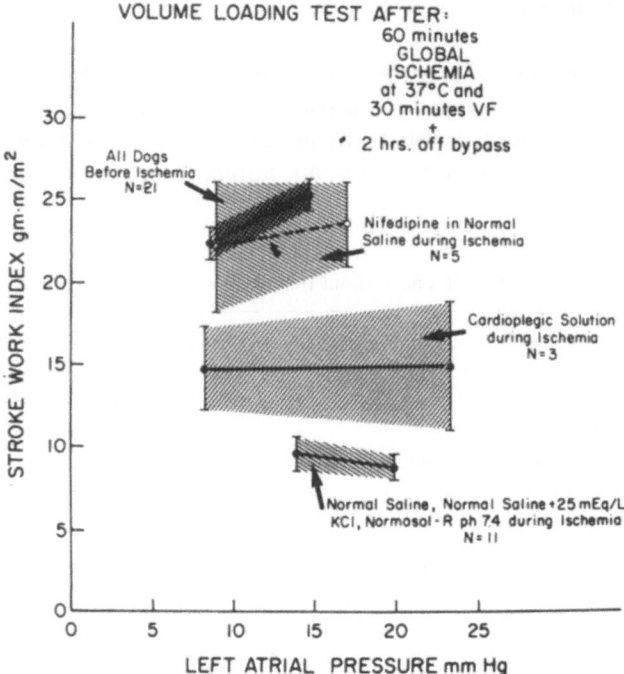

Fig. 7

chloride, ouabain) were unsuccessful. In contrast, dogs treated with nifedipine showed a remarkable preservation of cardiac function, compatible with survival.

The protective effects of nifedipine on the globally ischemic heart were also evident in dogs subjected to 1 h of normothermic cardiopulmonary bypass. Hemodynamic measurements 2 h after bypass for animals treated with nifedipine and other regimens are summarized in Table 3. Figure 7 illustrates that nifedipine-treated dogs responded to volume-loading with fluid from the reservoir of the oxygenator with a near-normal increase in stroke work, whereas control dogs exhibited no elevation. Dogs treated with cardioplegic solution showed an intermediate response.

Discussion

The present study demonstrates that rabbit hearts with surgically damaged A-V nodal area exhibit no mechanical manifestation of ventricular automaticity and remain asystolic. During standstill and maintained perfusion, ventricular wall stresses generated by balloon pulsing resulted in no change in diastolic pressure or ventricular structure. Apparently, myocardium in these instances is completely relaxed and applied stresses in the physiologic range have no ill effect. In contrast, passive pulsing during ischemic ventricular standstill produced a decrease in ventricular contracture pressure and marked alterations in structure, including cell ruptures. One way to explain these findings is to assume that ischemia results in increased cellular stiffness and fragility. As a result, wall stresses corresponding to physiologic systolic peak pressures may disrupt and fracture the myocardial cells. Globally ischemic muscle characteristically undergoes a contracture. On the other hand, during experimental myocardial infarction there is no evidence that ischemic segments undergo contracture [15]. Absence of segmental contracture in regional ischemia may reflect the fact that ischemic muscles subjected to pulsatile stresses generated by the rest of the intact myocardium may prevent contracture and disrupt cellular architecture. In recent experiments, we have observed in dogs that temporary myocardial ischemia followed by reperfusion produces cellular disarray somewhat similar to that observed in pulsed ischemic rabbit hearts. (Unpublished observation.) Results of the present experiments suggest that the occurrence of myocardial contracture and stiffness may be an important determinant of myocardial injury. Explosive deterioration of myocardial structure and function following temporary asystole due to ischemia [5,9] or withdrawal of calcium [8] may reflect the disruptive effects of active pulsatile stresses on cells with decreased deformability. These findings further emphasize the importance of preventing myocardial compliance changes during cardiopulmonary bypass.

Results of the bypass experiments demonstrate that nifedipine may prevent or delay the functional deterioration of the severely ischemic heart. The striking preservation of cardiac performance after cardiopulmonary bypass suggests that this agent may be potentially useful as an adjunctive measure for the protection of the heart during cardiopulmonary bypass.

In previous experiments with isolated perfused hearts, nifedipine has been shown to inhibit postischemic accumulation of intracellular calcium [10]. Therefore, it is tempting to attribute salutory effects of the drug to a blockade of calcium uptake by injured cells. It is well known that the hypoxic and ischemic myocardium releases potassium [16] and norepinephrine [17]. Recent experiments in our laboratory indicate that hypoxic release of potassium plays an important role in stimulating the exocytotic release of endogenous norepinephrine [18]. Catecholamines have been shown to produce regenerative, propagated action potentials in myocardium exposed to elevated potassium concentrations [19]. According to current concepts, the inward current responsible for these regenerated slow responses are predominantly carried by calcium and therefore may be expected to be sensitive to the inhibitory effects of slow channel inhibitors such as nifedipine, (−)-verapamil, and fendiline [20]. Previous studies in rats have demonstrated that myocardial necrosis and calcium accumulation may be largely inhibited by pretreatment with verapamil [6] of fendiline [21]. Accordingly, the possibility must be considered that calcium antagonists protect ischemic myocardium partly by exerting indirect antiadrenergic effects.

In summary, the present experiments demonstrate that ischemic myocardial stiffness may result in increased cellular fragility. In addition, they suggest that calcium antagonists may be useful agents for myocardial preservation during open heart surgery.

References

1. Gergely J (1976) Excitation-contraction coupling − cardiac muscle events in the myofilaments. Fed Proc 35:1283 − 1287
2. Mayer SE (1974) Effect of catecholamines on cardiac metabolism. Circ Res 35:129 − 135

3. Lehninger AL (1974) Ca^{2+}-transport by mitochondria and its possible role in the cardiac contraction-relaxation cycle. Circ Res 35:83 – 88
4. Carafoli E, Lehninger AL (1971) A survey of the interaction of calcium ions with mitochondria from different tissues and species. Biochem J 122:681 – 690
5. Shen AC, Jennings RB (1972) Kinetics of calcium accumulation in acute myocardial ischemic injury. Am J Pathol 67:417 – 440
6. Fleckenstein A (1970) Die Zügelung des Myocardstoffwechsels durch Verapamil. Arzneim Forsch 20:1317 – 1322
7. Flear CT, Riemersma RA, Nandra A, Nandra G, Talbot R (1976) Changes in myocardial water and solutes after ischemia. Adv Cardiac Structure Metab 7:307 – 312
8. Holland CE Jr, Olson RE (1975) Prevention by hypothermia of paradoxical calcium necrosis in cardiac muscle. J Mol Cell Cardiol 7:917 – 928
9. Henry PD, Shuchleib R, Davis J, Weiss ES, Sobel BE (1977) Myocardial contracture and accumulation of mitochondrial calcium in ischemic rabbit heart. Am J Physiol 233:H677 – H684
10. Reuter H (1974) Exchange of calcium ions in the mammalian myocardium. Circ Res 34:599 – 605
11. Henry PD, Shuchleib R, Borda LJ, Roberts R, Williamson JR, Sobel BE (1978) Effects of nifedipine on myocardial perfusion and ischemic injury in dogs. Circ Res 43:372 – 380
12. Cooley DA, Reul GJ, Wukasch DC (1972) Ischemic contracture of the heart: "stone heart". Am J Cardiol 29:575
13. Ross J Jr, Sonnenblick EH, Covell JW, Kaiser GA, Spiro D (1967) The architecture of the heart in systole and diastole – technique of rapid fixation and analysis of left ventricular geometry. Circ Res 21:409 – 421
14. Clark RE, Ferguson TB, West PN, Shuchleib RC, Henry PD (1977) Pharmacological preservation of the ischemic heart. Ann Thorac Surg 24:307 – 314
15. Théroux P, Ross J Jr, Franklin D, Covell JW, Bloor CM, Sasayama S (1977) Regional myocardial function and dimensions early and late after myocardial infarction in the unanesthetized dog. Circ Res 40:158 – 165
16. Downar E, Janse MJ, Durrer D (1977) The effect of ischemic blood on transmembrane potentials of normal porcine ventricular myocardium. Circulation 55:455 – 462
17. Shahab L, Wollenberger A, Haase M, Schiller U (1969) Noradrenalinabgabe aus dem Hundeherzen nach vorübergehender Okklusion einer Koronararterie. Acta Biol Med Ger 22:135 – 143
18. Borda LJ, Shuchleib R, Henry PD (1979, to be published) Hypoxic contraction of isolated coronary artery: mediation by potassium-dependent exocytosis of norepinephrine. Circ Res
19. Corabeuf E (1978) Ionic basis of electrical activity in cardiac tissues. Am J Physiol 234:H101 – H116
20. Kaufmann R (1977) Differenzierung verschiedener Kalzium-Antagonisten. Muench Med Wochenschr [Suppl 1] 119:6 – 11
21. Ciplea AG, Bock PR (1976) Kardioprotektion durch perorale Anwendung des Calcium-Antagonisten Fendilin. Arzneim Forsch 26:1819 – 1826

Calcium-Antagonismus, ein Grundprinzip der Vasodilatation[1]

G. Fleckenstein-Grün und A. Fleckenstein

Die entscheidende Rolle der Ca^{++}-Ionen als Mittlersubstanz zwischen Membranerregung und Kontraktion ist auch für die glatte Muskulatur gesichert. Daher sind alle spontan auftretenden oder elektrisch ausgelösten Kontraktionen ebenso wie die mit pharmakologischen Mitteln induzierten Verkürzungen der glatten Muskulatur durch Ca^{++}-Entzug oder Ca^{++}-Antagonisten blockierbar. Ca^{++}-Entzug oder Ca^{++}-Antagonisten stellen dabei die glatte Muskulatur meist sogar in doppelter Hinsicht ruhig; denn die Ca^{++}-verarmten oder mit Ca^{++}-Antagonisten behandelten glatten Muskelfasern verlieren außer ihrer Kontraktilität meistens auch die bioelektrische Spontan-Aktivität. Dieses für viele glatte Muskelzellen charakteristische Verhalten beruht darauf, daß hier die Ca^{++}-Ionen – ähnlich wie in den cardialen Schrittmacher-Zellen – auch für die automatische Bildung von Aktionspotentialen benötigt werden. Die Ca^{++}-Ionen sind offenbar neben den Na^{+}-Ionen als Träger des transmembranären depolarisierenden Einwärtsstroms an der Elektrogenese des Aktionspotentials glatter Muskelzellen obligatorisch beteiligt.

Die höchste Empfindlichkeit gegenüber Ca^{++}-Antagonisten besitzt die glatte Gefäßmuskulatur speziell aus Coronararterien, Pfortadern, Hirn-, Nieren- und Mesenterial-Arterien. Minimale Konzentrationen dieser Stoffe blockieren hier – teilweise noch in Milliarden-facher Verdünnung – nicht nur die phasische, sondern auch die tonische Gefäßkontraktilität. Auch die durch Dehnung der Gefäßwand bedingte autoregulatorische Vasokonstriktion bei Steigerung des intravasalen Drucks wird durch Ca^{++}-Antagonisten ausgeschaltet (vgl. [1, 8]). Die relaxierenden Gefäßwirkungen der Ca^{++}-Antagonisten treten dabei meist schon in einem Konzentrationsbereich zutage, der die Myocardkontraktilität noch nicht reduziert, d. h. nach Gabe von $\frac{1}{3} - \frac{1}{10}$ der Herz-wirksamen Dosis. Es ist daher nicht überraschend, daß die – später von Fleckenstein als Ca^{++}-Antagonisten klassifizierten – Stoffe, wie z. B. Prenylamin (Lindner [9]), Verapamil (Haas u. Härtefelder [10]), D 600 (Haas u. Busch [11]), Perhexilin (Hudak, Lewis u. Kuhn [12]), Diltiazem (Sato, Nagao, Yamaguchi, Nakajima u. Kiyomoto [13]) und Nifedipin (Vater, Kroneberg, Hoffmeister, Kaller, Meng, Oberdorf, Puls, Schlossmann u. Stoepel [14]), das primäre Interesse der genannten Autoren hauptsächlich auf Grund auffälliger coronardilatatorischer Potenzen erweckten.

Hemmung der elektro-mechanischen Koppelung an K^{+}-depolarisierter Coronarmuskulatur durch Ca^{++}-Antagonisten

Die wissenschaftliche Begründung der Gefäß-Therapie mit Ca^{++}-Antagonisten ist schon aus einfachen in-vitro-Versuchen an isolierter Gefäßmuskulatur ersichtlich.

---

1 Darstellungen der fundamentalen Gefäßwirkungen von Ca^{++}-Antagonisten sind in folgenden Publikationen gegeben worden: Grün u. Fleckenstein [1]; Fleckenstein u. Mitarb. [2, 3, 4, 6]; Fleckenstein u. Fleckenstein-Grün [5]; Häusler [7]

Als Beispiel ist in Abb. 1 ein Modell-Experiment an einem – aus der Wand einer
großen Coronararterie excidierten – glatten Muskelstreifen wiedergegeben. Hierbei
wurde zunächst in vitro durch Überführung in eine K^+-reiche Ringer- oder Tyrode-
lösung eine Dauerdepolarisation (d. h. Dauererregung) erzeugt, die bekanntlich einen für viele Stunden anhaltenden Dauerspasmus des Gefäß-Streifens zur Folge hat.
Der erzielte Verkürzungsgrad hängt von der Menge an extracellulären Ca^{++}-Ionen
ab, die durch die erregte Membran ins Innere der glatten Muskelzellen eindringt.
Überführt man das kontrahierte Coronar-Präparat in eine Ca^{++}-freie Lösung, so
kommt es infolge des Sistierens der elektro-mechanischen Koppelungsprozesse zu einer raschen Relaxation, obwohl die K^+-bedingte Depolarisation unverändert fortbe-
steht. Nach Rückkehr in normale Ca^{++}-haltige Tyrodelösung entwickelt sich sofort
wieder die volle Kontraktur. Es überrascht nach diesen Ergebnissen nicht, daß auch
Ca^{++}-Antagonisten, die den Ca^{++}-Influx in die glatten Gefäßmuskelzellen unterbin-
den, ebenfalls eine rasche Relaxation erzwingen. Abbildung 2 zeigt derartige Experimente an Coronar-Streifen von Schweinen mit Fendilin, Prenylamin, Verapamil
und Nifedipin. Ein einziges Molekül eines solchen Ca^{++}-Antagonisten kann bei dieser Versuchsanordnung unter Umständen den elektro-mechanischen Koppelungs-
effekt von mehreren Tausend Ca^{++}-Ionen blockieren. In Abb. 3 ist eine Auswertung
von Experimenten an annähernd 1000 Coronar-Streifen von Schweinen mit verschiedenen Ca^{++}-Antagonisten gegeben. Auf der Ordinate sind die jeweiligen Hem-
mungen der elektro-mechanischen Koppelung – gemessen an K^+-kontrahierten
Coronar-Streifen – in Prozent aufgetragen. Die Abszisse zeigt die dabei angewand-

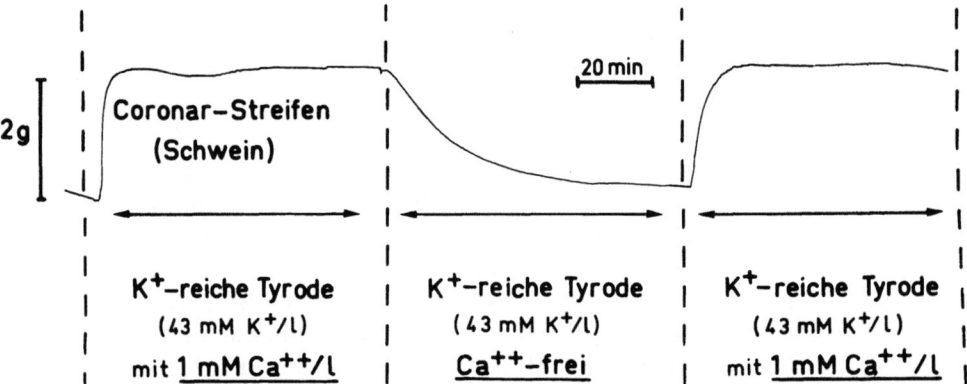

Abb. 1. Aufhebung der Kalium-Kontraktur eines isolierten Coronar-Gefäß-Streifens vom Schwein durch
Überführung des Präparates in eine Ca^{++}-freie Lösung. Kontraktur-Erzeugung mittels isotonischer K^+-
reicher Tyrode-Lösung, enthaltend 43 mM K^+/l (unter Reduktion von Na^+) und 1 mM Ca^{++}/l. Die Aktivierung des kontraktilen Systems in den glatten Gefäßmuskelzellen erfolgt bei dieser Versuchsanordnung
durch den Einstrom von extrazellulären Ca^{++}-Ionen durch die K^+-depolarisierte Membran ins Zellinnere.
Bei Entzug des extrazellulären Ca^{++} geht daher die Fähigkeit zur Verkürzung trotz Fortbestandes der K^+-
Depolarisation verloren. Nach Rückkehr in ein Ca^{++}-haltiges Milieu wird die Kontraktilität rasch restituiert. Vor Anwendung der K^+-reichen Lösung wurde der Coronar-Gefäß-Streifen in einer Tyrode-
Lösung mit normalem K^+-Gehalt (Konzentrationen in mM/l: NaCl 155; KCl 4; $NaHCO_3$ 11,9; $CaCl_2$
1,0; NaH_2PO_4 0,48; Glukose 5,6) für die Zeit von 60 min unter einer Belastung von 2,0 g gehalten. Die
Lösungen wurden während des gesamten Experimentes mit einem Gasgemisch von 97% O_2 und 3% CO_2
durchperlt (Temperatur 35 °C; pH 7,4). Die fortlaufende Registrierung der isometrischen Spannung erfolgte mittels eines mechano-elektronischen Transducers

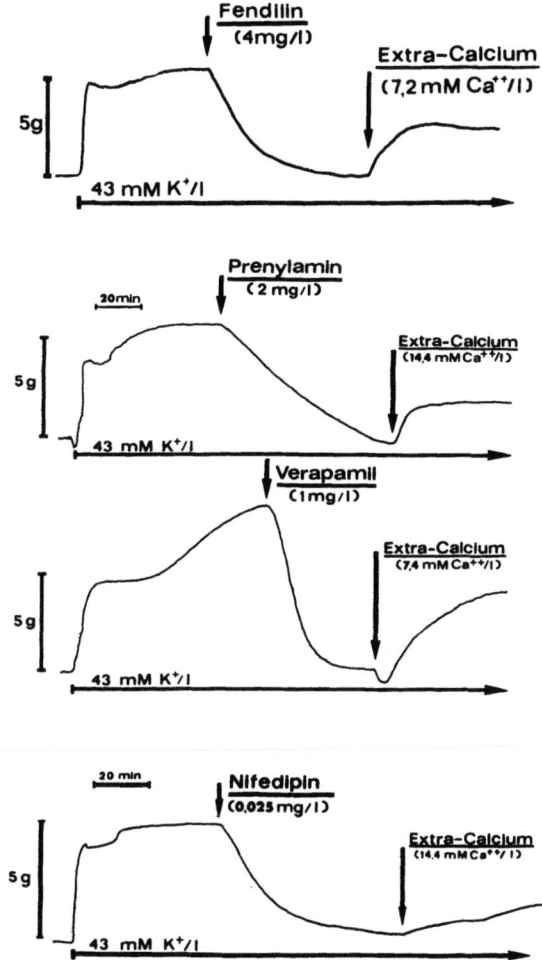

Abb. 2. Aufhebung der Kalium-Kontraktur isolierter Coronargefäß-Streifen aus dem R. descendens anterior vom Schwein durch die Ca^{++}-Antagonisten Fendilin, Prenylamin, Verapamil und Nifedipin. Diese Stoffe hemmen den transmembranären Ca^{++}-Einstrom in die K$^+$-depolarisierten Gefäßmuskelzellen, so daß es trotz Fortbestandes der Depolarisation zu einer Erschlaffung infolge elektro-mechanischer Entkoppelung kommt. Durch Zusatz von Extra-Ca^{++} läßt sich auch hier die kontraktile Funktion zumindest partiell regenerieren. Kontraktur-Erzeugung und sonstige Versuchsanordnung wie in Abb. 1

ten Konzentrationen der Ca^{++}-Antagonisten. Die so erhaltenen Dosis-Wirkungs-Kurven lassen unschwer erkennen, daß Nifedipin, d.h. Adalat, mit Abstand die stärkste Ca^{++}-antagonistische Wirkung entfaltet. Die coronar-relaxierende Potenz von Nifedipin ist dabei etwa 3000mal größer als diejenige der Vergleichssubstanz Papaverin. D 600 − ein Methoxyderivat von Verapamil − ist beinahe so wirksam wie Nifedipin (Adalat). Verapamil übertrifft das Papaverin rund um das 100fache. Prenylamin, Fendilin und Bencyclan sind an der glatten Coronarmuskulatur etwa 5- bis 10mal stärker als Papaverin. Ganz ähnliche Dosis-Wirkungs-Kurven wie an der glatten Coronarmuskulatur haben sich auch bei der Prüfung der verschiedenen Ca^{++}-Antagonisten gegenüber K$^+$-induzierten Spasmen von Hirngefäßen ergeben (vgl. Abb. 4). Solche quantitativen Wirkungsunterschiede zwischen den einzelnen

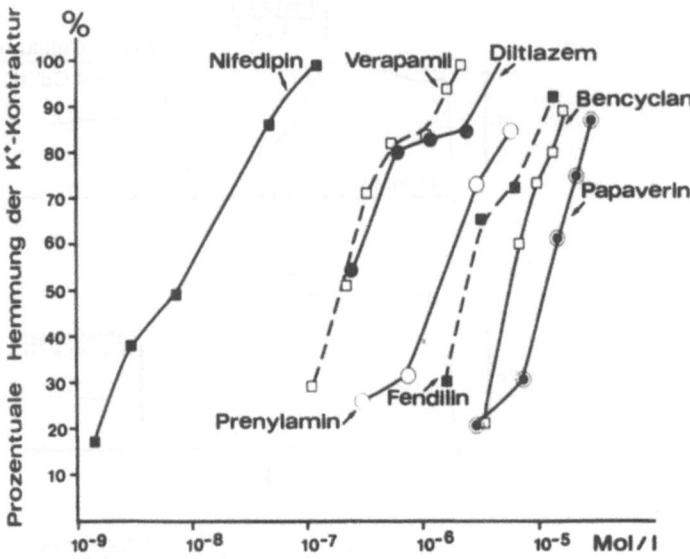

Abb. 3. Aufhebung K^+-induzierter Kontrakturen an Coronargefäß-Streifen von Schweinen durch Ca^{++}-antagonistische Inhibitoren der elektromechanischen Koppelung. Die Streifen wurden zunächst durch Depolarisation in einer K^+-reichen Tyrode-Lösung (43 mM KCl; Einwirkungsdauer jeweils 40 min) zu einer Dauerverkürzung gebracht. Anschließend wurden die Ca^{++}-Antagonisten in jeweils verschiedenen Konzentrationen zugegeben. Das hierdurch erzielte Ausmaß der Erschlaffung ist in Prozent der maximalen Gipfelspannung ausgedrückt, die kurz vor dem Zusatz der Ca^{++}-Antagonisten erreicht worden war. Vor Anwendung der K^+-reichen Tyrode-Lösung wurden die Coronar-Streifen für 60 min unter einer Belastung von 2,0 g in Tyrode-Lösung mit normalem K^+-Gehalt inkubiert (Zusammensetzung sowie sonstige Versuchsanordnung wie in Abb. 1)

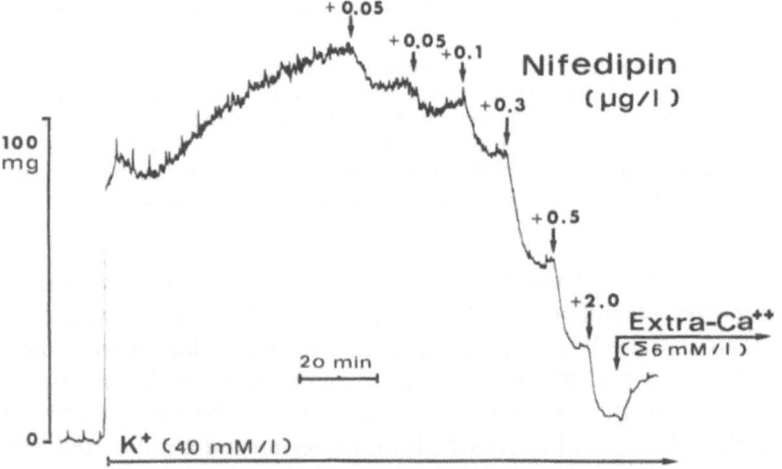

Abb. 4. Basilar-Arterie des Kaninchens: Beseitigung der Kalium-Kontraktur eines Gefäß-Streifens durch minimale Nifedipin-Dosen. Die Erschlaffung beginnt bereits nach Zusatz von 0,05 µg Nifedipin/l und ist nach Gabe von insgesamt 3 µg Nifedipin/l komplett. Versuchsanordnung wie in Abb. 1 (Nakajama u. Fleckenstein, unveröffentlicht)

Ca^{++}-Antagonisten sind allerdings kein entscheidendes Bewertungskriterium für die Praxis, da sie in der Regel durch entsprechende Dosierung wieder ausgeglichen werden können.

Der K^+-induzierte Spasmus der glatten Gefäßmuskulatur verdient in zweifacher Hinsicht besonderes Interesse, (a) als pharmakologischer Test und (b) wegen seiner möglicherweise pathophysiologischen Relevanz:

Der Wert als Test beruht darauf, daß die – durch Membrandepolarisation in K^+-reicher Lösung erzeugten – Verkürzungen der glatten Gefäßmuskulatur eine Klassifizierung vasodilatatorischer Pharmaka nach ihrem Wirkungsmechanismus erlauben; denn nur solche Stoffe sind zur Durchbrechung eines K^+-Spasmus befähigt, die in die elektro-mechanischen Koppelungsprozesse blockierend eingreifen. Physiologische Agentien dieser Art sind z. B. die H^+-Ionen, die bei Eintritt einer Gewebsazidose die elektro-mechanische Koppelungsfunktion der Ca^{++}-Ionen kompetitiv hemmen und dadurch auch bei K^+-Kontrakturen eine Relaxation erzwingen können [15, 16]. Als pharmakologische Relaxantien gegenüber K^+-Spasmen kommen dagegen nur Ca^{++}-Antagonisten in Frage oder solche Stoffe, die auf Grund einer Ca^{++}-antagonistischen Wirkungskomponente die elektro-mechanische Koppelung wenigstens partiell auszuschalten vermögen wie z. B. Nitroglycerin und Verwandte, Molsidomin oder Nitroprussid-Natrium (vgl. hierzu [17]).

Darüber hinaus liegt die Vermutung nahe, daß K^+-bedingte spastische Gefäßreaktionen an kleineren intramuralen Coronar-Ästen und Arteriolen möglicherweise eine zusätzliche pathogenetische Bedeutung bei gewöhnlicher Belastungs-Angina besitzen. Wird z. B. ein Angina-pectoris-Anfall durch frequentes Pacing ausgelöst, so ist in dieser Situation mit einer beträchtlichen Freisetzung von K^+-Ionen aus dem hypoxischen Myocard zu rechnen. Die gleichzeitig bestehende Minderperfusion begünstigt dabei natürlich eine kritische Anreicherung von K^+-Ionen im perivaskulären Raum und eine dadurch bedingte Tonussteigerung an den intramuralen Widerstandsgefäßen. Hierdurch würde die Durchblutung im Angina-pectoris-Anfall noch weiter im Sinne eines circulus vitiosus gedrosselt. Pharmakotherapeutisch würde sich natürlich in dieser Situation die Gabe von Ca^{++}-Antagonisten speziell zur Prophylaxe und von Nitroglycerin zur raschen Spasmolyse empfehlen. Andere „Coronardilatatoren" (Dipyridamol, Chromonar u. a.) sind gegenüber K^+-bedingten Gefäß-Spasmen wirkungslos. Dagegen können solche K^+-bedingten Tonusanstiege der glatten Gefäßmuskulatur auf physiologische Weise spontan behoben werden, wenn es im hypoxischen Myocard zu einer verstärkten Produktion von H^+-Ionen kommt. Auf dieser Basis könnte sich z. B. das bekannte „Walk-through-Phänomen" erklären.

Neutralisation der coronar-konstrictorischen Effekte von Acetylcholin, Serotonin, Histamin bzw. Noradrenalin (nach β-Receptoren-Blockade) durch Ca^{++}-Antagonisten

Ein zweiter Typ von experimentellen in-vitro-Spasmen – mit einem ausgeprägten phasischen Verlauf – ist an der isolierten Coronarmuskulatur durch Acetylcholin, Serotonin und Histamin hervorzurufen. Auch diese Kontrakturen werden durch Ca^{++}-Antagonisten prompt neutralisiert. Abbildung 5 zeigt die kontraktilen Reaktionen von 2 Schweine-Coronarstreifen nach Zusatz von 50, 100, und 200 µg Acetyl-

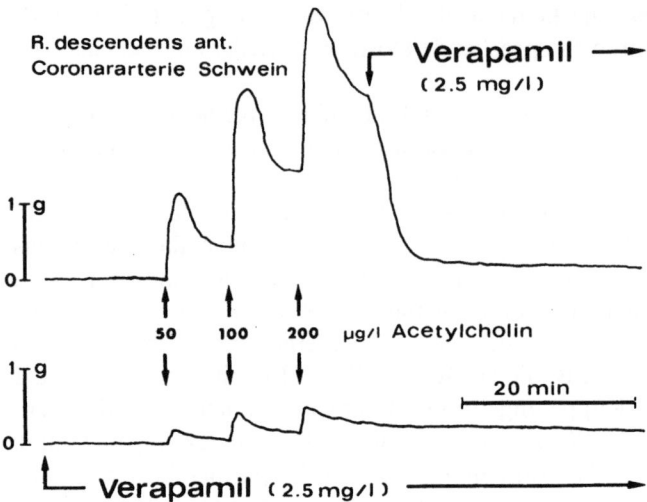

Abb. 5. Unterdrückung Acetylcholin-induzierter Kontrakturen bei zwei Streifenpräparaten aus einer Coronararterie vom Schwein. Acetylcholin wurde in steigender Dosis (50, 100 und 200 µg/l) gegeben. Mit Hilfe von Verapamil (2,5 mg/l) vor den Acetylcholin-Gaben (untere Zeile) oder nach der Acetylcholin-Verabreichung (obere Zeile) wurde eine weitgehende Neutralisation der Acetylcholin-Effekte erzielt

cholin/l. Offensichtlich reagiert die glatte Muskulatur aus größeren extramuralen Coronarästen unter dem Einfluß des parasympathischen Transmitters Acetylcholin mit einer beträchtlichen Tonus-Steigerung. Durch Injektion von Metacholin, einem Acetylcholin-Verwandten, ließen sich z. B. auch im Experiment am Menschen Coronarspasmen erzeugen und Anfälle von Prinzmetal-Angina provozieren. Solche spastischen Formen von Angina pectoris treten ganz offensichtlich auch in der Klinik dann bevorzugt auf, wenn der Parasympathikus dominiert, d. h. im Zustand körperlicher Ruhe nach vorausgegangener Belastung, infolge opulenter Mahlzeiten oder im Schlaf. Ca^{++}-Antagonisten können nicht nur in dem hier gezeigten in-vitro-Versuch solche Acetylcholin-bedingten Spasmen unterdrücken. Auch die klinische Erfahrung zeigt, daß die − unter Parasympathikus-Dominanz auftretende − spastische Ruheangina auf Ca^{++}-Antagonisten hervorragend reagiert.

Ein Überwiegen des Sympathikus bzw. der sympathischen Überträgerstoffe Adrenalin und Noradrenalin führt dagegen normalerweise an der glatten Muskulatur aus größeren extramuralen Coronararterien zur Erschlaffung. Dieses Verhalten der großen Coronaräste steht − worauf Langendorff schon 1907 [18] hinwies − im diametralen Gegensatz zu allen anderen Körperarterien. Eine Erklärung hierfür ist aus heutiger Sicht nicht schwierig: Normalerweise überwiegen nämlich in der glatten Wandmuskulatur der großen extramuralen Coronararterien die adrenergen β-Receptoren quantitativ über die α-Receptoren − ähnlich wie an den Bronchien. Normalerweise wirken daher Adrenalin und Noradrenalin durch überwiegende Stimulation von β-Receptoren an den großen Coronarästen − ähnlich wie an den Bronchien − relaxierend. Blockiert man jedoch, wie die in Abb. 6 wiedergegebenen Experimente zeigen, die β-Receptoren mit Pindolol, d. h. Visken, so kommt es zu einem Überwiegen der α-Receptoren, so daß die glatte Coronarmuskulatur plötzlich nicht nur auf Acetylcholin, sondern auch auf Adrenalin und Noradrenalin mit Spasmen reagiert. Die Verabreichung von β-Receptoren-Blockern bei vasospastischen Formen von Angina pectoris ist daher schon aus theoretischer Sicht absolut kontraindiziert. Auch klinische Erfahrungen haben dies bestätigt. Ca^{++}-Antagonisten sind dagegen selbst gegenüber solchen Noradrenalin-bedingten Coronarspasmen nach β-Receptoren-Blockade hochwirksam. In Abb. 6 wurden z. B. die Noradrenalin-Spasmen des Pindolol-behandelten Coronarstreifens in der oberen Zeile mit Hilfe von Fendilin, in der unteren Zeile mit Nifedipin weitgehend neutralisiert. Verapamil sollte hier in praxi nur zurückhaltend verwendet werden, da sich die Wirkungen von β-Receptoren-Blockern und Verapamil am AV-Knoten manchmal in schlecht vorausschaubarer Weise potenzieren können.

Auch die Muskulatur peripherer Körperarterien reagiert auf Ca^{++}-Antagonisten mit Relaxation. Während hier K^+-induzierte Kontrakturen meist sehr schnell aufgehoben werden, tritt die volle Hemmung von Noradrenalin-, Serotonin- und Histamin-bedingten Verkürzungen meist erst nach einer gewissen Latenzzeit ein. Abbildung 7 zeigt als Beispiel in der unteren Zeile die − über 2 Std progrediente − Blockierung von Noradrenalin-Spasmen an einem Streifenpräparat aus der A. femoralis nach Zusatz von Verapamil. Ca^{++}-Antagonisten setzen jedoch nicht nur die Kontraktilität größerer Körperarterien herab, sondern reduzieren auch den Tonus der peripheren Widerstandsgefäße im großen Kreislauf. Hieraus erklären sich die anti-hypertensiven Effekte, die speziell bei Verapamil und Nifedipin besonders auffällig sind. Ca^{++}-Antagonisten können auf diese Weise, d.h. durch Senkung des „Afterload", den O_2-Bedarf des Herzens auch indirekt senken.

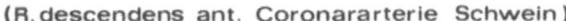
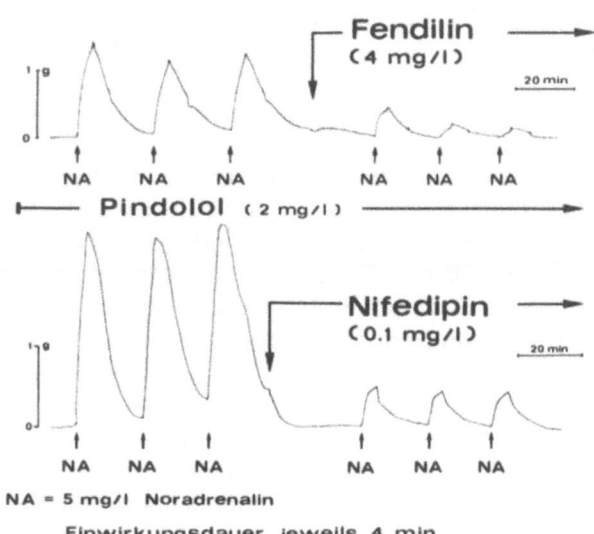

Abb. 6. Weitgehende Unterdrückung Noradrenalin-bedingter Coronarspasmen an 2 Pindolol-vorbehandelten Coronarstreifen mit Hilfe der Ca^{++}-Antagonisten Fendilin (oben) und Nifedipin (unten)

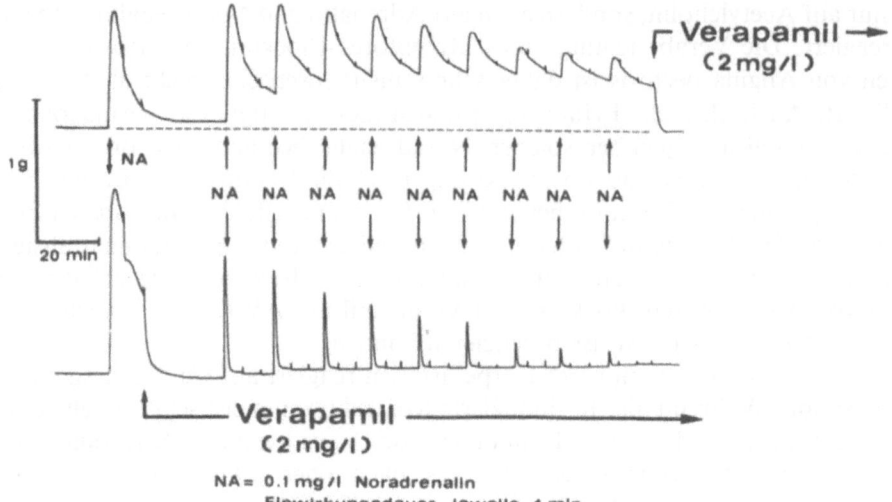

Abb. 7. Unterdrückung von Noradrenalin-bedingten Spasmen an Streifen-Präparaten aus peripheren Körperarterien (A. femoralis) von Kaninchen durch den Ca^{++}-Antagonisten Verapamil.
Obere Zeile: Verapamil (2 mg/l) – am Ende einer Serie von Noradrenalin-Kontrakturen gegeben – führt zu einer sofortigen Beseitigung der Fußpunkt-Anstiege bis herab zum Ausgangsniveau (Tonus-Senkung).
Untere Zeile: Verapamil (2 mg/l) – während der ganzen Versuchsdauer einwirkend – führt im Laufe von 2 Stunden zu einer progredienten Unterdrückung der phasischen Noradrenalin-Kontrakturen bis zur völligen Auslöschung. Tonus-Steigerungen werden durch Verapamil von Anfang an verhindert.
Die beiden Gefäß-Streifen wurden aus der gleichen A. femoralis exzidiert

Potenzierung der phasischen und tonischen Gefäß-Kontraktilität durch Ca^{++}-antagonistische Herzglykoside.
Neutralisation der vaskulären Glykosid-Effekte durch Ca^{++}-Antagonisten

Ausgedehnte Untersuchungen unseres Arbeitskreises haben in den letzten Jahren gezeigt, daß Herzglykoside schon in relativ niedriger Dosierung die Kontraktions-Bereitschaft der Coronar-, Gehirn- und Mesenterial-Arterien potenzieren [2 – 5]. Wiederholte elektrische Reize oder mechanische Irritation wie z. B. plötzliche Dehnung führen dann an Digitalis- oder Strophanthin-behandelten Gefäß-Streifen zu stark vergrößerten Kontraktionsamplituden und Steigerungen des Basaltonus. In Abb. 8 ist ein Experiment an zwei elektrisch gereizten Gefäß-Streifen aus der gleichen Coronararterie eines Schweines wiedergegeben. Hier kam es unter dem Einfluß von 10 µg Strophanthin/l im Laufe von Stunden in typischer Weise zu einer fortschreitenden Kontraktur, während sich das Mechanogramm des Kontroll-Präparates ohne Strophanthin während der 4stündigen Beobachtungszeit nicht veränderte. Auch die Kontraktur-Effekte coronar-konstriktorischer Agentien wie Histamin und Serotonin werden unter dem Einfluß von Herzglycosiden ganz wesentlich erhöht (vgl. Abb. 9).

Die Kontraktions-verstärkende Wirkung der Herzglykoside ist in Anlehnung an das klassische Konzept von Otto Loewi [19] darauf zurückzuführen, daß diese Pharmaka die Ca^{++}-Versorgung des kontraktilen Systems verbessern. Dieser Einfluß er-

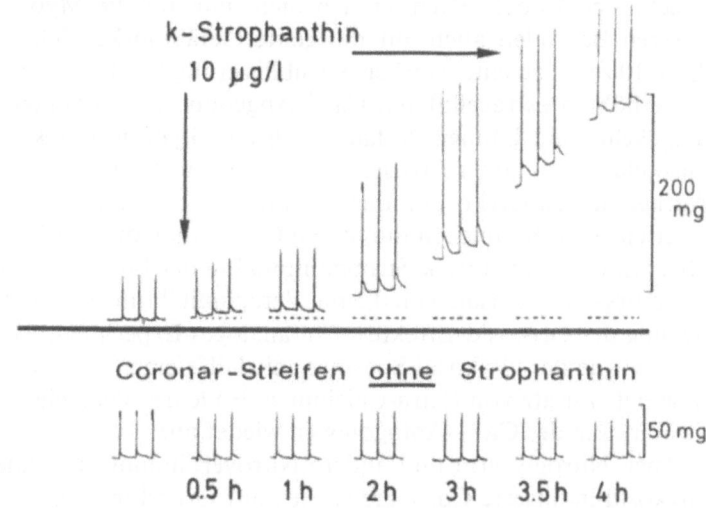

Abb. 8. Coronar-Streifen vom Kaninchen: Zunahme der Kontraktionsamplitude und des Grund-Tonus bei intermittierender elektrischer Reizung unter dem Einfluß von 10 µg k-Strophanthin/l. Keine Änderung des kontraktilen Verhaltens beim Kontrollstreifen ohne Strophanthin. Reizung mit alternierenden Rechteck-Stromstößen von 10 Hz. Reizstärke 10 V/cm. Reizdauer jeweils 8 sec. Intervall zwischen den Reizperioden jeweils 5 min. Ca^{++}-Gehalt der Tyrode-Lösung 2 mM/l. Feuchtgewicht der − aus der gleichen Coronar-Arterie stammenden − Streifen 2,2 und 2,0 mg. Temperatur 35 °C [2−4]

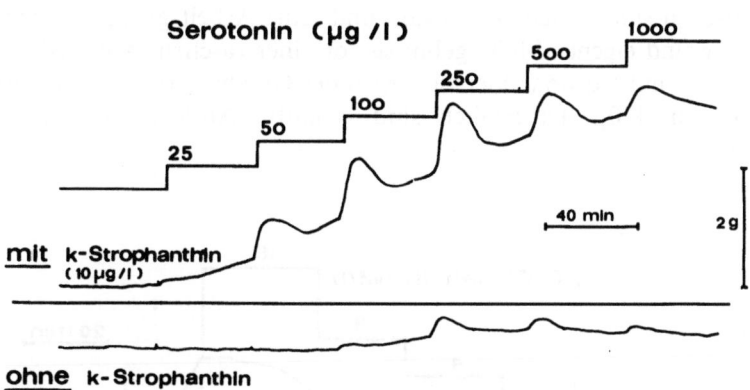

Abb. 9. Kontraktur-Wirkung steigender Dosen von Serotonin (25 − 1000 µg/l an 2 Gefäß-Streifen aus der gleichen Coronar-Arterie (R. descendens ant.) eines Schweines. *Unten* Schwache Tonus-Anstiege beim Kontroll-Streifen ohne Strophanthin. *Oben* Potenzierung des Kontraktur-Effektes durch k-Strophanthin (10 µg/l)

streckt sich jedoch offensichtlich nicht nur auf die Myocardfaser, sondern nach unseren Befunden auch auf die glatte Gefäßmuskel-Zelle. Dabei kommt es, wie Abb. 10 zeigt, zu einer starken Sensibilisierung für die Tonus-steigernden Effekte eines erhöhten extracellulären Ca^{++}-Angebots. Ca^{++}-Antagonisten wirken dagegen umgekehrt und können deshalb auch die Glykosid-Effekte an der glatten Gefäßmuskulatur mit hoher Effizienz neutralisieren. In Abb. 11 ist als Beispiel die rasche Aufhebung der Glykosid-induzierten Kontraktur eines elektrisch gereizten Coronar-Streifens vom Kaninchen durch den Ca^{++}-Antagonisten Verapamil wiedergegeben. Hier waren schon 3 µg k-Strophanthin/l in der Lage, eine hochgradige Kontraktur zu verursachen. Zusatz von 0,5 mg Verapamil/l führte dann zu einer prompten Aufhebung des Glykosid-Effektes. Ein analoges Experiment ist in Abb. 12 dargestellt. Hier wurde der Glykosid-Spasmus mit Hilfe einer zweimaligen Gabe von Fendilin beseitigt. Zusatz von Extra-Calcium zu Ende des Versuchs hob dann die relaxierende Wirkung des Ca^{++}-Antagonisten wieder auf.

Auch Nitroglycerin und andere Nitroverbindungen können im in-vitro-Versuch Glykosid-induzierte Coronarspasmen auf Grund ihrer Ca^{++}-antagonistischen Wirkungskomponente sehr schnell partiell neutralisieren. Der Relaxationseffekt derartiger Nitroverbindungen ist allerdings relativ rasch spontan reversibel. Dagegen sind eine Reihe von anderen „Coronardilatatoren" (Adenosin, Dipyridamol, Chromonar, Theophyllin, Coffein, Lidoflazin) gegenüber Glykosid-bedingten Spasmen der glatten Wandmuskulatur extramuraler Coronar-Äste sehr wenig wirksam. Die gleichen Stoffe ließen auch an der K^+-depolarisierten Coronarmuskulatur keine Ca^{++}-antagonistische Grundwirkung erkennen.

Die vorliegenden Befunde lassen keinen Zweifel, daß Herzglykoside schon im oberen therapeutischen Dosierungsbereich als potentielle Coronarkonstriktoren anzusehen sind. Auch Braunwald und seine Arbeitsgruppe in den USA haben daher aufgrund eigener Meßergebnisse vor einer raschen Digitalisierung von älteren Patienten mit Coronarsklerose wegen der Gefahr coronar-vaskulärer Komplikationen gewarnt [20]. Tatsächlich sind gehäufte Anfälle von Angina pectoris, einge-

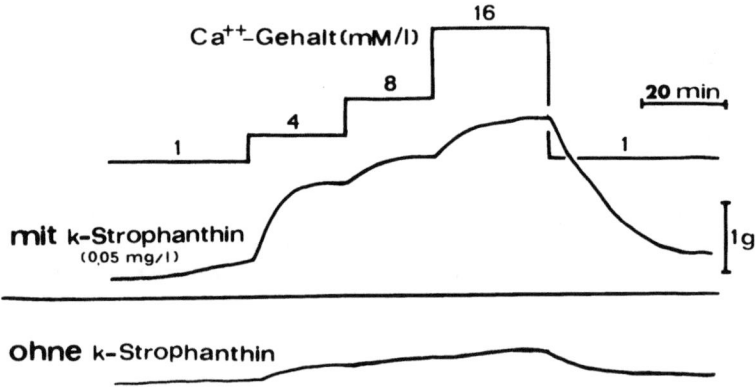

Abb. 10. Exzessive Tonussteigerung der Coronargefäß-Muskulatur bei Erhöhung der extrazellulären Ca^{++}-Konzentration nach vorheriger Sensibilisierung mit k-Strophanthin. Ca^{++}-Zusätze zu normaler Tyrode-Lösung (Zusammensetzung siehe Abb. 1)

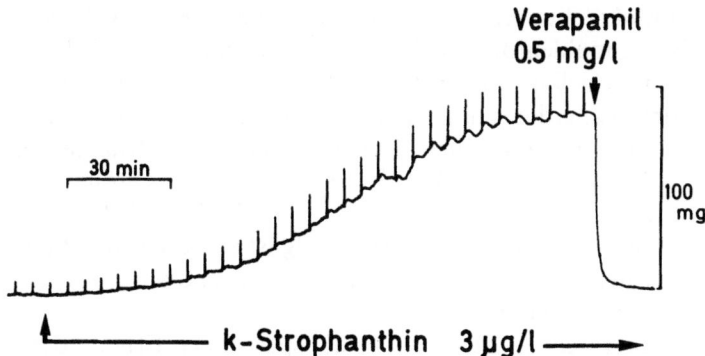

Abb. 11. Coronar-Streifen vom Kaninchen: Zunahme der Kontraktionsamplitude und des Grund-Tonus bei intermittierender elektrischer Reizung unter dem Einfluß von 3 μg k-Strophanthin/l. Sofortige totale Relaxation nach Zusatz von 0,5 mg Verapamil/l. Reizung wie in Abb. 8. Ca^{++}-Gehalt der Tyrode-Lösung 2 mM/l. Feuchtgewicht des Coronar-Streifens 1,3 mg. Temperatur 35 °C [2 – 4]

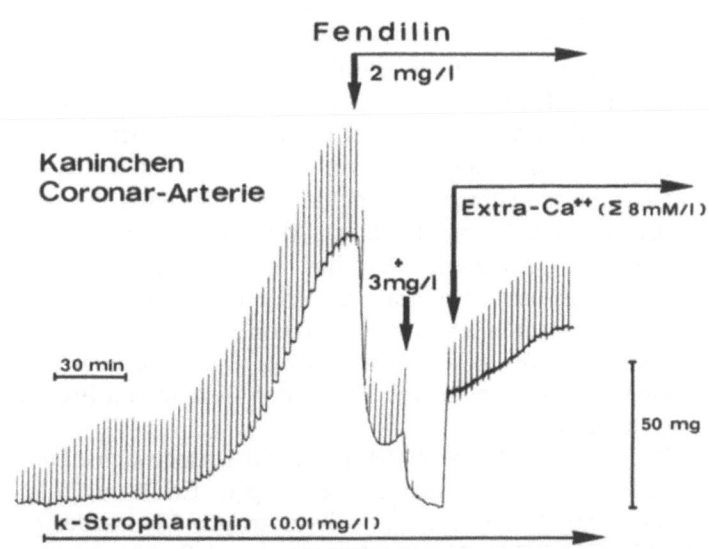

Abb. 12. Coronar-Streifen vom Kaninchen: Zunahme der Kontraktionsamplitude und des Grund-Tonus bei intermittierender elektrischer Reizung unter dem Einfluß von 10 μg k-Strophanthin/l. Reizung wie in Abb. 8. Nach $2\frac{1}{2}$ Stunden Einwirkung des Glykosids wird Fendilin (2 mg/l) zugesetzt. Daraufhin kehrt der gewaltig erhöhte Tonus beinahe zur Norm zurück. Eine weitere Gabe von Fendilin (3 mg/l) führt zur vollen Relaxation und schaltet die Kontraktilität des Coronar-Streifens vollständig aus. Mit Hilfe von Extra-Calcium läßt sich die Fendilin-Wirkung auch in diesem Fall partiell neutralisieren. Ca^{++}-Gehalt der Tyrode-Lösung (vor Zusatz von Extra-Calcium) 2 mM/l. Feuchtgewicht des Coronar-Streifens – aus dem R. descendens anterior der linken Coronararterie stammend – beträgt 1,0 mg. Temp. 35 °C (Nakajama u. Fleckenstein)

schränkte Leistungsbreite im Belastungs-EKG, Abflachung oder Umkehr der T-Zacke, muldenförmige Senkung der ST-Strecke als Folge einer kräftigen Digitalisierung speziell bei Patienten mit Altersherz oft beobachtet worden. Diese Phänomene wurden allerdings nur selten als Ischämie-Reaktion gedeutet, sondern vorzugsweise als „toxisch" angesehen. Trotzdem haben viele Kliniker seit jeher in der kombinierten Anwendung von Herzglykosiden und Coronardilatatoren gerade bei älteren Patienten eine sinnvolle Behandlungsmethode erblickt. Voraussetzung für einen befriedigenden therapeutischen Erfolg ist allerdings die Wahl des richtigen vasodilatatorischen Partners, wobei, wie vorausgehend dargelegt, den Ca^{++}-Antagonisten die Präferenz gebührt.

Überraschend ist, daß sich die spastischen Effekte der Herzglykoside – ebenso wie die Relaxation durch Ca^{++}-Antagonisten – keineswegs auf das Coronarsystem beschränken. So ist nach unseren eigenen Beobachtungen an der A. basilaris von Kaninchen die glatte Muskulatur dieses Gehirngefäßes sowohl gegenüber Herzglykosiden als auch gegenüber Ca^{++}-Antagonisten hochgradig empfindlich. Es ist erwägenswert zu prüfen, ob sich hieraus möglicherweise Kausalzusammenhänge zwischen der vasokonstriktorischen Potenz und gewissen cerebralen Nebenwirkungen von Herzglykosiden ergeben. Zu besonders verhängnisvollen Konsequenzen kann eine Digitalis-Intoxikation an der A. mesenterica superior führen: Hier kamen bei Patienten von über 70 Jahren unter der Glykosidtherapie tödliche Darminfarkte ohne einen autoptisch nachweisbaren Gefäßverschluß gehäuft zur Beobachtung. In einer Serie von klinischen Publikationen wurde seit 1960 auf dieses alarmierende Krankheitsbild aufmerksam gemacht [21 – 24 u.a.]. Veranlaßt durch eine Reihe solcher Zwischenfälle am eigenen Patientengut haben Brobmann u. Mitarb. [25] den vasokonstriktorischen Effekt von k-Strophanthin an der A. mesenterica des Hundes angiographisch geprüft. Dabei kam es gleichzeitig mit der Senkung der ST-Strecke im EKG zu lokalen ringförmigen Abschnürungen oder generalisierten Tonussteigerungen der Gefäßwand, begleitet von einer Erhöhung des mittleren Strömungswiderstandes um ein Vielfaches. Mit Hilfe des Ca^{++}-Antagonisten Verapamil wurden diese Spasmen schon innerhalb von 3 min beseitigt. Gleichzeitig stieg das Stromvolumen der A. mesenterica superior um 50% über die Ausgangswerte vor der Strophanthin-Gabe an (vgl. hierzu den Beitrag von Brobmann, S. 230 – 242 in diesem Bericht).

Das vaskuläre Risiko hoher Glykosid-Dosen wächst beim Menschen offenbar mit zunehmendem Lebensalter. Die gängige Erklärung war bislang, Herzglykoside könnten auf Grund ihrer positiv-inotropen Myocardeffekte den Sauerstoffbedarf des Herzmuskels u. U. so sehr steigern, daß sich eine bestehende Coronarerkrankung deutlicher manifestiert. Unsere neueren Befunde sprechen jedoch dafür, daß sich an atherosklerotisch verengten extramuralen Coronararterien möglicherweise ein zusätzlicher Vasospasmus superponiert. Eine solche Superposition von Atherosklerose und Vasospasmus liegt besonders dann im Bereich des Möglichen, wenn bei exzentrischer Plazierung des atherosklerotischen Intima-Prozesses beträchtliche Anteile der glatten Wandmuskulatur funktionell intakt, d.h. vasokonstriktorisch und vasodilatatorisch beeinflußbar bleiben.

Zu wenig berücksichtigt hat man bisher auch, daß die Neigung zu einem Glykosid-induzierten Vasospasmus wahrscheinlich mit zunehmendem Lebensalter wächst. So wurden tödliche Darminfarkte nach Glykosid-Intoxikation fast nur bei Patienten im Alter über 70 Jahren beobachtet. Dies könnte nach Untersuchungen von Fleckenstein, Janke und Frey damit zusammenhängen, daß der natürliche Alterungsprozeß über die gesamte Lebensspanne hinweg zu einer immer stärkeren Beladung der Gefäßwände mit Calcium führt, während sich die Magnesium-Werte nur wenig ändern[1]. In den Abb. 13 – 15 sind Analysendaten – nach Altersgruppen geordnet – wiedergegeben, die diese dramatische Ca^{++}-Akkumulation in der Arterienwand an autoptisch entnommenen Gewebsproben aus dem R. descendens ant. der linken Coronararterie (n = 86), der A. mesenterica sup. (n = 134) und der Aorta (n = 141) überzeugend demonstrieren. Dagegen bleibt, wie Abb. 16 an 122 Papillarmuskeln zeigt, das Myocard bis zum 90. Lebensjahr von dieser Verschiebung des Ca/Mg-Quotienten unberührt. Es ist nicht von der Hand zu weisen, daß diese progrediente Ca^{++}-Überladung der alternden Gefäßwände die glatte Muskulatur der Media in einen – für die Auslösung von Glykosid-Spasmen konditionierten – Zustand versetzt (soweit dies der Ionisationsgrad des gestapelten Ca^{++} gestattet), während das Myocard nicht in dieser Weise reagiert. Die klinische Empirie hat dieser prekären Situation schon lange Rechnung getragen, indem beim Altersherzen Zurückhaltung in der Glykosid-Dosierung wegen der Gefahr vaskulärer Komplikationen empfohlen wird. Es ist zu erwarten, daß nunmehr mit Hilfe der Ca^{++}-Antagonisten eine weitere Verminderung unerwünschter Gefäßreaktionen bei der Glykosidtherapie gelingt; denn in der Kombination von Ca^{++}-Antagonist und Herzglykosid wächst offenbar der – in der Glykosidbehandlung des Altersherzens praktikable – Dosierungsspielraum. Ob darüber hinaus mit Hilfe geeigneter Ca^{++}-Antagonisten auch die Alters-bedingte Ca^{++}-Überladung der Gefäßwände selbst gehemmt werden kann, ist zur Zeit Gegenstand weiterer Untersuchungen (vgl. hierzu den Beitrag von Frey, Janke u. Fleckenstein in diesem Bericht).

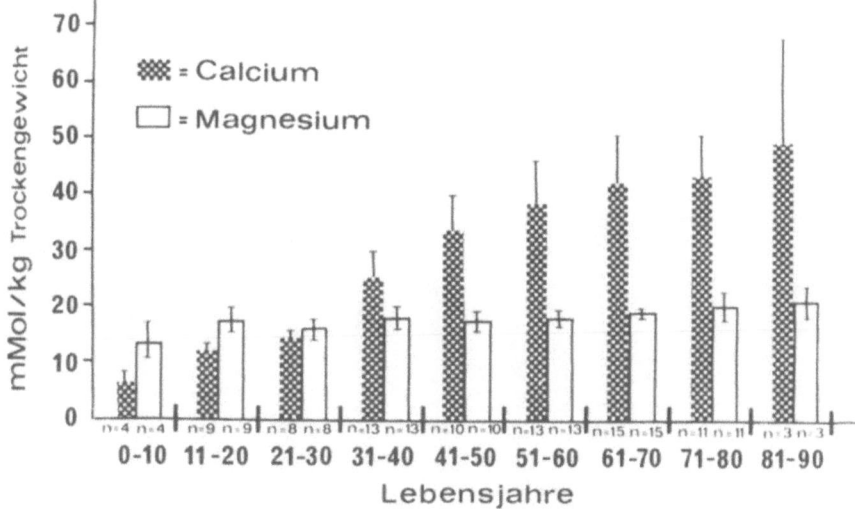

Abb. 13. Progrediente Calcium-Überladung der Arterienwand (R. descendens ant. der linken Coronar-Arterie) beim Menschen mit zunehmendem Lebensalter nach der Analyse von 86 Autopsie-Fällen mit dem Atomabsorptionsspektrometer (Fleckenstein, Janke u. Frey (1977))

---

1 Eine vorläufige Mitteilung dieser Ergebnisse ist im Rahmen der Arbeit Fleckenstein u. Mitarb. [6] erfolgt

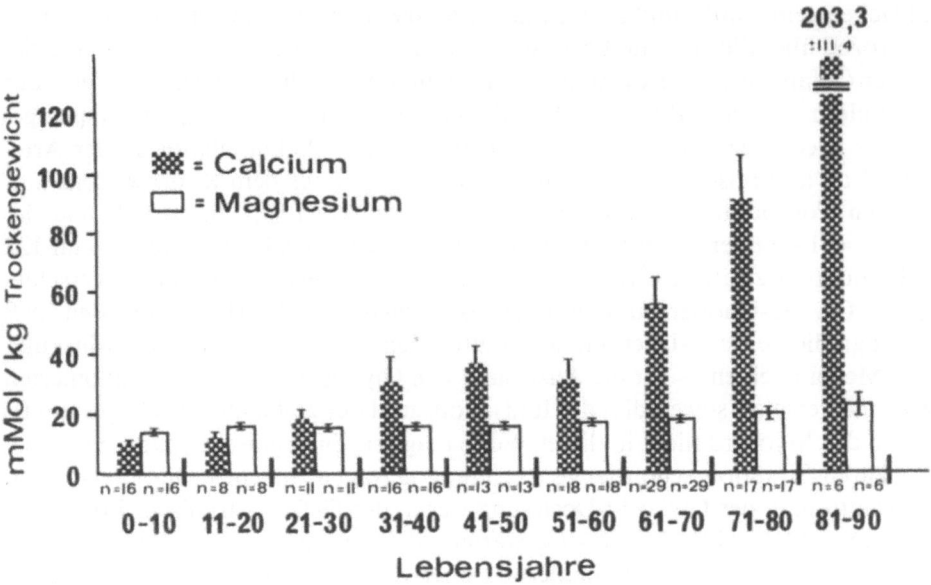

Abb. 14. Progrediente Calcium-Überladung der Arterienwand (A. mesenterica superior) beim Menschen mit zunehmendem Lebensalter nach der Analyse von 134 Autopsie-Fällen (Fleckenstein, Janke u. Frey (1977))

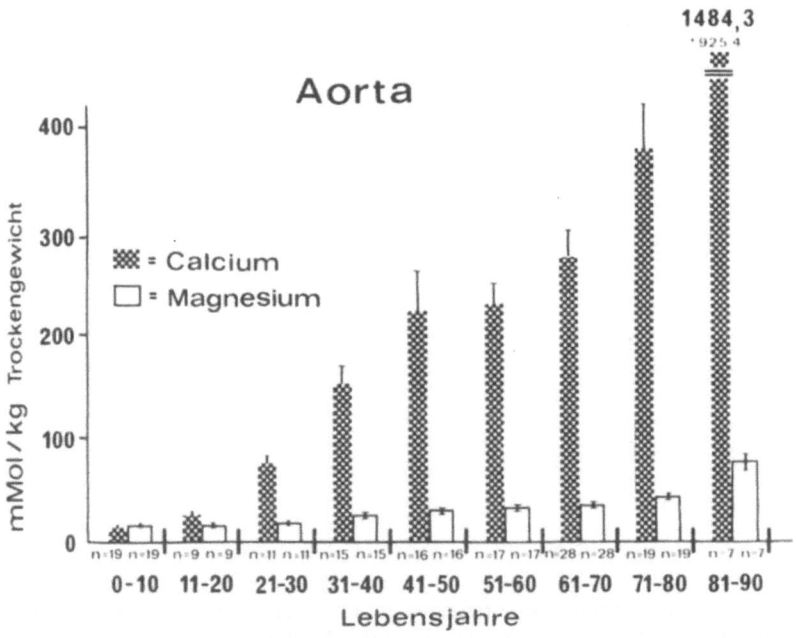

Abb. 15. Progredient fortschreitende, exzessive Calcium-Überladung der Wand der Aorta beim Menschen mit zunehmendem Lebensalter nach der Analyse von 141 Autopsie-Fällen (Fleckenstein, Janke u. Frey (1977))

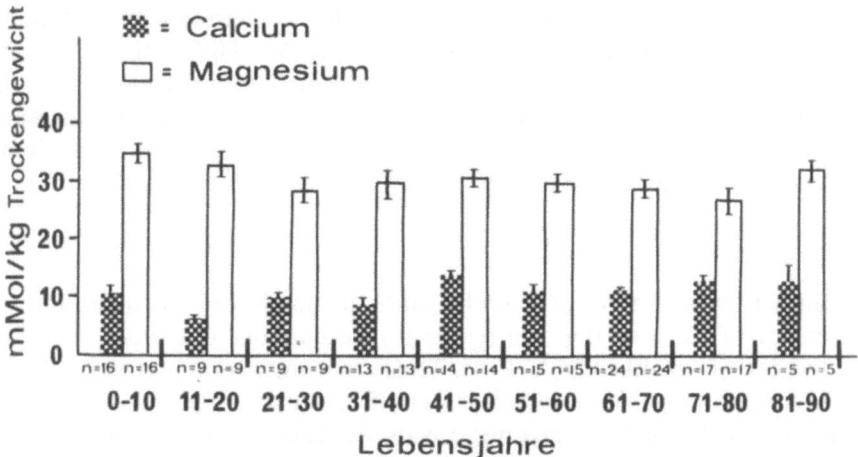

Abb. 16. Konstanz der Ca^{++}- und Mg^{++}-Konzentrationen im Myocardgewebe des Menschen unabhängig vom Lebensalter. Ergebnisse an 122 Gewebsproben aus 140 Autopsie-Fällen nach Fleckenstein, Janke u. Frey (1977)

Zusammenfassung

Ca^{++}-Ionen werden auch in den glatten Gefäßmuskel-Zellen als Mittlersubstanz zwischen Membranerregung und Kontraktion benötigt: Ca^{++}-Ionen aktivieren die Ca^{++}-abhängige Myofibrillen-ATPase und steuern damit quantitativ Kontraktilität und Tonus der Gefäßwand. Dementsprechend führt ein erhöhtes Ca^{++}-Angebot zu Vasokonstriktion, während ein Ca^{++}-Mangel vasodilatatorisch wirkt. H^+-Ionen sind physiologische Ca^{++}-Antagonisten. Eine verstärkte Produktion von H^+-Ionen im hypoxischen Gewebe hebt dementsprechend den vasokonstriktorischen Einfluß der Ca^{++}-Ionen an der glatten Gefäßmuskulatur wieder auf. Ein neuer Weg, mit pharmakologischen Mitteln die vasokonstriktorischen Ca^{++}-Wirkungen auszuschalten, wurde neuerdings durch den Einsatz von Ca^{++}-Antagonisten (Verapamil, D 600 (ein Methoxyderivat von Verapamil), Nifedipin, Diltiazem, Fendilin, Prenylamin, Perhexilin, Bencyclan u. a.) eröffnet. Diese Verbindungen hemmen – ähnlich wie am Myocard – die transmembranäre Ca^{++}-Versorgung des kontraktilen Systems. Dadurch werden die vasokonstriktorischen Effekte einer überhöhten extracellulären K^+-Konzentration sowie der Kontrakturstoffe Histamin, Serotonin, Acetylcholin und Noradrenalin (nach β-Receptorenblockade) an isolierten Streifenpräparaten aus großen extramuralen Coronargefäßen unterdrückt. Die glatte Gefäßmuskulatur aus Coronar- und Hirn-Arterien (A. basilaris) reagiert auf vasodilatatorische Ca^{++}-Antagonisten teilweise über 1000mal empfindlicher als auf Papaverin. Von Interesse ist, daß auch die Gefäß-Relaxation nach Gabe von Nitroglycerin und verwandten Verbindungen auf einem Eingriff in die Ca^{++}-abhängigen elektro-mechanischen Koppelungsprozesse beruht, obwohl in diesem Fall der spezielle Wirkungs-Modus noch unklar ist. Dagegen sind Herzglykoside auf Grund ihrer Ca^{++}-synergistischen Wirkungen in der Lage, die Ca^{++}-abhängige mechanische Spannungsentwicklung der glatten Gefäßmuskulatur zu potenzieren. Dementsprechend verstärken alle – praktisch interessierenden – Herzglykoside noch in sehr niedriger Konzentration (unter 10 μg/l) die kontraktilen Reaktionen der glatten Coronarmuskulatur auf elektrische Reize, mechanische Irritation (plötzliche Dehnung) oder vasokonstriktorische Agentien. Gleichzeitig steigt der basale Coronartonus beträchtlich an – bis zur Entwicklung langdauernder Kontrakturen. Mit Hilfe von Ca^{++}-Antagonisten sind diese vasokonstriktorischen Glykosid-Effekte leicht neutralisierbar ohne Beeinträchtigung der therapeutisch erwünschten positiv-inotropen Wirkung auf das Myocard. Die überragende Effizienz von Ca^{++}-Antagonisten in der Behandlung von Vasospasmen aller Art wird aus diesen Befunden gut verständlich.

Summary

Contractility and tone of vascular smooth muscle depend quantitatively on the presence of Ca ions that are required in excitation-contraction coupling for the activation of myofibrillar ATPase. Thus vasoconstriction occurs if the extracellular Ca concentration rises whereas vasodilation is produced by Ca-deficiency. Physiologically, a Ca-antagonistic action is exerted by H ions. Accordingly, the natural constrictor effect of Ca on vascular smooth muscle disappears if more H ions are produced during hypoxia. A pharmacologic way of interfering with the basic action of Ca on vascular smooth muscle was opened by the discovery of the powerful Ca-antagonistic effects of some drugs, such as verapamil, D 600 (a methoxy-derivative of verapamil), nifedipine, diltiazem, fendiline, prenylamine, perhexiline, or bencyclane. These compounds – in analogy to their cardiac action – inhibit the transmembrane Ca supply to the contractile system so that the vasoconstrictor effects of an elevated extracellular K concentration or of histamine, serotonine, acetylcholine, and noradrenaline (after adrenergic β-receptor blockade) on isolated tissue preparations from large extramural coronary stem arteries disappear. Vascular smooth muscle cells from coronary as well as from brain arteries (A. basilaris) are 1000 times more susceptible to the relaxing effect of some of these Ca-antagonistic drugs than to that of papaverine. Interestingly enough, the well-known vascular dilation produced by nitroglycerin and other compounds of the nitrite group is also due to interference with excitation-contraction coupling, although, in this case, the specific mode of action is still to be clarified. Conversely, cardiac glycosides, due to their Ca-synergistic effect, are capable of potentiating the Ca-dependent smooth muscle reactions. Thus all cardiac glycosides of practical interest increase, even in a concentration of less than 10 μg/l, the contractile responses of coronary smooth muscle to electric stimuli, mechanical stretch or to certain vasoconstrictor agents. Simultaneously, basal coronary smooth muscle tone is considerably augmented and even long-lasting contractures develop. With the help of Ca-antagonistic compounds the glycoside effects on vascular smooth muscle can be easily neutralized without restricting the therapeutic glycoside action on the myocardium. The observations explain the outstanding efficacy of Ca-antagonists in the treatment of practically all types of vasospasm in man.

References

1. Grün G, Fleckenstein A (1972) Die elektromechanische Entkoppelung der glatten Gefäß-Muskulatur als Grundprinzip der Coronardilatation durch 4-(2'-Nitrophenyl)-2,6-dimethyl-1,4-dihydropyridin-3,5-dicarbonsäure-dimethylester (Bay a 1040, Nifedipin). Arzneim Forsch 22:334–344
2. Fleckenstein A, Nakayama K, Fleckenstein-Grün G, Byon YK (1975) Interactions of vasoactive ions and drugs with Ca-dependent excitation-contraction coupling of vascular smooth muscle. In: Carafoli E, Clementi F, Drabikowski W, Margreth A (eds) North Holland, Amsterdam Oxford, American Elsevier, New York, pp 555–566

3. Fleckenstein A, Nakayama K, Fleckenstein-Grün G, Byon YK (1976) Mechanism and sites of action of calcium-antagonistic coronary therapeutics. In: Lichtlen PR (ed) Coronary angiography and angina pectoris. Thieme, Stuttgart, pp 297–316

4. Fleckenstein A, Nakayama K, Fleckenstein-Grün G, Byon YK (1976) Interactions of H ions, Ca-antagonistic drugs and cardiac glycosides with excitation-contraction coupling of vascular smooth muscle. In: Betz E (ed) Ionic actions on vascular smooth muscle. Springer, Berlin Heidelberg New York, pp 117–123

5. Fleckenstein A, Fleckenstein-Grün G (1977) Zur kombinierten Anwendung von Herzglykosiden und Ca^{++}-Antagonisten. Arzneim Forsch 27:736–742

6. Fleckenstein A, Fleckenstein-Grün G, Janke J, Frey M (1977) Kardiovaskuläre Grundwirkungen der Ca^{++}-Antagonisten und deren therapeutischer Wert in Kombination mit Herzglykosiden. Z Praeklin Klin Geriatr 7:269–284

7. Häusler G (1972) Differential effect of verapamil on excitation-contraction coupling in smooth muscle and on excitation-secretion coupling in adrenergic nerve terminals. J Pharmacol Exp Ther 180:672–682

8. Ono H, Kokubun H, Hashimoto K (1974) Abolition by calcium antagonists of the autoregulation of renal blood flow. Naunyn Schmiedebergs Arch Pharmacol 285:201–207

9. Lindner E (1960) Phenyl-propyl-diphenyl-propyl-amin, eine neue Substanz mit coronargefäß-erweiternder Wirkung. Arzneim Forsch 10:569–573

10. Haas H, Härtfelder G (1962) α-Isopropyl-α-(N-methyl-homoveratryl)-γ-aminopropyl)-3,4-di-methoxyphenyl-acetonitril, eine Substanz mit coronargefäßerweiternden Eigenschaften. Arzneim Forsch 12:549–558

11. Haas H, Busch E (1967) Vergleichende Untersuchungen der Wirkung von α-Isopropyl-α(N-methyl-homoveratryl)-γ-aminopropyl)-3,4-dimethoxyphenyl-acetonitril, seiner Derivate sowie einiger anderer Coronardilatatoren und β-Receptor-affiner Substanzen. Arzneim Forsch 17:257–271

12. Hudak WJ, Lewis RE, Kuhn WL (1970) Cardiovascular pharmacology of perhexiline. J Pharmacol Exp Ther 173:371

13. Sato M, Nagao T, Yamaguchi I, Nakajima H, Kiyomoto A (1971) Pharmacological studies on a new 1.5-benzothiazepine derivative (CRD-401 = Diltiazem). Arzneim Forsch 21:1338–1343

14. Vater W, Kroneberg G, Hoffmeister F, Keller H, Meng K, Oberdorf A, Puls W, Schlossmann K, Stoepel J (1972) Zur Pharmakologie von 4-(2-Nitrophenyl)-2,6-dimethyl-1,4-dihydropyridin-3,5-di-carbonsäuredimethyl-ester (Nifedipin, Bay a 1040). Arzneim Forsch 22:1–14

15. Grün G, Bayer M, Fleckenstein A (1972) Der Einfluß des pH auf den Ca^{++}-abhängigen Tonus der Coronar-Gefäßmuskulatur. Naunyn Schmiedebergs Arch Pharmacol [Suppl] 274:R43

16. Grün G, Weder U, Fleckenstein A (1972) The mutual antagonism between H and Ca ions in the control of vascular tone and autoregulation. Pfluegers Arch [Suppl] 335:R10

17. Fleckenstein-Grün G, Fleckenstein A, Späh F, Assmann R (1979) Beeinflussung der elektromechanischen Koppelungsprozesse in der isolierten Herz- und Gefäßmuskulatur durch Molsidomin und den Metaboliten SIN-1. In: Lochner W, Bender F (Hrsg) Molsidomin. Neue Aspekte in der Therapie der ischämischen Herzerkrankung. 1. Molsidomin-Symposium, München, 20./21. Januar 1978. Urban u. Schwarzenberg, München Wien Baltimore, S 56–68

18. Langendorff O (1907) Über die Innervation der Koronargefäße. Zentralbl Physiol 21:551–557

19. Loewi O (1917) Über den Zusammenhang zwischen Digitalis- und Calciumwirkung. Naunyn Schmiedebergs Arch Exp Pathol Pharmakol 82:131

20. Vatner SF, Higgins CB, McKown DP, Franklin D, Braunwald E (1970) Coronary vasoconstriction due to digitalis in the concious dog. Clin Res 18:526

21. Gazes PC, Holmes CR, Moseley V, Pratt HR (1961) Acute hemorrhage and necrosis of the intestines associated with digitalization. Circulation 23:358

22. Hess T, Stucki P (1975) Mesenterialinfarkt bei Digitalisintoxikation. Schweiz Med Wochenschr 105:1237–1240

23. Muggia FM (1967) Hemorrhagic necrosis of the intestine: its occurrence with digitalis intoxication. Am J Med Sci 253:263

24. Polansky BJ, Berger RL, Byrne JJ (1964) Massive nonocclusive intestinal infarction associated with digitalis toxicity. Circulation [Suppl] 29/30:3

25. Brobmann GF, Barth K, Strecker EP, Schmidt-Hieber M, Schmidt HA (1975) Die Wirkung von Strophanthin auf die intestinale Durchblutung. Ein Beitrag zur Pathophysiologie der haemorrhagischen Enteropathie. Langenbecks Arch Chir [Suppl] 291–295

Response of Large and Small Coronary Arteries to Adenosine, Nitroglycerin, Cardiac Glycosides, and Calcium Antagonists

R. M. Berne, L. Belardinelli, D. R. Harder, N. Sperelakis, and R. Rubio

Summary

Some electric membrane properties of isolated large (>1.0 mm) and small (<500 μm) coronary arteries of the dog were studied with intracellular microelectrodes. The resting membrane potential was not significantly different in large and small arteries (average -56 mV and -53 mV, respectively). Spontaneous action potentials were not present in either sized vessels, and action potentials could not be induced upon electric stimulation. Addition of tetraethylammonium ion (TEA, 10 mM) permitted overshooting action potentials to be elicited by electric stimulation. The relationship between action potential amplitude and $\log[Ca^{++}]_0$ was linear (between 0.5 to 5.0 mM) with a slope of 30 mV decade; the action potential amplitude was unaffected by removal of Na^+. This suggests that the inward current during the action potential is primarily carried by Ca^{++}. We tested two categories of vasoactive agents for their ability to affect the TEA-induced action potentials; relaxants of smooth muscle (adenosine, nitroglycerin, verapamil, and Mn^{++}) and smooth muscle constrictors (the cardiac glycosides, ouabain and digoxin). Adenosine (10^{-5} M) blocked the Ca^{++}-dependent action potentials in small coronary arteries, but had no effect on the action potential in large arteries. In contrast, nitroglycerin (10^{-5} M) blocked the action potential in large coronary arteries, but not in small ones. Verapamil (5×10^{-6} M) and Mn^{++} (1 mM) blocked the action potential irrespective of the size of the vessel. The cardiac glycosides (4×10^{-9} M to 1×10^{-7} M) increased the frequency, amplitude and maximal rate of rise of the TEA-induced action potentials in small (<500 μm) coronary arteries in a dose-dependent manner. In the presence of a subthreshold concentration of TEA (5 mM) the cardiac glycosides induced spontaneous action potentials. The effects of cardiac glycosides occurred before any significant depolarization, and the effects were not mimicked by phenylephrine (α-agonist) nor reduced by phentolamine (α-antagonist). Verapamil (10^{-5} M) and Mn^{++} (2 mM) abolished all spike activity produced by the cardiac glycosides. The results suggest that several vasoactive agents have the ability to affect the inward slow Ca^{++} current in coronary artery smooth muscle cells. Such an action could help to explain [1] the differential relaxation of large and small coronary arteries produced by adenosine and nitroglycerin, [2] the general relaxing effect of Ca^{++}-antagonists such as verapamil and Mn^{++}, and [3] the coronary vasoconstriction produced by cardiac glycosides that may be a factor in digitalis toxicity and could be blocked by Ca^{++}-antagonists. In view of the possible role of adenosine as a local regulator of coronary blood flow, the present results may suggest a mechanism whereby adenosine controls coronary vascular resistance.

Introduction

In some blood vessels, the contraction of smooth muscle is mediated by regenerative electric responses (action potentials) and/or changes in the level of the resting potential [1]. This process is referred to as electromechanical coupling. In some cases the contraction of smooth muscle produced by vasoactive agents is not associated with a change in membrane potential [2,3]. This is a nonelectrogenic mechanism and has been termed pharmaco-mechanical coupling [2]. However, in those cases in which neurotransmitters produce contractions without changes in membrane potential, there are still changes in membrane conductance [3]. In all cases there is an increase in the free myoplasmic calcium concentration. Thus, vascular smooth muscles (VSM) can be divided into two categories, those that generate action potentials (spiking VSM) and those that normally do not (nonspiking VSM) [1,4]. As an example of the first type, spiking VSM, the portal vein is the most extensively studied. An example of the second type, nonspiking VSM, is the large conductance vessels [1,4,5]. However, some resistance vessels also do not seem to generate action potentials physiologically [6].

The fact that spontaneous action potentials accompanied by phasic mechanical activity can be elicited in some of the nonspiking VSM after treatment with tetraethylammonium ion (TEA) [3,7–9], a known inhibitor of the K^+ outward current [10,11], suggests that an inward regenerative current can be produced, but that this inward current is normally suppressed or opposed by a large K^+ outward current. Droogmans et al. [3] have found that in the rabbit ear artery, the spontaneous action potentials induced by TEA are accompanied by contractions and are calcium dependent. We have recently [8,9] shown that the amplitude of TEA-induced action potentials in dog coronary arteries are mainly dependent on $[Ca^{++}]_0$. Thus, the TEA-induced action potential in arterial smooth muscle provides a useful preparation for study of the inward Ca^{++} current and its relationship to excitation-contraction coupling.

Based on mechanical recordings, it has been suggested [12,13] that the mechanism of action of the coronary dilation caused by adenosine, nitroglycerin and verapamil is inhibition of Ca^{++}-influx. In concert with these findings, Fleckenstein et al. [12] have suggested that the coronary constriction caused by cardiac glycosides is mediated by an increase in Ca^{++}-influx. The purpose of the present study was to test two types of vasoactive agents (relaxants of VSM such as adenosine, nitroglycerin, and verapamil) and (constrictors of VSM such as ouabain and digoxin) for their ability to affect the TEA-induced action potentials in isolated strips of large (>1.0 mm o.d.) and small (<0.5 mm o.d.) dog coronary arteries.

Resting Membrane Properties

From impalements with microelectrodes the resting membrane potential E_m in the VSM of the large coronary arteries averaged -56 ± 2 mV, and that of the small coronary arteries -53 ± 2 mV. The input resistance, measured as the slope of the steady-state voltage/current curve through the origin, averaged 9.0 ± 0.4 MΩ in the large arteries and 10 ± 1.0 MΩ in the small arteries. None of these differences were statistically significant.

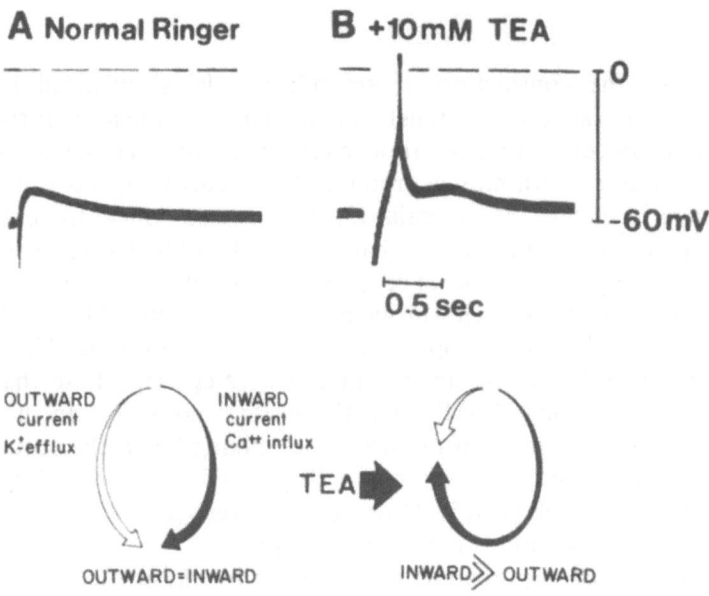

Fig. 1A – B. Induction of excitability by tetraethylammonium (TEA) in the smooth muscle of a small coronary artery of the dog. *Upper row,* **A** Control in normal Ringer's solution showing inexcitability. **B** Record from the same cell in **C** *(upper row)* 10 min after addition of 10 mM TEA, illustrates a large overshooting action potential in response to electric stimulation. *Lower row:* Illustration depicts a hypothetical mechanism for TEA induction of regenerative spikes. Normally (without TEA), the outwart K^+ current that flows upon depolarizing stimuli has comparable magnitude to the inward Ca^{++} current (open and closed arrows are equal); thus, the VSM cells are inexcitable. Addition of TEA might alter the balance of inward and outward current either by reducing the outward K^+ current *(smaller open arrow)* and/or increasing the inward Ca^{++} current *(larger closed arrow)*. In either case, sufficient net inward current would flow to allow generation of action potentials. (Adapted from Circ Res [8] by permission of the American Heart Association.)

Induction of Excitability by TEA

The VSM cells in both large and small coronary arteries were quiescent and had stable resting potentials of -55 ± 1 mV. No action potentials were observed upon application of intracellular or extracellular current pulses (Fig. 1a). Addition of 10 mM TEA allowed overshooting action potentials to be elicited upon electric stimulation (10 V, 2 impulses/min, 10 – 30 ms duration) (Fig. 1b). The TEA (10 mM) caused only a small depolarization of about 4 mV.

The mean action potential amplitude was 55 ± 1 mV in the smooth muscle of the large arteries and 54 ± 1 mV in the smooth muscle of the small arteries. The maximal rate of rise ($+\dot{V}_{max}$) of the TEA-induced action potential was 5 ± 1 V/s in the large arteries and 6 ± 1 V/s in the small arteries.

Ca^{++} Dependency of the TEA-Induced Action Potentials

The amplitude of the TEA-induced action potentials varied as a function of $[Ca^{++}]_0$, that is, the action potential amplitude increased as the $[Ca^{++}]_0$ was

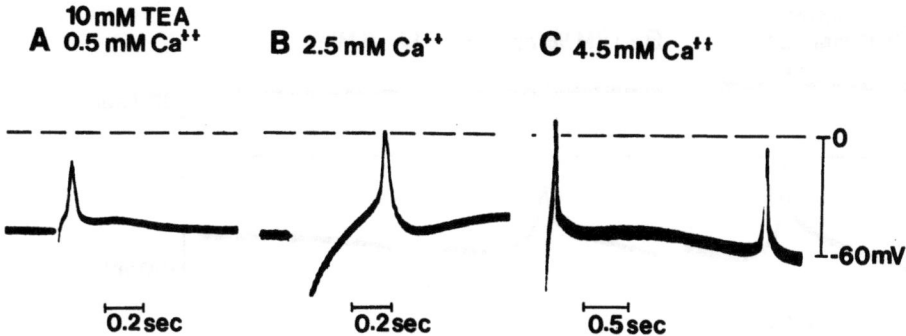

Fig. 2A – C. Illustration of the Ca^{++}-dependency of the tetraethylammonium (TEA, 10 mM)-induced action potential in a small coronary artery of the dog. **A** Record illustrates production of an undershooting action potential (in response to electrical stimulation 10 V, 2 impulses/min. 10–30 ms duration) in solutions containing only 0.5 mM Ca^{++}. **B** Record shows an increase in amplitude of the action potential upon increase in $[Ca^{++}]_0$ to 2.5 mM. **C** In 4.5 mM Ca^{++}, there was a further increase in action potential amplitude; in addition a second spontaneous action potential is shown. Voltage calibration in **C** applieds to all records. The horizontal broken line gives the zero potential. (Reproduced from Circ Res [8] by permission of the American Heart Association)

increased (Fig. 2). The relationship between action potential amplitude and the log of $[Ca^{++}]_0$ was linear and had a slope of 30 mV/decade (between 0.5 and 5.0 mm $[Ca^{++}]_0$) in the large arteries and 31 mV/decade in the small arteries (Fig. 3). These values agree with the theoretically predicted value from the Nernst equation of 30.5 mV/decade for a membrane purely selective for calcium ions. These data suggest that the inward current during the action potential is carried primarily by calcium ions.

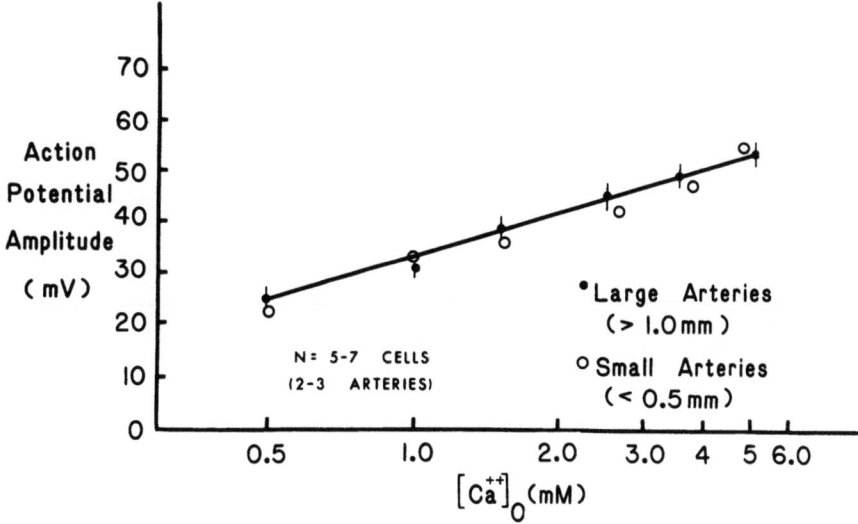

Fig. 3. Effect of increase of the external Ca^{++} concentration ($[Ca^{++}]_0$) on the amplitude of the TEA-induced action potentials in large *(closed circles)* and small *(open circles)* coronary arteries of the dog. Each point plotted is the mean value (± SE) for 5–7 cells impaled in 2–3 arteries. The average slope of the action potential amplitude vs. log $[Ca^{++}]_0$ is 30 mV/decade between 0.5 and 5.0 mM Ca^{++} in the large arteries and 31 mV/decade in the small arteries. The curves were fitted by linear regression analysis

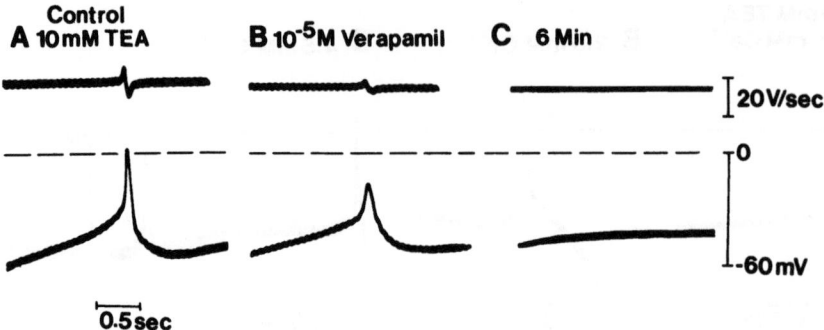

Fig. 4A – C. Verapamil blockade of the TEA-induced action potentials in the smooth muscle of small coronary arteries of the dog. A Control action potential induced by 10 mM TEA upon electric stimulation. B Record shows depression of the action potential 1 min after 10^{-5} M verapamil was added. C Record shows complete blockade of the action potential 6 min after the verapamil addition. The shock artifacts are not shown in these records because they occurred at the beginning of each sweep. The reason for the long delay in the response is not known, but may be caused by an anodal-break type of excitation. The upper trace gives dV/dt; the peak excursion of this trace is proportional to the maximal rate of rise of the action potential. (Circ Res [8] by permission of the American Heart Association)

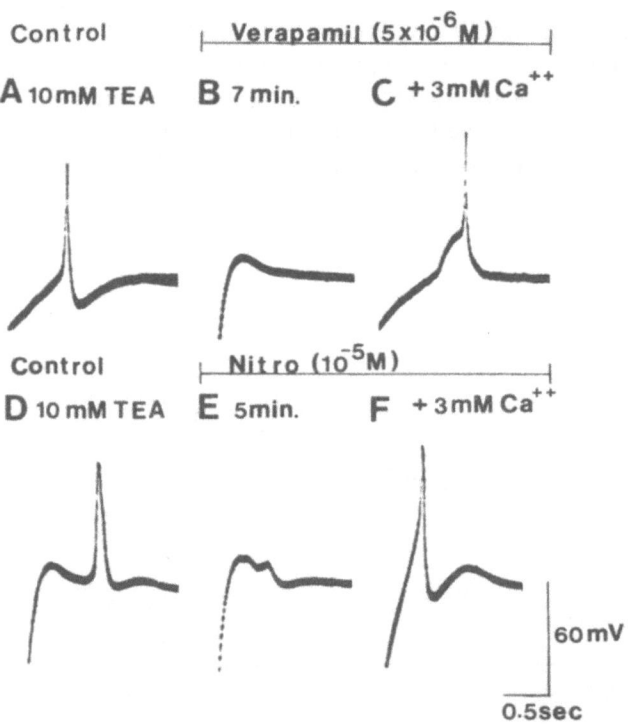

Fig. 5A – F. Reversal of the inhibitory effects of verapamil and nitroglycerin by elevation of $[Ca^{++}]_0$. A Control action potential induced by 10 mM TEA upon electrical stimulation. B Record shows blockade of the action potential 7 min after addition of verapamil. C Restoration of the action potential by addition of 3 mM Ca^{++}. D Control action potential induced by 10 mM TEA upon electric stimulation. E Blocking effects of nitroglycerin. F Reversal of the inhibitory effects of nitroglycerin by addition of 3 mM Ca^{++}. Voltage and time calibration in F apply throughout

Verapamil-HCl ($10^{-5}\,M$), a known blocker of Ca^{++} inward current [14], rapidly depressed the TEA-induced action potentials in both large and small coronary arteries (Fig. 4). Thus, verapamil abolished the TEA-action potential irrespective of the artery size. The verapamil blockade is also consistent with the Ca^{++}-dependency of the action potential. In addition, the inhibitory effects of verapamil can be overcome by elevation of $[Ca^{++}]_0$ (Fig. 5A – C). Effects similar to those obtained with verapamil were observed with $1-2\,mM\,Mn^{++}$.

Effects of Adenosine and Nitroglycerin

Adenosine ($10^{-5}\,M$) blocked the Ca^{++}-dependent, TEA-induced action potentials in small coronary arteries (Fig. 6), but had no effect on the action potential in large arteries (Fig. 7). The blockade of the action potential in small coronary arteries produced by adenosine was promptly reversed by adenosine deaminase (Fig. 6). Adenosine had no significant effect on the resting potential.

In contrast, nitroglycerin ($10^{-5}\,M$) blocked the TEA-induced action potential in large coronary arteries (Fig. 7) but not in the small arteries (Fig. 6). Addition of 3.0 $mM\,[Ca^{++}]_0$ restored the action potentials depressed by nitroglycerin (Fig. 5D – F). Thus, the inhibitory effects of nitroglycerin is antagonized by calcium ions.

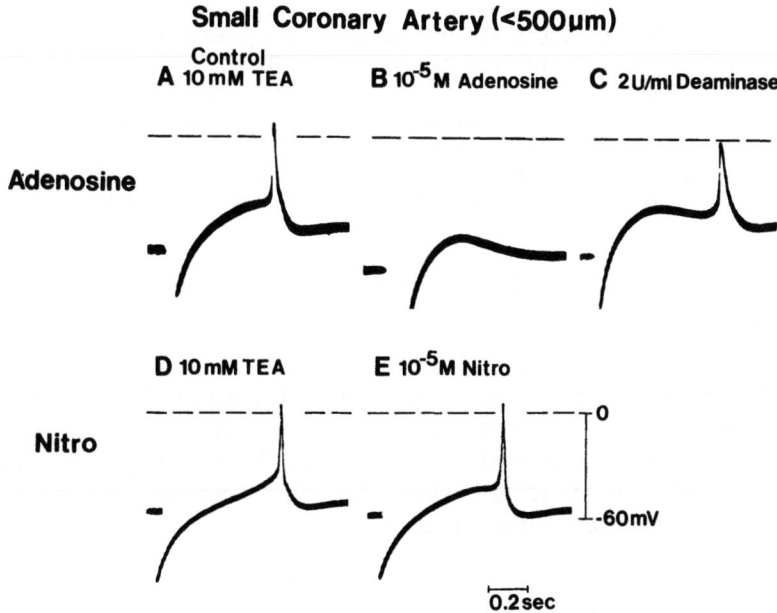

Fig. 6A – E. Illustration of the effects of adenosine (**A – C**) and of nitroglycerin (Nitro) (**D – E**) on the TEA-induced action potentials in the smooth muscle of small (< 500 μm) coronary arteries of the dog. **A – C** Blocking effect of adenosine (all records taken from the same cell). **A** Control action potential produced by electric stimulation in the presence of 10 mM TEA. **B:** $10^{-5}\,M$ adenosine completely blocked the action potential within 30 s. **C** Partial recovery of the action potential following addition of adenosine deaminase (2 units/ml). **D – E** Lack of effect of nitroglycerin (records from one cell). **D** Control action potential produced by electrical stimulation in 10 mM TEA. **E** Addition of $10^{-5}\,M$ nitroglycerin had no effect on the action potential amplitude or overshoot. Voltage and time calibrations in **E** apply throughout. (Circ Res [8] by permission of the American Heart Association)

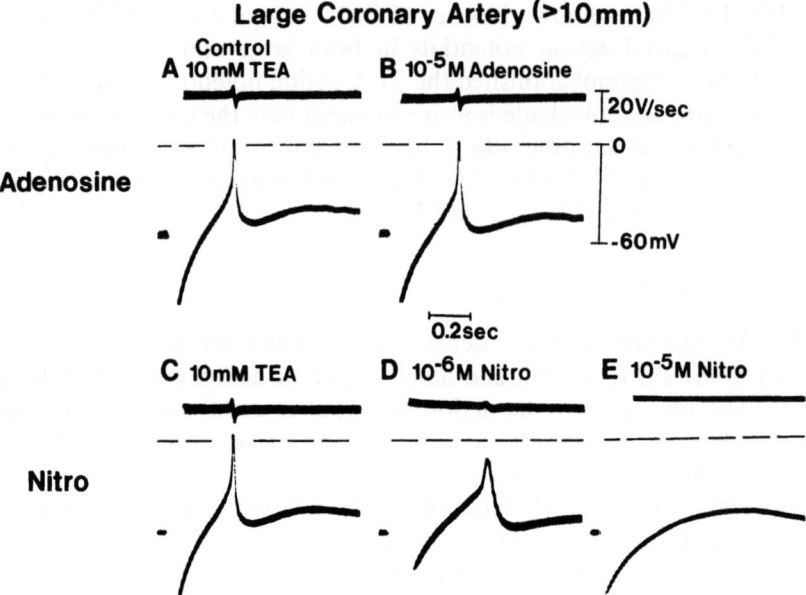

Fig. 7A – E. Illustration of the effects of adenosine (**A, B**) and of nitroglycerin (Nitro) (**C – E**) on the TEA-induced action potentials in the smooth muscle of large (>1.0 mm) coronary arteries of the dog. **A, B** Lack of effect of adenosine. **A** Control action potential produced by electric stimulation in the presence of 10 mM TEA. **B** Record from same cell impaled in **A** shows the lack of effect of 10^{-5} M adenosine on the action potential. Note that the amplitude, overshoot and rate of rise were not altered. **C – E** Blocking effect of nitroglycerin (all records from one cell). **C** Control action potential induced by 10 mM TEA. **D** Depression of the action potential by 10^{-6} M nitroglycerin (record depicted taken at 5 min after addition). **E** Record shows complete abolition of the action potential when nitroglycerin was raised to 10^{-5} M (record depicted taken at 5 min). Voltage and time calibrations in **B** apply throughout. Upper trace gives dV/dt. (Circ Res [8] by permission of the American Heart Association)

Effect of the Cardiac Glycosides on the Resting Potential of Small Coronary Arteries

The cardiac glycoside, ouabain, in concentrations ranging from 4×10^{-9} to 1×10^{-8} M had no significant effect on resting E_m within 15 min (Table 1). However, ouabain at 1×10^{-7} M produced a significant depolarization (from a control value of -54 mV ± 1.3 to -50 ± 0.8 mV) (Table 1). At 1×10^{-6} M, ouabain depolarized the VSM cells by 12 mV within the 15 min period. Digoxin was less potent in producing depolarization (Table 1).

Effect of the Cardiac Glycosides on the TEA-Induced Action Potentials of Small Coronary Arteries

Ouabain

In the absence of TEA, ouabain did not induce spontaneous action potentials in small (<500 µm o.d.) coronary arteries. However, in the presence of 5 mM TEA, addition of ouabain to the bathing solution produced spontaneous oscillations in membrane potential (E_m) (Fig. 8B,C). By 8 – 12 min after addition of ouabain, these

Table 1. Effects of cardiac glycosides on resting membrane potential in the vascular smooth muscle of dog coronary arteries

Digoxin			Ouabain		
Dose (M)	N^a	E_m (mV)	Dose (M)	N^a	E_m (mV)
0	35/16	-55 ± 1.0	0	33/12	-54 ± 1.3
4×10^{-9}	8/5	-55 ± 0.8	4×10^{-9}	7/3	-54 ± 1.0
1×10^{-8}	9/5	-55 ± 0.9	1×10^{-8}	12/6	-53 ± 0.7
1×10^{-7}	8/5	-54 ± 0.6	1×10^{-7}	10/6	-50 ± 0.8^b
1×10^{-6}	10/4	-51 ± 1.0^b	1×10^{-6}	11/4	-42 ± 1.1^b

Source: Reproduced by permission from J Pharmacol Exp Therap [9]. Values given are the mean ± 1 SE, measured 15–20 min after addition of digoxin or ouabain.
[a] Numerator gives number of cells penetrated, denominator gives number of arteries.
[b] Significantly different from control in glycoside-free solution at $p < 0.05$.

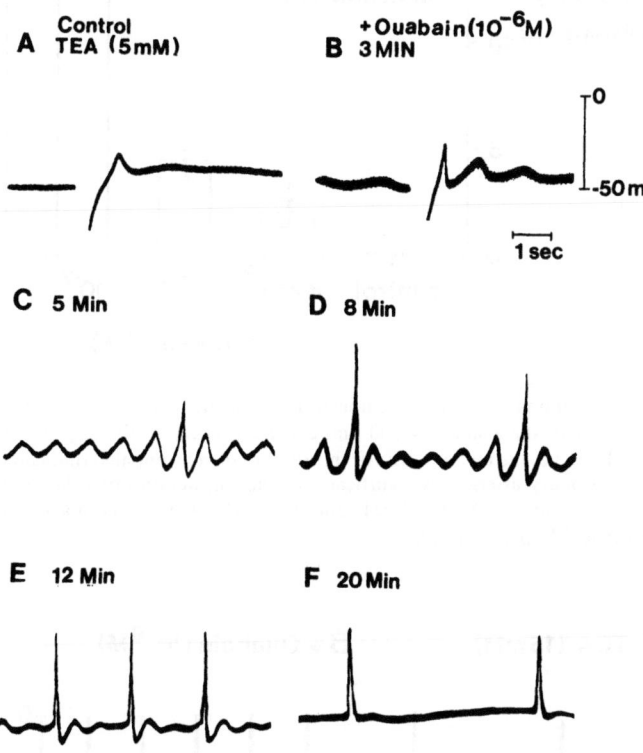

Fig. 8A–F. Induction of spontaneous electrical activity by ouabain in a small (< 500 µm) coronary artery pretreated with a subthreshold dose of TEA. **A** Control record demonstrates only a small graded response to electrical stimulation 20 min after addition of TEA 5 mM. **B,C** Initiation of spontaneous oscillations in resting potential 3 min **B** and 5 min **C** after addition of ouabain (10^{-6} M). **D,E** Records show the ouabain-induced spontaneous oscillations that give rise to overshooting action potentials; records taken 8 min **D** and 12 min **E** following addition of the ouabain. **F** After 20 min of exposure to ouabain, a significant depolarization occurred with a concomitant decrease in action potential amplitude and frequency. All recordings were taken from the same cell. Voltage and time calibrations in **B** apply throughout. (By permission from J Pharmacol Exp Therap [9])

spontaneous oscillations reached threshold and elicited action potentials (Fig. 8D, E). By 15 – 20 min, significant depolarization (10 mV) had occurred, and only then was a decrease in action potential frequency and amplitude observed (Fig. 8F). The data with respect to the frequency of the action potentials induced by various doses of ouabain in previously quiescent cells (pretreated with 10 mM TEA, but not stimulated) is depicted in Fig. 9. Note that low doses of ouabain ($4 \times 10^{-9}\,M$) had a significant effect and that $10^{-6}\,M$ had a marked effect. The effects of ouabain on the frequency of the spontaneous action potentials occurred prior to any significant depolarization (Fig. 10).

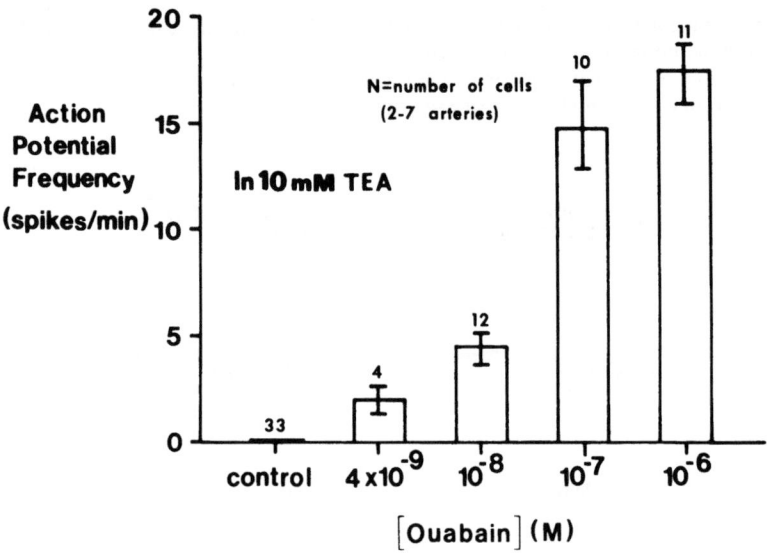

Fig. 9. Summary of data demonstrating the dose-dependency of ouabain on the action potential frequency of the a small ($< 500\ \mu\mathrm{m}$) coronary artery of the dog. Tissue was exposed to TEA (10 mM). Each bar gives the mean $\pm$ SE for the number of cells impaled (indicated by the numbers over the bars) in $2 - 7$ coronary arteries. A significant increase in action potential frequency was observed even at low doses of ouabain ($4 \times 10^{-9}\,M$), and $10^{-6}\,M$ gave a very marked increase. (By permission from J Pharmacol Exp Therap [9])

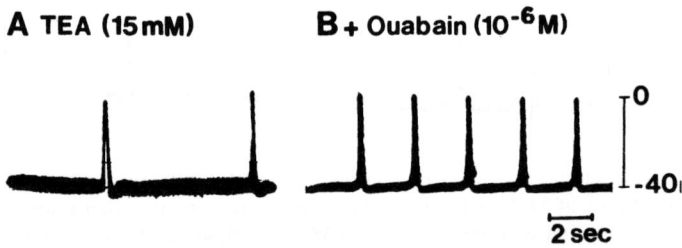

Fig. 10A, B. Increase in frequency of TEA-induced action potentials produced by ouabain. **A** Control record in the presence of TEA (15 mM) shows the spontaneous action potentials; resting potential was -40 mV (compared to the control value in the absence of TEA of -54 mV. **B** Record taken from the same cell shows a marked increase in action potential frequency within 30 s after addition of ouabain ($10^{-6}\,M$) in the absence of depolarization. (By permission from J Pharmacol Exp Therap [9])

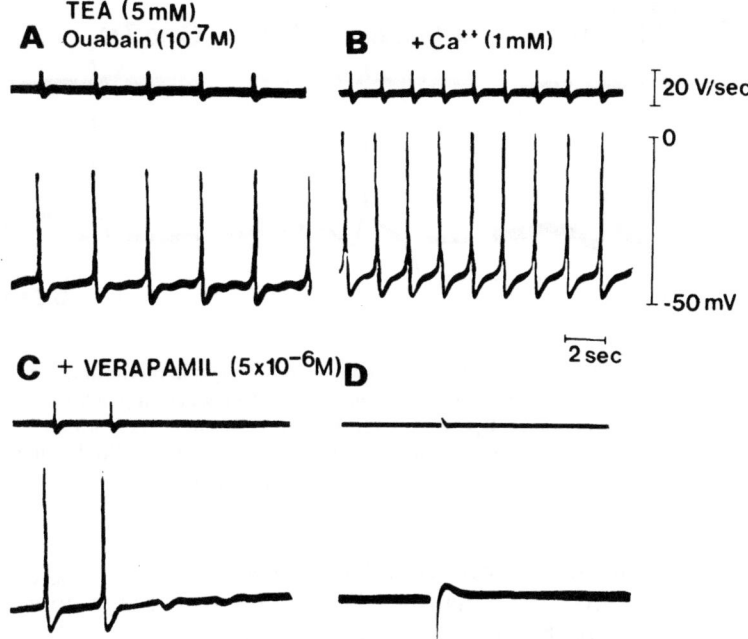

Fig. 11A – D. Effect of extracellular Ca^{++} concentration on the ouabain-induced spontaneous action potentials in a small (<500 μm) coronary artery of the dog. **A** Spontaneous action potentials induced by TEA (5 mM). **B** Record shows a marked increase in amplitude, maximal rate of rise and frequency of the action potentials within 30 s after increasing $[Ca^{++}]_0$ by 1 mM (from 2.5 to 3.5 mM). **C** Record shows abolition of spontaneous action potentials after 5×10^{-6} M verapamil was added. **D** Record shows complete blockade of the action potentials 5 min after the verapamil addition. Records were taken from the same cell. The upper trace in panels A – C give dV/dt, the peak excursion of which is proportional to the maximal rate of rise of the action potential. The dV/dt calibration is given in **B** (Adapted from Pharmacol Exp Therap [9])

To examine the interaction between ouabain and calcium, the following experiments were carried out. Spontaneous action potentials were induced by 5 mM TEA plus 10^{-7} M ouabain, and as can be seen in Fig. 11, elevation of $[Ca^{++}]_0$ by 1 mM caused a marked increase in amplitude, rate of rise, and frequency of the action potentials. Thus, it appears that calcium and ouabain act synergistically. Verapamil (5×10^{-6} M) abolished the spontaneous action potentials (Fig. 11C) as well as those elicited by electric stimulation (Fig. 11D).

Digoxin

The effects of digoxin were similar to those of ouabain. The main difference between the two cardiac glycosides was that ouabain was more potent in the induction of spontaneous action potentials. However, when spontaneous action potentials were already present digoxin increased their frequency of firing.

In those preparations in which 5 mM TEA produced undershooting action potentials upon electric stimulation (Fig. 12A), addition of digoxin produced a dose-dependent increase in amplitude and rate of rise of the action potential without affecting the resting potential (Fig. 12B, C). Figure 13 summarizes the data with

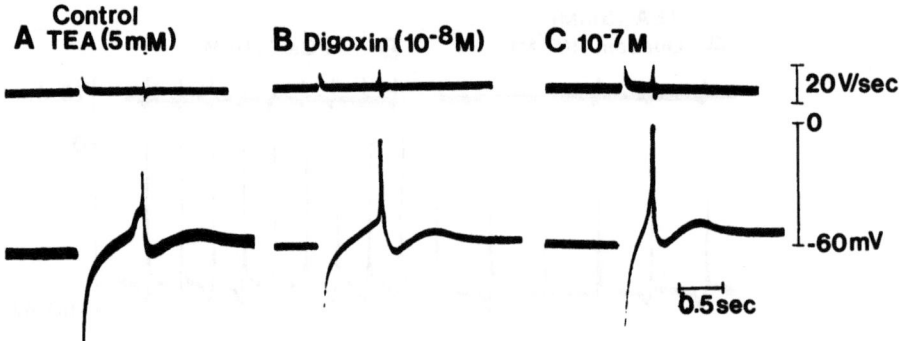

Fig. 12A – C. Illustration of the potentiating effect of digoxin on the amplitude and maximal rate of rise of the action potential. **A** Elicitation of an undershooting action potential by electric stimulation in the presence of TEA (5 mM). **B, C** Records from same cell as in **A** taken within 2 min after addition of 10^{-8} M **B** and 10^{-7} M **C** digoxin, showing a marked increase in the amplitude and maximal rate of rise of the action potentials. Upper trace gives dV/dt. (By permission from J Pharmacol Exp Therap [9])

respect to the dose-dependent effect of digoxin on the $+\dot{V}_{max}$ and amplitude of the action potential. Note that the effects of digoxin at high doses (10^{-6} M) were less, and this was probably due to a depolarizing action (Table 1).

Since it has been suggested [15] that the coronary vasoconstriction caused by the cardiac glycosides could be mediated through α-adrenergic receptor stimulation, we investigated this possibility. The α-adrenergic blocker, phentolamine, did not prevent the action of the cardiac glycosides. In addition, the α-adrenergic agonist, phenylephrine did not mimic the effects of the glycosides. Thus, while some evidence indicates an involvement of α-receptor stimulation in cardiac glycoside-induced coronary vasoconstriction, the cardiac glycosides also appear to exert a direct action on the VSM, possibly mediated through stimulation of the slow inward current.

Conclusions

The results demonstrate that the quiescent and inexcitable VSM cells of dog coronary arteries can generate action potentials upon addition of TEA. The TEA-induced action potentials in both large and small coronary arteries are Ca^{++}-dependent and are abolished by verapamil and/or $MnCl_2$.

The fact that adenosine abolished the Ca^{++}-dependent action potentials in small (but had no effect on the action potentials in large) coronary arteries contrasts with the results with nitroglycerin that blocked the action potentials in large coronary arteries, but not in small ones. These findings may provide a mechanism that is responsible for the differential relaxing effects of adenosine and nitroglycerin on the coronary vascular bed such as a higher concentration of adenosine receptors in the smaller coronary arteries. In view of the possible role of adenosine as a local regulator of coronary blood flow [16], the present results may suggest a means whereby adenosine controls vascular resistance.

The ability of the cardiac glycosides to produce coronary vasoconstriction could be related to an augmentation of the inward calcium current. Consistent with this

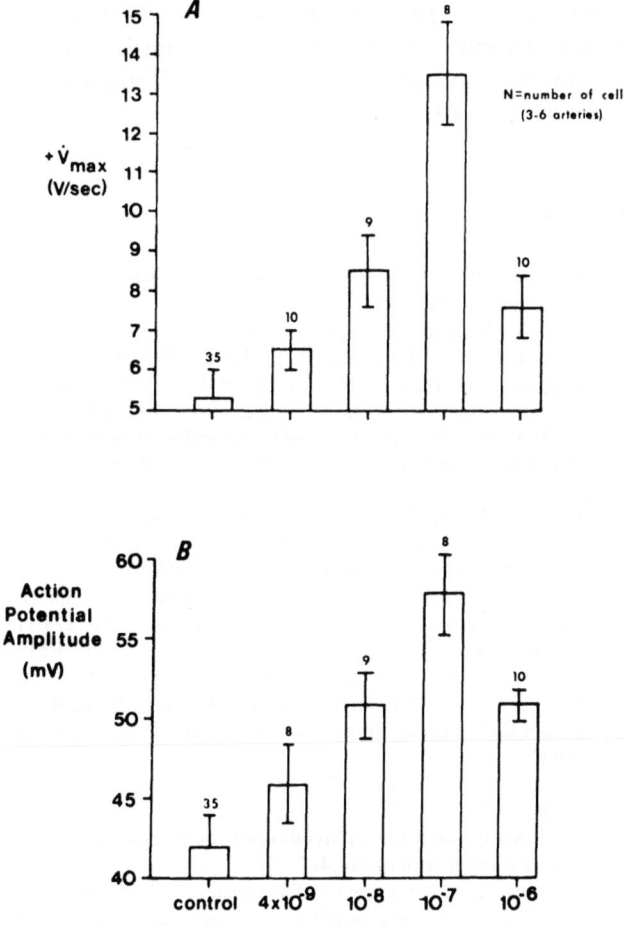

Fig. 13A, B. Summary of data demonstrating the dose-dependency of digoxin on the maximal rate of rise **A** and amplitude **B** of the action potential. The tissue was bathed in 5 mM TEA to allow the elicitation of action potentials. Each bar gives the mean ± 1 SE for the number of cells impaled (indicated by the number over the bars) in 3–6 coronary arteries. Significant increases in both maximal rate of rise and amplitude occurred at 10^{-8} M, and the peak effect occurred at 10^{-7} M. At higher doses of digoxin (10^{-6} M), there was a significant decrease in maximal rate of rise and amplitude. (By permission from J Pharmacol Exp Therap [9])

view, known calcium antagonists such as verapamil, fully inhibit the ouabain-induced contraction [12] and also abolish the action potentials induced by TEA plus ouabain [9]. Finally, since coronary vasoconstriction could be another factor in digitalis toxicity, verapamil may be useful in antagonizing the glycoside-induced coronary vasoconstriction.

Acknowledgements

This research was supported by a grant from the National Institute of Health (HL 19242). Dr. Belardinelli was supported by this grant and is a recipient of a fellowship (No. 1112 – 1273/76) from CNPq and Fundaçao Imoversotaroa de Cardiologia do Rio Grande do Sul, Brasil. Dr. Harder's present address is Department of Physiology, College of Medicine, East Tennessee State University, Johnson City, Tennessee, 37061.

References

1. Johansson B (1971) Electromechanical and mechanoelectrical coupling in vascular smooth muscle. Angiologia 8:129 – 143
2. Somlyo AV, Somlyo AP (1968) Electromechanical and pharmacomechanical coupling in vascular smooth muscle. J Pharmacol Exp Therap 159:129 – 145
3. Droogmans G, Raeymakers L, Casteels R (1977) Electro- and pharmacomechanical coupling in the smooth muscle cells of the rabbit ear artery. J Gen Physiol 70:129 – 148
4. Somlyo AP, Somlyo AV (1968) Vascular smooth muscle. I. Normal structure, pathology, biochemistry and biophysics. Pharmacol Rev 20:197 – 272
5. Johansson B (1978) Vascular smooth muscle: Byophysics. In: Kaley G, Altura BM (eds) Microcirculation. University Park Press, Baltimore London Tokyo
6. Von Loh D, Bohr DF (1973) Membrane potentials of smooth muscle cells of isolated resistance vessels. Proc Soc Exp Biol Med 144:513 – 516
7. Harder D, Sperelakis N (1978) Membrane electrical properties of vascular smooth muscle from the guinea pig superior mesenteric artery. Pfluegers Arch 378:111 – 119
8. Harder D, Belardinelli L, Sperelakis N, Rubio R, Berne RM (1979) Differential effects of adenosine and nitroglycerin on the action potentials of large and small coronary arteries. Circ Res 44:176 – 182
9. Belardinelli L, Harder D, Sperelakis N, Rubio R, Berne RM (1979) Cardiac glycoside stimulation of inward Ca^{++} current in vascular smooth muscle of canine coronary artery. J Pharmacol Exp Therap 209:62 – 66
10. Kumamoto M, Horn L (1970) Voltage clamping of smooth muscle from taenia coli. Microvasc Res 2:188 – 201
11. Ito Y, Kuriyama H (1971) Membrane properties of the smooth muscle fibers of the guinea-pig portal vein. J Physiol (Lond) 214:427 – 449
12. Fleckenstein A, Nakayama K, Fleckenstein-Grün G, Byon YK (1975) Interactions of vasoactive ions and drugs with Ca-dependent excitation-contraction coupling of vascular smooth muscle. In: Carafoli E (ed) Calcium transport in contraction and secretion. North Holland, Amsterdam Oxford, pp 555 – 564
13. Schnaar RC, Sparks HV (1972) Response of large and small coronary arteries to nitroglycerin, $NaNO_2$ and adenosine. Am J Physiol 223:223 – 228
14. Kohlhardt M, Bauer B, Krause H, Fleckenstein A (1972) Differentiation of the transmembrane Na^+ and Ca^{++} channels in mammalian cardiac fibers by use of specific inhibitors. Pfluegers Arch 307:190 – 203
15. Hamlin NP, Willerson JT, Garan H, Powell WJ Jr (1974) The neurogenic vasoconstrictor effect of digitalis on coronary vascular resistance. J Clin Invest 53:288 – 296
16. Berne RM (1963) Cardiac nucleotides in hypoxia: possible role in regulation of coronary blood flow. Am J Physiol 204:317 – 322

Blockade of Renal Autoregulatory Vasoconstriction by Calcium Antagonists

K. Hashimoto, H. Ono, and N. O'Hara

Introduction

Autoregulation of blood flow is defined as the intrinsic regulatory mechanism of a vascular bed to maintain the blood at a constant flow rate. It is affirmed by observing the lack of proportional changes in the blood flow to those in the perfusion pressure.

Among various parts in the peripheral circulation, renal vascular bed is known to possess a distinct potency of autoregulation. Thus many studies have been performed on this phenomenon using excised and in situ perfused kidney and the mechanism has been discussed from various aspects. Since some vasoactive compounds were proved to abolish the autoregulation of the renal vascular beds, it has been accepted that the vascular smooth muscle itself regulates the blood flow against the change in the perfusion pressure. In this study, further evidence is presented on the myogenic nature of the renal autoregulation.

Methods

Adult mongrel dogs of either sex, weighing 10 to 20 kg, were anesthetized intravenously with 30 mg/kg of sodium pentobarbital. The left renal artery was exposed retroperitoneally, cannulated, and perfused with blood conducted from the femoral artery by means of a Harvard peristaltic pump. An initial dose of 500 Units sodium heparin per kg was given and 100 Units/kg was added at 1 h intervals. Perfusion pressure was maintained by a Starling pneumatic resistance through which excess blood was conducted to the femoral vein. A desired level of perfusion pressure was obtained by changing the pressure of the pneumatic resistance by opening the communication to the air reservoir, the atmospheric pressure of which was adjusted beforehand to a desired level (Fig. 1). Perfusion pressure and systemic blood pressure in the femoral artery were measured with electric manometers (transducers: Stetham P23Db and carrier amplifiers: San-ei 1206 B). Renal blood flow was measured by use of an electromagnetic flowmeter (Narco RT-500). These parameters were recorded on ink-writing oscillographs (San-ei 8S-11). The drug solution was infused into a rubber tube connected close to the shank of the renal arterial cannula by the aid of an infusion pump (Harvard Apparatus 901).

Drugs used in these experiments were nifedipine (Bayer AG), verapamil hydrochloride (Eisai), dilitiazem hydrochloride (Tanabe), perhexiline hydrochloride (Merrell), papaverine hydrochloride (Tokyo Kasei), aminophylline (Sanko) and glyceryl trinitrate (Nippon Kayaku). The desired concentration of drugs except perhexiline was obtained by dilution with 0.9% saline. Perhexiline was dissolved in distilled water. Doses of drugs are expressed as their base.

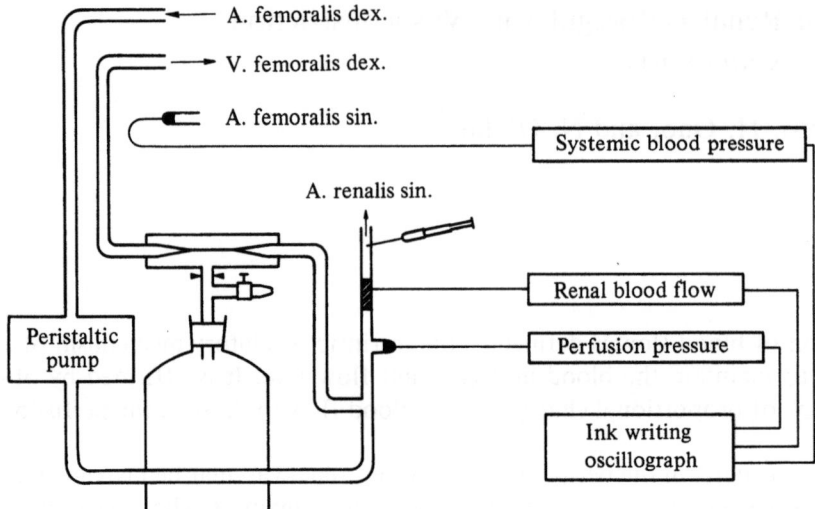

Fig. 1. Diagram of the perfusion system

Results

Autoregulatory Response in the Control Experiments and Effects of Ca^{++}-antagonists (Nifedipine, Verapamil, Dilitiazem, and Perhexiline)

The basal condition of renal blood flow at perfusion pressure of 100 mmHg became stable within 30 min after experimental set-up. The response of blood flow to step-wise changes by 20 mmHg of the perfusion pressure was observed, varying in the range from 60 to 220 mmHg in the control trial. The autoregulation of the renal vascular bed was confirmed by maintenance of stable level of the blood flow in spite of change in the perfusion pressure in the range between 100 and 200 mmHg.

The drug was infused intra-arterially and the effect of the drug on autoregulation was observed in the same range of perfusion pressure as done in the control trial. The autoregulatory response was abolished partially at the rate of infusion of 3 µg/min and completely at that of 10 µg/min of nifedipine. Simultaneous infusion of CaCl$_2$ at the rate of 30 mg/min protected the autoregulation to be impaired by 3 µg/min of nifedipine as shown in Fig. 2.

The similar results with abolition of autoregulation were obtained by infusion of verapamil, 30 and 100 µg/min (Fig. 3), dilitiazem 30 µg/min (Fig. 4), and perhexiline, 500 µg/min (Figs. 5 and 6). Simultaneous infusion of CaCl$_2$ at the rate of 30 mg/min antagonized the effects of these compounds on the autoregulation (Figs. 3, 4, 5, and 6).

Effects of Infusion of Papaverine and Aminophylline

The renal blood flow was regulated at nearly constant rate against step-wise changes in perfusion pressure in control trials; meanwhile the autoregulation of blood flow was abolished by papaverine 5 mg/min, and by aminophylline, 5 mg/min.

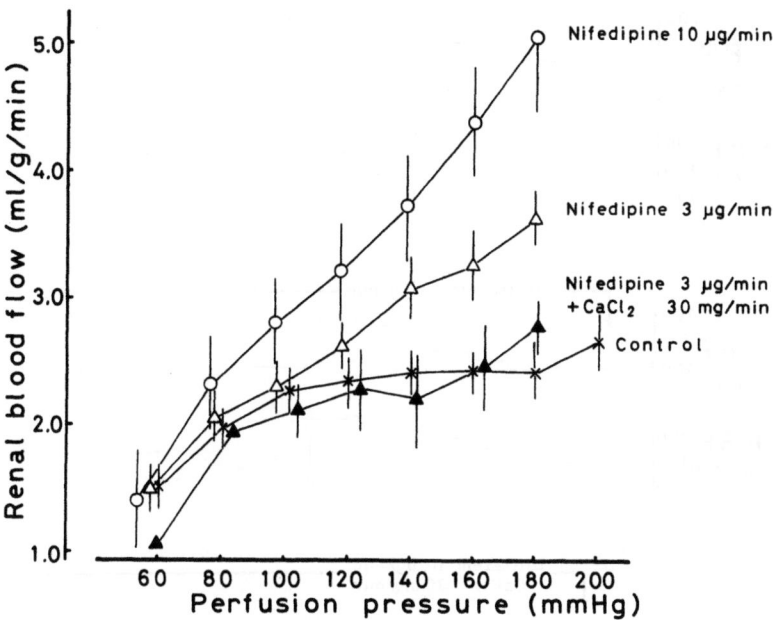

Fig. 2. Effect of nifedipine on the autoregulation of renal blood flow. Summary of 6 experiments. Symbols and vertical bars represent means ± S.E.'s, respectively. Control pressure-flow curve (×———×) shows that strict autoregulation existed in the range of 100 to 200 mmHg of perfusion pressure. Pressure-flow relation during infusion of 3 μg/min of nifedipine (△———△) showed that the autoregulation was partially impaired, and infusion of 10 μg/min of nifedipine (○———○) completely abolished the renal autoregulation. Simultaneous infusion of CaCl₂, 30 mg/min, with 3 μg/min of nifedipine (▲———▲) cancelled the effect of the calcium-antagonist

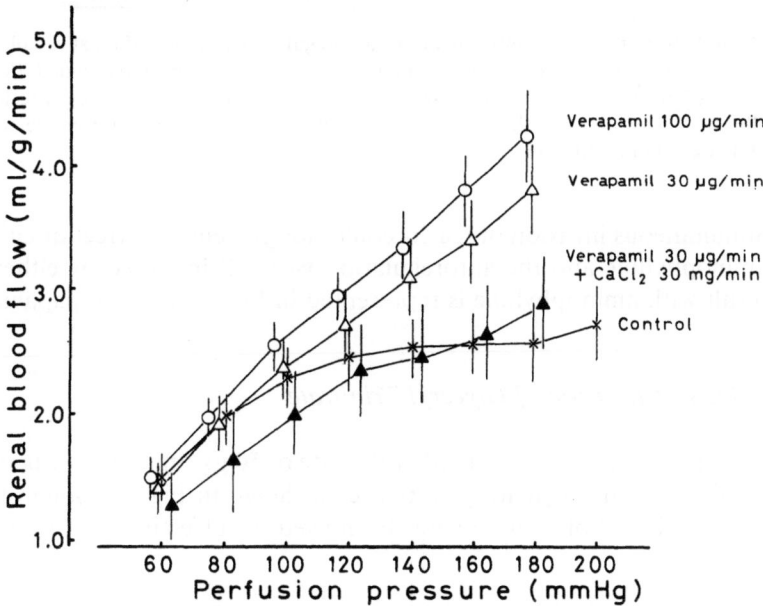

Fig. 3. Effect of verapamil on the autoregulation of renal blood flow. Summarized results of 5 experiments. Symbols and vertical bars represent means ± S.E.'s. Pressure-flow curves of control observation (×———×), during infusion of 30 μg/min (△———△) and 100 μg/min (○———○) of verapamil, and simultaneous infusion of 30 mg/min of CaCl₂ and 30 μg/min of verapamil (▲———▲)

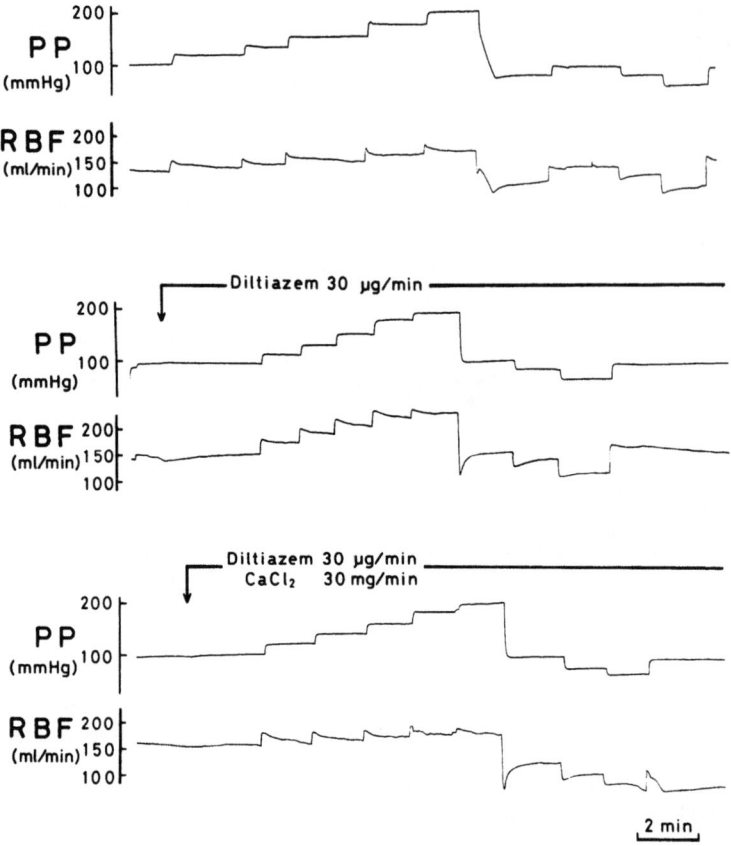

Fig. 4. Effect of diltiazem infusion on the autoregulatory response of renal vascular bed. The upper two traces show changes of the perfusion pressure (PP) and the renal blood flow (RBF) in control observation. The middle part shows abolition of the autoregulation by infusion of 30 µg/min of diltiazem. The lower part shows the preventive effect of $CaCl_2$ infusion from the impairment by infusion of 30 µg/min of diltiazem

Simultaneous infusion of $CaCl_2$ could not prevent the effect of either papaverine or aminophylline and the autoregulation was still impaired by either drug. A typical result with aminophylline is represented in Fig. 7 and with papaverine in Fig. 8.

Effects of Infusion of Glyceryl Trinitrate

Glyceryl trinitrate was infused at the rate of 50 µg/min. The drug infusion could not abolish the autoregulatory response as shown in Fig. 9, though the change in the systemic blood pressure obviously showed the effectiveness of the drug.

Discussion

The autoregulation of blood flow is generally accepted as one of the mechanisms responsible for the maintenance of a stable level of the blood flow in spite of

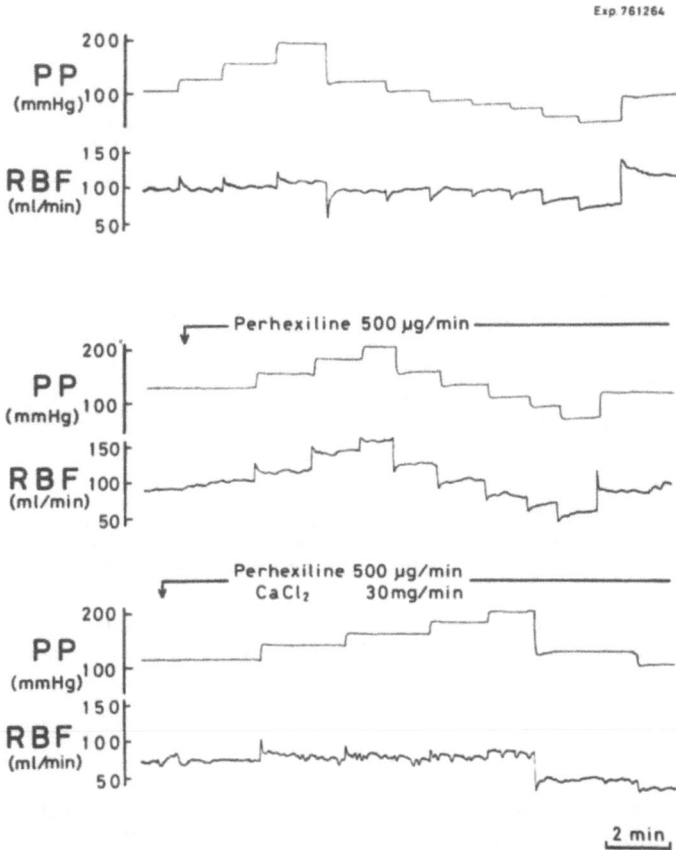

Fig. 5. Effect of infusion of 500 µg/min of perhexiline on the renal autoregulation. The abbreviations and the protocol are the same as in Fig. 4

fluctuation in the arterial blood pressure. Many studies have been performed in order to elucidate its mechanism by use of excised and in situ perfused kidney. Various theories including the tissue-pressure and the myogenic theories have been presented; however, at present, it is doubtless that the vascular smooth muscle plays an essential role in the autoregulatory mechanism, since the myogenic nature of the renal autoregulation was recognized first by Thurau and Kramer in 1959 [1] by using a smooth muscle relaxant, papaverine. The present authors have confirmed their results and added to a knowledge of myogenic nature the similar effect of aminophylline [2]. Later on, the new aspect has been opened since calcium antagonists such as nifedipine and verapamil were found to impair the autoregulatory response [3,6,7]. The effects of calcium antagonists were further examined with diltiazem and perhexiline in this study and similar results were obtained.

A unique characteristic of calcium antagonists is that by simultaneous administration of excess calcium, the renal autoregulation was protected against the effect of Ca^{++}-antagonists. This allows a differentiation of the mode of action of "general" smooth muscle relaxants from that of calcium antagonists on the basis of

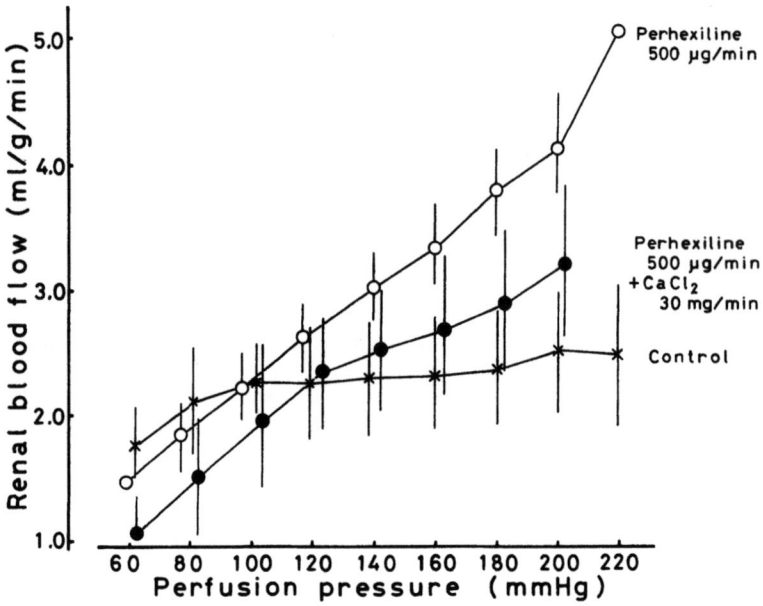

Fig. 6. Summarized results of effect of perhexiline infusion (N = 5). ×————×: control pressure-flow relation, ○————○: that during infusion of 500 μg/min of perhexiline, and ●————●: that during simultaneous infusion of CaCl₂ and perhexiline

their influence on renal autoregulation: The infusion of excess calcium failed to antagonize either papaverine or aminophylline. Both drugs produce a potent inhibition of phosphodiesterase which is understood as the basic mode of action of these drugs, and adenyl nucleotide such as cyclic-AMP is expected to be an intrinsic mediator of the relaxation. It seems to be very important that glyceryl trinitrate failed to impair the autoregulation, because glyceryl trinitrate and related compounds were found to interfere with calcium-dependent, excitation-contraction coupling of vascular smooth muscle, although the kinetics of nitrite-induced vascular relaxation proved to be rather different [4]. Previously Imai and Takeda [5] observed that glyceryl trinitrate failed to produce the relaxation of potassium-contracture teniae coli while papaverine and aminophylline maintained their relaxant actions. All of these compounds relaxed the teniae coli associated with an inhibition of spontaneous spike discharge and a hyperpolarization. In the present study, calcium antagonists, papverine and aminophylline increased the renal blood flow but stabilized at a certain level when perfusion pressure was kept at 100 mmHg, while glyceryl trinitrate induced the vasodilation but returned to the initial level even with the continuation of infusion. The absence of the impairment of autoregulation with glyceryl trinitrate may be ascribed to these differences in the vascular responses.

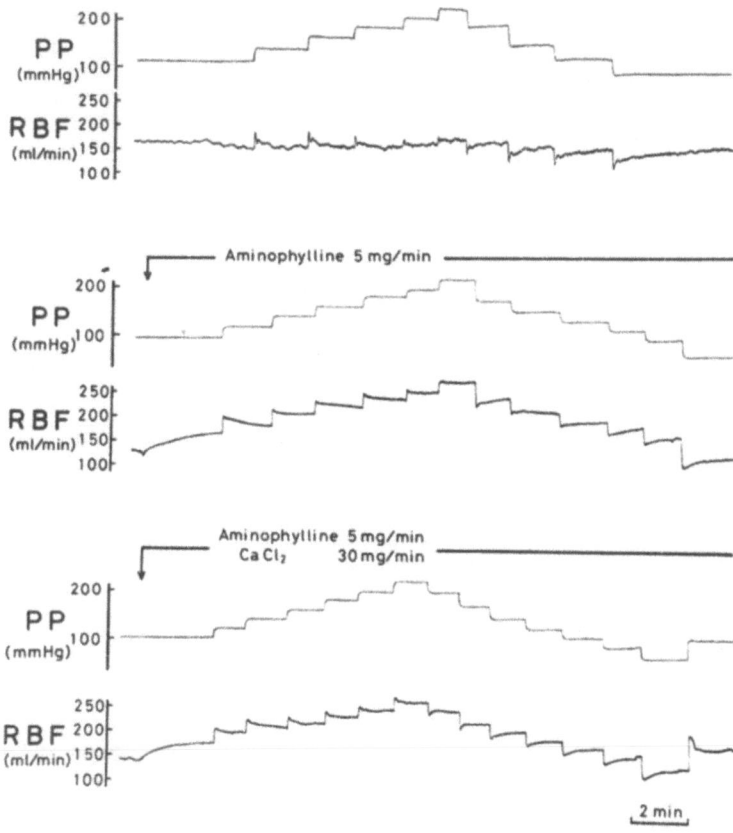

Fig. 7. Effect of aminophylline infusion on the renal blood flow. Control autoregulatory response was strict as shown in the upper part of the figure. Autoregulation was impaired by infusion of 5 mg/min of aminophylline *(middle)*, and simultaneous infusion of 30 mg/min of $CaCl_2$ failed to prevent the impairment with aminophylline *(lower)*. PP: perfusion pressure, RBF: renal blood flow

It is concluded that the nature of the autoregulation of the renal blood flow is essentially myogenic: it depends on the spontaneous activity of the vascular smooth muscle, which develops the tension and regulates the vascular caliber according to the transmural pressure (i.e., the pressure difference between the blood pressure and the tissue pressure).

Acknowledgments

The authors express their gratitude to Miss S. Suzuki for her help in preparing the manuscript.

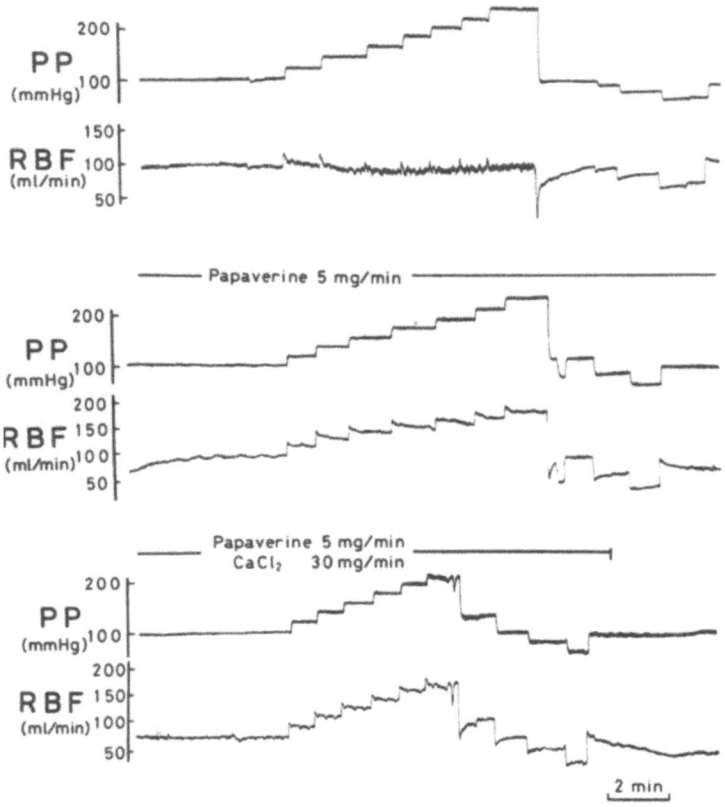

Fig. 8. Effect of infusion of papaverine, 5 mg/min, on the renal autoregulation. Autoregulation of blood flow as shown in the upper part of the figure was impaired by infusion of papaverine as shown in the middle part, and the impairment was not cancelled with simultaneous infusion of $CaCl_2$, as obvious from the result shown in the lower part of the figure

References

1. Thurau K, Kramer K (1959) Weitere Untersuchung zur myogenen Natur der Autoregulation des Nierenkreislaufes. Pfluegers Arch 269:77–93
2. Ono H, Inagaki K, Hashimoto K (1966) A pharmacological approach to the nature of the autoregulation of the renal blood flow. Jpn J Physiol 16:625–634
3. Ono H, Kokubun H, Hashimoto K (1974) Abolition by calcium antagonists of the autoregulation of renal blood flow. Naunyn Schmiedebergs Arch Pharmacol 285:201–207
4. Fleckenstein A (1977) Specific pharmacology of calcium in myocardium, cardiac pacemakers, and vascular smooth muscle. Annu Rev Pharmacol Toxicol 17:149–166
5. Imai S, Takeda K (1967) Effect of vasodilators upon the isolated taenia coli of the guinea pig. J Pharmacol Exp Ther 156:557–564
6. Grün G, Fleckenstein A (1972) Die elektromechanische Entkoppelung der Gefäßmuskulatur als Grundprinzip der Koronardilatation durch 4-(2'-Nitrophenyl)-2,6-dimethyl-1,4-dihydropyridin-3,5-dicarbonsäuredimethylester (BAYa1040, Nifedipine). Arzneim Forsch 22:334–344
7. Hashimoto K, Taira N, Chiba S, Hashimoto K Jr, Endoh M, Kokubun M, Kokubun H, Iijima T, Kimura T, Kubota K, Oguro K (1972) Cardiohemodynamic effects of BAYa1040 in the dog. Arzneim Forsch 22:15–21

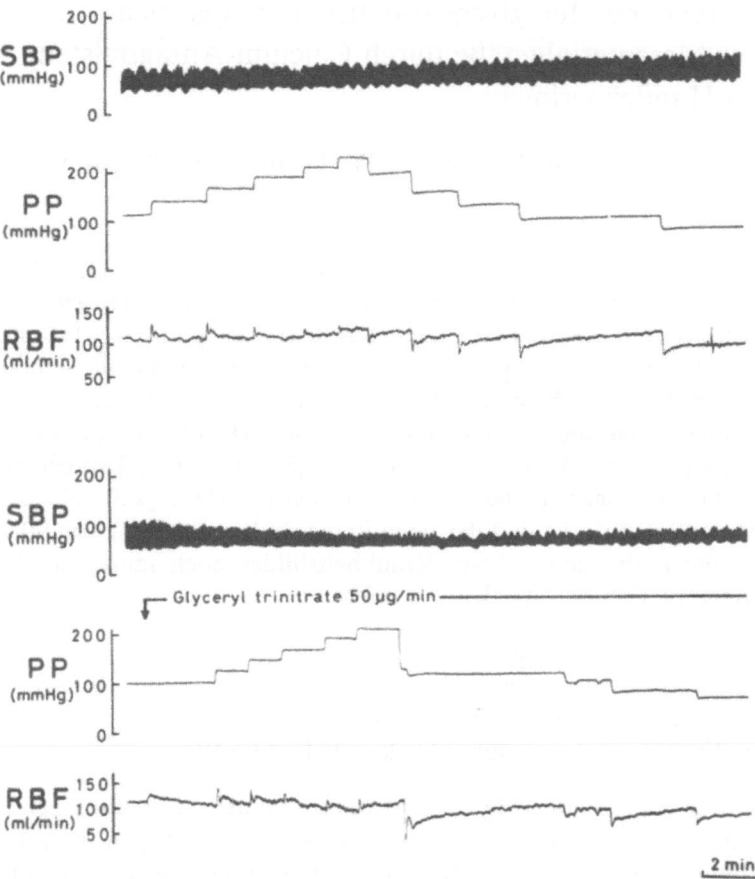

Fig. 9. Effect of intra-arterial infusion of glyceryl trinitrate on the renal blood flow (RBF) and the systemic blood flow (SBP). Infusion of 50 µg/min of glyceryl trinitrate did not influence the autoregulatory response of the blood flow to changes of the perfusion pressure (PP), though decrease of systolic blood pressure revealed effectiveness of the infused drug

Aufhebung Herzglycosid-induzierter Spasmen der Mesenterialgefäße durch Calcium-Antagonisten im Hundexperiment

G. F. Brobmann, M. Mayer, W. Grimm und A. Safer

Nicht nur organische Gefäßprozesse wie Embolie und/oder Thrombose können zu klinisch relevanten Durchblutungsstörungen im Bereich der mesenterialen Strombahn führen. Seit der Erstbeschreibung durch Moulonget [1] im Jahre 1931 ist das Krankheitsbild der sog. non occlusive mesenteric ischemia – besonders in den letzten Jahren – mehr und mehr in das Interesse der Kliniker gerückt. Fogarty [2] berichtete 1966 über ca. 600 gesicherte Fälle (Häufigkeit bei der Verdachtsdiagnose Mesenterialinfarkt 35 – 40%). Minami [3] und Silen [4] sprechen in neueren Untersuchungen sogar von 60 – 80%. Trotz der rel. Häufigkeit bei der Verdachtsdiagnose Mesenterialinfarkt und der noch immer hohen Letalität von 90 – 100% (Tabelle 1) ist die Pathogenese dieses Krankheitsbildes noch immer unklar und umstritten. Mehrere Theorien werden diskutiert:

a) Hämokonzentration [2, 5],
b) Herzinsuffizienz mit und ohne kardiogenem Schock [6, 10],
c) Intoleranz-Schock-Theorie [11, 12],
d) Vasokonstriktion durch Glykoside [2, 13 – 19].

Soweit heute zu überblicken scheint insbesondere von klinischen Beobachtungen her eine Kombination mehrerer dieser Theorien vorzuliegen. Es erkranken meist ältere Patienten mit kardialer oder peripherer Kreislaufinsuffizienz, die über längere Zeit mit Digitalisglykosiden behandelt wurden [2, 6 – 10, 20 – 23]. Price [24], Fogarty [2], Freiman [16] und Habboushe [21] sehen in der Digitalisbehandlung zumindest einen potenzierenden Faktor. Daß Glykoside eine erhebliche vasokonstriktorische Komponente haben, wurde in zahlreichen experimentellen Untersuchungen nachgewiesen [15, 19, 25 – 30]. Glykosidbedingte Gefäßspasmen lassen sich tierexperimentell nicht nur hämodynamisch, sondern auch angiographisch nachweisen [15, 31, 32]. Diese angiographischen Veränderungen ähneln denen von Patienten mit sog. non occlusive mesenteric ischemia.

In den vorliegenden Untersuchungen verwendeten wir verschiedene Digitalisglykoside (Strophanthin, Digoxin und Proscillaridin), um eine Vasokonstriktion im Mesenterialkreislauf auszulösen. Digitalisglykoside sind Calcium-Synergisten (Tabelle 2). Es lag also nahe, die Calcium-synergistischen Glykosideffekte durch Calcium-Antagonisten zu blockieren bzw. aufzuheben.

Tabelle 1. Nicht okklusive mesenteriale Ischämie

Häufigkeit bis 80%	bei Verdachtsdiagnose Mesenterialinfarkt
Letalität ~100%	

Tabelle 2. Wirkung auf die glatte Muskelzelle

Glykoside	Ca^{++}-Antagonisten
Steigerung des transmembranären Ca^{++}-Influx	Hemmung des transmembranären Ca^{++}-Influx
↓	↓
mehr freie intrazelluläre Ca^{++}-Ionen	weniger freie intrazelluläre Ca^{++}-Ionen
↓	↓
Aktivierung der elektromechanischen Koppelung	elektro-mechanische Entkoppelung
↓	↓
Vasokonstriktion	Vasodilatation

Methodik

Wir verwendeten Bastardhunde beiderlei Geschlechts mit einem Körpergewicht von 12 – 45 kg. Die Narkoseeinleitung erfolgte mit Chloralose/Urethan. Alle Tiere wurden endotracheal intubiert, relaxiert (Alloferin 0,2 mg/kg) und während des Versuchs beatmet (positive Druckbeatmung, $N_2O:O_2$ = 2:1, Atemfrequenz 16 – 18/min). Der Versuchsaufbau ist in Abb. 1 skizziert. Der zentralvenöse Druck

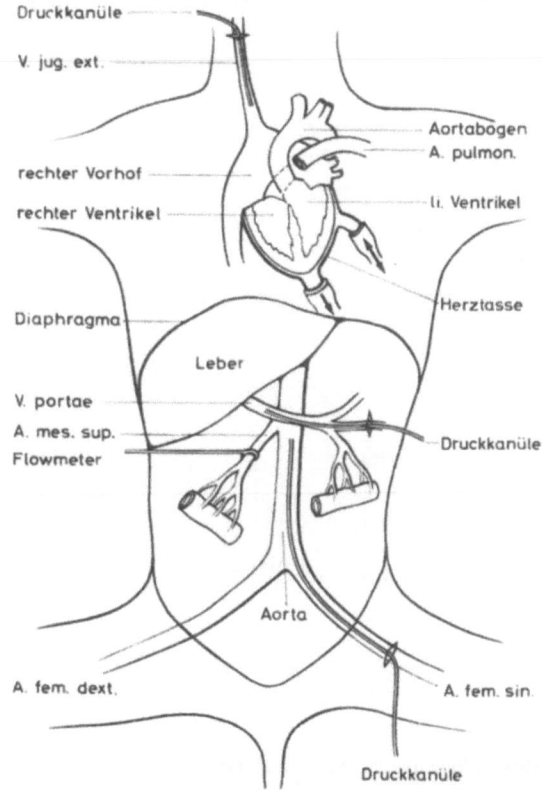

Abb. 1. Skizze des Versuchsaufbaus

wurde (via V. jugularis ext.) im rechten Vorhof gemessen, der portale Druck (via Mesenterialvene) vor der Leber und der arterielle Druck (via A. femoralis) in der Aorta abdominalis. Alle Druckkatheter wurden mit Statham-Druckreglern verbunden. Die Durchblutung im Bereich der A. mesenterica sup. wurde mit einem „square wave type flowmeter" (Typ 3765-M) der Fa. Devices Instr., Ltd. gemessen. Die Flowmeßköpfe wurden um den Stamm der Mesenterialarterie vor dem Abgang der ersten Jejunaläste implantiert. Die Glykosidwirkung wurde elektrokardiographisch (Extremitätenableitung) kontrolliert. Durchblutung, Drucke und EKG wurden kontinuierlich auf einem Mehrfachschreiber aufgezeichnet.

Zur Ausschaltung kardialer Glykosideffekte verwendeten wir die intrathorakale mechanische Herzmassage [33, 36] nach Anstadt (Abb. 2) bei einer Frequenz von 150/min und einer Systolendauer von 45 – 46%. Die Perfusionsrate kann so von kardialen Faktoren unabhängig gehalten werden. Hinsichtlich methodischer Einzelheiten dürfen wir auf frühere Veröffentlichungen verweisen [15, 37, 38].

Folgende Glykoside wurden verwendet:

1. Strophanthin 0,05 mg/kg als Bolusinjektion i.v.
2. Digoxin 0,06 mg/kg über Perfusor i.v.
3. Proscillaridin 0,05 mg/kg über Perfusor i.v.

Als Calcium-Antagonisten verwendeten wir Verapamil in einer Dosierung von 0,5 mg/kg (Strophanthinversuche) und 0,2 mg/kg (übrige Versuche).

Die statistische Auswertung erfolgte mit Hilfe der verteilungsfreien Varianzanalyse.

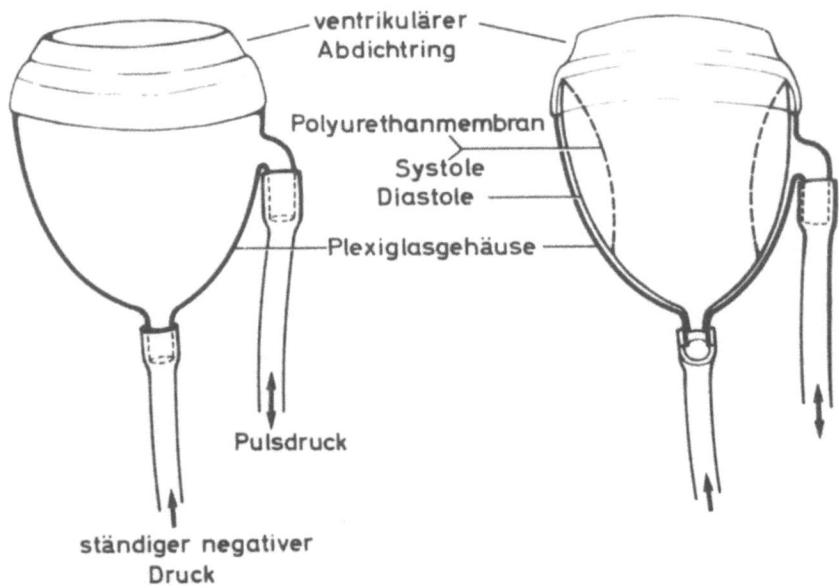

Abb. 2. Schema der Anstadt-Herztasse

Ergebnisse

Die Injektion von 0,05 mg/kg Strophanthin führt bereits nach wenigen Minuten zu einer deutlichen Steigerung des arteriellen Druckes, während die Infusion von 0,06 mg/kg Digoxin und 0,05 mg/kg Proscillaridin nur eine geringe nicht signifikante arterielle Drucksteigerung hervorruft. In keinem Fall und zu keinem Zeitpunkt kommt es zu einer statistisch auffälligen Änderung des portalen Druckes. Die Herzfrequenz sinkt zwar bei Gabe der verschiedenen Glykoside ab, signifikante Änderungen konnten aber wegen der großen Streuung nicht beobachtet werden.

Die Durchblutung im Bereich der mesenterialen Strombahn (Flow A. mesenterica sup. − Abb. 3) sank nach Glykosidgabe in jedem Fall signifikant. Die Werte lagen nach 20 min um 25% (Strophanthin), um 29% (Proscillaridin) und um 17% (Digoxin) unter dem Ausgangswert (= Beginn der Glykosidgabe). Der aus Druckgradient und Flow errechnete periphere Gefäßwiderstand (Abb. 3) stieg entsprechend signifikant an. Die Widerstandserhöhung nach Strophanthingabe war am deutlichsten, da in diesen Versuchen auch der arterielle Druck signifikant (bei konstantem portalen Druck) anstieg.

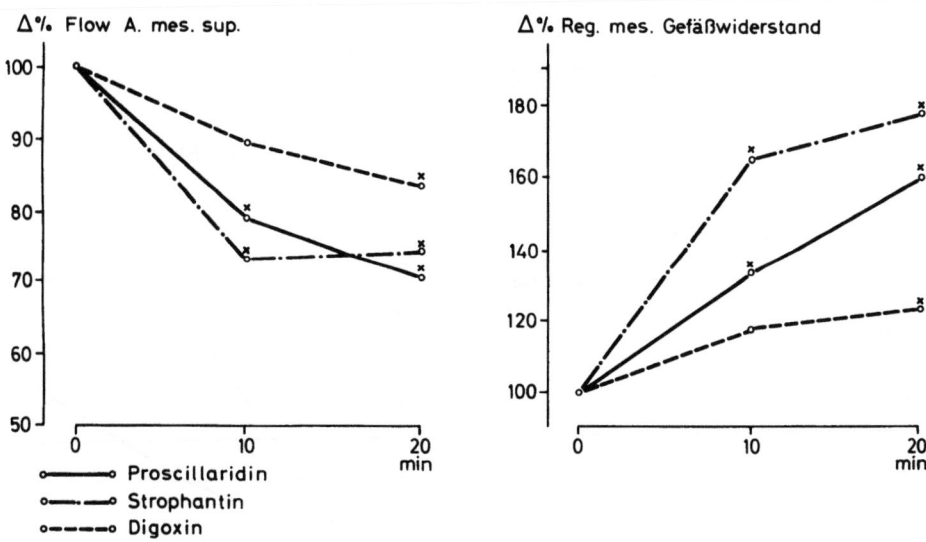

Abb. 3. Glykosideffekt an der mesenterialen Strombahn

Auch unter den Bedingungen der mechanischen Herzmassage (Abb. 4) kommt es zu einer Vasokonstriktion im Splanchnikusgebiet. Nach Bolusinjektion von Strophanthin bzw. nach Infusion von Proscillaridin kommt es nach 20 min zu einem signifikanten Abfall der Durchblutung um 27%. Der Anstieg des arteriellen Druckes von 116 auf 129 mmHg (nach Strophanthin) ist stat. signifikant ($p < 0,01$), während der Anstieg von 110 auf 117 mmHg nach Proscillaridininfusion nicht signifikant ist. Der zentralvenöse Druck ändert sich weder nach Strophanthin- noch nach Proscillaridinapplikation. Der kalkulierte periphere Gefäßwiderstand ist nach Gabe beider Glykoside sowohl nach 10 min als auch nach 20 min (Abb. 4) signifikant erhöht. Der graduelle Unterschied zwischen Strophanthinbehandlung (Anstieg um 78%) und Proscillaridin (Anstieg um 48%) erklärt sich aus dem Verhalten des arteriellen Drucks.

20 min nach Glykosidgabe bzw. zum Ende der Glykosidinfusion wird als Calcium-Antagonist Verapamil injiziert bzw. über 20 min infundiert. In einer Kontrollgruppe (Proscillaridin NaCl) wird statt Verapamil physiol. Kochsalzlösung in identischer Menge infundiert. Als Ausgangswert gilt jetzt der Endwert der Glykosidgabe. Unter NaCl-Infusion fällt der arterielle Druck von 200 auf 188 mmHg (nach 30 min), d.h. um 6%; jedoch sind diese Änderungen zu keinem Zeitpunkt signifikant (Abb. 5). Unter Verapamilinfusion sinkt der arterielle Druck dagegen (nach Proscillaridinvorbehandlung) schon nach 10 min signifikant von 180 auf 155 mmHg (14%) und nach 20 min auf 149 mmHg (17%) ab. Nach Digoxinvorbehandlung ist unter Verapamilinfusion nur nach 5 min eine signifikante Abnahme des arteriellen

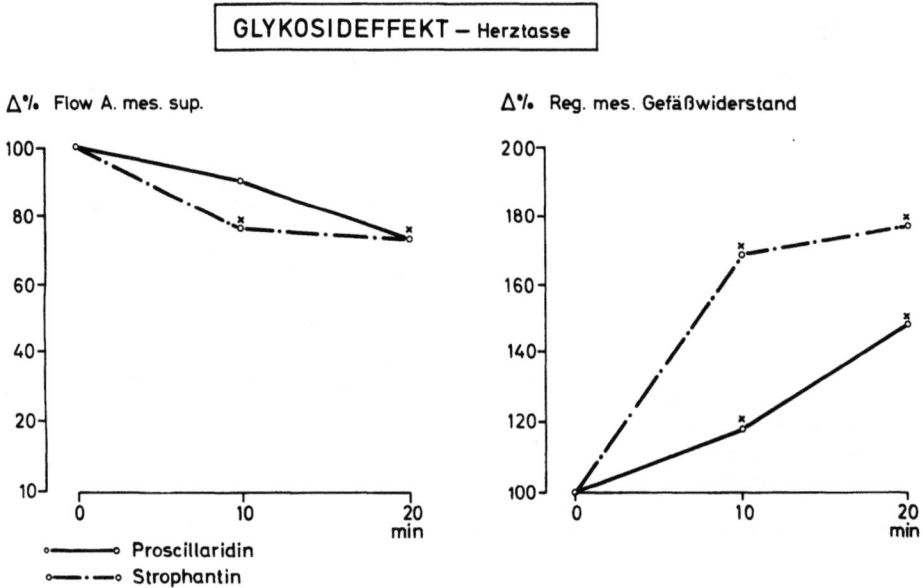

Abb. 4. Glykosideffekt an der mesenterialen Strombahn unter mech. Herzmassage

Drucks von 166 auf 149 mmHg (10%) festzustellen. Nach 30 min ist der Druck wieder auf 156 mmHg angestiegen (Abb. 5). Der portale Druck bleibt unter NaCl-Infusion unverändert (Abb. 5 *rechts*), steigt aber unter Verapamilinfusion sowohl bei Digoxin- als auch bei Proscillaridinvorbehandlung zu allen Zeitpunkten signifikant an (Abb. 5 *rechts*). Die höchsten Werte werden mit 25% (Proscillaridin vorbehandelt) bzw. 37% (Digoxin vorbehandelt) nach 20 min (Ende der Verapamilinfusion) erreicht.

NaCl-Infusion führt weder zu einer statistisch auffälligen Änderung des mesenterialen Flow noch zu einer signifikanten Änderung des errechneten peripheren Widerstandes (Abb. 6). Verapamilinfusion führt dagegen zu einer zu allen Zeitpunkten signifikanten Steigerung der Durchblutung (Abb. 6 *links*) und zu einem zu allen Zeitpunkten signifikanten Abfall des peripheren Widerstandes (Abb. 6 *rechts*), wobei die Vorbehandlung keine Rolle spielt. Die mit Proscillaridin vorbehandelten Tiere zeigen bereits nach 5 min eine Durchblutungssteigerung von 29% (von 243 auf 313 ml/min), die mit Digoxin vorbehandelten Tiere einen Anstieg um 41% (von 202

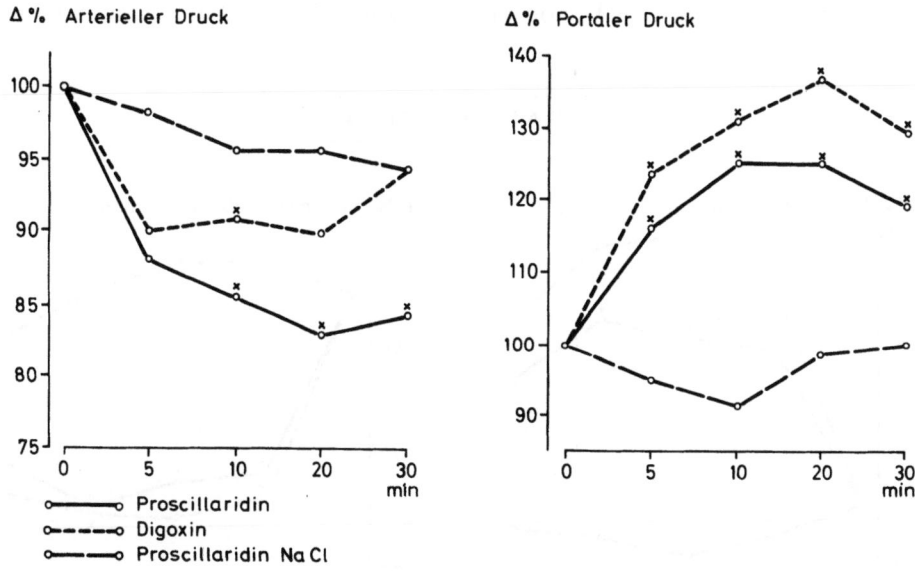

Abb. 5. Verapamilwirkung auf den arteriellen und venösen Druck

auf 284 ml/min). 10 min nach Ende der Infusion fallen die Werte gering, bleiben jedoch gegenüber dem Ausgangswert signifikant erhöht (Abb. 6 *links*). Der periphere Gefäßwiderstand verhält sich umgekehrt proportional zum Flow. Hier findet sich nach 5 min bereits ein Abfall von 33% (Proscillaridin vorbehandelt) bzw. von 38% (Digoxin vorbehandelt). Die höchsten Werte werden mit 40% (Proscillaridinvorbehandlung) und mit 41% (Digoxinvorbehandlung) nach 20 min erreicht (Abb. 6 *rechts*).

Ähnliche Veränderungen ruft die Gabe des Calcium-Antagonisten unter den Bedingungen der mechanischen Herzmassage hervor (Abb. 7). Nach Strophanthinvorbehandlung steigt die Durchblutung im Bereich der A. mesenterica sup. bereits nach 5 min (Bolusinjektion von 0,5 mg/kg Verapamil!) um rund 100% an, während der Anstieg nach Proscillaridinvorbehandlung nach 5 min (0,2 mg/kg Verapamil per infusionem) „nur" bei 47% ($p < 0,05$) liegt. Nach 30 min ist die Flowsteigerung mit 33% (Proscillaridin) bzw. 39% (Strophanthin) mehr oder weniger identisch (Abb. 7 *links*). Der periphere Gefäßwiderstand fällt nach Strophanthinvorbehandlung 5 min nach Bolusinjektion von 0,5 mg/kg Verapamil um 65% ($p < 0,05$), nach Digoxinvorbehandlung unter Infusion von 0,2 mg/kg Verapamil (über 20 min) um 30% ($p < 0,05$). Auch hier ist die Änderung nach 20 min mit 42% (Proscillaridin) und 46% (Digoxin) fast identisch (Abb. 7 *rechts*). Die mit Strophanthin vorbehandelten Tiere zeigen 5 min nach Bolusinjektion von 0,5 mg/kg Verapamil einen erheblichen Abfall des arteriellen Drucks von 119 auf 79 mmHg ($p < 0,01$), während die Infu

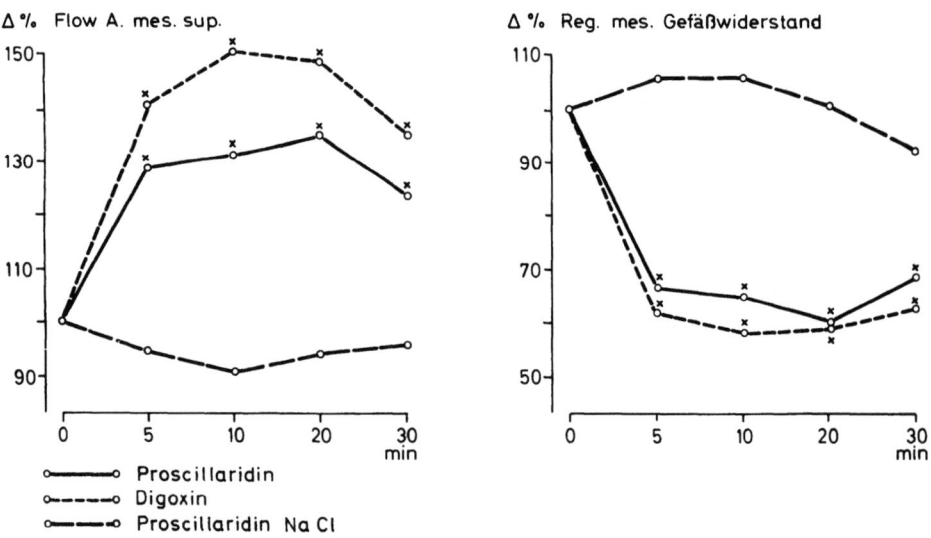

Abb. 6. Verapamilwirkung auf den mesenterialen Flow und Widerstand

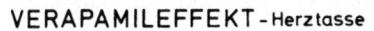

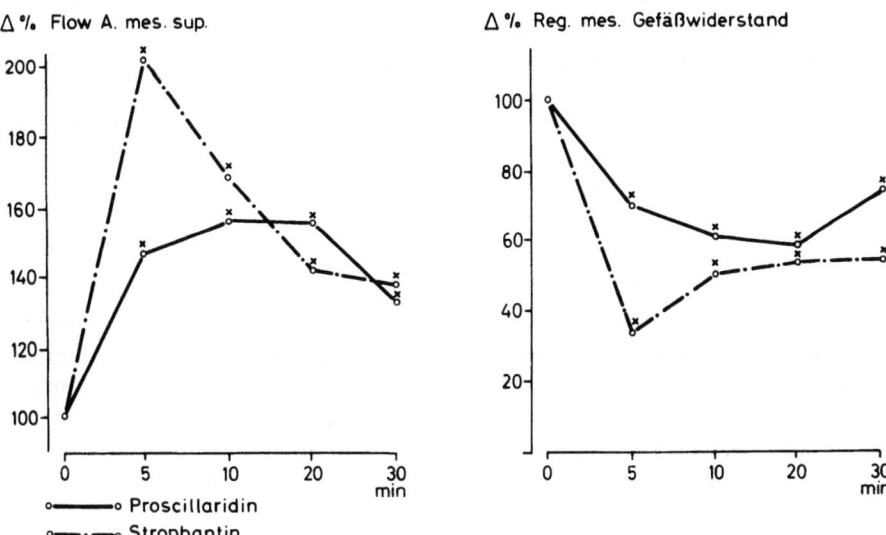

Abb. 7. Verapamileffekt an der mesenterialen Strombahn unter mech. Herzmassage

sion von 0,2 mg/kg Verapamil über 20 min bei den mit Proscillaridin vorbehandelten Tieren nach 5 min nur zu einem geringen Druckabfall von 117 auf 114 mmHg führt. Der zentralvenöse Druck steigt nach Bolusinjektion von Verapamil (0,5 mg/kg) nur um ca. 3% (Strophanthin vorbehandelt), während die Infusion von 0,2 mg/kg Verapamil über 20 min Drucksteigerungen von ca. $10-15\%$ ($p < 0,05$) hervorruft (Proscillaridin vorbehandelt).

Diskussion

Sicherlich ist es nicht ganz unproblematisch, hämodynamische Untersuchungen an Hunden durchzuführen. Der Hund ist jedoch in der Mehrzahl der früheren Untersuchungen [31, 39 – 42] das Versuchstier gewesen. Weiterhin haben Studien an Rhesusaffen [19] gezeigt, daß hinsichtlich der Glykosidwirkung im Splanchnikusgebiet keine Speziesunterschiede zwischen Hund und Affe bestehen.

Die von uns beobachtete Abnahme der mesenterialen Durchblutung nach Glykosidgabe wird nicht nur durch zahlreiche tierexperimentelle Untersuchungen [19, 30, 39 – 42] bestätigt, sondern sie steht auch in Einklang mit Beobachtungen von Bynum [43] an herzgesunden Probanden. Vorbestehende Veränderungen im Splanchnikusgebiet z. B. im Sinne einer schockbedingten Vasokonstriktion [20, 44] können nicht verhindern, daß Glykoside zu einer weiteren Intensivierung dieser Veränderungen führen können.

Die Untersuchungen von Higgins [45], der zeigen konnte, daß Glykosidgabe nur bei narkotisierten Hunden eine Vasokonstriktion hervorruft, bei wachen Tieren jedoch eher eine Vasodilatation, dokumentieren, daß noch viele Probleme bezüglich der Pathogenese ungeklärt sind und daß sich Tierexperimente nicht ohne weiteres auf die menschliche Situation übertragen lassen. Bynum [43] fand bei herzgesunden wachen Probanden nach einmaliger Glykosidgabe eine 30%ige Durchblutungsminderung im Splanchnikusgebiet. Braunwald [46] stellte bei Patienten, bei denen Operationen mit Hilfe eines kardiopulmonalen Bypass durchgeführt wurden, nach Gabe von Strophanthin eine erhebliche Vasokonstriktion fest.

Die in-vitro-Untersuchungen von Fleckenstein [47, 48] zeigen, daß Glykoside nicht nur am Mesenterialkreislauf zu einer Vasokonstriktion führen, sondern auch im Bereich der Koronararterien. Diese Ergebnisse wurden inzwischen von Steiness [29] durch tierexperimentelle Untersuchungen bestätigt. Sie fand nach akuter und chronischer Digitalisierung eine Abnahme der myokardialen Durchblutung (Messung mit Radioisotopen). Treat [30] konnte nachweisen, daß Strophanthin intraarteriell appliziert zu einer Vasokonstriktion im Bereich der A. carotis führt. In eigenen Untersuchungen konnten wir zeigen (unveröffentlicht), daß Digoxin intravenös gegeben ebenso eine Durchblutungsminderung im Bereich der A. carotis bis 30% zur Folge hat.

Die Durchblutung im Bereich der A. mesenterica sup. hängt nicht nur vom peripheren Gefäßwiderstand ab, sondern auch vom Herzminutenvolumen. Herzglykoside beeinflussen beide Parameter, wenn auch in antagonistischer Weise [49]. Cotten [50] fand jedoch bei narkotisierten herzgesunden Hunden mit intaktem Kreislauf nach Digitalisgabe einen geringen Abfall des Herzminutenvolumens. Wir beobachteten in früheren Untersuchungen [15] einen ähnlichen Effekt. Um kardiale von extrakardialen Glykosideffekten sicher unterscheiden zu können, wiederholten wir unsere jetzigen Experimente unter den Bedingungen der mechanischen Herzmassage. Auch bei dieser Versuchsanordnung führte die Gabe von Glykosiden zu einer signifikanten Abnahme der mesenterialen Durchblutung und zu einem signifikanten Anstieg des peripheren Gefäßwiderstandes, so daß die glykosidbedingte Vasokonstriktion durch eine direkte Glykosidwirkung auf die glatte Gefäßmuskulatur erklärt werden muß.

In der Behandlung glykosidbedingter Gefäßspasmen wurden schon viele Pharmaka untersucht. Einige sind in Tabelle 3 aufgelistet. An das optimale Pharmakon muß man jedoch einige Voraussetzungen knüpfen:

1. Es muß in Hinsicht auf die mesenterialen Verhältnisse nicht nur die Ischämie, sondern auch die Hypoxie [51] aufheben.
2. Da die intestinale Ischämie immer im Bereich der Mukosa und Submukosa beginnt [52], muß der Vasodilatator besonders die Durchblutung im Bereich von Mukosa und Submukosa steigern und nicht nur im Bereich der Muskularis.
3. Das Pharmakon muß in Form einer Langzeittherapie in Kombination mit einem Glykosid gegeben werden können, da die sog. non occlusive intestinal ischemia meist ältere herzinsuffiziente Patienten betrifft.

Papaverin ist zwar ein potenter Dilatator im Bereich des Intestinum, beeinflußt die Hypoxie jedoch eher negativ [53]. Glucagon hebt die glykosidbedingte Hypoxie im Mesenterialbereich auf und steigert gleichzeitig die Durchblutung in allen Wand-

Tabelle 3. Therapie glykosidbedingter Gefäßspasmen

Ca^{++}-Antagonisten
Papaverin
Glucagon
Histamin
Phenoxybenzamin
Prostaglandin E_1

schichten [52], hier fehlt jedoch die klinische Erfahrung insbesondere in der Kombination mit Glykosiden. Histamin führt zwar zu einer Aufhebung der Hypoxie und zu einer selektiven Flowsteigerung, ohne jedoch den Mukosa-Submukosa-Flow auf den Ausgangswert anzuheben [52]. Phenoxybenzamin [7,54] ist erst in wenigen Fällen klinisch erprobt worden [54], hier meist in Form intraarterieller Infusionen über den liegenden Angiographiekatheter. Tierexperimentelle Untersuchungen liegen nur von Britt [7] vor. Auch hier wurde Phenoxybenzamin intraarteriell gegeben. Die Durchblutung im Bereich der A. mesenterica sup. wurde jedoch ohne Angaben über den fraktionierten Flow und den Sauerstoffverbrauch gemessen. Prostaglandin E_1 [31] führt nach intraarterieller Gabe zwar zu einer Vasodilatation und Aufhebung der intestinalen Hypoxie, jedoch fehlt auch hier die klinische Erfahrung [51], speziell in der Langzeittherapie und Kombination mit Glykosiden. Von den in Tabelle 3 aufgelisteten Pharmaka erfüllen zur Zeit nur die Calcium-Antagonisten alle Forderungen. Wir konnten in unseren Untersuchungen nachweisen, daß Verapamil unabhängig vom Injektionszeitpunkt [15] und unabhängig davon, mit welchem Glykosid vorbehandelt wurde, immer zu einer Aufhebung glykosidbedingter Gefäßspasmen führt. Perhexilin (ein anderer Calcium-Antagonist) führt nach Untersuchungen von Schwaiger [52] neben der Aufhebung der Hypoxie auch zu einer Steigerung der Durchblutung in allen Wandschichten, insbesondere im Bereich von Mukosa und Submukosa. Klinische Erfahrungen mit Kombinationspräparaten (Glykosid + Calcium-Antagonist) liegen in reichlicher Zahl vor. Daß die bekannten und häufig beschriebenen negativ inotropen und negativ chronotropen Eigenschaften der Calcium-Antagonisten [48,55 − 59] nicht für die beobachtete Vasodilatation verantwortlich gemacht werden können, haben unsere Versuche mit der mechanischen Herzmassage gezeigt. Unter diesen Versuchsbedingungen läßt sich der beobachtete Blutdruckabfall weder durch Frequenzminderung noch durch Abnahme der Kontraktionskraft erklären. Es muß sich um einen Effekt direkt an der glatten Gefäßmuskulatur handeln.

Literatur

1. Hortholmei N, Burghelle T (1938) Darminfarkte durch Intoleranz-Schock-Wirkung. Zentralbl Chir 65:85 − 91
2. Fogarty TJ, Fletcher WS (1966) Genesis of nonocclusive mesenteric ischemia. Am J Surg 111:130 − 137

3. Minami T, Sousa Dias JC, Matos Sipahi H: Intestinal lesion of ischemic origin. VI. Weltkongreß für Gastroenterologie, Madrid, 1978 (in press)
4. Silen W: Ischemic intestinal syndromes. VI. Weltkongreß für Gastroenterologie, Madrid, 1978 (in press)
5. Adar R, Franklin A, Salzman EW (1974) Letter: Hemoconcentration in acute nonocclusive mesenteric ischemia. JAMA 228:27
6. Berger RL, Byrne JJ (1961) Intestinal gangrene associated with heart disease. Surg Gynecol Obstet 112:529–533
7. Britt LG, Cheek RC (1969) Nonocclusive mesenteric vascular disease. Clinical and experimental observations. Ann Surg 169:704–711
8. Corday E (1961) Mesenteric vascular insufficiency. Editorial. JAMA 175:235
9. Ende N (1958) Infarction of the bowel in cardiac failure. N Engl J Med 258:879–881
10. Larsen A (1970) Nonocclusive intestinal gangrene. Acta Chir Scand 136:227–234
11. Hortholmei N, Burghele T (1938) Darminfarkte durch Intoleranz-Schock-Wirkung. Zentralbl Chir 65:85–91
12. LeVine S (1959) Intestinal infarction without vascular occlusion. Am J Proctol 10:257–265
13. Adar R, Salzman EW (1974) Letter: Intestinal ischemia and digitalis. JAMA 229:1577
14. Brobmann GF, Barth K, Strecker EP, Schmidt-Hieber M, Schmidt HA (1975) Die Wirkung von Strophanthin auf die intestinale Durchblutung. Ein Beitrag zur Pathophysiologie der hämorrhagischen Enteropathie. Langenbecks Arch Chir [Suppl.] 291–295
15. Brobmann GF (1977) Die hämorrhagische Enteropathie. Tierexperimentelle und klinische Untersuchungen zur Pathogenese. Habilitationsschrift, Freiburg
16. Freiman DG (1965) Hemorrhagic necrosis of the gastrointestinal tract. Circulation 32:329–331
17. Pierce GE, Brockenbrough EC (1970) The spectrum of mesenteric infarction. Am J Surg 119:233–239
18. Polansky BJ, Berger RL, Byrne JJ (1964) Massive nonocclusive intestinal infarction associated with digitalis toxicity. Circulation 30:III–141
19. Shanbour LL, Jacobson ED, Brobmann GF, Hinshaw LB (1971) Effects of ouabain on splanchnic hemodynamics in the rhesus monkey. Am Heart J 81:511–515
20. Ferrer MI, Bradley SE, Wheeler HO, Enson Y, Preisig R, Harvey RM (1965) The effect of digoxin in the splanchnic circulation in ventricular failure. Circulation 32:524–537
21. Habboushe F, Wallace HW, Nusbaum M, Baum S, Dratch P, Blakemore WS (1974) Nonocclusive mesenteric vascular insufficiency. Ann Surg 180:819–822
22. Hoffman FG, Zimmerman SL, Cardwell ES Jr (1959) Massive intestinal infarction without vascular occlusion associated with aortic insufficiency. N Engl J Physiol 197:757–760
23. Watt-Boolsen S (1977) Non-occlusive intestinal infarction. Acta Chir Scand 143:365–369
24. Price WE, Rohrer GV, Jacobson ED (1969) Mesenteric vascular diseases. Gastroenterology 57:599–604
25. Fleckenstein A, Döring H-J, Janke J, Byon KY (1975) Basic actions of ions and drugs on myocardial high-energy phosphate metabolism and contractility. In: Schmier J, Eichler D (eds) Heart and circulation. Springer, Berlin Heidelberg New York (Handbuch der experimentellen Pharmakologie, Vol XVI/3, pp 345–505)
26. Fleckenstein A, Fleckenstein-Grün G, Janke J, Frey M (1977) Kardiovaskuläre Grundwirkungen der Ca-Antagonisten und deren therapeutischer Wert in Kombination mit Herzglykosiden. Geriatrie 6:3–24
27. Grün G, Weder U (1974) Augmentation of coronary smooth muscle tone and sensitization to Ca by cardiac glycosides. Naunyn Schmiedebergs Arch Pharmacol [Suppl] 282:28
28. Grün G, Fleckenstein A, Weder U (1974) Changes in coronary smooth muscle tone produced by Ca, cardiac glycosides and Ca-antagonistic compounds (Verapamil, D 600, Prenylamine etc.). Pfluegers Arch [Suppl] 347:1
29. Steiness E, Bille-Brahe NE, Hansen JF, Lomholt N, Ring-Larsen H (1978) Reduced myocardial blood flow in acute and chronical digitalization. Acta Pharmacol Toxicol (Kbh) 43:29–35
30. Treat E, Ulano HB, Jacobson ED (1971) Effects of intraarterial ouabain on mesenteric and carotid hemodynamics. J Pharmacol Exp Ther 179:144–148
31. Davis LJ, Anderson J, Wallace S, Jacobson ED (1975) Experimental use of prostaglandin E_1 in nonocclusive mesenteric ischemia. Am J Roentgenol Radium Ther Nucl Med 125:99–110

32. Siegelman SS, Sprayregen S, Boley SJ (1974) Angiographic diagnosis of mesenteric arterial vasoconstriction. Radiology 112:533 – 542
33. Anstadt GL, Blakemore WS, Baue AE (1965) A new instrument for prolonged mechanical cardiac massage. Circulation [Suppl] 32:II – 43
34. Anstadt GL, Schiff P, Baue AE (1966) Prolonged circulatory support by direct mechanical ventricular massage. Trans Am Soc Artif Intern Organs 12:72 – 79
35. Anstadt GL, Britz WE Jr (1968) Continued studies in prolonged circulatory support by direct mechanical ventricular assistance. Trans Am Soc Artif Intern Organs 14:297 – 303
36. Skinner DB, Newman MH, Squire RA (1970) Preservation and transplantation of dog organs maintained in vivo for 24 hours by mechanical ventricular assistance. J Surg Res 10:287 – 294
37. Brobmann GF, Mikosch H, Mayer M (1976) Therapeutische Beeinflussung strophanthinbedingter Durchblutungsstörungen des Darmes. Langenbecks Arch Chir [Suppl] 257 – 261
38. Brobmann GF, Mikosch H, Mayer M (1976) Glykosidbedingte Durchblutungsstörungen des Darmes und Möglichkeiten therapeutischer Beeinflussung. Med Klin 71:2066 – 2071
39. Harrison LA, Plaschke J, Phillips RS, Price WE, de Cotten MV, Jacobson ED (1969) Effects of ouabain on the splanchnic circulation. J Pharmacol Exp Ther 169:321 – 327
40. Pawlik W, Jacobson ED (1974) Effects of digoxin on the mesenteric circulation. Cardiovasc Res Cent Bull 12:80 – 84
41. Pawlik W, Shepherd AP, Mailman D, Jacobson ED (1974) Effects of ouabain on intestinal oxygen consumption. Gastroenterology 67:100 – 106
42. Ulano HB, Treat E, Shanbour LL, Massion W, Jacobson ED (1971) Mesenteric vasoconstriction with ouabain. Fed Proc 30:321
43. Bynum TE, Hanley HG, Cole JS (1973) Effect of digitalis glycosides on splanchnic blood flow in man. Clin Res 21:509
44. Ulano HB, Treat E, Chang ACK, Jacobson ED (1971) Splanchnic circulatory responses to ouabain in shock. Surgery 70:678 – 684
45. Higgins ChB, Vatner SF, Braunwald E (1972) Regional hemodynamic effects of a digitalis glycoside in the conscious dog with and without experimental heart failure. Circ Res 30:406 – 417
46. Braunwald E, Bloodwell RD, Goldberg LI, Morrow AG (1961) Studies on digitalis. IV. Observations in man on the effects of digitalis preparations on the contractility of the non-failing heart and on total vascular resistance. J Clin Invest 40:52 – 59
47. Fleckenstein A Neuere Ergebnisse zur Physiologie, Pharmakologie und Pathologie der elektromechanischen Koppelungsprozesse am Warmblütermyokard. In: Keidel WD, Plattig KH (Hrsg) Vorträge der Erlanger Physiologentagung 1970. Springer, Berlin Heidelberg New York, S 13 – 15
48. Fleckenstein A (1971) Specific inhibitors and promotors of calcium action in the excitation-contraction coupling of heart muscle and their role in the prevention or production of myocardial lesions. In: Harris P, Opie L (eds) Calcium and the heart. Academic Press, London, pp 135 – 188
49. Bynum TE, Jacobson ED (1975) Shock, intestinal ischemia, and digitalis. Circ Shock 2:235 – 237
50. Cotten M de V, Stopp PE (1958) Action of digitalis on the non-failing heart. Am J Physiol 192:114 – 120
51. Lanciault G, Jacobson ED (1976) The gastrointestinal circulation. Gastroenterology 71:851 – 873
52. Schwaiger M, Fondacaro JD, Jacobson ED Effects of glucagon, histamine and perhexiline on the ischemic canine mesenteric circulation
53. Lanciault G, Fang WF, Jacobson ED, Bowen JC (1976) Evaluation of potential agents for treatment of nonocclusive mesenteric ischemia in the dog. Circ Shock 3:239
54. Athanasoulis CA, Wittenberg J, Bernstein R, Williams LF (1975) Vasodilatory drugs in the management of nonocclusive bowel ischemia. Gastroenterology 68:146 – 150
55. Döring H-J, Kammermeier H, Fleckenstein A (1966) Zur wechselseitigen Beeinflussung der Kontraktionskraft und der Frequenz des Herzens durch Proscillaridin und α-Isopropyl-α-[(N-methyl-N-homoveratryl)-γ-amino-propyl]-3,4-dimethoxyphenylacetonitril. Arzneim Forsch 16:1197 – 1202
56. Fleckenstein A, Kammermeier H, Döring H-J, Freud HJ, Grün G, Kienle A (1967) Zum Wirkungsmechanismus neuartiger Koronardilatatoren mit gleichzeitig Sauerstoff-einsparenden Myokardeffekten, Prenylamin und Iproveratril. Z Kreislaufforsch 56:1 – 48
57. Fleckenstein A, Byon KY (1974) Prevention by Ca-antagonistic compounds (Verapamil, D 600) of coronary smooth muscle contracture due to treatment with cardiac glycosides. Naunyn Schmiedebergs Arch Pharmacol [Suppl] 282:20
58. Raff WK, Kosche F, Lochner W (1972) Untersuchungen mit Nifedipine, einer coronargefäßerweiternden Substanz mit schneller sublingualer Wirkung. Arzneim Forsch 22:33 – 39

59. Vater W, Kroneberg G, Hoffmeister F, Kaller H, Meng K, Oberdorf A, Puls W, Schlossmann K, Stoepel K (1972) Zur Pharmakologie von 4-(2′-Nitrophenyl)-2,6-dimethyl-1,4-dihydropyridin-3,5-dicarbonsäuredimethylester (Nifedipine, BAYa1040). Arzneim Forsch 22:1 – 14

Application of Calcium Antagonists in Patients with Vasospastic Angina Pectoris

A. Maseri, S. Severi, O. Parodi, A. Distante, and A. Biagini

Coronary vasospasm appears to be "a proved hypothesis for 'variant' angina" [1]. However, "variant" angina appears to be only one extreme of a continuous spectrum of vasospastic acute myocardial ischemia [2].

Vasospastic angina pectoris characterized by S-T segment elevation or depression may be rather frequent when appropriately searched for [3]. The therapy of this form of angina remains symptomatic until the causes of vasospasm will be discovered. Empirically, favorable results were reported in some patients with beta-blockers administered at doses much higher than those required for effective beta-blocking [4]. Our experience indicates that the evaluation of the treatment is rather complex because of the frequent spontaneous waning and waxing of symptoms and because the mechanisms responsible for vasospasm may differ in individual patients.

Medical Trials

In order to evaluate the consistency of the drug response in each individual patient, we decided to perform our studies in a double crossover design with placebo, according to the scheme R (Run-in), T (Treatment), P (Placebo), T, P, rather than in the traditional double-blind group study.

This protocol has allowed us to establish that about 90% of these patients respond consistently to i.v., nitrates infusion [5], and to oral verapamil [6] with a dramatic reduction of the number of attacks during treatment periods and with recurrence of symptoms during placebo periods.

Trial 1

In 12 patients with frequent transient ischemic episodes at rest with variable degree of coronary atherosclerosis, one to three vessel disease, and evidence of vasospastic origin of angina (good exercise tolerance, ^{201}Tl studies during angina at rest, ergonovine maleate test, and angiographic study), we performed a continuous i.v. infusion of isosorbide dinitrate, $(1.25 - 5.0 \text{ mg/h})$ during 2 periods (T_1 and T_2) of 24 h (4 patients) or 12 h (8 patients) alternated with 2 equal periods (T_1, P_1, T_2, P_2). Continuous electrocardiographic monitoring revealed that the total number of transient ischemic attacks at rest characterized by S-T segment elevation (4 patients), depression (2 patients), and by S-T depression or elevation (6 patients), with or without pain, was 100, 104, and 91 respectively during run-in period, P_1 and P_2, but were reduced to 13 and 20 respectively during T_1 and T_2 ($p = .002$). Transient ischemic attacks at rest were completely prevented during both T_1 and T_2

in 4 patients; during T_1 or T_2 in 3 patients, and were not abolished, but significantly reduced in T_1 and T_2 in the other 5 patients. The reduction was similar for episodes characterized by S-T segment elevation or depression with or without pain.

Trial 2

In 12 patients admitted to our coronary care unit because of frequent daily attacks of angina at rest with a variable severity of coronary atherosclerosis and with evidence of vasospastic origin of angina, verapamil 480 mg/day and placebo were administered orally during four randomized alternated 48-h-periods. The incidence of transient ischemic attacks with S-T segment elevation or depression, with or without pain, documented by continuous electrocardiographic monitoring, were 128, 123, and 130 respectively during the run-in and the two placebo periods, and 31 and 23 during the verapamil periods ($p = 0.006$ and $p = 0.003$). Only in one patient the number of attacks was not reduced during T_1 and T_2.

Therefore, both drugs appear to be remarkably effective in preventing transient ischemic episodes at rest, although to a variable extent in the individual patients.

Short and Long-Term Clinical Results

Notwithstanding the proven efficacy of these treatments in some patients, even the combined use of these two drugs at high doses was not effective in preventing the development of myocardial infarction or sudden death. In 74 patients with crescendo angina with S-T segment elevation under optimal medical treatment, during the initial 1-month follow-up we observed 9 myocardial infarctions (two fatal) and two sudden deaths. Complete 1-year follow-up in all remaining 70 patients under medical treatment showed two sudden deaths and one myocardial infarction. These patients had a variable duration in the onset of symptoms, 27% had an old myocardial infarction, 85% had a limitation of their exercise tolerance with typical exertional angina besides their angina at rest caused by vasospasm [7 – 9].

Coronary Vasospasm and Myocardial Infarction

Myocardial infarction was documented by persisting S-T changes, by development by serum enzymes elevation. In all patients the infarction developed in the heart wall corresponding to the location of the electrocardiographic changes during the angina attacks.

Even a posteriori we were unable to find any clue suggesting that the onset of the ischemic episode that evolved into myocardial infarction was in any way different from the previous ones that were reversible and that were characterized by transient S-T changes in the same electrocardiographic leads where the signs of infarction developed.

A small fresh thrombus found in the stenotic portion of the circumflex coronary artey at the site of an occlusive spasm documented angiographically [10] indicates that, under some circumstances, blood stagnation caused by vasospasm may result in thrombus deposition at the site of damaged intima. Thromboxane A_2 released from platelet aggregation may further potentiate coronary vasospasm that tends to spread along the vessel, thus closing a vicious circle.

Thus, symptomatic treatment with nitrates and calcium antagonists, while effective on other occasions, under some yet obscure circumstances, is unable to prevent the onset of ischemia or to interrupt the ischemic attack. Prevention of myocardial infarction in these patients requires understanding of the mechanisms responsible for the variable duration of vasospasm in transient ischemic episodes.

References

1. Meller J, Pichard A, Dack S (1976) Coronary arterial spasm in Prinzmetal's angina: a proved hypothesis. Am J Cardiol 37:938–940
2. Maseri A, Severi S, De Nes M, L'Abbate A, Chierchia S, Marzilli M, Ballestra AM, Parodi O, Biagini A, Distante A (1978) "Variant" angina: One aspect of a continuous spectrum of vasospastic myocardial ischemia. Pathogenetic mechanisms, estimated incidence, clinical and coronary arteriographic findings in 138 patients. Am J Cardiol 42:1019–1041
3. Hillis LD, Braunwald E (1978) Coronary-artery spasm. N Engl J Med 299:695–702
4. Guazzi M, Fiorentini C, Polese A, Magrini F, Olivari MT (1978) Use of betareceptor antagonists in spontaneous angina pectoris. In: Maseri A, Klassen GA, Lesch M (eds) Primary and secondary angina pectoris. Grune & Stratton, New York, pp 373–382
5. Distante A, Maseri A, Severi S, Biagini A (1979) Management of vasospastic "crescendo" angina by continuous infusion of isosorbide dinitrate. 44:533–539
6. Parodi O, Maseri A, Simonetti I (1979) Management of unstable angina at rest by verapamil. A double-blind cross-over study in CCU. Br Heart J 41:167–174
7. Maseri A, Mimmo R, Chierchia S, Marchesi C, Pesola A, L'Abbate A (1975) Coronary spasm as a cause of acute myocardial ischemia in man. Chest 68:625–633
8. Maseri A, Parodi O, Severi S, Pesola A (1976) Transient transmural reduction of myocardial blood flow, demonstrated by thallium-201 scintigraphy, as a cause of variant angina. Circulation 54:280–288
9. Maseri A, Severi S, Chierchia S, Parodi O, Biagini A (1978) Characteristics and pathogenetic mechanism of "primary" angina at rest. In: Maseri A, Klassen GA, Lesch M (eds) Primary and secondary angina pectoris. Grund & Stratton, New York, pp 265–273
10. Maseri A, L'Abbate A, Baroldi G, Chierchia S, Marzilli M, Ballestra AM, Severi S, Parodi O, Biagini A, Distante A, Pesola A (1978) Coronary vasospasm as a possible cause of myocardial infarction. A conclusion derived from the study of "preinfarction" angina. N Engl J Med 229:1271–1277

Application of Calcium Antagonists in Patients with Prinzmetal Angina Pectoris

H. Kishida

The variant angina pectoris is a type of angina pectoris that was first described by Prinzmetal et al. in 1959. In Japan numerous cases of this disease have been reported and several studies have been made concerning the medical treatment of variant angina. Nifedipine [1,2] and diltiazem [3,4] have been observed to be most effective in suppression of the attacks of variant angina.

Subjects

The subjects are 243 males and 43 females diagnosed as variant angina in 11 cardiology institutes in Japan. In addition, the cases with unstable angina pectoris in our department were also added to this study.

Results

Table 1 shows the results obtained in 11 cardiology institutes in Japan. With nifedipine, attacks of variant angina were completely eliminated in 115 of 149 cases, or in 77.2%, and in 25 cases, or in 16.8%, the number of attacks decreased to less

Table 1. Effect of antianginal agents on variant angina (11 institutes[a])

	Total number of cases	Complete elimination of attacks	Decrease of attacks to less than half	No effects	% of effective cases
Nifedipine	149	115	25	9	94.0
Diltiazem	87	70	9	8	90.8
Nifedipine + Diltiazem	15	11	4	0	100.0
Verapamil	28	3	21	4	85.7
Anticoagulants	52	21		31	40.4
β-blockers	81	9		72	11.1

[a] Third Department of Internal Medicine, Kurume University (Dr. H. Toshima), Research Institute of Angiocardiology, Kyushu University (Dr. A. Kuroiwa), Institute of Balneotherapeutics, Kyushu University (Dr. T. Yanaga), Surgical Department, Kobe University (Dr. S. Asada), Division of Internal Medicine, Shizuoka City Hospital (Dr. H. Yasue), Second Department of Internal Medicine, University of Tokyo (Dr. S. Murao), Third Department of Internal Medicine, Showa University (Dr. H. Niitani), Department of Cardiovascular Disease, Toranomon Hospital (Dr. H. Yamaguchi), The Cardiovascular Institute, Tokyo (Dr. K. Kato), Department of Internal Medicine, Jichi Medical School (Dr. S. Hosoda) and First Department of Internal Medicine, Nippon Medical School (Dr. E. Kimura)

than half. It was ineffective only in 9 cases, or in 6.0%. In total, beneficial effects were obtained in 94.0% of the cases.

Diltiazem was markedly effective in 70 of 87 cases, or in 80.5%, and produced results similar to nifedipine. It was effective in 90.8% of the cases. The attacks were completely suppressed by combination of these drugs. Verapamil was effective in 21 of 28 cases, or in 85.7%, but seldom produced complete elimination of the attacks.

Formerly, anticoagulants have been used for treatment of variant angina. Although they were effective sometimes, only 40% of patients were improved by anticoagulants.

β-blockers were effective only 11.1%, but in a few cases, in which nifedipine and diltiazem were not effective, β-blocker was effective.

Table 2 shows the relationship between the effects of drugs and severity of organic coronary lesion as observed by arteriography. In the group with normal coronary arteries nifedipine was effective in 13 of 14 cases, or in 92.9%, and in the group with coronary artery stenosis in 15 of 17 cases, or in 88.2%. Diltiazem was effective in 11 of 12 cases, or in 91.7% and 4 of 6, or 66.7%, respectively. There was no significant difference between groups with and without coronary artery disease. These results show that the effect of nifedipine and diltiazem was independent of the presence or absence of coronary artery stenosis.

Table 3 shows the effects of the drugs on variant angina and on classical angina at rest in our department. Nifedipine was effective not only in treatment of variant angina, but also in classical angina at rest. However, β-blocker was not effective in either, especially in angina at rest. Warfarin was more effective in angina at rest than in variant angina, although the number of cases is not sufficient for statistical analysis. Other drugs in both groups were effective in more than half of the cases.

Table 2. Effect of calcium antagonists and severity of organic coronary lesion (Nippon Medical School)

	Nifedipine		Diltiazem	
	Effective	Not effective	Effective	Not effective
Normal or near-normal	13	1	11	1
Stenosis more than 50%	15	2	4	2

Table 3. Effects of the drugs on variant angina and on classical angina at rest (Nippon Medical School)

	Variant angina			Classical angina at rest		
	Effective	Not effective	%	Effective	Not effective	%
Nifedipine	26	3	89.7	6	2	75.0
β-blocker	1	2	33.3	0	4	0.0
Warfarin	7	9	43.8	3	2	60.0
Other drugs[a]	8	7	58.3	7	6	53.8

[a] Diltiazem, verapamil, perhexiline, molsidomine, etc.

Table 4 shows the incidence of arrhythmia in patients with variant angina in our department. Variant angina is associated with high incidence of various kinds of arrhythmias. Of particular importance are the serious life-threatening arrhythmias, such as ventricular fibrillation or AV block, which occurred in a few cases.

Figure 1 shows an actual example. As seen in the left side of this figure, the ECG taken at the intermittent stage showed WPW pattern. On ECG in the center taken during anginal attack, significant ST elevation was observed, an example of a very rare association of WPW syndrome and variant angina. As seen in the right side, ventricular fibrillation occurred abruptly immediately after admission to our Coronary Care Unit.

Figure 2 shows the time course of this patient from 6^{00} to 16^{00} on the day of admission. Intravenous infusion of lidocaine could not suppress the frequently occurring ventricular premature beats, and ventricular fibrillation occurred 13 times. DC countershock was required 3 times. However, nifedipine given intravenously at 1 PM was very effective. Ventricular premature beats and ventricular fibrillation were completely suppressed. The patient was discharged without complaints after hospitalization of about 1 month. We postulate that nifedipine

Table 4. Incidence of arrhythmias

	Variant Angina	Angina at rest with ST depression
Total cases	50	33
Cases with arrhythmias	33 (66.0%)	5 (15.2%)
Ventricular fibrillation	7	0
Premature beats	26	5
Marked sinus bradycardia	2	0
AV block	6	0

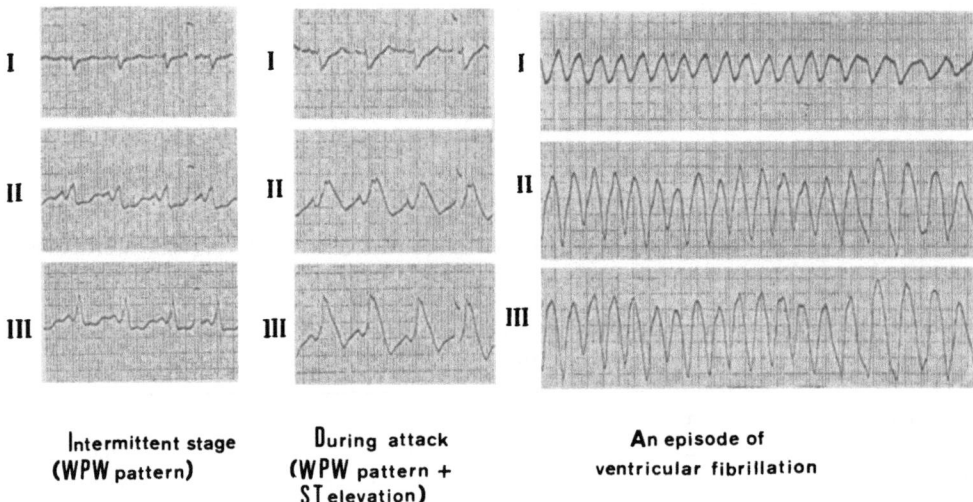

Intermittent stage
(WPW pattern)

During attack
(WPW pattern +
ST elevation)

An episode of
ventricular fibrillation

Fig. 1. G.T. 64 yrs. male: Variant angina pectoris with episodes of ventricular fibrillation

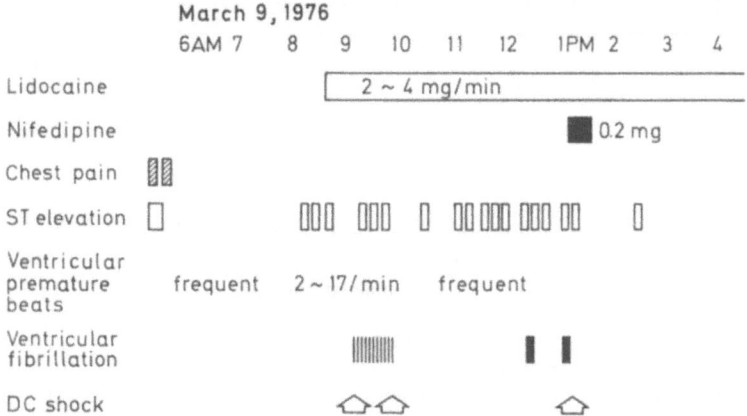

Fig. 2. Clinical course of this case during the period of repeated attacks of ventricular fibrillation

effectively controlled the arrhythmia indirectly through the inhibition of coronary spasm, rather than by a direct action on arrhythmia.

Table 5 shows the summary of AC-bypass surgery for variant angina reported until March, 1977. The effectiveness of AC-bypass operation was 14 of 22 cases, 63.6% in Japan and 30 of 51 cases, 58.8% in Western countries. The remaining cases had recurrent anginal attacks, myocardial infarction, or sudden death.

Table 6 compares the effect of calcium antagonistic drugs and AC-bypass surgery on variant angina with coronary artery disease in Japan. Calcium antagonistic drugs were effective in 20 of 24 cases, 83.3%. On the other hand, AC-bypass operation was effective in 14 of 22 cases, 63.6%. There was no significant difference between

Table 5. A-C bypass surgery for variant angina (Reported before March 31, 1977)

	No. of patients	Effective cases	% of effective cases
Japan	22	14	63.6
USA, Canada, etc.	51	30	58.8
Total	73	44	60.3

Table 6. Comparison of effect between calcium antagonistic drugs and A-C bypass surgery for variant angina in Japan

	Effective Cases	No Effective Cases	Total
Calcium antagonistic drug	20 (83.3%)	4	24
A-C bypass surgery	14 (63.6%)	8	22

Table 7. Effects of drugs on unstable angina (Nitrates are excluded)

		Unstable angina (n = 39)	
		With ST depression (n = 22)	With ST elevation (variant) (n = 17)
Nifedipine	effective	9	10
	pain eliminated but AMI developed	2	1
	not effective	1	2
Nifedipine not effective but with β-blocker	effective	1	
	not effective	1	
Diltiazem	effective	1	1
β-blocker	not effective	3	
No medication	due to spontaneous improvement	2	
	due to prompt development of AMI	2	2
	due to prompt development of VF		1

% of effective cases 70.4% to 85.2%.
AMI: acute myocardial infarction.
VF: ventricular fibrillation.

these two groups. However, because attacks of variant angina can be effectively suppressed by calcium antagonistic drugs, surgical treatment is not required in most cases of variant angina.

Table 7 shows the effects of drugs in 39 cases of unstable angina diagnosed according to Fulton's criteria [5]. Of 22 cases with ST depression nifedipine was used in 14, and was effective in 9 cases. In two cases pain was eliminated by nifedipine, but these cases were followed by acute myocardial infarction. In one case, nifedipine alone was ineffective, but a combination of β-blocker and nifedipine was effective. Diltiazem was effective in one case. In three cases, the use of β-blocker alone had no effect.

Of the remaining 17 cases of unstable angina with ST elevation during attack, anginal attacks were suppressed in 10 by nifedipine and in one case by diltiazem. In one case pain was eliminated by nifedipine, but acute infarction developed. In two cases nifedipine was ineffective. These results show that nifedipine is very effective in treatment of unstable angina. Diltiazem also had a similar effect. It is noteworthy that there were few cases in which nifedipine did not prevent the development of infarction, although this drug suppressed the anginal pain effectively.

Conclusion

Coronary arterial spasm might play role in variant angina pectoris, angina pectoris, and acute myocardial infarction. The excellent effectiveness in variant angina has been ascribed to the antispastic action of calcium antagonists [6]. However, the effect on exertional angina can also be due to dilatation of coronary arteries and decrease of myocardial O_2 consumption.

Recently some investigators reported [7,8] that coronary spasm plays an important role in producing acute myocardial infarction. In such cases, myocardial infarction may be prevented when calcium antagonistic drugs are used.

The fact that nifedipine did not prevent the development of infarction in some cases suggests that spasm of coronary artery might not have been directly related to the pathogenesis of myocardial infarction.

Accordingly further investigation is required to understand the mechanism of coronary spasm and the mode of action of drugs that are dramatically effective in variant angina.

References

1. Kimura E, Mabuchi G, Kikuchi H (1972) The clinical effect of 4-(2'-nitrophenyl)-2,6-dimethyl-3,5-dicarbomethoxy-1,4-dihydropyridine (BAY a 1040) on angina pectoris evaluated by sequential analysis. Arzneim Forsch 2:365
2. Hashimoto K, Kimura E, Kobayashi T (1975) 1st International nifedipine-adalat symposium. Bayer Yakuhin, Osaka
3. Yasue H, Omote S, Takizawa A (1978) Pathogenesis and treatment of angina pectoris at rest as seen from its response to various drugs. Jap Circul J 42:1
4. Kusakawa R, Kinoshita M, Shimono Y (1977) Haemodynamic effects of a new anti-anginal drug, diltiazem hydrochloride. Arzneim Forsch 27:878
5. Fulton M, Duncan B, Lutz W, Morrison SL, Donald KW, Kerr F, Kirby BJ, Julian DG (1972) Natural history of unstable angina. Lancet I:860
6. Fleckenstein A (1970) Specific inhibitors and promotors of calcium action in the excitation-contraction coupling of heart muscle and their role in the prevention of production of myocardial lesions. In: Harris P, Opie LH (eds) Calcium and the heart. Academic Press, London New York, p 135
7. Oliva PB, Breckinridge JC (1977) Arteriographic evidence of coronary arterial spasm in acute myocardial infarction. Circulation 56:366
8. Wiener L, Kasparian H, Duca PR, Walinsky P, Gottlieb RS, Hanckel F, Brest AN (1976) Spectrum of coronary arterial spasm. Clinical, angiographic and myocardial metabolic experience in 29 cases. Am J Cardiol 38:945

Einfluß der Calcium-Antagonisten Verapamil, Nifedipin und Fendilin auf Blutdruck und Herzfrequenz

H. F. Spies, W. Schulz, H. Werner, E. Appel, H. J. Becker, und M. Kaltenbach

Die Angina pectoris gilt als Hauptindikation für die Calcium-Antagonisten. Durch die relaxierende Wirkung an der glatten Muskulatur der Gefäßwand ist jedoch auch eine blutdrucksenkende Wirkung vorhanden [1]. Dieser Effekt ist seit 1969 beim Verapamil bekannt [2], wobei er jedoch nur in der Akutbehandlung von hypertensiven Krisen breitere Anwendung gefunden hat, obwohl einzelne Hinweise vorlagen, daß auch eine orale Behandlung blutdrucksenkend wirkt [3]. Vor allem im Akutversuch ist auch vom Nifedipin in seiner oralen und parenteralen Applikationsform von Blutdrucksenkungen berichtet worden [4, 5].

Das Ziel der durchgeführten Untersuchungen ist es, die Wirkung des Calcium-Antagonisten Verapamil auf Blutdruck und Herzfrequenz, sowie die Plasma-Katecholamine bei Hypertonikern in Ruhe und bei Belastung zu überprüfen. Darüber hinaus soll noch kurz von dem akuten antihypertensiven Effekt des parenteral verabfolgten Nifedipins sowie von dem Einfluß von Fendilin auf Blutdruck und Herzfrequenz im Akutversuch sowie unter der Langzeitbehandlung berichtet werden.

Bezüglich des Verapamil wurden 9 Patienten mit arterieller Hypertonie untersucht. Das Durchschnittsalter der 6 männlichen und 3 weiblichen Patienten betrug 52 Jahre und es schwankte zwischen 33 und 76 Jahren. Bei 2 Patienten bestand ein Stadium I, bei 6 Patienten ein Stadium II und bei einem ein Stadium III der arteriellen Hypertonie. Ein Patient hatte eine renale, 8 Patienten eine essentielle Hypertonie. Nach einer 4wöchigen Vorperiode wurde in randomisierter Reihenfolge 3mal 160 mg Verapamil, 3mal 100 mg Metoprolol pro die und ein Placebo-Präparat gegeben. Bei 3 Patienten erfolgte während der gesamten Beobachtungszeit eine konstante Diuretikatherapie, 4 Patienten waren digitalisiert. Dreimal täglich wurde vom Patienten der Ruhe-Blutdruck im Sitzen gemessen. Dabei wurden einmal die in den letzten 2 Beobachtungswochen eines jeden Behandlungsabschnittes gemessenen Blutdruckwerte verglichen. Zum anderen stand am Ende jeder Beobachtungsperiode ein Arbeitsversuch am Fahrradergometer im Sitzen, wobei Blutdruck, Herzfrequenz und Ruhe- und Belastungs-EKG kontrolliert wurden. Die Messung des Blutdruckes erfolgte nach Riva Rocci. Vor Beginn und am Ende der Belastung fand eine Kontrolle des Adrenalins und Noradrenalins im Plasma statt. Die Belastungshöhe schwankte zwischen 50 und 70 Watt.

Bei einer Patientin konnte wegen leichter gastrointestinaler Beschwerden die Verapamildosis nicht auf die vorgesehene Höhe gesteigert werden. Bei einer weiteren, insgesamt schwer einstellbaren Patientin, sprach die angesetzte Verapamil-Therapie nicht an, so daß die Behandlung kurzfristig abgebrochen werden mußte.

Unter Ruhe-Bedingungen verminderte sich der Blutdruck in den letzten 2 Behandlungswochen durch Verapamil von 169/101 auf 148/98 mmHg. Die unter Metoprolol beobachtete Senkung von 168/103 auf 149/94 mmHg fiel vergleichbar aus. Ein verwertbarer Unterschied in der Blutdruckwirkung des hochdosierten Verapamils mit dem Metoprolol fand sich nicht. Ebensowenig bestand ein signifikanter Unterschied zwischen Placebo und der Vorperiode.

Unter Belastung verminderte Verapamil den Blutdruck von 213/109 auf 168/87 mmHg. Die Ruhe-Frequenz verminderte sich gering von 90 auf 84/min, wobei diese geringe Frequenzsenkung im Vergleich zum Placebo nicht mehr signifikant nachweisbar ist. Deutlich ist jedoch der Abfall der Belastungsfrequenz von 131 auf 102/min (Abb. 1).

Unter Metoprolol verminderte sich der Blutdruck bei Belastung von 210/109 auf 172/97 mmHg. Typisch für die Beta-Rezeptorenblockade fiel die Herzfrequenz in Ruhe von 83 auf 62/min deutlich ab. Dazu passend zeigte sich ein Abfall der Belastungsherzfrequenz von 131 auf 94/min (Abb. 2).

Vor Beginn und am Ende des Belastungsversuchs wurde noch das Adrenalin und Noradrenalin im Plasma bestimmt. In der Vorperiode kam es durch die Belastung zu einem Anstieg des Noradrenalins von 269 auf 490 ng/l. Durch die Verapamil-Behandlung ließ sich eine verwertbare Änderung dieses Anstiegs nicht nachweisen. Entsprechend der niedrigen Belastungsstufe zeigte sich nur ein geringer Plasma-Adrenalinanstieg. In der Vorperiode erhöhte sich durch die Ergometrie der Wert von 102 auf 131 ng/l. Verapamil führte demgegenüber zu einer deutlicheren Steigerung von 123 zu 178 ng/l. Diese deutlichere Anhebung des Adrenalin-Spiegels ist auffallend, ist jedoch statistisch nicht eindeutig sicherbar (Abb. 3).

Nach diesen Untersuchungsbefunden senkt Verapamil in der vergleichsweise hohen Dosis von 3mal 160 mg pro die auch in der Langzeitbehandlung den arteriellen

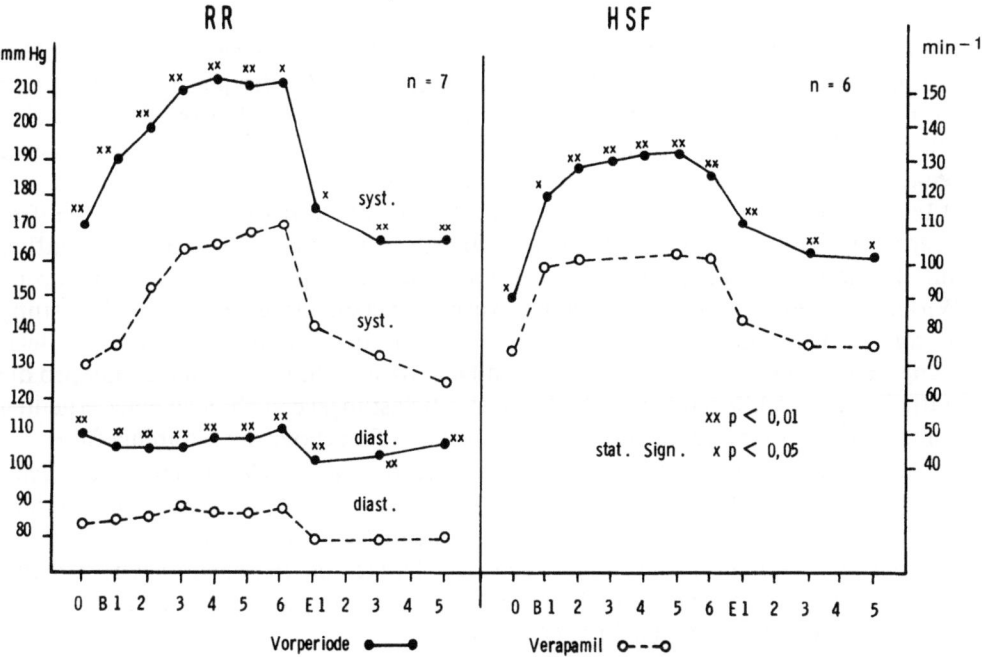

Abb. 1. Blutdruck- und Herzfrequenzverhalten im Arbeitsversuch am Fahrradergometer im Sitzen nach 4wöchiger Behandlung mit 3mal 160 mg Verapamil pro die im Vergleich zur Vorperiode. Auf der linken Seite der Abbildung ist das Blutdruckverhalten (RR), auf der rechten Seite das Herzfrequenzverhalten (HSF) aufgezeichnet

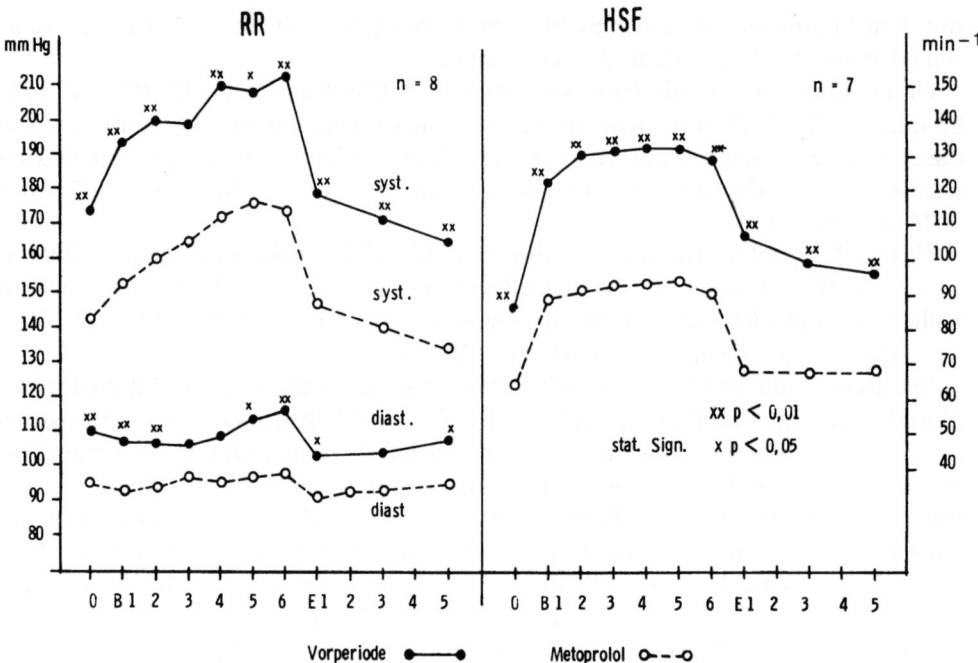

Abb. 2. Blutdruck- und Herzfrequenzverhalten nach 4wöchiger Behandlung mit 3mal 100 mg Metoprolol pro die im Vergleich zur Vorperiode. Auf der linken Seite ist das Blutdruckverhalten (RR), auf der rechten Seite das Herzfrequenzverhalten (HSF) aufgezeichnet

Blutdruck, wobei die Blutdrucksenkung etwa der des Beta-Rezeptorenblockers Metoprolol vergleichbar ist. Bezüglich des Verhaltens der Herzfrequenz verhielten sich die beiden Medikamente unterschiedlich. Im Gegensatz zum Verapamil zeigte sich erwartungsgemäß eine deutliche Frequenzsenkung in Ruhe. Beide Medikamente senkten die Belastungsfrequenz, der Beta-Blocker jedoch ausgeprägter.

Ich möchte noch kurz über den Einfluß des Fendilin auf Blutdruck und Herzfrequenz bei 20 Patienten ohne arterielle Hypertonie berichten, bei denen der Einfluß auf Blutdruck und Herzfrequenz im Rahmen der Überprüfung der antianginösen Wirkung gemessen wurde. Nach einem Ausgangsversuch folgte die zweite Belastung 95 min nach der Gabe einer Einzeldosis von 300 mg Fendilin. Der nächste Belastungsversuch fand nach einer 4wöchigen Dauerbehandlung mit 3mal 50 mg pro die statt. Daran anschließend erfolgte der fünfte Belastungsversuch nach einer erneuten Gabe von 300 mg Fendilin. Zusätzlich wurde ein Placeboversuch durchgeführt.

Die Ausgangswerte von 137/85 mmHg in Ruhe und 175/98 mmHg unter Belastung werden weder durch die akute noch die chronische Applikation von Fendilin verwertbar verändert. Genausowenig läßt sich eine Verschiebung der Ruhe- und Belastungsherzfrequenz nachweisen. Nach den gemachten Beobachtungen ist somit eine Wirkung von Fendilin auf Blutdruck und Herzfrequenz unter den genannten Bedingungen nicht zu beobachten (Abb. 4).

Abschließend möchte ich noch die Akutwirkung des Nifedipin auf Blutdruck und Herzfrequenz bei der intravenösen Applikation darstellen, wobei Patienten mit koronarer Herzkrankheit und arterieller Hypertonie anläßlich der Herzkatheteruntersuchung überprüft wurden.

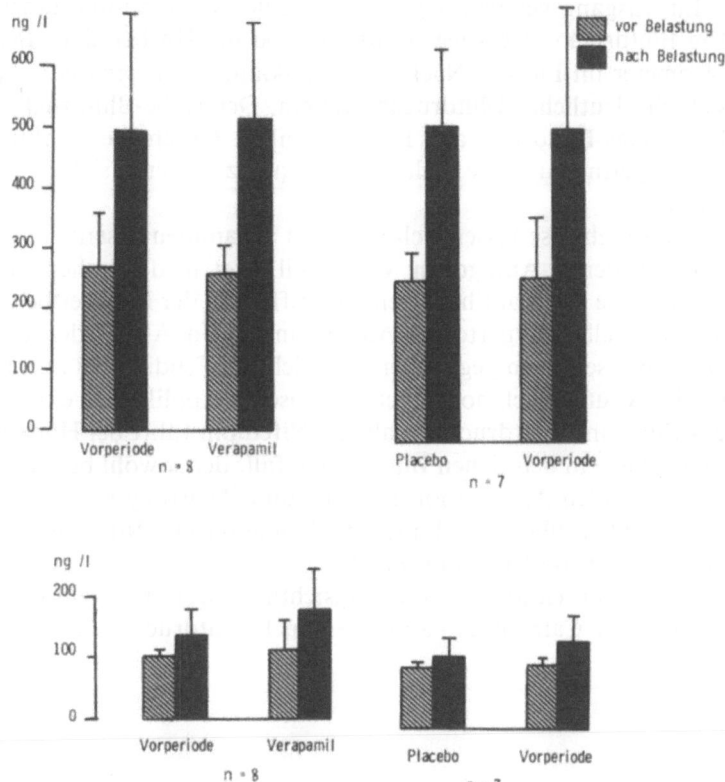

Abb. 3. Plasma-Noradrenalin- und Adrenalin-Konzentrationen vor und nach Belastung am Fahrradergometer im Sitzen nach 4wöchiger Behandlung mit 3mal 160 mg Verapamil pro die im Vergleich zur Vorperiode und einer Behandlungsphase mit Placebo

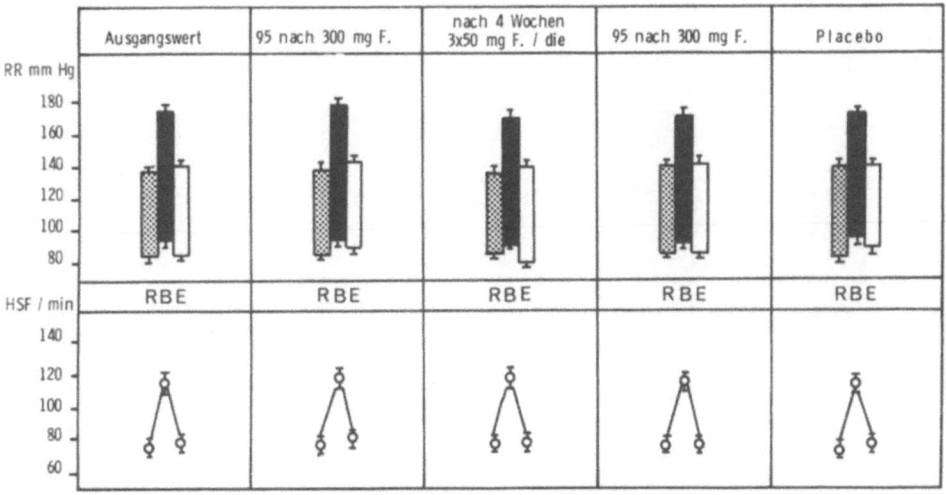

Abb. 4. Das Blutdruck- und Herzfrequenzverhalten in Ruhe und bei Belastung nach akuter Gabe von 300 mg Fendilin, nach 4wöchiger Behandlung mit 3mal 50 mg Fendilin pro die, nach erneuter Akutgabe von 300 mg Fendilin sowie nach Placebo. Im oberen Anteil der Abbildung ist das Blutdruckverhalten (RR), im unteren Anteil das Herzfrequenzverhalten (HSF) in Ruhe (R), unter Belastung (B) und während der Erholungsphase (E) aufgezeichnet (n = 20)

Im Ausgangsversuch zeigten sich vor der Medikation Blutdruckwerte von 175/91. Die Blutdruckwerte stiegen auf 193/100 mmHg bei einer Belastung am Fahrradergometer im Liegen. Nach der Applikation von 1 mg Nifedipin intravenös stellte sich ein deutlicher Blutdruckabfall ein. Der Ruhe-Blutdruck sank auf 138/78, der Belastungs-Blutdruck auf 171/89 mmHg. Durch die Injektion stieg die Herzfrequenz gering an. Die Belastungsfrequenz änderte sich jedoch nicht verwertbar (Abb. 5).

Die Ergebnisse lassen sich wie folgt zusammenfassen:

Der Calcium-Antagonist Verapamil zeigt in der hohen oralen Dosis von 3mal 160 mg/die einen antihypertensiven Effekt in der Langzeitbehandlung bei Patienten mit arterieller Hypertonie. Außerdem ist ein Abfall der Belastungsherzfrequenz nachzuweisen. Demgegenüber zeigt sich mit Fendilin bei normotonen Patienten weder im Akutversuch noch nach chronischer Applikation eine verwertbare Änderung des Puls- und Blutdruckverhaltens. Nifedipin führt bei Hypertonikern im Akutversuch zu einem deutlichen Blutdruckabfall, der sowohl bei der intravenösen als auch bei der oralen Applikation in Ruhe und Belastung sichtbar ist. Größere Untersuchungsreihen über eine Langzeitbehandlung mit Nifedipin bestehen bezüglich des antihypertensiven Effektes nicht.

Es wird erkennbar, daß die hinsichtlich ihrer antianginösen Wirkung heterogene Gruppe der Calcium-Antagonisten auch Blutdruck und Herzfrequenz unterschied-

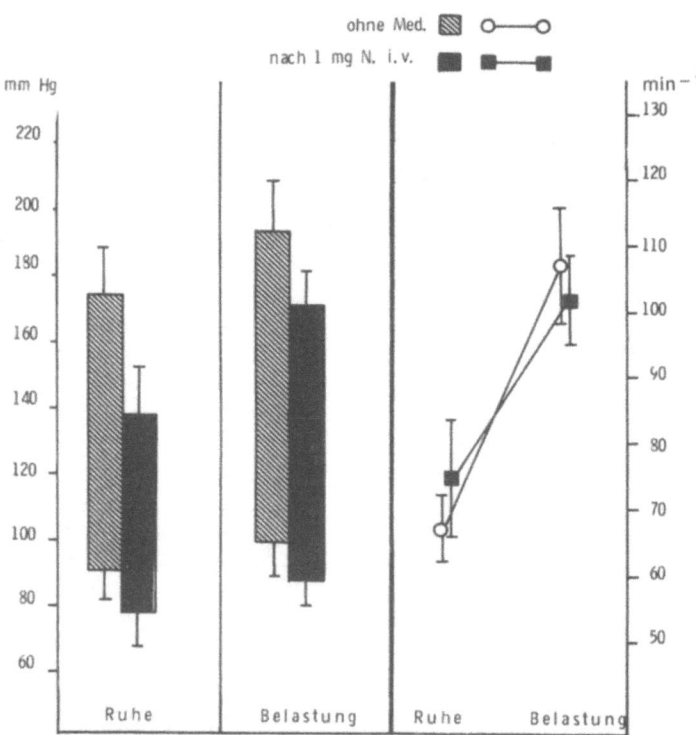

Abb. 5. Aortendruck und Herzfrequenz nach intravenöser Injektion von 1 mg Nifedipin. Im linken Anteil der Abbildung ist das Blutdruckverhalten, im rechten Anteil das Herzfrequenzverhalten aufgezeichnet (n = 6)

lich beeinflussen. Nach den Erfahrungen mit Verapamil muß zum Erreichen einer antihypertensiven Wirkung die bei der Angina pectoris-Behandlung vorgeschlagene Dosis erheblich gesteigert werden. Unter Berücksichtigung dieser Dosierungsfrage sollte überprüft werden, welche Rolle neben dem Verapamil den übrigen wirksamen Calcium-Antagonisten im Rahmen der zur Zeit üblichen antihypertensiven Therapie zukommt.

Literatur

1. Fleckenstein-Grün G, Fleckenstein A (1975) 2nd international adalat symposium. 66
2. Brittinger DW, Strauch M, Huber W, Koch WD, von Henning GE, Willenmeier KW, Trittendorf WD (1969) Dtsch Med Wochenschr 94:945
3. Bachour G, Bender F, Wessels F, Losse H (1976) Verh Dtsch Ges Inn Med 82:1334
4. Bartorelli C, Guazzi M (to be published) International adalat panel discussion, Tokyo 1978
5. Laaser U, Meurer KA, Krüger H, Kaufmann W (1973) 2nd international adalat symposium. 283

Verhütung experimenteller Gefäßverkalkungen (Mönckebergs Typ der Arteriosklerose) durch Calcium-Antagonisten bei Ratten[1]

M. Frey, J. Keidel und A. Fleckenstein

Nach früheren Untersuchungen von Selye [1] kommt es im Tierexperiment bei gleichzeitiger Verabreichung von Dihydrotachysterol (AT 10) und Natriumphosphat nicht nur zu schweren Herzmuskelnekrosen, sondern auch zu arteriosklerotischen Gefäßprozessen vom sog. Mönckeberg-Typ. Diese Mönckeberg-Arteriosklerose ist charakterisiert durch Nekrotisierung und Calcifizierung der glatten Gefäßmuskulatur. Selye hat diese Befunde vornehmlich unter morphologischem Aspekt ausführlich dargestellt, wobei der pathophysiologische Entstehungs-Mechanismus jedoch noch unklar blieb.

Das Interesse des Freiburger Physiologischen Instituts an experimentellen Gefäßverkalkungen reicht 10 Jahre zurück. Der damalige Ausgangsbefund war, daß Ca^{++}-Ionen für die Myocardfasern zu einem gefährlichen Nekrose-Faktor werden können, falls der Ca^{++}-Einstrom ins Faserinnere aus irgendeinem Grunde exzessive Werte erreicht [2 – 6]. Dies gilt z. B. für die Pathogenese von Myocardnekrosen infolge Überdosierung von Vitamin D, von Dihydrotachysterol (AT 10) oder von β-adrenergen Catecholaminen. Hieraus ergab sich die Vermutung, daß auch die Nekrotisierung der glatten Gefäßmuskulatur bei der Mönckeberg-Arteriosklerose *primär* durch eine intrazelluläre Überladung mit Ca^{++}-Ionen verursacht sein könnte und daher möglicherweise auf die gleiche prophylaktische Behandlung mit organischen Ca^{++}-Antagonisten (Verapamil, Prenylamin) bzw. Ca^{++}-antagonistischen K^+- oder Mg^{++}-Salzen anspricht, die sich auch gegenüber Ca^{++}-bedingten Herznekrosen als wirksam erwiesen hatten. Die erste Bestätigung dieses Konzeptes ergab sich in Untersuchungen von Janke u. Mitarb. [7] an AT 10- und NaH_2PO_4-behandelten Ratten. Hierbei ließ sich unter Verwendung von radioaktivem ^{45}Ca zeigen, daß tatsächlich unter dem äußeren Erscheinungsbild der experimentellen Mönckeberg-Sklerose eine massive Potenzierung der Ca^{++}-Aufnahme in die Gefäßwände erfolgt (Abb. 1). In den damaligen Versuchen erhielten Ratten 10 Tage lang täglich peroral 0,5 mg/kg AT 10 und 20 mMol/kg NaH_2PO_4. Am 11. Tag wurden 10 μCi ^{45}Ca/kg intraperitoneal appliziert. Sechs Std später wurden die Tiere getötet und die Radioaktivität in der Aorta und A. mesenterica gemessen. Wie der linke Bildabschnitt zeigt, ist bei unbehandelten Kontroll-Ratten die ^{45}Ca-Inkorporation relativ gering. Die Radioaktivität in 1 g Gefäßwand entspricht normalerweise der Radioaktivität von 1 ml Blutplasma (= 100%). Nach 10 Tagen Vorbehandlung der Ratten mit AT 10 plus Natriumphosphat änderte sich jedoch die Situation von Grund auf; denn wie der rechte Bildabschnitt zeigt, verlief die Radiocalcium-Aufnahme in die genannten Gefäße nunmehr mit einer 50- bis 70mal höheren Geschwindigkeit als bei den unbehan-

---

1 Vorläufige Mitteilungen der Ergebnisse sind bereits anläßlich der 47. Tagung (Herbsttagung der Deutschen Physiol. Ges., 13. – 18. Sept. 1976 in Regensburg) und der 50. Tagung (Herbsttagung, 3. – 6. Okt. 1978 in Göttingen) erfolgt; siehe Pflügers Arch Eur J Physiol [Suppl] 365:R6 (1976) und [Suppl] 377:R9 (1978)

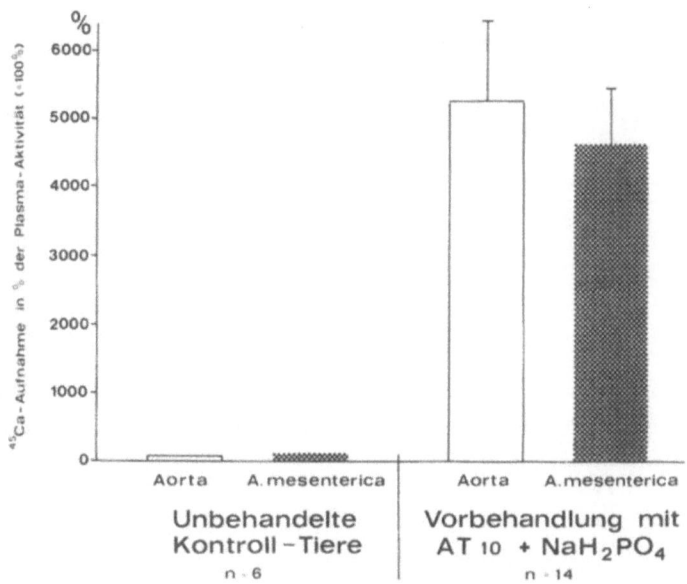

Abb. 1. Exzessive Steigerung der Netto-Aufnahme von Radiocalcium in die Wand der Aorta und A. mesenterica von Ratten nach 10tägiger peroraler Vorbehandlung mit Dihydrotachysterol (AT 10) + NaH_2PO_4. Dosierung: Täglich 0,5 mg/kg Dihydrotachysterol + 20 mMol NaH_2PO_4/kg Körpergewicht. Nach intraperitonealer ^{45}Ca-Injektion am 11. Versuchstag wurde die während 6 Std in 1 g Gefäßwand aufgenommene Radioaktivität bestimmt und in Prozent der gleichzeitig gemessenen Aktivität von 1 ml Plasma (= 100%) ausgedrückt (nach Janke u. Mitarb. [7])

delten Kontroll-Tieren. Kalium- und Magnesiumchlorid sowie die organischen Calcium-Antagonisten Verapamil und Prenylamin konnten diese exzessive Radiocalcium-Inkorporation in die Gefäßwände hochsignifikant hemmen.

Unsere neueren Untersuchungen, über die im folgenden berichtet wird, wurden mit Vitamin D_3 in Form von Vi-De 3 Hydrosol[1], einem wasserlöslichen Cholecalciferol, durchgeführt. Dieses Vitamin D_3-Präparat hat den Vorteil, *intramuskulär* injizierbar zu sein. Hierdurch werden die Zufälligkeiten der Darmresorption ausgeschaltet. Schon eine einzige Injektion von 50000 bzw. 90000 I.E. führt bei Ratten innerhalb von wenigen Tagen zu schweren nekrotisierenden Herzmuskel- und Gefäßcalcinosen. Abbildung 2 demonstriert die Steigerung der Radiocalcium-Nettoaufnahme in die Wand der Aorta und der Arteria mesenterica am 4. Tag nach einer einzigen Injektion von Vitamin D_3. Verabreicht man die niedrigere Dosis von 50000 I.E., so kommt es in der Aorta zu einem Anstieg der Geschwindigkeit der ^{45}Ca-Aufnahme auf das 5- bis 6fache, in der A. mesenterica auf das 13- bis 14fache des — bei unbehandelten Kontroll-Ratten gefundenen — Normalwertes. Steigert man die Vitamin D_3-Dosis weiter auf 90000 I.E., so wird die Potenzierung der ^{45}Ca-

---

1 Hersteller: Wander AG., Bern, Schweiz

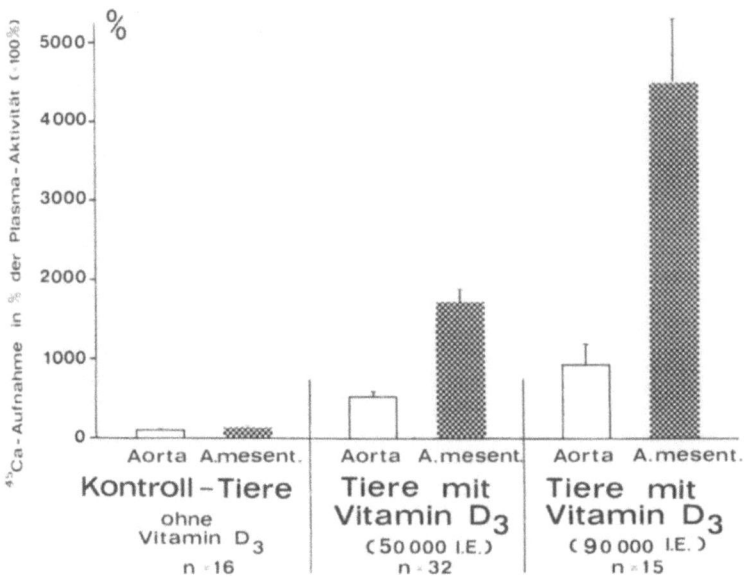

Abb. 2. Steigerung der Netto-Aufnahme von Radiocalcium in die Wand der Aorta und A. mesenterica von Ratten am 4. Tag nach einer einmaligen intramuskulären Injektion von Vitamin D_3 (50000 bzw. 90000 I.E.). Nach einer 80stündigen Einwirkungsdauer dieser Vitamin D_3-Dosen erhielten die Tiere intraperitoneal ^{45}Ca und wurden dann 6 Std später zur Bestimmung der zwischenzeitlich in die Gefäßwände inkorporierten Menge an Radiocalcium getötet

Nettoaufnahme, besonders in der A. mesenterica sup., noch exzessiver. Die Inkorporation des intraperitoneal injizierten Radiocalcium in die Wand der A. mesenterica verlief z. B. unter dem Einfluß dieser höheren D_3-Dosis während der üblichen Meßperiode von 6 Std 35- bis 40mal rascher als normal. Unsere Untersuchungen haben weiterhin gezeigt, daß die Vitamin D_3-induzierte Ca^{++}-Überladung der Arterienwände wochenlang bestehen bleibt, also spontan kaum reversibel ist.

In Abb. 3 ist der Effekt einer einmaligen Vitamin D_3-Injektion von 50000 I.E. auf den ^{45}Ca-Einbau in die arteriellen Gefäße und in den Rippenknochen vergleichend gegenübergestellt. Hierbei fällt zunächst auf, daß das injizierte Radiocalcium von den normalen Kontroll-Ratten *(im linken Bildabschnitt)* am schnellsten ins Knochengewebe aufgenommen wird. So ist im Normalfall der Radiocalcium-Gehalt der Rippe (6 Std nach der ^{45}Ca-Injektion) etwa 70mal höher als der des Plasmas, während die Arterienwände gerade das Niveau der Plasmaaktivität erreichen. Nach Vorbehandlung der Ratten mit Vitamin D_3 gleicht sich dagegen *(im rechten Bildabschnitt)* der hohe Markierungs-Unterschied zwischen Gefäß- und Knochengewebe weitgehend aus. Dies kommt dadurch zustande, daß unter Vitamin D_3 die ^{45}Ca-Inkorporation in die Gefäßwände dramatisch ansteigt, während überraschenderweise die Geschwindigkeit der ^{45}Ca-Aufnahme in die Rippe auf annähernd $\frac{1}{3}$ der Norm zurückgeht. Offensichtlich wird also markiertes Calcium unter dem Einfluß hoher Dosen von Vitamin D_3 bevorzugt in den Gefäßen und nicht mehr, wie normal, im

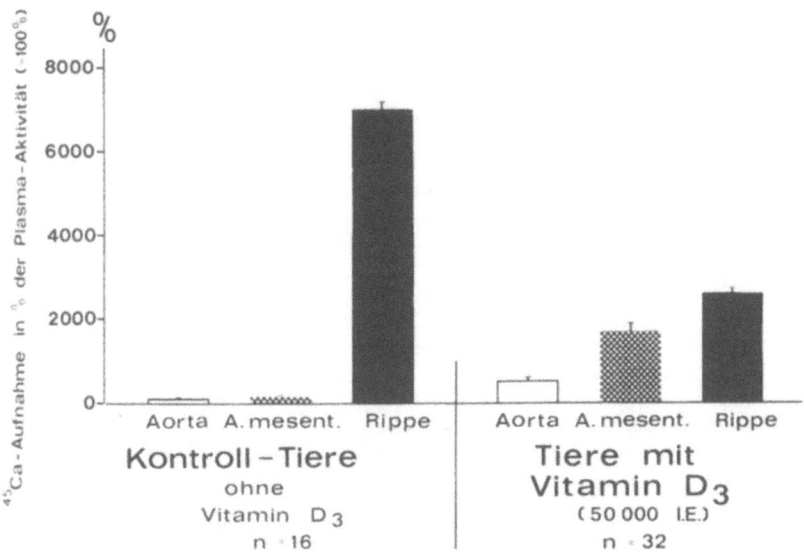

Abb. 3. Steigerung der Netto-Aufnahme von Radiocalcium in die Wand der Aorta und A. mesenterica von Ratten am 4. Tag nach einer einmaligen intramuskulären Injektion von Vitamin D_3 (50000 I.E.). Umgekehrt wird die Radiocalcium-Inkorporation in das Knochengewebe (Rippe) durch Vitamin D_3 erheblich reduziert. Sonstige Versuchsanordnung wie in Abb. 2

Knochen abgelagert. Diese exzessive Stimulation der Ca^{++}-Aufnahme in die glatten Gefäßmuskelzellen – bei gleichzeitiger Einschränkung der Calcium-Bindung im Knochen – ist offenbar der entscheidende Grund für die Entstehung der Media-Calcinose vom Mönckeberg-Typ.

Ein noch klareres Indiz für die primäre pathogenetische Bedeutung der Ca^{++}-Ionen als Zerstörer der glatten Gefäßmuskelzellen, ist jedoch die Tatsache, daß die experimentelle Mönckeberg-Sklerose nach hohen Gaben von Dihydrotachysterol (AT 10) oder Vitamin D_3 verhütet werden kann, wenn es gelingt, die Radiocalcium-Aufnahme in die Gefäßwand durch prophylaktische Verabreichung von $MgCl_2$ oder Verapamil zu normalisieren und dadurch die deletäre Ca^{++}-Überladung der glatten Gefäßmuskelzellen zu verhindern. Abbildung 4 zeigt, daß unter dem Einfluß einer mehrtägigen oralen Magnesium-Verabreichung die Absolut-Werte an Calcium trotz der Vitamin D_3-Gabe nur noch wenig über die Norm ansteigen. Hierdurch werden Beobachtungen von Selye erklärt, der aufgrund histologischer Studien schon früher über die Prophylaxe Dihydrotachysterol-induzierter Gefäßsklerosen von Ratten mit Hilfe von $MgCl_2$ berichtet hat. Abbildung 4 demonstriert aber auch die hohe Effizienz des organischen Ca^{++}-Antagonisten Verapamil, der die Vitamin D_3-bedingte Gefäßcalcinose sowohl bei subkutaner als auch bei peroraler Verabreichung fast noch wirksamer als $MgCl_2$ verhindern kann. Die subkutane Gabe betrug dabei 2mal täglich 30 mg/kg, die orale Gabe 2mal täglich 100 mg/kg über einen Zeitraum von 4 Tagen, wobei die erste Verapamil-Dosis jeweils 12 Std vor der einmaligen Injektion von 50000 I.E. Vitamin D_3 verabreicht wurde.

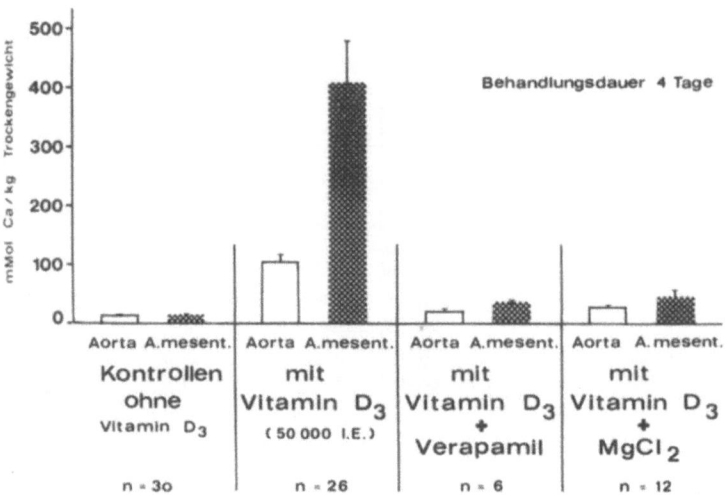

Abb. 4. Verhütung der Vitamin D_3-induzierten Ca^{++}-Überladung der Gefäßwände von Aorta und A. mesenterica von Ratten durch perorale Gabe von Verapamil bzw. $MgCl_2$. Dosierung: Einmalige intramuskuläre Injektion von 50 000 I.E. Vitamin D_3 am 1. Versuchstag. Perorale Gaben von 2mal 100 mg Verapamil/kg bzw. 2mal 15 mMol $MgCl_2$/kg am 1., 2. und 3. Versuchstag sowie 1mal 100 mg Verapamil/kg bzw. 1mal 15 mMol $MgCl_2$/kg am 4. Versuchstag. Bestimmung des absoluten Ca^{++}-Gehalts der Gefäßwände (mMol Ca^{++}/kg Trockengewicht) 80 Std nach der Verabreichung von Vitamin D_3

Eine statistische Auswertung aller mit Verapamil durchgeführten Experimente ist in den Tabellen 1 und 2 wiedergegeben. Tabelle 1 zeigt dabei das Endergebnis unserer Versuche mit Radiocalcium. Hierbei ist berechnet, um wieviel Prozent die Vitamin D_3-stimulierte Radiocalcium-Aufnahme ins Myocard und in die Gefäßwände durch die verwendeten Verapamil-Dosen gehemmt wurde. Tatsächlich wird durch diese Daten belegt, daß Verapamil das Ventrikelmyocard und die Arterien-Wände annähernd gleichstark vor der Vitamin D_3-bedingten Ca^{++}-Überladung schützt. Dabei wird der Vitamin D_3-Effekt bei peroraler und subkutaner Verabreichung von Verapamil im Mittel zu etwa 75 – 95% neutralisiert. Zu einem analogen Ergebnis führten auch die in Tabelle 2 zusammengestellten Resultate. In diesen Experimenten wurden die protektiven Wirkungen von Verapamil gegenüber der Vitamin D_3-bedingten Herz- und Gefäßcalcinose nicht mit Hilfe von Radiocalcium, sondern durch Bestimmung des *absoluten* Calcium-Gehaltes quantifiziert. Offensichtlich läßt sich auch der absolute Anstieg der Calcium-Konzentration in Herz- und Gefäßmuskulatur mit Hilfe von Verapamil im gleichen hohen Ausmaß von 75 – 95% hemmen wie die D_3-stimulierte Radiocalcium-Aufnahme. Auch hierbei zeigt Verapamil in entsprechender Dosis subkutan oder peroral verabreicht – als Prototyp einer Ca^{++}-antagonistisch wirksamen Substanz – erstaunliche cardiovaskuläre Schutzeffekte.

Tabelle 1. Prozentuale Hemmung der Vitamin D_3-stimulierten Radiocalcium-Nettoaufnahme in die Herz- und Gefäßmuskulatur (Vit. D_3 50 000 I.E.)

	% Hemmung durch 2 × 30 mg Verapamil/kg (subcutan)	% Hemmung durch 2 × 100 mg Verapamil/kg (peroral)
rechter Ventrikel	94,0 (± 2,2)	87,0 (± 8,4)
linker Ventrikel (Innenschicht)	94,1 (± 2,4)	86,5 (± 7,7)
linker Ventrikel (Außenschicht)	90,5 (± 2,5)	80,1 (± 9,9)
Aorta	79,4 (± 5,9)	71,7 (± 11,7)
A. mesenterica sup.	77,9 (± 8,7)	87,6 (± 5,2)
	n = 13	n = 9

Subkutane Dosierung: 2mal tägl. 30 mg/kg Verapamil während 4 Tagen.
Orale Dosierung: 2mal tägl. 100 mg/kg Verapamil während 4 Tagen.

Tabelle 2. Prozentuale Hemmung der Vitamin D_3-stimulierten Steigerung des Calcium-Gehaltes in der Herz- und Gefäßmuskulatur (Vit. D_3 50 000 I.E.)

	% Hemmung durch 2 × 30 mg Verapamil/kg (subcutan)	% Hemmung durch 2 × 100 mg Verapamil/kg (peroral)
rechter Ventrikel	88,5 (± 3,8)	81,9 (± 6,8)
linker Ventrikel (Herzspitze)	86,2 (± 4,0)	72,7 (± 11,2)
linker Ventrikel (Herzbasis)	84,6 (± 4,4)	78,3 (± 8,5)
Aorta	81,4 (± 9,0)	91,7 (± 3,3)
A. mesenterica sup.	81,5 (± 9,5)	93,8 (± 1,2)
	n = 14	n = 6

Subkutane Dosierung: 2mal tägl. 30 mg/kg Verapamil während 4 Tagen.
Orale Dosierung: 2mal tägl. 100 mg/kg Verapamil während 4 Tagen.

Zusammenfassung

Vorausgegangene Studien haben gezeigt, daß eine mehrtägige orale Behandlung mit Dihydrotachysterol (AT 10) + NaH_2PO_4 oder eine einmalige intramuskuläre Injektion von Vitamin D_3 (50 000 – 90 000 I.E.) bei Ratten eine sog. Mönckeberg-Arteriosklerose erzeugen kann. Charakteristisch ist hierbei eine gewaltige Potenzierung der Ca^{++}-Aufnahme in die arteriellen Gefäßwände. So wurde 4 Tage nach Gabe von 50 000 I.E. Vitamin D_3 eine Zunahme der Radiocalcium-Nettoaufnahme in die Wand der Aorta auf das 5- bis 6fache und in die Wand der A. mesenterica auf das 13- bis 14fache der Norm gefunden. Damit erreichte die Vitamin D_3-induzierte [45]Ca-Aufnahme in die Wand der A. mesenterica nahezu die Geschwindigkeit der

^{45}Ca-Inkorporation in das Knochengewebe (Rippe). Eine prophylaktische Behandlung mit oralen MgCl$_2$-Gaben kann umgekehrt die Ca^{++}-Überladung beinahe vollständig verhindern. Darüberhinaus erwiesen sich auch organische Ca^{++}-Antagonisten wie z. B. Verapamil (2mal 30 mg/kg subcutan oder 2mal 100 mg/kg oral während 4 Tagen verabfolgt) als hochwirksam; Verapamil konnte dabei die Vitamin D$_3$-bedingte Stimulation der ^{45}Ca-Inkorporation und den Anstieg des Ca^{++}-Absolutgehaltes der Gefäßwände zu 80–90% verhindern. Offensichtlich schützt also Verapamil nicht nur die Myocardfasern, sondern auch die glatte Gefäßmuskulatur vor den deletären Folgen einer intracellulären Ca^{++}-Überladung.

Summary

Previous investigations have shown that daily oral doses of dihydrotachysterol plus NaH$_2$PO$_4$ or a single intramuscular injection of vitamin D$_3$ (50 000 – 90 000 I.U.) produce an arteriosclerosis of the so-called "Mönckeberg's type" in rats, which is characterized by a large potentiation of Ca uptake into the arterial walls. Thus, following administration of 50 000 I.U. vitamin D$_3$, the radiocalcium incorporation into the aortic wall was increased within 4 days by 5 to 6 times, and into that of the mesenteric artery even by 13 to 14 times. Hence the D$_3$-induced ^{45}Ca uptake into the wall of the mesenteric artery was nearly as fast as the labeling of bone tissue (ribs). Prophylactic oral administration of MgCl$_2$ prevented arterial Ca overload almost completely. Moreover organic Ca antagonists such as verapamil (2 × 30 mg/kg subcutaneously or 2 × 100 mg/kg orally administered over a period of 4 days) proved to be capable of blocking the promoter effects of vitamin D$_3$ on both vascular ^{45}Ca uptake and absolute Ca content by 80% – 90%. Obviously verapamil not only protects the myocardium but also vascular smooth muscle from deleterious Ca overload.

Literatur

1. Selye H (1958) Prophylactic treatment of an experimental arteriosclerosis with magnesium and potassium salts. Am Heart J 55:805–809
2. Fleckenstein A (1968) Myokardstoffwechsel und Nekrose. In: Heilmeyer L, Holtmeier HJ (Hrsg) Herzinfarkt und Schock. Thieme, Stuttgart, S 94–109
3. Fleckenstein A (1971) Specific inhibitors and promoters of calcium action in the excitation-contraction coupling of heart muscle and their role in the prevention or production of myocardial lesions. In: Harris P, Opie L (eds) Calcium and the heart. Academic Press, London New York, pp 135–188
4. Fleckenstein A, Janke J, Döring HJ, Leder O (1971) Die intrazelluläre Überladung mit Kalzium als entscheidender Kausalfaktor bei der Entstehung nicht-coronarogener Myokard-Nekrosen. Verh Dtsch Ges Kreislaufforsch 37:345–353
5. Fleckenstein A, Janke J, Döring HJ, Leder O (1974) Myocardial fibre necrosis due to intracellular Ca overload – a new principle in cardiac pathophysiology. In: Dhalla NS (ed) Myocardial biology. Recent advances in studies on cardiac structure and metabolism, vol 4. University Park Press, Baltimore London Tokyo, pp 563–579
6. Fleckenstein A, Janke J, Döring HJ, Leder O (1975) The key-role of Ca in the production of non-coronarogenic myocardial necroses. In: Fleckenstein A, Rona G (eds) Pathophysiology and morphology of myocardial cell alterations. Recent advances in studies on cardiac structure and metabolism, vol 6. University Park Press, Baltimore London Tokyo, pp 21–32
7. Janke J, Hein B, Pachinger O, Leder O, Fleckenstein A (1972) Hemmung arteriosklerotischer Gefäßprozesse durch prophylaktische Behandlung mit MgCl$_2$, KCl und organischen Ca^{++}-Antagonisten (Quantitative Studien mit Ca^{45} bei Ratten). In: Betz E (Hrsg) Vascular smooth muscle. Springer, Berlin Heidelberg New York, S 71–72

Therapeutische Wirkung von Calcium-Antagonisten auf den globalen myokardialen Blutfluß

M. Tauchert, D. W. Behrenbeck, B. Niehues und H. H. Hilger

Unter dem Einfluß calciumantagonistisch wirksamer Pharmaka wird im kontraktilen System weniger ATP-gebundene Energie in mechanische Arbeit überführt [1]. Dies muß zu einer Abnahme des myokardialen Sauerstoffverbrauches führen. Gleichzeitig wird der Tonus der glatten Wandmuskulatur der Widerstandsgefäße gesenkt; hieraus ergibt sich eine Verminderung des Koronarwiderstandes und damit eine Steigerung der Koronardurchblutung. Wir haben das Ausmaß dieser Wirkungen an den beiden Präparaten Verapamil (V) und Nifedipin (N) untersucht.

Methodik

Die Verapamil-Untersuchungen wurden an 10 Patienten mit angiographisch gesicherter koronarer Herzkrankheit durchgeführt. Es handelte sich um 8 Männer und 2 Frauen im Alter zwischen 33 und 53 Jahren, im Mittel 42 Jahre. Die Behandlung mit koronarwirksamen Medikamenten war vor der Untersuchung für mindestens 24 Std unterbrochen; es erfolgte keinerlei sedierende oder analgetische Prämedikation.

Folgende Ausgangsparameter wurden bestimmt: Herzfrequenz, Drucke im großen und kleinen Kreislauf, Herzzeitvolumen (mit der Farbstoffverdünnungsmethode), Koronardurchblutung (mit der Argon-Methode [2]), Koronarwiderstand, arterieller und koronarvenöser Sauerstoffgehalt und myokardialer Sauerstoffverbrauch. Anschließend erhielten die Pat. 0,1 mg pro Kilogramm Körpergewicht Verapamil in 2 min i.v.; die Injektion wurde dann mit 0,005 mg pro Kilogramm pro Minute während der folgenden 25 min fortgesetzt. Bei Ende der Injektion wurden alle Prüfparameter erneut bestimmt. Nifedipin wurde an 8 Patienten geprüft, von denen 4 einen hämodynamisch unbedeutenden Herzfehler hatten, die übrigen 4 eine durch Angiogramm gesicherte coronare Herzkrankheit (Abb. 1). Das Alter lag in dieser Gruppe zwischen 18 und 49 Jahren und betrug im Mittel 38 Jahre (5 Männer, 3 Frauen). Die Patienten erhielten nach den Kontrollmessungen 20 mg Nifedipin buccal (Zerbeißen von 2 Kapseln zu je 10 mg); die Wiederholung der Messungen erfolgte zum Zeitpunkt des Maximums des durch Nifedipin induzierten Anstiegs der koronarvenösen Sauerstoffsättigung. Das übrige Protokoll entsprach dem der Verapamil-Untersuchung.

Ergebnisse (vgl. Abb. 2 – 4)

Die in Ruhe normale Herzfrequenz wurde durch Verapamil nicht beeinflußt (75 ± 12 Schläge/min vorher, 74 ± 14 Schläge/min nachher).

Durch das Nifedipin wurde sie um 14% angehoben (von 81 ± 15/min auf 92 ± 14/min).

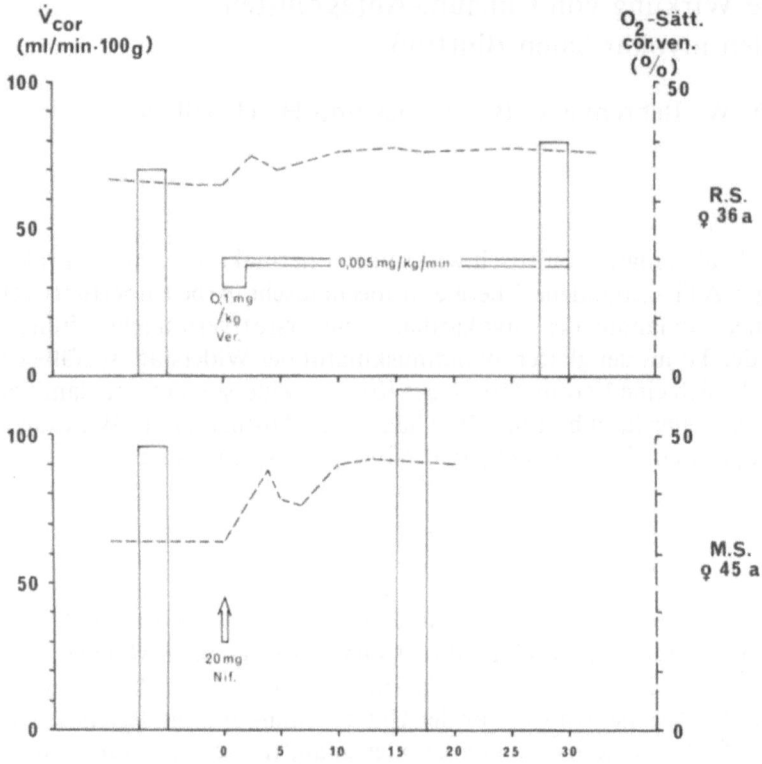

Abb. 1. Schema des Untersuchungsprotokolls für Verapamil (oben) und Nifedipin (unten). Der Zeitplan der Verapamil-Untersuchung war bei allen 10 Patienten gleich. Bei der Nifedipin-Studie (8 Patienten) fand die 2. Messung je nach Erreichen des Maximums der koronarvenösen O_2-Sättigung zwischen der 15. und der 30. min nach Zerbeißen der beiden 10-mg-Kapseln statt

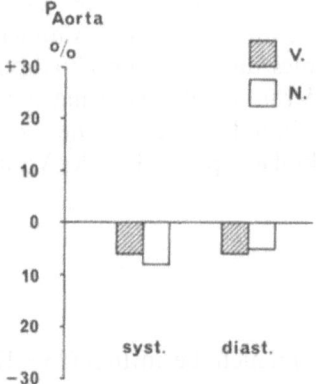

Abb. 2. Prozentuale Änderung des systolischen und diastolischen Aortendruckes unter dem Einfluß von Verapamil (V.) und Nifedipin (N.)

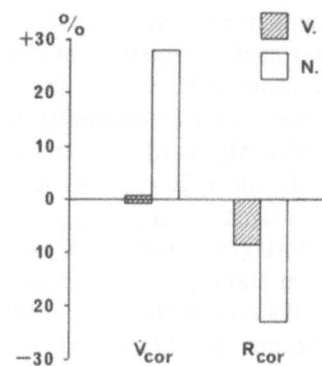

Abb. 3. Veränderungen der Koronardurchblutung ($\dot{V}_{cor}$) und des Koronarwiderstandes unter Verapamil und Nifedipin

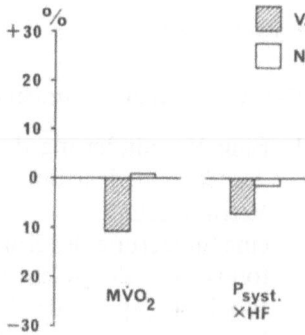

Abb. 4. Einfluß von Verapamil und Nifedipin auf den myokardialen Sauerstoffverbrauch ($M\dot{V}O_2$) und das Produkt aus systolischem Aortendruck und Herzfrequenz

Der systolische Druck in der Aorta sank nach Verapamil um 6% (von 135 ± 16 auf 127 ± 17 mmHg) bzw. nach Nifedipin um 8% (von 132 ± 15 auf 121 ± 7 mmHg).

Der diastolische Aortendruck nahm nach Verapamil ebenfalls um 6% ab (von 77 ± 5 auf 72 ± 5 mmHg), nach Nifedipin um 5% (von 73 ± 8 auf 69 ± 9 mmHg). Systolischer und diastolischer Druck in der Arteria pulmonalis zeigten in beiden Gruppen keine wesentliche Veränderung. Der Herzindex stieg nach Verapamil nur ganz gering an (im Mittel um 3%); nach Nifedipin war der Anstieg mit 12% deutlicher (von $3,69 \pm 0,83$ auf $4,12 \pm 84$ l/min/m^2).

Das Schlagvolumen nahm nach Gabe des Verapamil um 9% zu (von 61 ± 17 auf 67 ± 15 ml); unter Nifedipin-Einfluß betrug der Anstieg 5% (von 81 ± 20 auf 85 ± 22 ml). Die koronarvenöse Sauerstoffsättigung zeigte unter Verapamil einen Anstieg um 5,1 Sättigungsprozent (von 29,6 auf 34,7%); nach Nifedipin war dieser Anstieg mit 11,9 Sättigungsprozent (von 37,2 auf 49,1%) sehr viel deutlicher. Entsprechend verringerte sich die arterio-koronarvenöse Differenz des Sauerstoffgehaltes nach Verapamil um 8% (von $11,67 \pm 2,14$ auf $10,69 \pm 2,23$ Vol.%), nach Nifedipin um 19% (von $11,98 \pm 1,43$ auf $9,72 \pm 2,06$ Vol. %). Die Koronardurchblutung blieb unter Verapamileinfluß unverändert (vorher und nachher je 75 ml/min × 100g Myokard); unter Nifedipin stieg sie um 28% an (von 85 ± 18 auf 109 ± 34 ml/min × 100 g). Der Koronarwiderstand zeigte unter Verapamil regelmäßig einen geringen Rückgang, der im Mittel 9% betrug (von $1,17 \pm 26$ auf $1,07 \pm 0,26$ mmHg/ml/min × 100 g). Die koronardilatierende Wirkung des Nifedipin war deutlich stärker; es senkte den Koronarwiderstand bei allen Patienten, im Mittel um 23% (von $0,96 \pm 0,31$ auf $0,74 \pm 0,33$ mmHg/ml/min × 100 g). Der Sauerstoffverbrauch des Myokards wurde durch Verapamil im Mittel um 11% gesenkt (von $8,81 \pm 3,46$ auf $7,87 \pm 1,92$ ml/min × 100 g); das Nifedipin hatte auf diesen Parameter keinen gerichteten Einfluß (vorher $10,03 \pm 1,61$, nachher $10,16 \pm 1,82$ ml/min × 100 g). Das Produkt aus systolischem Aortendruck und Herzfrequenz, ein Parameter zur Abschätzung des myokardialen Sauerstoffverbrauches, gab die direkt gemessene Veränderung des Sauerstoffverbrauches recht gut wieder (für Verapamil −7%, für Nifedipin −2%).

Folgerungen

Den Calcium-Antagonisten werden zwei kardiale Hauptwirkungen zugeschrieben:

1. Eine Verminderung des myokardialen Sauerstoffverbrauches durch Hemmung des Calciumeinstromes in die erregte Myokardfaser und durch eine „afterload"-Verminderung,
2. eine Steigerung der Koronardurchblutung durch Abnahme des koronaren Gefäßtonus. Im Vergleich zu den Nitraten [3] und zu den kardioselektiven Beta-Blockern [4] ist die Verminderung des Sauerstoffverbrauches nach Gabe von Verapamil jedoch verhältnismäßig gering (vgl. Abb. 5); für das Nifedipin ist sie nicht nachweisbar, möglicherweise infolge der nach Applikation von Nifedipin

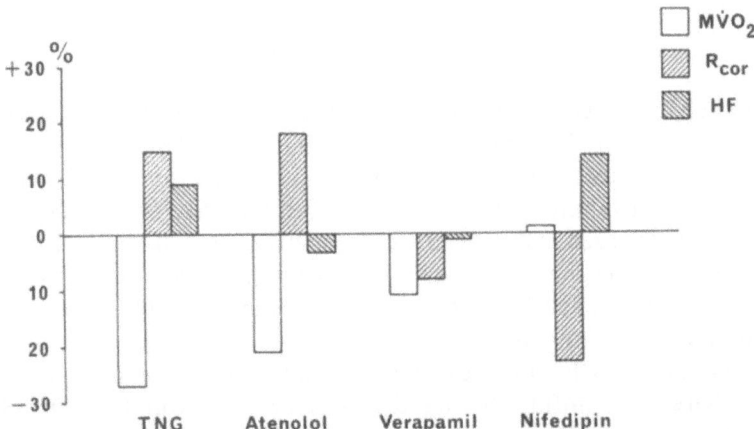

Abb. 5. Vergleich der Wirkungen von Nitroglyzerin (TNG, nach [3]), Atenolol (nach [4]), Verapamil und Nifedipin auf myokardialen Sauerstoffverbrauch (MV̇O$_2$), Koronarwiderstand (R$_{cor}$) und Herzfrequenz

häufigen Steigerung der Herzfrequenz. Im Gegensatz zu den Nitraten und den Beta-Blockern setzen beide Präparate den Koronarwiderstand herab, ohne daß die auch bei koronarkranken Patienten noch vorhandene Koronarreserve annähernd ausgeschöpft wird.

Da einerseits die durch die beiden untersuchten Calcium-Antagonisten erzielte Sauerstoffeinsparung kaum ins Gewicht fällt, andererseits aber das Prinzip „Koronardilatation" therapeutisch von zweifelhaftem Wert ist, fällt es schwer, den antianginösen Effekt von Verapamil und Nifedipin anhand der untersuchten Parameter zu erklären. Die beiden Substanzen können jedenfalls nach Art und Ausmaß ihrer Wirkungen mit den in der Koronartherapie etablierten Nitraten und Beta-Blockern nicht gleichgesetzt werden.

Literatur

1. Fleckenstein A (1971) Neuere Ergebnisse zur Physiologie, Pharmakologie und Pathologie der elektro-mechanischen Koppelungsprozesse im Warmblütermyokard. In: Keidel WD, Plattig KH (Hrsg) Vorträge der Erlanger Physiologentagung 1970. Springer, Berlin Heidelberg New York, S 13
2. Tauchert M, Kochsiek K, Heiss HW, Probst R, Bretschneider HJ (1971) Technik der Organdurchblutungsmessung mit der Argon-Methode. Z Kreislaufforsch 60:871
3. Tauchert M, Behrenbeck DW, Hilger HH (1977) Der Einfluß von Nitraten auf Hämodynamik und myokardialen Sauerstoffverbrauch. In: Schettler G, Horsch A, Mörl H, Orth H, Weizel A (Hrsg) Der Herzinfarkt. Schattauer, Stuttgart New York, S 332
4. Tauchert M, Behrenbeck DW, Niehues B, Hötzel J, Jansen W, Hombach V, Hilger HH (1978) Der Sauerstoffverbrauch des Herzens bei Koronarkranken in Ruhe und unter Belastung vor und nach Gabe von Atenolol. Z Kardiol [Suppl] 5:76

The Effect of the Calcium-Antagonistic Drug Nifedipine on Coronary and Left Ventricular Dynamics in Patients with Coronary Heart Disease

P. R. Lichtlen, H.-J. Engel, R. Wolf, and I. Amende

The antianginal effect of the so-called "calcium-antagonistic" drugs has been demonstrated beyond doubt through numerous clinical studies [1]. However, their mode of action, both with regard to coronary and left ventricular as well as peripheral dynamics, still needs further analysis. Various "calcium-antagonists" are in clinical use today. The investigations reported here were performed exclusively with Nifedipine, the calcium antagonist with the strongest action on the coronary system and on left ventricular hemodynamics among those accepted for clinical use. Accordingly, mainly two problems are discussed: the effect of Nifedipine on the coronary system, and its action on left ventricular hemodynamics.

Effect of Nifedipine on the Coronary Circulation in the Presence of Coronary Artery Disease

Changes of Poststenotic Flow at Rest After Sublingual Administration of Nifedipine

Methods

Flow measurements were performed by the use of the regional precordial Xenon clearance technique (for details see [2]). Under fluoroscopic control 10 to 20 mCi Xenon 133, dissolved in 5 cc of saline, were injected selectively into the main left or right coronary artery. Washout of the isotope was recorded by a Phogamma 3 camera (Nuclear Chicago) using a 64×64 matrix, approximately 400 to 600 matrix points covering the area of the heart. All flow recordings were performed in a left anterior oblique projection of 40 degrees. Calculations were done by a CDC 1700 computer, based on a monoexponential model, concerning mainly the first 30 s of washout after global peak activity had been reached, the frame rate being 2 s. Washout was followed for another 90 s with a frame rate of 4 s. Standard deviations of the washout curves were calculated for each matrix point; curves with standard deviations exceeding 30% of the flow value as well as matrix points reaching their maximum activity later than $10-15$ s after global peak activity, or displaying a maximum of less than 10% global peak activity, were rejected. Flow values were expressed both numerically in ml/min/100 g myocardium for each matrix point, for larger areas of 25 matrix points and for myocardial regions perfused by the left anterior descending or left circumflex artery. In addition, flow was displayed in an analog way, as so-called "flow image", indicating the flow values in different colors, highest flow values being demonstrated in red, the lowest once in green and blue (typical example in Fig. 1).

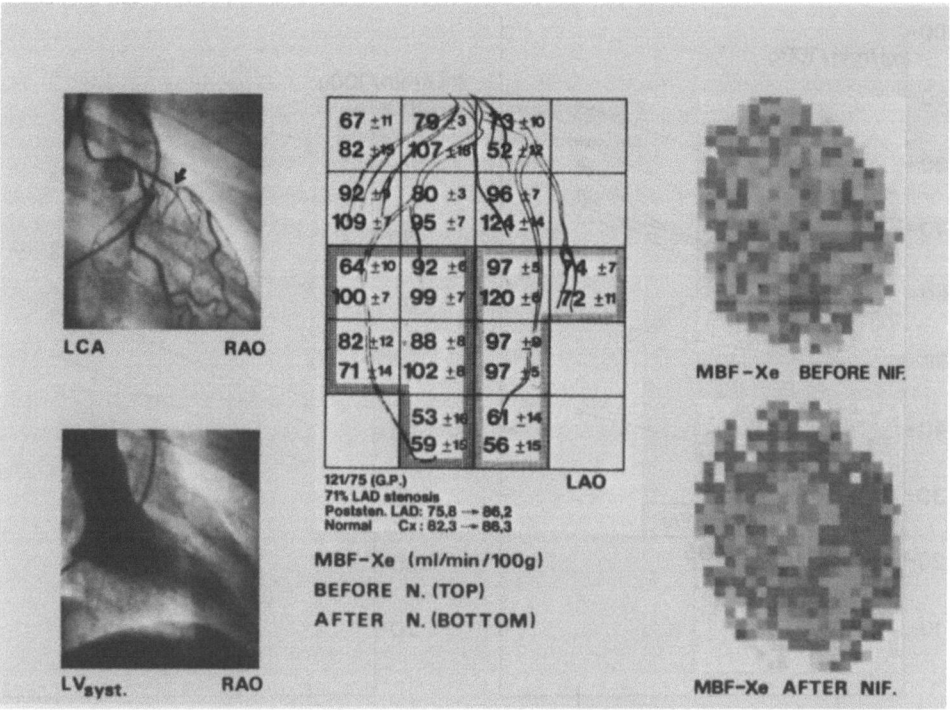

Fig. 1. Regional myocardial blood flow before and 10 min after sublingual administration of 20 mg Nifedipine.

Upper left: left coronary angiogram (RAO-projection, 40°), demonstrating a 70% obstruction of the left anterior descending branch (LAD).

Lower left: left ventricular angiogram (RAO-projection, 40°), endsystolic silhouette. Note that wall motion was still within normal limits.

Middle: numerical printout for areas of 25 matrix points; *on top of each quadrant,* the control value and its standard deviation, *on the bottom,* the flow value after Nifedipine. The regions representing LAD-and LCX-flow are outlined especially by large quadrangles.

Right: the so-called "flow-image": red indicates the highest flow values — here present in the LCX area; in this example corresponding to approximately 100 ml/min/100 g myocardium, after Nifedipine to approximately 120 ml/min/100 g myocardium; blue and green demonstrate the lowest values, corresponding approximately to 50 ml/min/100 g myocardium. After Nifedipine, there was a clear and significant increase in flow both in the normal and the poststenotic area.

Results

A typical example of the regional coronary flow before and after Nifedipine is shown on Fig. 1. It is interesting to note that in this example resting myocardial blood flow was clearly lower in the poststenotic region of the left anterior descending artery than in the normal area of the left circumflex branch, a phenomenon observed in the majority of our cases with high-grade proximal coronary obstructions [2, 3]. After administration of Nifedipine, there was a clear increase in flow both in the normal and poststenotic area, in the latter from approximately 70 to 100 ml/min/100 g myocardium.

The changes in poststenotic flow observed in ten patients are shown in Fig. 2. In the poststenotic region, comprising in the majority of cases the left anterior descending artery, the increase in flow averaged 18.4% ($p < 0.001$) versus 11.2% in

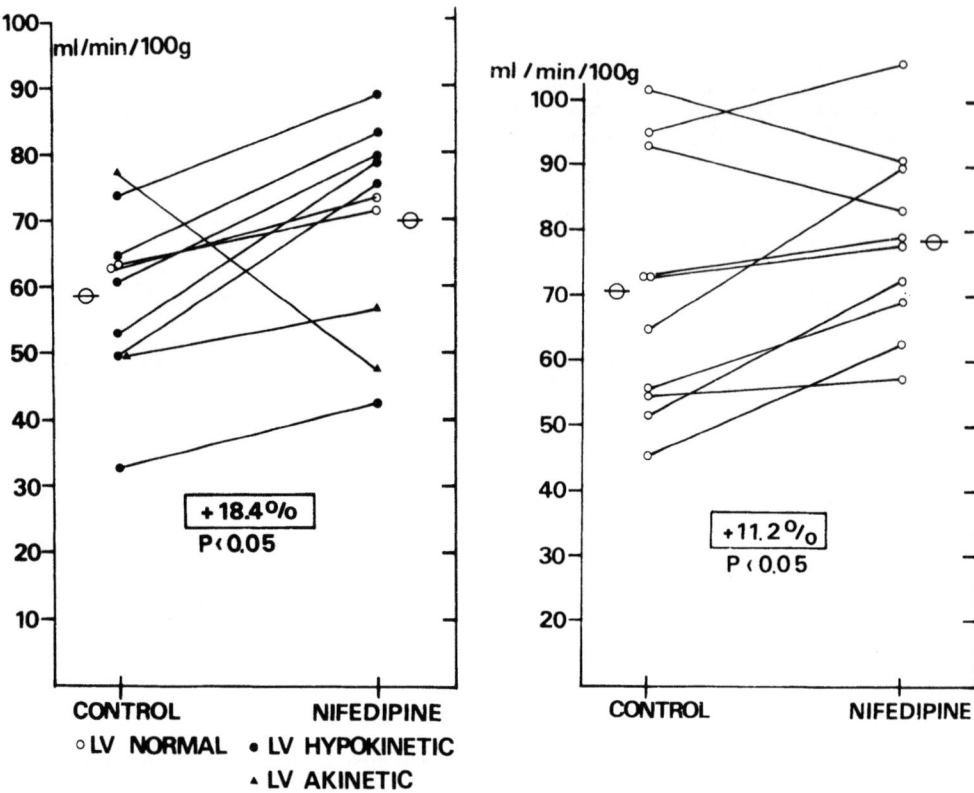

Fig. 2. Changes of regional myocardial blood flow in poststenotic and normal areas in ten patients after sublingual administration of Nifedipine (20 mg)

the normal area, i.e. in regions with angiographically normal or only minimally altered coronary arteries. The increase in poststenotic flow was independent of the degree of obstruction, most of the luminal narrowings being above 80%, as well as of the degree of impairment of poststenotic wall motion, occurring with equal frequency in normo- and hypokinetic regions. Hence, in the majority of cases (9 of 10), Nifedipine led to a marked increase in poststenotic resting flow of approximately 15% to 20%. However, as will be shown, this did not result in maximal coronary arteriolar dilatation and coronary reserve was not completely exhausted, as for example in the case of Dipyridamole [4]. Accordingly, the normal areas showed a decrease in coronary resistance of approximately 20%, i.e. from 1.5 to 1.1 units.

Changes in Poststenotic Flow at Rest After Intracoronary Administration of Nifedipine (0.1 mg) (Fig. 3, Table 1)

A considerably stronger increase in flow is reached by intracoronary administration of Nifedipine (0.1 mg). This change in flow is, however, of short duration, usually not exceeding 3 min, as was shown by repeated recordings with the Xenon-clearance-technique, as well as by continuous measuring of coronary sinus oxygen

Table 1a. Changes of regional myocardial blood flow after intracoronary injection of 0.1 mg Nifedipine

	Regional myocardial blood flow before and after intracoronary injection of nifedipine (0.1 mg) (n = 12)		
	Poststenotic Areas (>50% narrowings)	Normal Areas (<50% narrowings)	p
	ml/min/100 g Myocardium		
Control	50.3± 7.38	62.7± 9.96	<0.025
Nifedipine	102.4±25.2	125.8±21.34	n.s.
% Increase	+104%	+101%	
p	<0.0005	<0.0005	
n	7	5	

Table 1b. Changes of major hemodynamic parameters after intracoronary injection of 0.1 mg Nifedipine (n = 12)

	Control	Nifedipine	p
Mean Aortic Pressure (mmHg)	90.0±9.59	85.0±7.76 −5.6%	<0.005
Heart Rate (min^{-1})	66.1±5.51	74.0±6.89 +12.0%	<0.0025
Coronary Resistance (mmHg/ml/min/100 g)			
Poststenotic Areas	1.86±0.36	0.82±1.13	<0.0005
Normal Areas	1.39±0.23	0.66±0.13	<0.0005
	$p < 0.025$	$p < 0.05$	

content [5]. Figure 3 demonstrates flow changes 1 min after intracoronary administration, in a patient with an isolated proximal 75% obstruction of the LAD. In this case poststenotic flow increased from 50 to 110 ml/min/100 g myocardium; a similar increase in flow was also observed in the normal area perfused by the left circumflex artery where values after Nifedipine reached 120 ml/min/100 g. Measurements were done in 12 regions of six patients, in five normal and seven poststenotic areas. Also in these patients, average flow of the poststenotic area was with 50 ml/min/100 g significantly lower than in the normal regions, where it amounted to 63 ml/min/100 g ($p < 0.05$). Accordingly, the flow maximum reached after intracoronary administration of Nifedipine was with 126 ml/min/100 g clearly higher in normal than in poststenotic regions, where it averaged 102 ml/min/100 g; this difference, however, was not significant. Furthermore, intracoronary administration of Nifedipine led to a mild, yet significant increase in heart rate (+12%) and drop of mean aortic pressure (−5.6%) ($p < 0.005$); hence, coronary resistance of the normal areas dropped to minimal levels.

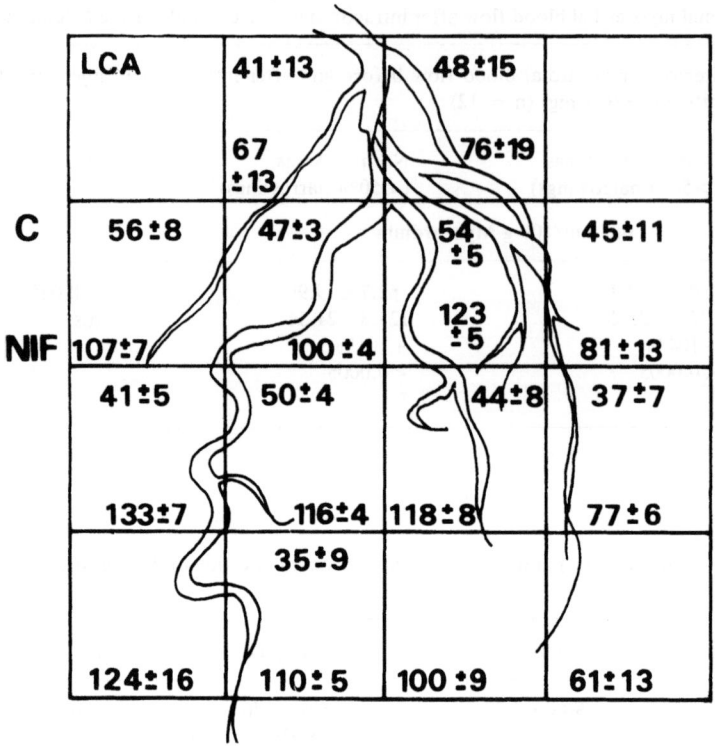

Fig. 3. Typical example of changes of coronary flow after intracoronary injection of Nifedipine (0.1 mg) in a patient with a high-grade, 75% proximal obstruction of the LAD. Flow values (mean ± standard deviation) – measured 1 min after injection – are demonstrated for areas of 25 matrix points. There was an approximately 100% increase in flow both in the poststenotic and normal area

The changes observed after intracoronary administration led to the following conclusion:

1. The considerable increase in flow observed also in those poststenotic areas where flow was significantly lower than in the normal zone, suggests that this decrease in poststenotic flow at rest, in the absence of angina, is not accompanied by complete arteriolar dilatation.
2. The absolute and percentage increase in flow was almost equal for normal and poststenotic areas, the former reaching only mildly higher values. The lack of a more significant increase in the normal zones might be due to a dose of Nifedipine (0.1 mg) too low to achieve complete arteriolar dilatation, flow in the normal zones not yet reaching maximal values; on the other hand, considerable coronary artery disease on the arteriolar level, angiographically not demonstrable, might have been present, prohibiting a maximal rise of flow also in the so-called normal zones. Anyhow, in no case did the intracoronary administration provoke angina pectoris so far, further suggesting that coronary reserve was not yet completely exhausted.
3. The mild, yet significant decrease in aortic pressure is a manifestation of the negative inotropic effect of Nifedipine, unmashed: by the intracoronary administration.

Changes in Global Flow in Coronary Patients During Bicycle Ergometry

From the flow recordings after intracoronary administration of Nifedipine, it becomes evident that sublingual or oral administration does indeed not lead to complete coronary arteriolar dilatation. This was already shown in previous studies recording flow under conditions of increased oxygen demand, that is, during bicycle ergometry [6] (Fig. 4). As measurements of regional flow during exercise still encounter serious technical difficulties when the gamma camera is used, these recordings in six patients with angiographically severe coronary artery disease (double or triple vessel disease) were performed with a single scintillation probe placed over the heart, i.e., in a global fashion (for details see [7]). The protocol was as follows: A control flow measurement performed at rest was followed by a flow recording during exercise of approximately 75 to 100 Watt, the flow increase from rest to exercise averaging 123%. After an interval of 30 min, 20 mg Nifedipine were administered sublingually, and 5 min later a second flow recording was performed at rest, demonstrating an increase of approximately 20% when compared with the control resting flow. Finally, approximately 20 min after administration of Nifedipine, a fourth flow measurement was performed, this time during exercise of

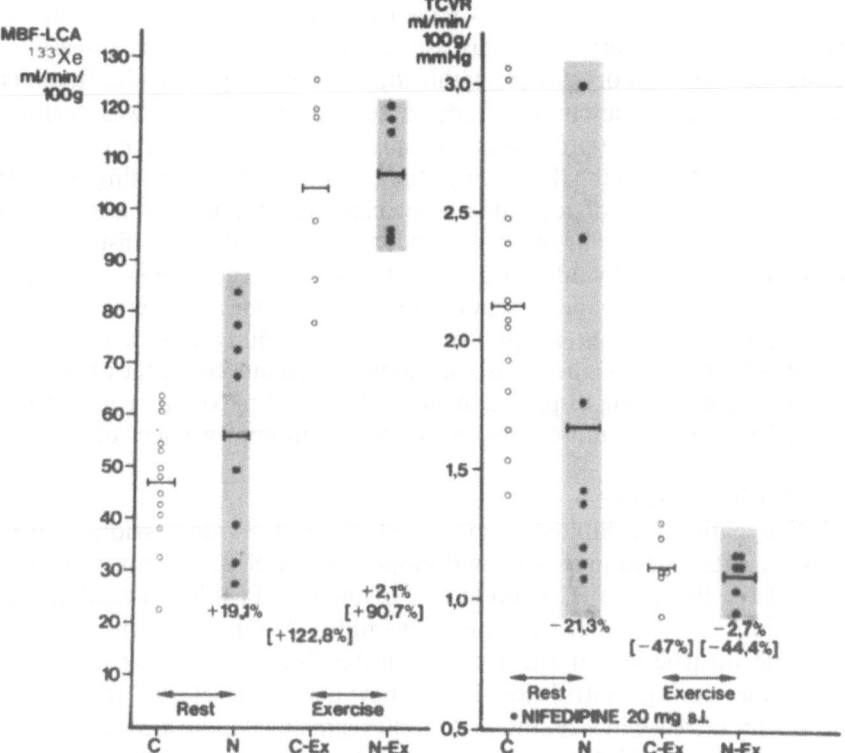

Fig. 4. Global myocardial blood flow at rest and during bicycle ergometry before and after sublingual administration of Nifedipine (20 mg).
Left: flow values (ml/min/100 g myocardium) at rest and during exercise; hatched areas represent flow after Nifedipine. *Right:* calculated global coronary resistance. (For details see text)

exactly the same workload as during the first exercise period; the second exercise flow values were identical with those observed before Nifedipine. The results demonstrate that in spite of Nifedipine, flow during exercise is still capable of increasing considerably, again indicating that the calcium antagonist did not lead to maximal arteriolar dilatation at rest and that coronary autoregulation was still preserved. This is in contrast to Dipyridamole, which was shown to lead to complete coronary arteriolar dilatation already at rest, i.e. to complete abolishment of coronary reserve [4].

Changes in Myocardial Perfusion During Exercise, Analyzed by the Use of 201 Thallium-Scintigraphy

Changes in coronary flow as measured by the precordial regional Xenon-clearance-technique do not necessarily reflect an improvement of perfusion in ischemic areas and by this, a true antianginal effect. Such an improvement of perfusion, associated with relief of angina, has been shown for Isosorbide dinatrate using 201 Thallium myocardial scintigraphy [8].

Methods

201 Thallium myocardial scintigraphy was performed during exercise (bicycle ergometry) and 4 h later at rest, in 5 patients with severe angina and angiographically proven severe coronary artery disease (double or triple vessel disease). Two days before the study, all drugs were withheld, none of the patients being under digitalis. Three weeks after the control study, a second investigation was performed under Nifedipine. The entire protocol, especially workload during exercise, the dosage of Thallium (2 mCi) and the time of injection, projections of recording (PA, 30° and 60° LAO) and beginning of recording (approximately 2 min after cessation of exercise) remained unchanged. The only difference consisted in the administration of 20 mg of Nifedipine sublingually 30 min before the study. In each patient six left ventricular segments, an anterior, apical, septal, inferior, posterior and lateral one, were studied, altogether 30 segments in the five patients. Scintigrams were analyzed on a semiquantitative basis, the areas with maximal counts being set as 100%, the other areas of the scan being displayed in steps of 10% of maximum count. Only increases in activity of 50% or more were considered as an improvement of perfusion.

Results (Fig. 5, Table 2)

All five patients exhibited angina and showed ST-depressions during control exercise. After Nifedipine, angina disappeared and ST-segments were normalized in three of the five patients, whereas two of them still exhibited mild angina and ST-depressions of 0.5 mm. A typical example of a patient with isolated, almost complete obstruction of the left circumflex branch is shown in Fig. 5. Before Nifedipine, during control exercise, 12 new defects developed and four old defects showed an increase in size; thus, 16 of 30 segments demonstrated a deterioration in perfusion. After Nifedipine, six of the twelve new defects were normalized and the four enlarged defects showed a significant reduction of size.

Thus, 10 of the 16 new defects showed a significant improvement of perfusion or were even normalized, the number of deteriorated segments being reduced to six of 30 (chi-square = 14.354; $p < 0.0005$).

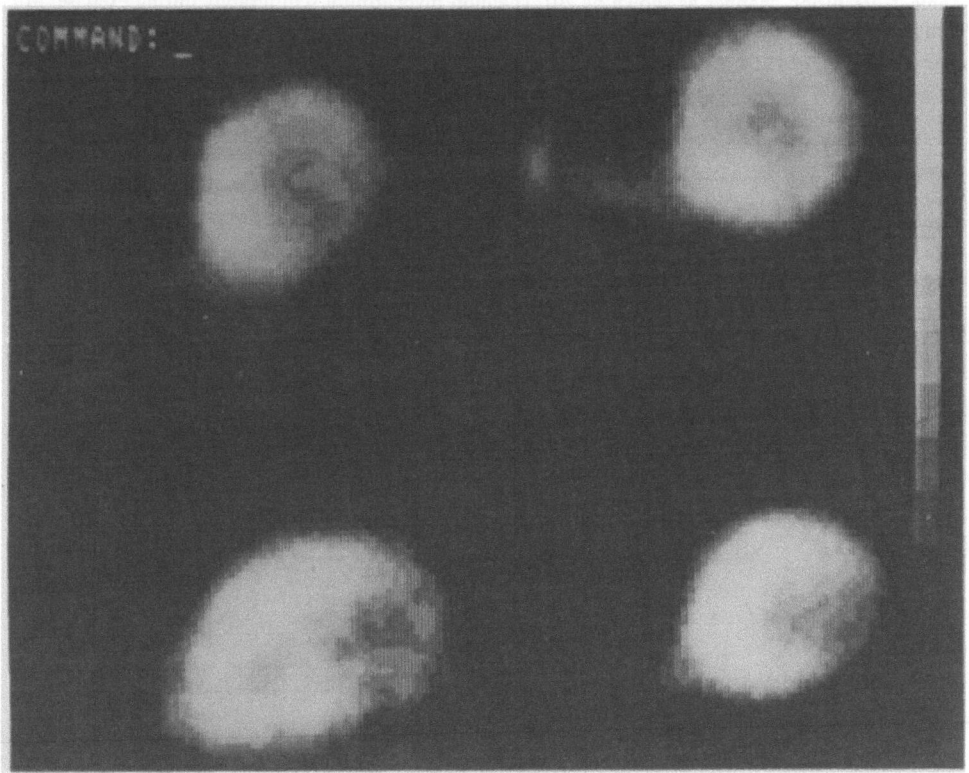

Fig. 5. 201 Thallium-scintigrams recorded in 30° and 60° LAO-projection *(upper and lower panels)* (immediatly after exercise).
Left: control exercise study; *Right:* exercise performed after 20 mg Nifedipine, performed 3 weeks after the control study. The patient showed an almost complete obstruction of the main left circumflex branch at angiography. Control exercise study shows a large perfusion defect in the posterolateral zone of the left ventricle. After administration of the drug, Thallium activity is almost completely restored, indicating a marked improvement, i.e. normalization of perfusion in this region. At the same time the patient was relieved from angina, and the exercise ECG was normalized

In summary, the calcium-antagonist Nifedipine, when administered sublingually, leads to a 20% increase in poststenotic flow at rest, whereas intracoronary administration is followed by 100% increase in flow, also in myocardial areas supplied by coronary arteries with severe, 75% or greater luminal obstruction. Most importantly, sublingual administration of Nifedipine does not inhibit an exercise-induced flow rise, leaving coronary autoregulation intact. To which extent these flow changes are involved in the antianginal effect of the drug is still open to discussion. Nevertheless, 201 Thallium myocardial scintigraphy demonstrates that in the majority of patients, perfusion is restored to normal or almost normal levels in the poststenotic area, perfusion by this becoming homogenous throughout the heart, a phenomenon accompanied by a normalization of the exercise ECG and relief from angina.

Table 2. Perfusion changes as shown by 201 Thallium myocardium scintigraphy during exercise, after sublingual administration of Nifedipine

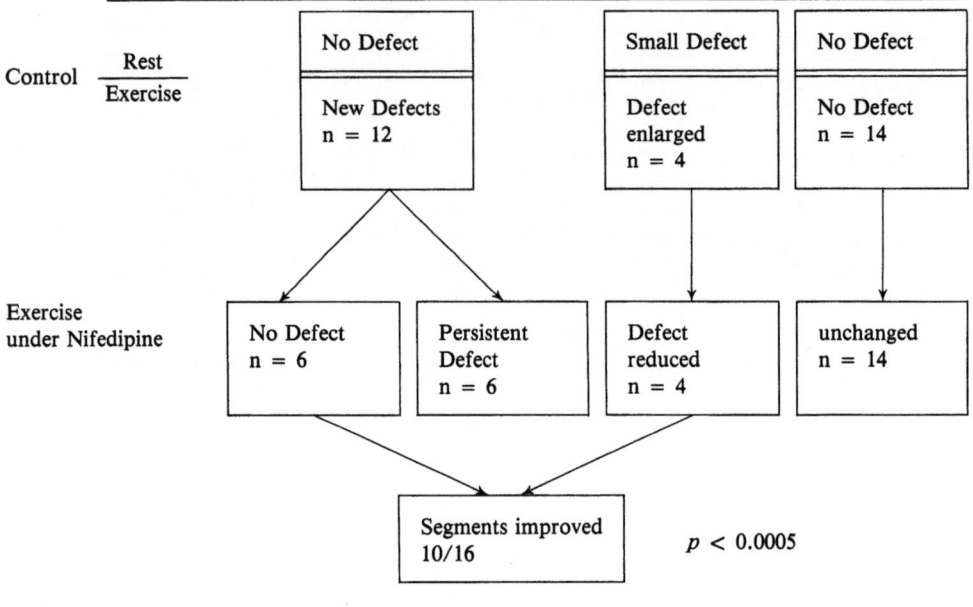

Effect of nifedipine (20 mg p.os) on coronary perfusion in the 201-Thallium-Myocardial-Scintigram during exercise (5 patients, each with 6 segments = 30 segments)

Improvement of Perfusion = Increase of Activity $\geq 50\%$.

Left Ventricular Hemodynamics

Methods

Left ventricular hemodynamics were recorded in seven patients with multiple vessel disease. Left ventricular angiograms revealed normal or hypokinetic wall motion in the poststenotic segment, patients with akinetic or dyskinetic segments being excluded. High fidelity pressure measurements (Millar-Tip-Manometers) were performed before, during, and after injection of contrast medium (35 ml Urografin 65%) into the left ventricle. Recordings were done at rest and repeated 10 min after 20 mg Nifedipine sublingually. Left ventricular angiograms were performed in 40 degree RAO-projection; wall motion was assessed by calculating percentage systolic shortening of six hemiaxes drawn perpendiculary to the longitudinal axis (aortic-mitral valve junction to the apex) at 25%, 50%, and 75% of its length (for details see [9,10]); in addition, V_{pm} and V_{CF} were calculated in the usual way; in some patients, pressure-volume relations during diastole, beginning with the point of lowest diastolic pressure and ending before the a-wave, were also analyzed.

Results (Table 3)

Nifedipine resulted in a significant, 22% increase in heart rate, a 25% rise of cardiac index and 17% decrease in total peripheral resistance ($p < 0.01$), whereas mean aortic pressure remained unchanged. Dp/dt_{max}, registered by tip manometry,

Table 3. Hemodynamic changes following nifedipine (n = 7)

	HR (min^{-1})	CO (l/min)	Mean AO (mmHg)	PVR (dyn sec cm^{-5})	dp/dt$_{max}$ (mmHg/sec)
Before	62.6	5.87	87.8	1217	1421
After	75.8	7.33	89.1	1011	1606
Diff.	+ 13.2	+ 1.46	+ 2.3	− 206	+ 185
$p<$	0.001	0.01	N.S.	0.005	0.05

showed a small, yet significant rise of 13% ($p < 0.05$), yet all other parameters of contractility, V_{pm} and V_{CF} as well as percentage systolic shortening of the hemiaxes showed no change. Furthermore, all volume parameters, i.e. enddiastolic and endsystolic volume, ejection fraction and mean normalized ejection rate, remained unaltered.

Thus, due to the decrease in afterload after Nifedipine, a mild increase in heart rate, accompanied by a small rise of contractility, was observed. On the other hand preload, in this study, remained unchanged; this was demonstrated by the pressure-

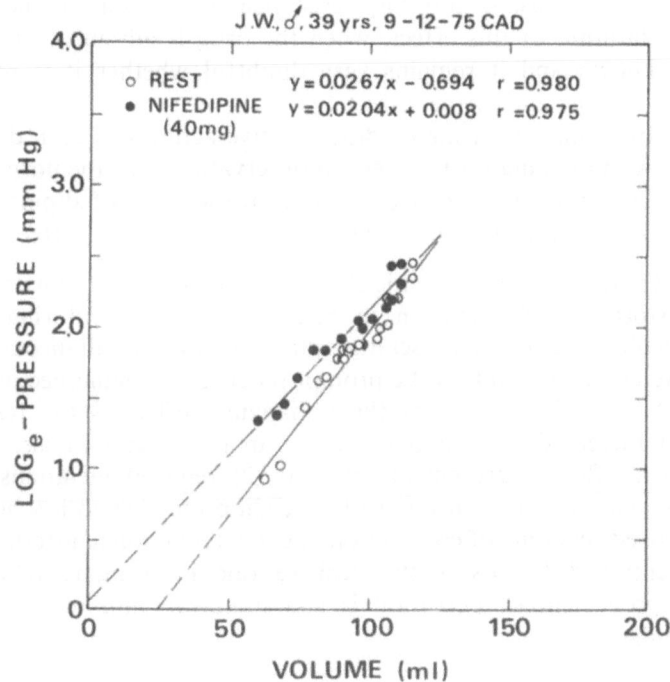

Fig. 6. Typical example of the diastolic pressure-volume-relation before and after Nifedipine in a patient with severe coronary artery disease (triple vessel disease). Changes in pressure throughout diastole are demonstrated on the ordinate in logarithmic fashion, volume changes on the abscissa. The pressure-volume-relation was analyzed frame by frame starting with the lowest diastolic pressure and ending before the a-wave. Nifedipine did not alter the slope of the pressure-volume-relation significantly, indicating no change in diastolic compliance, that is, in preload. (For details, see text)

volume-relation during diastole, a typical example being shown in Fig. 6. There was no change in the slope of the diastolic pressure-volume-relation after Nifedipine, indicating no alteration in diastolic compliance or stiffness nor in preload alone.

Discussion

Calcium-antagonists are known to have an inhibitory effect both on cardiac conduction especially in the AV node, as well as on the contractile system of the smooth muscle of the arterioles and of the working muscle of the heart. Prolongation of AV-conduction and negative inotropic action differ, however, in the various drugs. Verapamil, for instance, in human beings acts mainly on AV-conduction [11], Nifedipine predominantly on the arteriolar contraction, exhibiting a strong vasodilatory effect.

Nifedipine, thus, has mainly the following three effects:

1) By dilating the peripheral arterioles, it decreases afterload and by this, wall tension, resulting in a decrease in global myocardial oxygen consumption. This, however, is counterbalanced to some degree by a mild increase in heart rate, dp/dt_{max}, and cardiac output, brought about through a resetting of baroreceptor tone.

2) It leads to coronary vasodilatation, that is, to a mild increase in coronary flow and decrease in coronary resistance both in normal and poststenotic areas. The duration of this effect, when the drug is administered sublingually, is not yet known and it remains very doubtful whether it is responsible for the long standing antianginal effect.

3) In animals a strong cardioprotective action has been demonstrated [12, 13, 14]. Also in human beings certain observations like the normalization of the exercise ECG after intracoronary administration of Nifedipine at a time when flow is back to control levels, suggest such an additional effect (5).

Finally, the anti-ischemic effect of Nifedipine was proved beyond doubt by (1) the restoration of perfusion in poststenotic regions during exercise as shown by Thallium myocardial scintigraphy, (2) the simultaneous normalization of the exercise ECG, and (3) the prompt relief from angina pectoris.

So far, it seems that the antianginal effect is the result of several factors: (1) Increased flow in poststenotic areas during exercise, as it is suggested from Xenon-flow-measurements at rest; (2) reduced metabolism, that is, myocardial oxygen consumption due to the cardioprotective anti-ischemic effect, and (3) improved economy of contraction due to a reduction in afterload. Which of the above-mentioned factors is the decisive one in bringing relief from angina by an improvement of perfusion is still unknown and remains the object of further studies.

References

1. Ebner F, Dünnschede DHB (1976) Hemodynamics, therapeutic mechanism of action and clinical findings of adalat use based on world-wide clinical trails. In: Jatene AD, Lichtlen PR (eds) Third international adalat symposium. New therapy of ischemic heart disease. Excerpta Medica, Amsterdam Oxford, p 283

2. Lichtlen PR, Engel H-J, Hundeshagen H (1978) Clinical application and results of the assessment of coronary blood flow by the regional precordial Xenon residue detection technique. Nucl Med 17:161
3. Engel H-J, Lichtlen PR, Hundeshagen H (1977) Effects of coronary obstructions and segmental LV dysfunction on regional myocardial blood flow. Circulation 55/56:III – 10
4. Lichtlen P, Engel H-J, Amende I, Rafflenbeul W, Simon R (1976) Mechanisms of various antianginal drugs. Relationship between regional flow behaviour and contractility. In: Jatene AD, Lichtlen PR (eds) Third international adalat symposium. New therapy of ischemic heart disease. Excerpta Medica, Amsterdam Oxford, p 14
5. Kaltenbach M, Schultz W, Kober G (1979) Effects of Nifedipine after intravenous and intracoronary administration. Am J Cardiol 44:832
6. Lichtlen P (1975) Coronary and left ventricular dynamics under nifedipine in comparison to nitrates, betablocking agents and dipyridamole. In: Lochner W, Braasch W, Kroneberg G (eds) Second international adalat symposium. New therapy of ischemic heart disease. Springer, Berlin Heidelberg New York, p 212
7. Lichtlen P, Moccetti T, Halter J, Schönbeck M, Senning A (1972) Postoperative evaluation of myocardial blood flow in aorta-to-coronary artery vein bypass grafts using the xenon residue detection technique. Circulation 46:445
8. Wolf R, Pretschner BP, Engel H-J, Hundeshagen H, Lichtlen P (1979) Die Wirkung von Isosorbiddinitrat auf die belastungsinduzierte abnorme Myokardperfusion bei koronarer Herzkrankheit, objektiviert anhand der 201 Thallium-Belastungs-Szintigraphie. Z Kardiol 68:676
9. Karliner JS, Gault JH, Eckberg D, Mullins ChB, Ross J (1971) Mean velocity of fiber shortening. A simplified measure of left ventricular myocardial contractility. Circulation 44:323
10. Simon R, Amende I, Lichtlen P (1979) Das linksventrikuläre Angiogramm. In: Lichtlen, PR (ed) Koronarangiographie. Straube, Erlangen, p 249
11. Seipel L (1978) His-Bündel-Elektrokardiographie und intrakardiale Stimulation. Thieme, Stuttgart
12. Nayler WG, Fassold E, Yepez C (to be published) The pharmacological protection of mitochondrial function in hypoxic heart muscles. Effect of verapamil, propranolol and methylprednisolon. Cardiovasc Res
13. Henry PD (to be published) Chronotropic and inotropic effects of coronary vasodilators. In: International Adalat Panel Discussion, Tokio, Sept. 20, 1978
14. Clark RE, Henry PD (to be published) Protection of ischemic myocardium by nifedipine. In: International Adalat Panel Discussion, Tokio, Sept. 20, 1978
15. Engel H-J, Hundeshagen H, Lichtlen P (1978) Regionale Myokarddurchblutung bei koronarer Herzkrankheit – Auswirkung des Stenosegrades und der poststenotischen Ventrikelfunktion. Z Kardiol 67:205

Regional Wall Motion Following Intra-Bypass Injection of Nifedipine: Design of a Protocol and Initial Experience[1]

P. W. Serruys, M. v. d. Brand, H. J. ten Katen, and R. W. Brower

Introduction

It still remains unclear whether Nifedipine at therapeutic dosages has a direct inotropic effect on the myocardium or whether the change in function is the result of changes in loading conditions [1,2,3]. Kaltenbach and his group have demonstrated that intracoronary injections provoke practically no changes in heart rate, but a small drop in aortic pressure [4]. This result has been attributed to a direct and specific negative inotropic action of the drug independent of a vasodilator effect at the periphery.

We have the opportunity to verify this hypothesis with intrabypass injection of Nifedipine in patients with implanted radiopaque markers (regional function), while coronary sinus flow and beat-to-beat left ventricular performance were continuously monitored. Under the conditions of intrabypass injection of Nifedipine, we determined the regional and global inotropic properties of the drug before the appearance of its vasodilator effects on the coronary system itself.

Methodology

Regional Wall Motion of Bypassed Regions

The methodology for measuring regional shortening has been previously described [5]. Radiopaque markers were implanted during surgery on the epicardium in bypassed regions (Fig. 1), in pairs aligned transversely to the major axis of the heart, 2 cm apart and located from 0 to 3 cm distal to the coronary anastomosis. The technique was modified to measure the absolute distance between the marker pairs using synchronized biplane cinefluorography (50 frames/s), at 30° right anterior oblique and 60° left anterior oblique views of the heart, while the patient stops breathing; five consecutive heartbeats were filmed as a control run before intrabypass injection of Nifedipine, and afterwards at 30, 60, 120, and 180 s after injection. The three dimensional coordinates for each marker pair were determined and the absolute distances (L) between each marker pair were calculated. Calibration was obtained from exposures of a spherical ball of known diameter, and correction for X-ray and optical distortion was performed for each image intensifier. The acquisition system includes a digitizer with a reproducibility of 0.1 mm. All calculations are done on a PDP-11 computer. As shown in Fig. 2, marker pair separation is plotted from the frame prior to onset of the Q-wave of the ECG to the minimal separation. Shortening fraction (SF) is defined as SF =

---

1 This work was supported by the Dutch Heart Foundation, grant 76–067

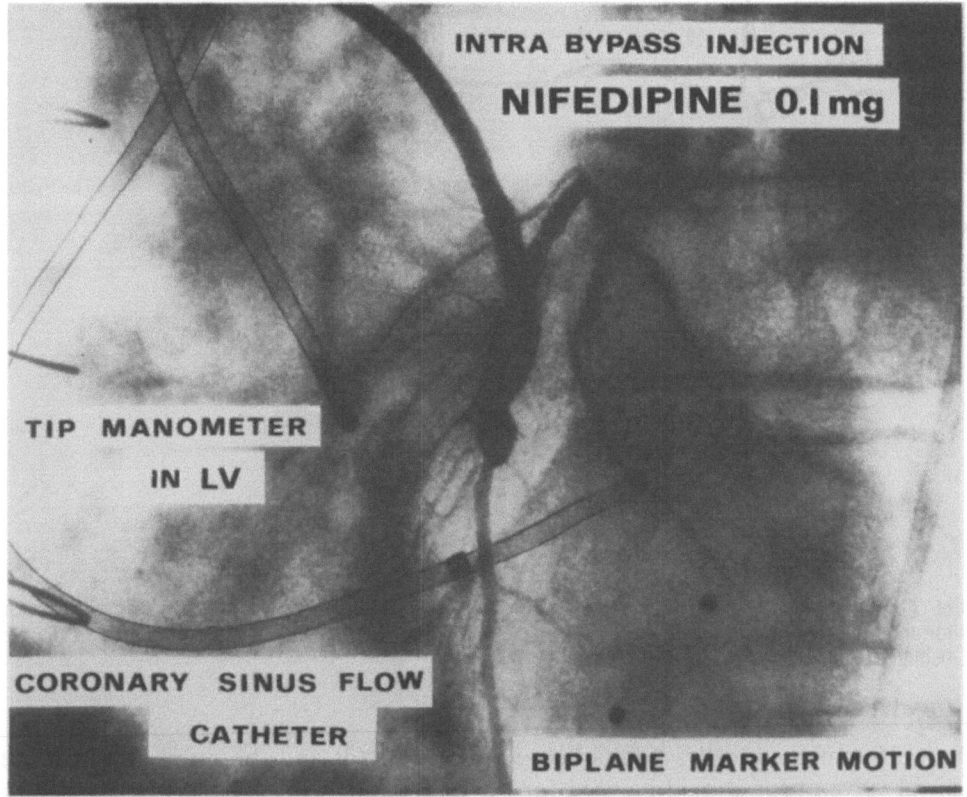

Fig. 1. Retouched photo from the original ciné angiogram showing the platinum markers *(lower right)* sutured to the left ventricular epicardium, the coronary sinus flow catheter *(center)*, and the LV tip manometer *(left center)*, together with the opacified graft

(Lmax-Lmin)/Lmax and expressed as a percentage, where Lmax is the maximal marker separation and Lmin the minimal marker separation. Mean shortening rate (SR) is defined as SR = (Lmax-Lmin)/(Lmax × Ts) where Ts is the time interval between Lmax and Lmin.

Beat-to-beat Analysis of Left Ventricular Function

The beat-to-beat analysis program of our catheterization laboratory system was used [6]. The left ventricular pressure from a catheter tip manometer (Millar) was sampled at a rate of 250 Hz for a period of 2 to 4 min. For every beat the following calculations were performed: end diastolic pressure (EDP), peak systolic pressure (LVP), peak positive rate of change of pressure (+ dP/dt), cycle length (end diastole to end diastole), and Vmax [7]. In addition, the isovolumic relaxation phase was quantified by the peak negative rate of change of pressure (− dP/dt) and by − dP/dt at 35 mmHg. The time constant of relaxation (T) was determined by a least squares fit of the equation $P = e^{At+B}$ (T = − 1/A) from the moment of − dP/dt to

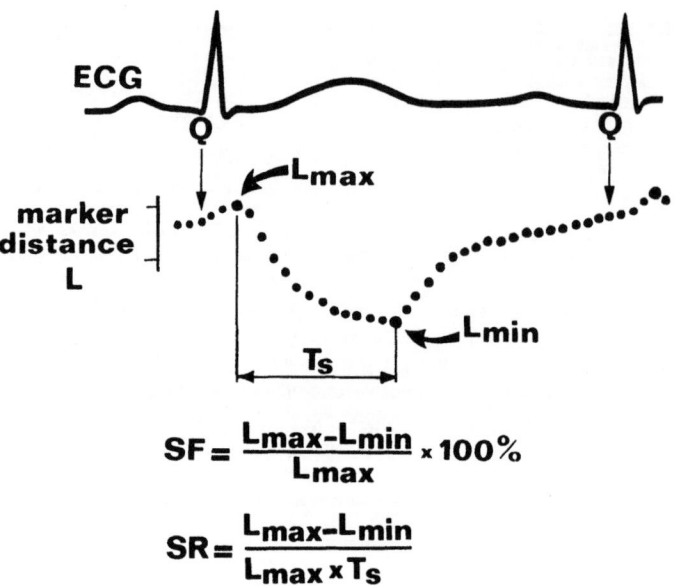

Fig. 2. Ciné frame markers are recorded simultaneously with the ECG to allow reconstruction of shortening pattern in relation to electric events. Shortening fraction (SF) and shortening rate (SR) are calculated as shown

P = 35 mmHg. Ideally, points between the − dP/dt and the point at which the mitral valve opens should be used for the calculation. However, it was decided to take the 35 mmHg point, since off-line tests showed that this made little difference, if any, to the slope and consequently the value of T.

Measurement of Coronary Sinus Blood Flow

Measurement of coronary sinus blood flow was performed by continuous thermodilution [8]. The main objective of this measurement was to detect rapid changes in the coronary flow following the intrabypass injection of Nifedipine. Catherization of the coronary sinus was performed from the right antecubital vein. In order to measure total coronary sinus flow, the catheter was carefully placed in such a way that the external thermistor was located near the ostium. After insertion, 3 ml of contrast material was therefore injected into the sinus for fluoroscopic identification of the ostium. Five percent dextrose at room temperature was infused at a constant rate of 38 ml/min for a period of 4 min. The computation of flow was based on the following formula:

$$FB = FI \left(\frac{SI \times CI}{SB \times CB} \right) \times \left(\frac{TM - TI}{TB - TM} \right) \text{ml/min}$$

FB and FI are the volume flows (in ml/min) of blood and infusate, participating in the process of mixing and heat exchange. TB, TI, and TM, the temperature of blood, infusate, and mixture in degrees Celsius, SB and SI, the density of blood and infusate, respectively, in g/cm^3; and CB and CI, the specific heat of blood and infusate, respectively in $cal/g/°C$. For computation of flow, the TB determined immediately after the end of infusion was used.

As demonstrated by Ganz et al. [8], the time constant of the method varies between 0.8 and 0.4 s in the range of flow between 100 and 200 ml/min. Since a time interval equal to three time constants is necessary to record 95% of a sudden change in flow, changes in flow due to Nifedipine can be detected within 2.4 s. Before the intrabypass injection of Nifedipine, a control run for flow, pressure, and biplane marker motion was recorded during 90 b.p.m. coronary sinus pacing (or 5 to 10 paced beats above basal heart rate). Constant paced heart rate facilitates the interpretation of changes in the different recorded parameters by excluding a chronotropic effect, although this is slight after intracoronary injection.

Intrabypass Injection of Nifedipine

Before intrabypass administration of Nifedipine, bypass injection of up to 3 ml contrast material was performed to verify selective positioning of the Sones' catheter, but no other angiographic investigation was done before the study. One ml of a solution containing 0.1 mg of Nifedipine is first introduced into the Sones' catheter (7.5 French, 70 cm length) of which the dead space is 1.2 ml. At the appropriate moment the catheter is flushed with 2 ml of physiologic saline, within 5 to 10 s. In order to establish the pharmacologic effects due to the solvent (ethanolic solution), in which Nifedipine is dissolved, we tested the solvent in the same way.

Case Report I

Twelve months after bypass surgery, patient H was recatheterized. Since surgery he has been asymptomatic and the single bypass on the left anterior descending was patent. Despite this successful and effective revascularization of the anterior wall, the postoperative study of this region with biplane cinefluoroscopy of marker motion has shown a persisting hypokinetic contraction pattern. This abnormal contraction pattern was confirmed during pacing-induced tachycardia, potentiation post tachycardia, and handgrip. During these different stresses, this region also exhibited an abnormal behavior.

The beat-to-beat analysis of regional and global myocardial function, and flow following intrabypass injection of Nifedipine are shown in Fig. 3. The influence of respiration on the pressure is clearly identified during the beat-to-beat analysis, but is less marked on the pressure-derived parameters which are less sensitive to this physiologic variation. There is a drop of about 15 mmHg in left ventricular peak systolic pressure occurring 15 to 20 beats after beginning of intrabypass injection. At the same time, the EDP increases on average from 9 mmHg to 15 mmHg. A plateau of 15 mmHg EDP is particularly apparent during the voluntary apnea (for filming of the marker motion). Simultaneously there is a decrease in Vmax (from mean $67 s^{-1}$ to $55 s^{-1}$) and an increase in time constant for the rate of relaxation (from 33 ms to 42 ms). All these changes are transient and after 3 min, all the hemodynamic parameters return to their basal values. As for the regional short-

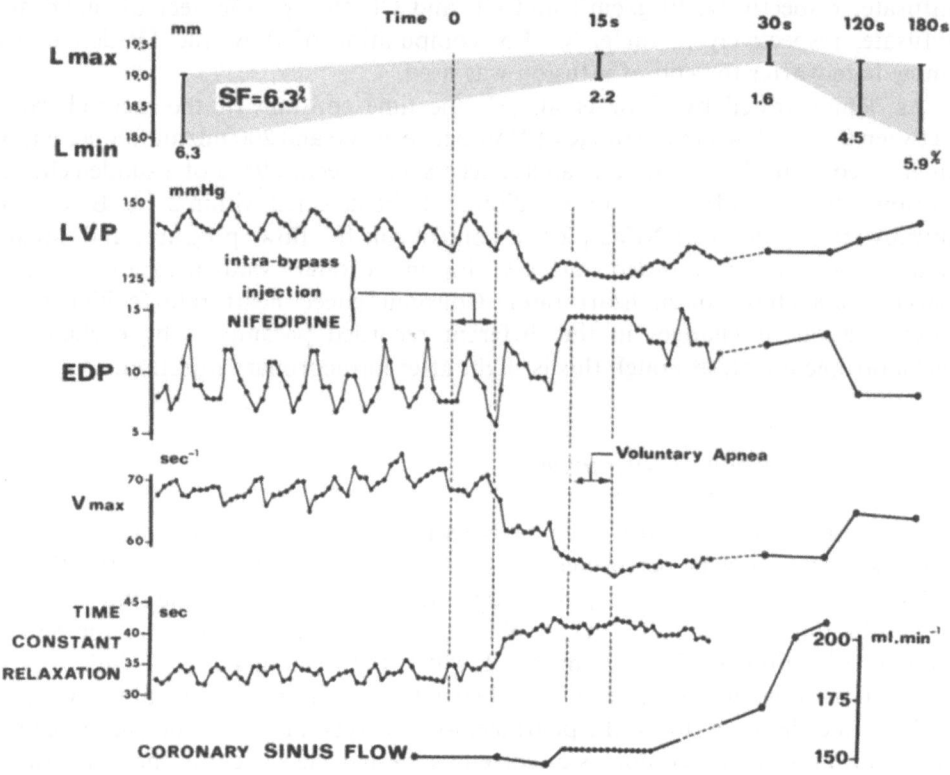

Fig. 3. The beat-to-beat analysis of regional and global myocardial function following a single intrabypass injection of Nifedipine is shown. *Lmax*, maximal marker separation; *Lmin,* minimal marker separation; *LVP*, peak left ventricular pressure; *EDP*, end diastolic pressure; *Vmax,* extrapolated maximum velocity of shortening of the contractile element

ening, before the Nifedipine injection, the bypass region already showed a hypokinetic contraction pattern with a shortening fraction of 6.3%. After injection, the region becomes practically akinetic (SF: 2.2% and 1.6%) with a striking increase in end systolic and end diastolic marker separation. Again the depressant effect of the drug on regional contraction disappears in less than 3 min.

While the pressure derived variables are already depressed (15 s after Nifedipine injection), the coronary sinus flow remains unchanged; this reaches its peak value (216 ml/min from 143 ml/min) only 30 to 45 s after the intrabypass injection. Therefore, it must be inferred that 15 s after the intrabypass injection of Nifedipine the vasodilator effect of the drug on the coronary system itself is not yet effective. In other words, under the condition of intrabypass administration of Nifedipine, we were able to demonstrate the regional and global negative inotropic properties of the drug before the appearance of any vasodilator effect which might affect the coronary system, the peripheral resistance, and therefore the afterload.

Case Report II

Twelve months after bypass surgery, patient ACM was recatheterized. This patient had three vessel disease and the three major coronary arteries were grafted (LAD,

RCA, obtuse marginal branch). Of these three bypasses, two (RCA and obtuse marginal) were found occluded at recatheterization and only the LAD bypass was patent and normal. During surgery two radiopaque epicardial marker pairs had been implanted in bypassed regions: in the LAD region and in the obtuse marginal (OM) region. In the postoperative period, a paradoxical systolic expansion of the marker pair implanted in the OM region occurred, whereas the LAD region showed a normal contraction pattern.

In this second case (Fig. 4), the hemodynamic changes are quite similar to the first case. Two consecutive injections were performed and they provoked *additive* effects. Nevertheless it must be noted that, after the first intrabypass injection, all the hemodynamic parameters tend to return to their basal values showing again the

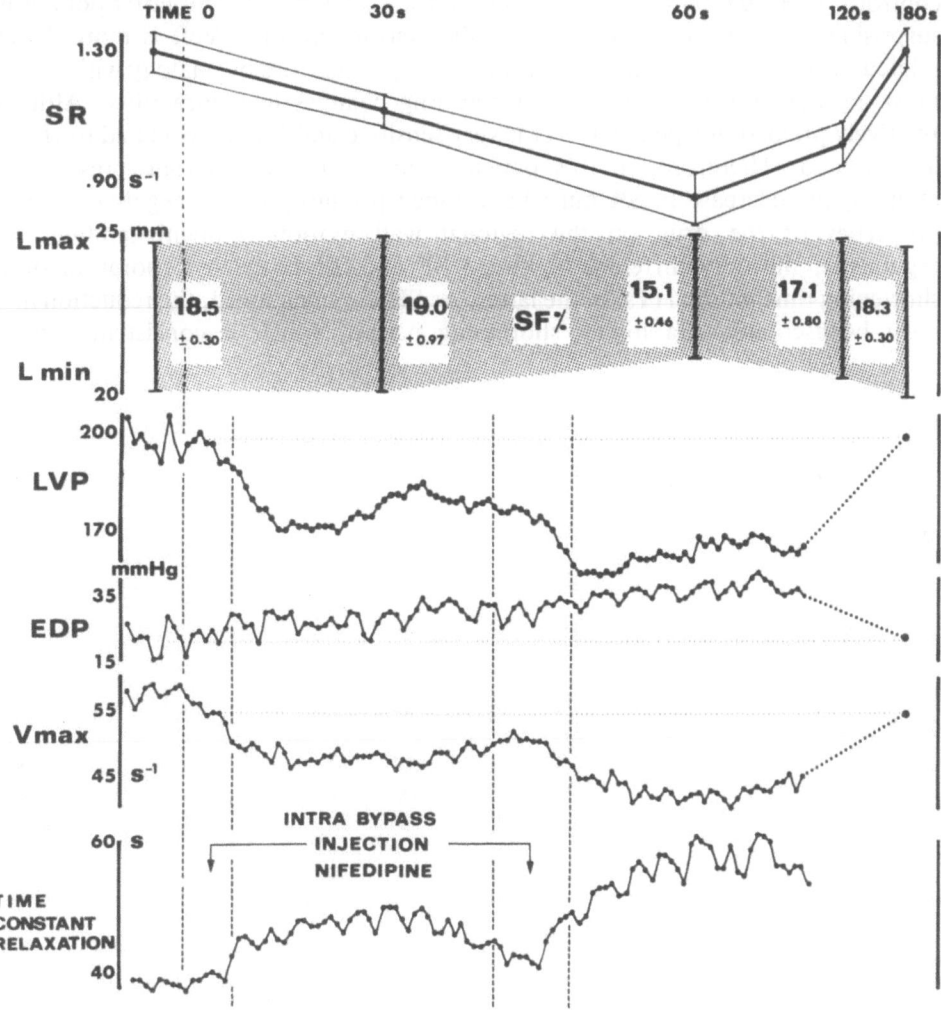

Fig. 4. The beat-to-beat analysis of regional and global myocardial function following a double intrabypass injection of Nifedipine is shown. See legend to Fig. 3 for definition of abbreviations

rapid *reversibility* and *transient* effect of alterations induced by the regional Nifedipine administration. After the two consecutive injections of 0.1 mg, the negative inotropic properties of the drug were manifest: we observed a 35 mmHg drop in peak systolic pressure (LVP), with a concomitant and significant increase in end diastolic pressure (EDP) from 20 mmHg to 40 mmHg. Following the Nifedipine injection, Vmax was reduced from 58 s^{-1} to 41 s^{-1} and T increased from 37.5 ms to 61 ms. In view of the fact that these measurements were performed at constant paced heart rate (113 b.p.m.) with a 531 ms cycle length, a direct slowing of the contractile process and mechanisms involved in relaxation must be inferred. The behavior of regional shortening is more complicated than in the previous case. After the first Nifedipine (N1) injection (0.1 mg) shortening fraction remains unchanged: Control (5 beats), 18.5% ± sd 0.30% versus Nifedipine (5 beats) 19.0 ± sd 0.97%. On the other hand, mean shortening rate (SR) is significantly decreased from control 1.30 ± sd 0.06 s^{-1} to Nifedipine, 1.12 ± sd 0.05 s^{-1}. This latter point is not surprising since mean circumferential fiber shortening rate (Vcf) is more directly related to contractility than ejection fraction [9]. Therefore by analogy with Vcf, SR must be more sensitive than SF in detecting changes in contractility. Although relatively preload independent, Vcf is very sensitive and *inversely* related to changes in afterload. Therefore, in this patient, where the peak systolic pressure was reduced, the decrease in SR must be ascribed primarily to the negative inotropic properties of the drug on the regional wall motion. Notwithstanding these arguments, the only difference between SF and SR is the incorporation of the shortening time interval (Ts) in the latter. As SF was unchanged, the reduction in SR must be ascribed to a longer shortening period, which is consistent with the

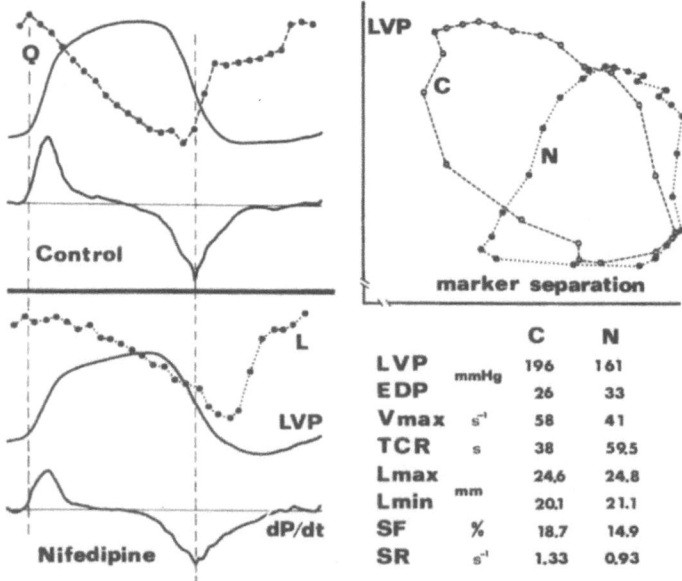

		C	N
LVP	mmHg	196	161
EDP		26	33
Vmax	s⁻¹	58	41
TCR	s	38	59.5
Lmax	mm	24.6	24.8
Lmin		20.1	21.1
SF	%	18.7	14.9
SR	s⁻¹	1.33	0.93

Fig. 5. Regional shortening in relation to left ventricular pressure is shown as simultaneously recorded *(left panel)* and the pressure-marker separation loop *(right panel)*. See legend to Fig. 3 for definition of abbreviations

somewhat slower contraction of the myocardium as demonstrated by the reduction in Vmax and increase in relaxation time constant T.

After the second Nifedipine (N2) injection (0.1 + 0.1 mg), mean shortening rate ($\overline{SR}$), calculated from five beats, is still more affected and falls to the value of 0.85 ± sd 0.88 s. At the same time and for the same beats, a significant reduction of SF is observed: Nifedipine (N1) 19.0 ± sd 0.97% versus Nifedipine (N2) 15.1 ± sd 0.50%. In fact, this reduction in shortening fraction results essentially from an increase in end systolic marker separation (N1: 20.1 ± sd 0.1 mm versus N2: 21.1 ± 0.09 mm) while the end diastolic marker separation remains constant (N1: 24.9 ± sd 0.1 mm versus N2: 24.9 ± 0.08 mm). If we analyze simultaneously the pressure data and the actual marker separation (Fig. 5), then it becomes apparent that the point of minimal marker separation after the second Nifedipine injection (N2) occurs very clearly (60 ms) after the aortic closure (end systolic pressure). In fact, the point of minimal marker separation coincides actually with a pressure of 22 mmHg. Thus, not only a reduction in SF and SR, but a real regional dyssynergy is observed. While the left ventricular pressure is falling down, the regional contraction is going on.

On the other hand, after two consecutive Nifedipine injections, the paradoxical systolic expansion observed in the adjacent region is unaffected: the contraction pattern, timing with regard to hemodynamic event, and extent of lengthening remain unchanged.

Discussion

In 1972, Fleckenstein et al. demonstrated that the isometric tension and the extra consumption of oxygen in the isolated, electrically stimulated papillary muscle of the rabbit after 10 – 100 µg/liter Nifedipine were reduced dose dependently [10]. In this isolated modified Langendorff heart preparation Raff et al. [11] showed that the systolic pressure and the left ventricle dP/dt max were also reduced dose dependently after 1 – 5 µg/l. In these experiments coronary blood flow increased whereas the myocardial oxygen consumption was reduced. Thus, a negative inotropic effect was clear. However, in studies carried out by Kober et al. on the human heart, decreases in left ventricular diastolic pressure, systolic, and diastolic aortic pressure were observed together with maintenance of heart rate and a slight increase in the quotient max dP/dt/P [12]. Lichtlen [13] found that Nifedipine brought about a significant decrease in left ventricular systolic and end diastolic pressure as well as a significant increase in heart rate and dP/dt max. In these different studies performed at rest and without adequate control of heart rate, it was not clear whether these effects were interrelated: was the higher peak dP/dt the result of an unsuspected positive inotropic action of Nifedipine independent of a concomitantly higher heart rate, or was it the result of the positive inotropic effect of the higher heart rate itself? Indeed, the vasodilation due to Nifedipine necessarily induces reflex baroreceptor activation and it has been suggested that beta adrenergic stimulation could easily abolish the expected negative inotropic action of a calcium antagonist. In addition, contractility should not be defined only by the measurement of max dP/dt, which is both preload and afterload dependent, but ought to be characterized by variables less sensitive to loading effects, such as Vmax.

Therefore, two years ago, in our laboratory we tried to define the way in which contractility was altered by peroral administration of Nifedipine, at a fixed heart rate of 90 [13]. Under these conditions a significant decrease was demonstrated in left ventricular systolic pressure, aortic systolic, and diastolic pressure persisting throughout the study (60 min). The value of Vmax showed a slight trend to increase, the rise being significant 60 min after Nifedipine administration. At this stage it became apparent that the effects of an antianginal drug had to be studied not only at rest but also under a stress situation. The global and regional LV function in many cases is only impaired during stress, when transient regional asynergy occurs provoked by localized imbalance between oxygen supply and demand. In addition coronary artery disease is essentially a regional disease where regional behavior and interaction between regions is of major interest. Therefore a means had to be developed to quantify regional shortening in areas newly perfused by the coronary artery bypass. This led to the introduction of implanting radiopaque marker pairs during surgery in every bypass region [5]. Using this method, regional left ventricular wall motion was recently studied in 11 patients during pacing induced tachycardia and following an intravenous administration of Nifedipine (1 mg within 3 min) [14].

LV pressure derived measurements were recorded simultaneously with a tip manometer. The dominant effect of Nifedipine at basal heart rate was a lowering of peak LV pressure (152 mmHg to 128) with an increase in heart rate (HR) from 70 b.p.m. to 86. During pacing, Nifedipine produced significant ($p < .02$) reduction in the pressure-rate product, suggesting a mechanism reducing or sparing myocardial oxygen consumption. At the highest paced rate, the maximal velocity (Vmax) of the contractile element was significantly ($p < .02$) increased from 61 s^{-1} to 68 s^{-1}. After Nifedipine infusion, SF was increased over the entire pacing range: basal HR, 13.7% to 14.6% ($p < .025$); HR 120, 11.6% to 13.5% ($p < .005$); max HR, 10.9% to 11.8% ($p < .05$). At a common heart rate of 120, the increase in shortening fraction was significantly correlated with an increase in end diastolic marker separation and not with the change in peak LV pressure. Conversely, at the highest paced rate, it was suggested that the main mechanism of increase in SF was a decrease of afterload with a concomitant reduction in end diastolic dimension.

At this stage, it still remained unclear whether we had measured the effects of loading changes or whether we had measured some specific action of the drug on the heart. Although up to now our experience with intrabypass injection is very limited (pilot study of six different left ventricular regions), our preliminary results clearly demonstrated the negative inotropic properties of the drug when regionally administrated. Conversely, it must be assumed that the negative inotropic effect of this calcium antagonist is completely masked by systemic effects when the drug is administrated peroral or intravenously. For the intravenous injection, one mg. (1000 µg) was infused over three min; the intrabypass injections (100 µg, eventually 200 µg) were performed within 10 to 15 s. These differences in dosage and rates of administration must be taken into account for the interpretation of the data. In anesthetised dogs, after intracoronary injection of Nifedipine (1 to 3 µg/kg in 20 s), myocardial oxygen consumption decreased dose dependently (25% and 42%) in the region supplied by the coronary branch selectively injected, while a slight drop in blood pressure (7% and 8%) was observed [15]. In view of the similar response in man and dog to Nifedipine, it may be assumed that a similar effect occurs in the human heart following a intracoronary injection of a quite comparable amount of Nifedipine (1.4 to 2.8 µg/kg within 15 s). To what extent the decrease in O_2 consumption is due to the drop in blood pressure or to a direct action of the drug on cardiac metabolism or the contractility of the muscle could not be established in our patients. On the basis of studies by Fleckenstein et al. [10] it may be assumed that the electromechanical decoupling occurring in the myocardium after administration of Nifedipine, and leading to a decrease in myocardial contraction, may be an essential cause of the experimentally observed fall in O_2 consumption. The negative inotropic effect on the heart which we recorded is probably an expression of that fundamental biochemical effect.

The difference of effects, observed following an intravenous or an intracoronary injection of Nifedipine, is partially due to the fact that the regulatory mechanism of the blood pressure, that is mediated by baroreceptors of the arterial system, is practically not solicited – or very transiently (less than 3 min) – after an intra-coronary injection of 100 µg Nifedipine. This latter point has been confirmed by Kaltenbach et al. [4] who did not observe any peripheral or central hemodynamic changes after an intravenous injection of 100 µg. Therefore, the transient drop in peak systolic pressure (less than 3 min) observed after intracoronary injection must be interpreted as the result of a negative inotropic effect on the myocardium whereas the long standing decrease of blood pressure (more than 60 min) observed after the intravenous injections is the result of a persistent decrease in peripheral resistance. Catecholamines are released from the sympathetic nerves and in the heart they counteract the negative inotropic effect of Nifedipine. In addition, the pressure relief on the heart conditioned by the lowering of the peripheral resistance also influences cardiac action; changes in loading condition definitely have an influence on the regional ventricular shortening. For all these reasons, it is concluded that the negative inotropic effect of Nifedipine is masked or even inhibited by the systemic effects.

Acknowledgement

We thank the Bayer Company for providing us with the Nifedipine samples.

References

1. Kaltenbach M, Becker HJ, Kober G, Loos A (1972) Veränderungen der Hämodynamik des linken Herzen unter der Wirkung von Nifedipine (BAY a 1040) im Vergleich mit Nitroglycerine. Arzneim Forsch 22:362
2. Lichtlen P, Engel HJ, Amende I, Rafflenbuel W, Simon R (1976) Mechanism of various antianginal drugs. Relationship between regional flow behaviour and contractility. In: Jatene AD, Lichtlen PR (eds) New therapy of ischemic heart disease. Excerpta Medica, Amsterdam-Oxford, p 14
3. Brand M van den, Remme WJ, Meester GT, Tiggelaar-de Widt I, Ruiter R de, Hugenholtz PG (1976) Changes in left and right ventricular haemodynamics in angina pectoris patients following adalat administration. In: Jatene AD, Lichtlen PR (eds) New therapy of ischemic heart disease. Excerpta Medica, Amsterdam-Oxford, p 69
4. Kaltenbach M, Schulz W, Kober G, Bamberg E (1978) Cardiac and peripheral action of a calcium inhibitive antianginal drug. Trans Eur Soc Cardiol 1:22
5. Brower RW, Katen HJ ten, Meester GT (1978) Direct methods for determining regional myocardial shortening after bypass surgery from radiopaque markers in man. Am J Cardiol 41:1223

6. Meester GT, Bernard N, Zeelenberg C, Brower RW, Hugenholtz PG (1975) A computer system for real time analysis of cardiac catheterization data. Cathet Cardiovasc Diagn 1:113

7. Meester GT, Zeelenberg C, Gorter S, Miller AC, Hugenholtz PG (1974) Beat-to-beat analysis of left ventricular function parameters. Eur J Cardiol 1:279

8. Ganz W, Tamura K, Marcus HS, Donoso R, Yoshida S, Swan HJC (1971) Measurement of coronary sinus blood flow by continuous thermodilution in man. Circulation 44:181

9. Mahler F, Ross J Jr, O'Rourke RA (1975) Effects of changes in preload, afterload, and inotropic state on ejection and isovolumic phase measures of contractility in the conscious dog. Am J Cardiol 35:626

10. Fleckenstein A, Tritthart H, Döring HJ, Byon KY (1972) BAY a 1040 ein hochaktiver Ca^{++}-antagonistischer Inhibitor des elektromechanischen Koppelungsprozesses in Warmblüter Myokard. Arzneim Forsch 22:22

11. Raff WK, Kosche F, Lochner W (1972) Untersuchungen mit Nifedipine, einer coronargefäßerweiternden Substanz mit schneller sublingualer Wirkung. Arzneim Forsch 22:33

12. Kober G, Becker HJ, Kaltenbach M (1975) Left ventricular hemodynamics in patients at rest before and after nifedipine. In: Lochner W, Braasch W, Kroneberg G (eds) New therapy of ischemic heart disease. Springer, Berlin Heidelberg New York, p 164

13. Lichtlen P (1973) The influence of nifedipine on left ventricular and coronary dynamics at rest and during exercise in patients with coronary artery disease. In: Hashimoto K, Kimura E, Kobayshi T (eds) New therapy of ischemic heart disease. University of Tokyo, Tokyo, p 144

14. Serruys P, Hugenholtz PG, ten Katen HJ, Brower RW (1978) Effect of nifedipine on regional ventricular shortening during pacing after coronary artery bypass grafting. Proceedings VIII world congress of cardiology, Tokyo, p 214

15. Vater W (1975) Myocardial oxygen consumption under the influence of nifedipine (adalat) in the anaesthetized dog. In: Lochner W, Braasch W, Kroneberg G (eds) New therapy of ischemic heart disease. Springer, Berlin Heidelberg New York, p 77

Der kalziumantagonistische Effekt auf die zentrale und periphere Haemodynamik, Ventrikelvolumina und die regionale Wandbewegung bei koronarer Herzkrankheit

W. Rutsch, M. Schartl, T. Krais und H. Schmutzler

Einleitung

Durch Hemmung des transmembranären Kalziumeinstromes und der intrazellulären Freisetzung von Kalzium-Ionen aus dem sarkoplasmatischen Retikulum beeinflussen Kalziumantagonisten die elektromechanische Kopplung. Da die Aktivierung der myofibrillären ATPase kalziumabhängig ist, werden weniger energiereiche Phosphate gespalten, was zu verminderter Spannungsentwicklung und Abnahme des Sauerstoffverbrauches führt [1]. Insbesondere ist der kalziumabhängige Tonus der glatten Gefäßmuskulatur und die Kontraktilität isolierter Papillarmuskelstreifen durch Kalziumantagonisten beeinflußbar [2]. Durch Abnahme des Arteriolentonus sinkt der koronare und totale periphere Gefäßwiderstand, was zum Abfall des Aortendruckes und zusammen mit einer Compliancezunahme der großen Gefäße zu einer Verminderung der kardialen Nachlast führt. Die über Barorezeptoren vermittelte Gegenregulation mit vermehrter Noradrenalinfreisetzung bewirkt eine Steigerung der Herzfrequenz, eine Zunahme der isovolumetrischen Druckanstiegsgeschwindigkeit und erhöht den venösen Rückstrom, wodurch teilweise der calciumantagonistische, sauerstoffsparende Effekt wieder zunichte gemacht wird. Die Verminderung der Nachlast und der relative Zuwachs an Kontraktilität führen zu einer Abnahme der Wandspannung mit Verkleinerung des Herzens, Verbesserung der Kontraktilitätsparameter der Auswurfphase und zu einem globalen Zuwachs der linksventrikulären Wandbewegung.

Methodik

Untersucht wurden 10 Patienten mit koronarer Herzkrankheit, die teilweise Myokardinfarkte erlitten hatten und unter einer Koronarinsuffizienz litten. Mit einem Millar-TIP-Manometer wurden die linksventrikulären Drucke, dp/dt_{max} und die Aortendrucke, sowie mit einem Swan-Ganz-Thermokatheter die Niederdruckdaten gemessen und das HZV mit dem Kälteverdünnungsverfahren nach einer Stabilisierungsphase von 30 min bestimmt. Nach monoplaner Ventrikulographie in 30°-RAO-Position erhielten die Patienten nach einer Pause von 30 min 20 mg Nifedipin sublingual. Nach einer Registrierzeit von 45 min erfolgte eine zweite Ventrikulographie unter gleichen Bedingungen und abschließend die Koronarangiographie. Die Ventrikulvolumina wurden nach der Methode von Sandler und Dodge ermittelt und die regionale Wandbewegung anhand einer kontinuierlichen, über die gesamte Ventrikelcircumferenz reichenden Kurve der mittleren Verkürzungsgeschwindigkeit bewertet [3]. Die Position der endsystolischen Kontur wurde nicht korrigiert, als Bezugspunkt für die Achsenverkürzung wurde der gemeinsame Flächenschwerpunkt gewählt. Eine ungestörte Wandbewegung wurde bei einer $\bar{V}_{CF}$ von mehr als

0,5 circ/sec angenommen, eine Hypokinesie bei einer $\bar{V}_{CF}$ kleiner als 0,5, eine Akinesie bei fehlender Achsenverkürzung und eine Dyskinesie bei paradoxer, systolischer Auswärtsbewegung mit negativer $\bar{V}_{CF}$.

Wir unterteilten die linksventrikuläre Kontur in fünf Segmente und ermittelten anhand der $\bar{V}_{CF}$-Kurve den zugehörigen Asynergiegrad.

Ein Patient wurde nicht in die Bewertung einbezogen, da er bei einer zugrundeliegenden schweren koronaren 2-Gefäßerkrankung mit subtotalen, proximalen Stenosen des RIVA und des RCX ohne Kollateralkreislauf als Folge des beträchtlichen diastolischen Blutdruckabfalls mit starkem Frequenzanstieg und Kontraktilitätszuwachs einen schweren Angina-pectoris-Anfall erlitt.

Ergebnisse

Haemodynamische Maximaleffekte nach einer einzelnen sublingualen Dosis werden verzögert in der 40. – 50. min nach Applikation beobachtet, während erste Effekte schon nach wenigen Minuten auftreten [4]. Nach 15 min hatte der Kreislaufwiderstand erst 51%, der systolische Aortendruck 40% und die Herzfrequenz 70% der maximalsten Veränderung erreicht. Erst ab etwa 30. Minute nach Applikation erreichten die Differenzen statistische Signifikanz auf dem 5%-Niveau.

Vergleicht man die haemodynamischen Daten der 45. Registrierminute mit den Kontrollwerten, so ergeben sich für folgende Parameter statistisch signifikante Abweichungen (Abb. 1):

1. Der totale, periphere Kreislaufwiderstand wurde um 28% hochsignifikant von 1253 ± 220 auf 905 ± 177 dyn · sec · cm^{-1} gesenkt,
2. systolischer, diastolischer und mittlerer Aortendruck wurden um 20, 15 bzw. 16% von 138 ± 15 auf 111 ± 13, von 75 ± 8 auf 64 ± 10 und von 100 ± 8 auf 84 ± 10 mmHg erniedrigt.
3. Als Folge der Herzfrequenzsteigerung um 11% von 65 ± 12 auf 73 ± 8 Schlägen/min nimmt das Herzminutenvolumen um 12% von $3,3 \pm 0,5$ auf $3,73 \pm 0,46$ L/min/m^2 zu. Das aus der HZV-Bestimmung mit der Kälteverdünnungsmethode errechnete Schlagvolumen blieb nahezu konstant, während das cineangiographisch aus der Volumendifferenz ermittelte einen tendenziellen Anstieg um 21% von 63 ± 15 auf 76 ± 20 ml/m^2 zeigte.
4. Die Kontraktilitätsparameter der Auswurfphase stiegen an, die Ejektionsfraktion um 16% von 52 ± 15 auf $62 \pm 11\%$, die $\bar{V}_{CF}$ um 23% von $0,79 \pm 0,26$ auf $1,03 \pm 0,24$ circ/sec. Lediglich die mittlere, auf das enddiastolische Volumen normalisierte Austreibungsstromstärke MNSER nahm nicht signifikant um 8% von $1,41 \pm 0,6$ auf $1,54 \pm 0,8$/sec zu.

dp/dt$_{max}$ zeigte als Kontraktilitätsparameter der isovolumetrischen Anspannungsphase mit 1377 ± 220 gegenüber 1318 ± 163 mmHg/sec keine wesentliche Änderung.

Im Niederdruckbereich gab es keine signifikanten Veränderungen. Verschlußplethysmographische Messungen des peripheren Venentonus zeigten eine kontinuierliche, prozentuale Zunahme der Venenkapazität und eine entsprechende Abnahme des Elastizitätskoeffizienten bis zur 45. min, ohne daß die Differenz zu irgendeinem Zeitpunkt statistisch signifikant gewesen wäre.

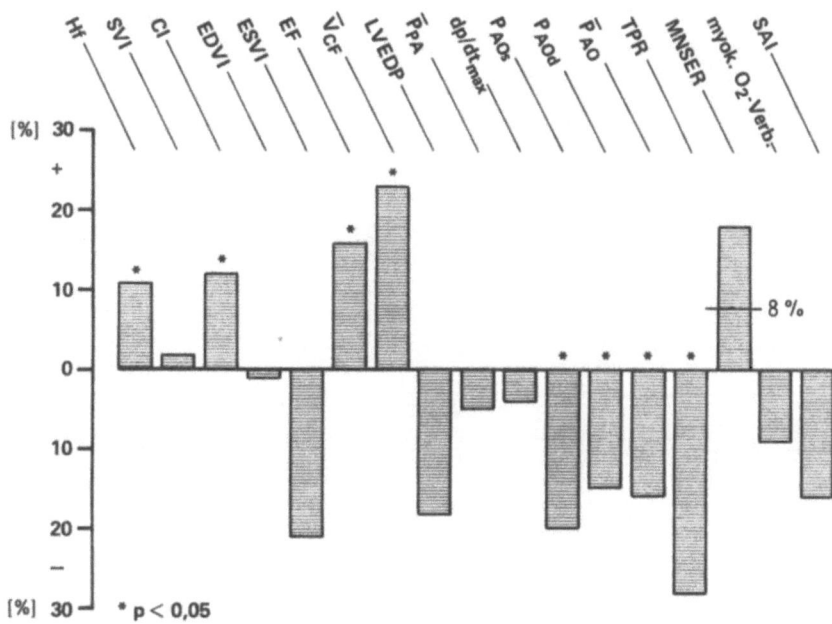

Abb. 1. Prozentuale Änderung der Mittelwerte der zentralen und peripheren Haemodynamik der Kontraktilitätsparameter der isovolumetrischen und Auswurfphase, des myokardialen Sauerstoffverbrauches (Bretschneider) und der Schlagarbeit nach 20 mg Nifedipin sublingual in der 45. Registrierminute

Wesentliche Abweichungen des Mitteldruckes in PC-Position, in der Arteria pulmonalis oder dem rechten Vorhof konnten nicht registriert werden. Der linksventrikuläre enddiastolische Druck fiel nicht signifikant um 18% von 17,7 ± 8,6 auf 14,6 ± 7,5 mmHg ab. Entsprechend der großen Streubreite der Einzelwerte lag der Mittelwert für das enddiastolische Volumen im Bereich des Kontrollwertes, in sechs von neun Fällen war es jedoch zu einer deutlichen Verkleinerung gekommen. Das endsystolische Volumen nahm tendentiell um 21% von 67 ± 33 auf 53 ± 28 ml/m² ab (Abb. 2).

Stellt man die den myokardialen Sauerstoffverbrauch bestimmenden Parameter den errechneten Äquivalenzwerten des tatsächlichen Sauerstoffverbrauches gegenüber, so erklärt sich die der verminderten Schlagarbeit entsprechende Abnahme des mit der Bretschneider-Formel und des Tension-Time-Indexes errechneten Sauerstoffverbrauches allein aus einer Abnahme der systolischen und diastolischen Wandspannung. Der durch Katecholaminfreisetzung bewirkte relative Zuwachs an Kontraktilität und der Anstieg der Herzschlagfolge beeinträchtigen den nach in-vitro-Versuchen vorstellbaren sauerstoffsparenden Effekt der Kalziumantagonisten (Tabelle 1, Abb. 3).

Beim Vergleich der kontinuierlichen $\bar{V}_{CF}$-Kurven über die gesamte Ventrikelcircumferenz zur Analyse der regionalen Wandbewegung fiel eine homogene Zunahme der Faserverkürzungsgeschwindigkeit mit Ausnahme der dys- und akinetischen Bereiche auf. Die bei 9 Patienten insgesamt bewerteten 45 Segmente zeigten in 25% eine Verbesserung der Verkürzungsgeschwindigkeit mit Verschiebung der Asynergie um einen Schweregrad. 53% der hypokinetischen (Abb. 4) Segmente zeigten nach

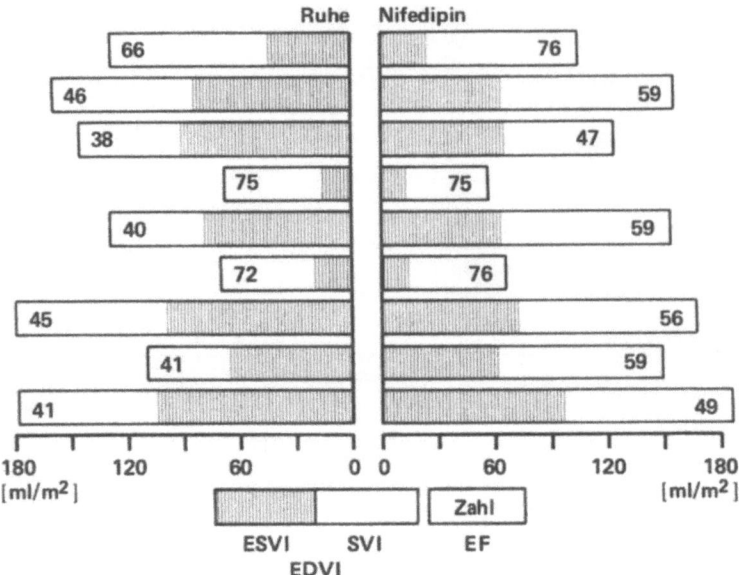

Abb. 2. Linksventrikuläre Volumina und Ejektionsfraktion nach 20 mg Nifedipin sublingual, 45. Registrierminute (n = 9)

Tabelle 1. Die wesentlichen Parameter des myokardialen Sauerstoffverbrauches vor und nach 20 mg Nifedipin sublingual (n = 9), 45. Registrierminute

	vor		nach
HF	65	+ 11% *	73 min^{-1}
LVEDP	17,7	− 18%	14,6 mmHg
EDVI	130	− 1%	129 ml/m^2
LVSP$_m$	117	− 18% *	96 mmHg
dp/dt$_{max}$	1377	− 4%	1318 mmHg · sec^{-1}
ET	317	− 1%	313 msec

* p 0,05

Nifedipin eine Normalisierung der Wandbewegung. Nur bei zwei Segmenten, Myokardareale mit zugehöriger subtotaler Koronarstenose ohne Kollateralkreislauf, kam es ohne Entwicklung einer Angina pectoris zu einer Verschlechterung der regionalen $\bar{V}_{CF}$, ohne daß jedoch der Grenzwert von 0,5 circ/sec erreicht wurde. Die globale Verbesserung normaler und hypokinetischer Myokardareale korreliert mit der verminderten kardialen Nachlast, ist also kein Effekt primären Kontraktilitätszuwachses. Aus dieser Beobachtung ist weiterhin zu schließen, daß es zu keiner wesentlichen Umverteilung des Koronarflusses mit Provokation eines Steal-Phänomens kommt. Eine Entwicklung hypo- oder akinetischer Wandbewegungsstörungen konnte nicht beobachtet werden, da trotz teilweise beträchtlicher Abnahme des Perfusionsdruckes eine kritische Verminderung des poststenotischen Koronarflusses offensichtlich nicht auftrat.

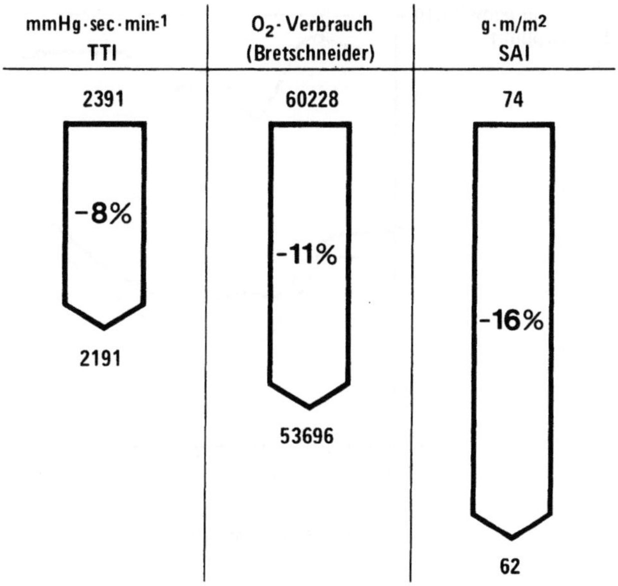

mmHg·sec·min⁻¹	O₂·Verbrauch	g·m/m²
TTI	(Bretschneider)	SAI
2391	60228	74
−8%	−11%	−16%
2191	53696	62

Abb. 3. Äquivalenzwerte des myokardialen Sauerstoffverbrauches und Schlagarbeitsindex vor und nach 20 mg Nifedipin (n = 9, 45. Registrierminute). Unterschiede der Daten statistisch nicht signifikant

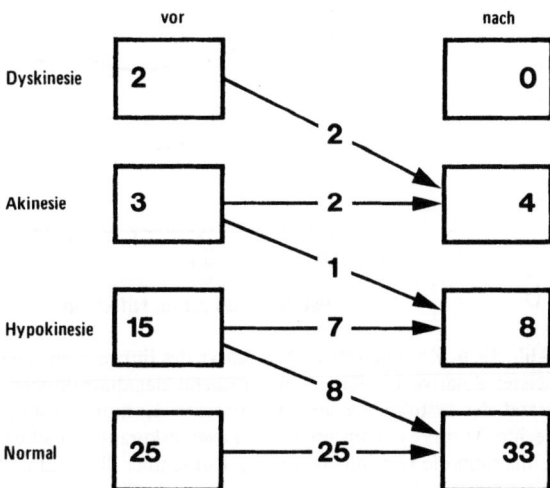

Abb. 4. Veränderung der segmentalen Wandbewegung des linken Ventrikels vor und nach 20 mg Nifedipin sublingual (n = 9), 45. Registrierminute

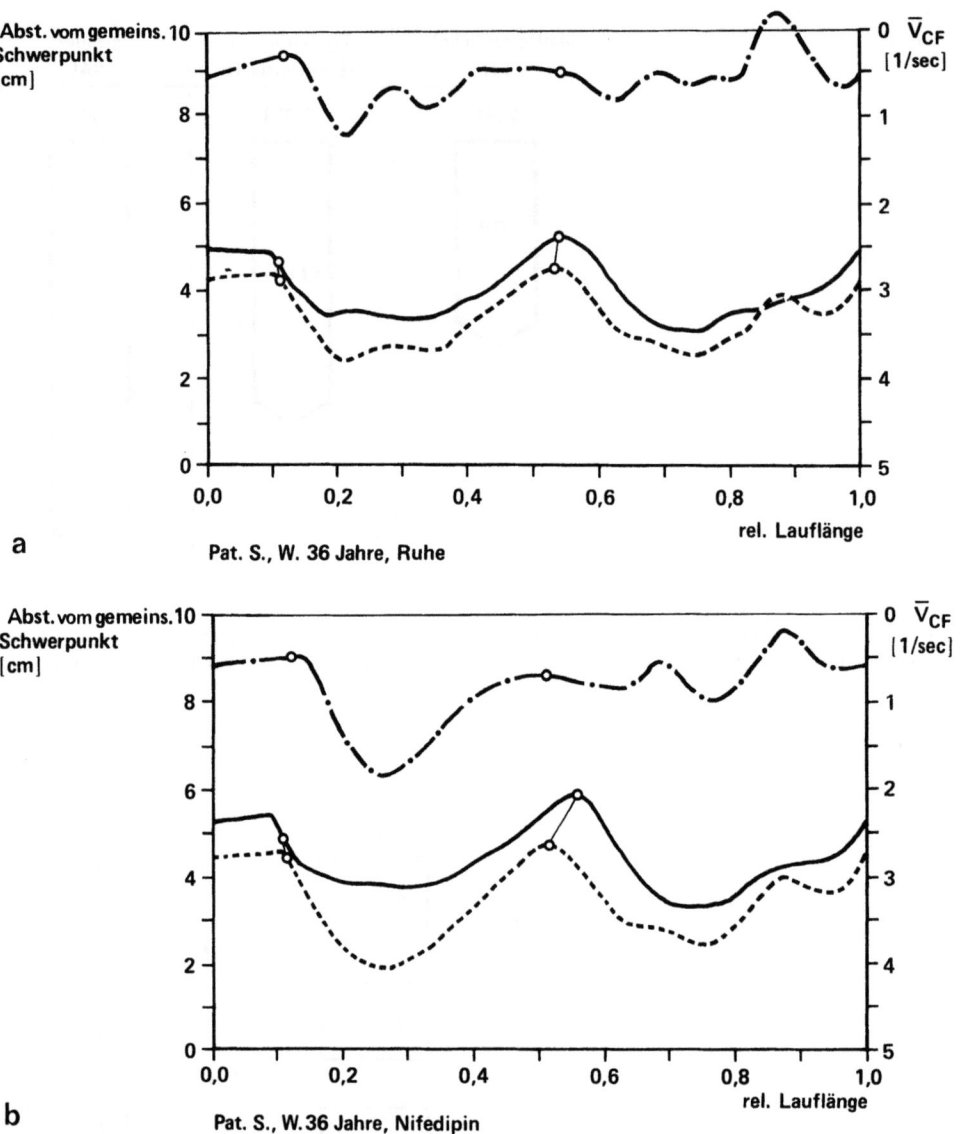

a   Pat. S., W. 36 Jahre, Ruhe

b   Pat. S., W. 36 Jahre, Nifedipin

Abb. 5a, b. Kontinuierliche V_{CF}-Kurve des linken Ventrikels vor und nach 20 mg Adalat sublingual. Abscisse: Relative Lauflänge entsprechend der diastolischen Ventrikelcircumferenz, Ordinate links: Abstand der systolischen und diastolischen Konturen vom gemeinsamen Flächenschwerpunkt, Ordinate rechts: Mittlere circumferenzielle Faserverkürzungsgeschwindigkeit, obere Abscisse $\bar{V}_{CF} = 0$. Die obere Linie stellt die kontinuierliche $\bar{V}_{CF}$-Kurve über die gesamte Ventrikelcircumferenz dar, die mittlere Linie die diastolische Ventrikelkontur, wobei links die Aortenklappe, in der Mitte die Herzspitze und rechts die Mitralklappe gelegen ist, unterste Linie systolische Ventrikelkontur, zwischen Fixpunkten auf die diastolische Länge aufgedehnt. Bis auf einen kleinen Abschnitt im diaphragmalen Hinterwandbereich globale Zunahme der circumferenziellen Faserverkürzungsgeschwindigkeit

Zusammenfassung

Kalziumantagonisten wirken vasodilatatorisch auf das koronare und periphere Gefäßsystem und sind negativ-inotrop. Der Tonus der systemischen Widerstandsgefäße wird deutlicher erniedrigt als der Tonus der venösen Kapazitätsgefäße. Die Blutdrucksenkung führt zu einer reaktiven gegenregulatorischen Katecholaminfreisetzung mit Anstieg der Herzfrequenz und Zunahme der Kontraktilität. Die Nachlastverminderung führt zu einer Verschiebung von Druck- zu Volumenarbeit, die mit geringerem myokardialem Sauerstoffverbrauch verbunden ist. Die Kontraktilitätsparameter der Auswurfphase werden nachlastabhängig verbessert. Entsprechend wird die regionale Wandbewegung mit Ausnahme von Narbenarealen als Folge der peripheren haemodynamischen Effekte des Kalziumantagonisten global verbessert. Ein primärer Kontraktilitätszuwachs im poststenotischen Areal durch Zunahme des Koronarflusses und eine Umverteilung des Koronarflusses mit Ausbildung eines Steal-Phänomens konnte nicht beobachtet werden. Die Herzarbeit und der myokardiale Sauerstoffverbrauch werden nur tendenziell als Folge verminderter kardialer Wandspannung reduziert.

Literatur

1. Fleckenstein A (1972) Arzneim Forsch 22:22
2. Raff WK (1972) Arzneim Forsch 22:334
3. Rutsch W (1976) Verh Dtsch Ges Kreislaufforsch
4. Rutsch W (1977) Herbsttagung der Dtsch Ges Kreislaufforsch

Hämodynamik und Kontraktilitätsreserve des linken Ventrikels während körperlicher Belastung bei Gesunden nach oraler Einnahme von Fendilin

P. Bubenheimer, J. Gabriel und H. Roskamm

Einleitung

Auf Grund experimenteller Untersuchungen, insbesondere von Fleckenstein [1,2], wurde zunächst angenommen, daß die negativ-inotrope Wirkung der Calcium-Antagonisten auf das Myocard über eine Verminderung des myokardialen Sauerstoffverbrauches eine wesentliche Rolle bei der antianginösen Wirkung dieser Substanzen spiele. Während heute periphere Angriffspunkte der Calcium-Antagonisten in den Vordergrund der Diskussion über ihren Wirkungsmechanismus gerückt sind, ist das Problem der negativen Inotropie bei der Diskussion über potentielle Nebenwirkungen von Calcium-Antagonisten für den Kliniker von Bedeutung. Er muß sich fragen, ob diese Substanzen bei manifester oder drohender Herzinsuffizienz gefahrlos angewandt werden können, insbesondere wenn gleichzeitig mit β-Blockern behandelt wird. Bei Nifedipin soll die geringe myocarddepressive Wirkung am Menschen durch einen reflektorisch erhöhten Sympathikotonus ausgeglichen werden, so daß allenfalls bei Patienten mit schwerer Herzinsuffizienz, bei denen die sympathische Kompensation bereits ausgeschöpft ist, Vorsicht geboten wäre. Für den Calcium-Antagonisten Fendilin ist die Relevanz der direkten myocardialen Wirkung am Menschen nicht untersucht. Diese Substanz wurde in unserer Studie an 9 herzgesunden jungen männlichen Probanden angewandt. Da wir davon ausgingen, daß möglicherweise vorhandene, aber nur geringe, negativ-inotrope Effekte mit klinisch anwendbaren Methoden unter Ruhebedingungen, in Folge von Kompensationsmechanismen (Sympathikusaktivierung, Frank-Starling-Mechanismus) nicht erfaßt werden, wurden unsere Messungen auch unter körperlicher Belastung durchgeführt. Da unter Belastung die Kontraktilitätsreserven in Anspruch genommen werden müssen, kann sich ein negativ-inotroper Effekt bei noch normalen Ruhewerten an einem verminderten Zuwachs an Kontraktilität unter Belastung zeigen, insbesondere dann, wenn bei hoher Belastung keine weitere sympathische Kompensation mehr möglich ist [3].

Methodik

Die Belastung wurde liegend am Fahrradergometer stufenweise mit 50, 100 und 150 Watt über je 4 – 5 min durchgeführt. In Ruhe vor Belastung, am Ende jeder Belastungsstufe, während Belastung und 4 min nach Belastung wurden folgende Meßgrößen bestimmt: Herzfrequenz aus dem EKG, systolischer und diastolischer arterieller Druck nach Riva-Rocci, enddiastolischer und endsystolischer Durchmesser des linken Ventrikels sowie systolische Verkürzungszeit im Echokardiogramm des linken Ventrikel. Davon abgeleitet wurden die Verkürzungsfraktion (relative systolische Durchmesserverkürzung) und die mittlere circumferentielle Faserverkürzungsgeschwindigkeit als Kontraktilitätsparameter der Auswurfphase sowie die hämodynamischen Parameter Schlagvolumen und Herzminutenvolumen.

Die Ableitung von Volumengrößen aus dem Echokardiogramm erschien uns zulässig, da es sich einerseits nur um gesunde, homogen kontrahierende Ventrikel handelte und andererseits jeder Proband als eigene Kontrolle diente. Jeweils im Abstand von 1 Woche wurden 3 Untersuchungen durchgeführt, wobei die erste und dritte Untersuchung als Kontrollen ohne Medikation dienten. Der Vergleich der Meßwerte von Kontrolltest 1 zu Kontrolltest 3 zeigte, daß die angewandte Methode – Echokardiographie – unter Belastung reproduzierbare Werte mit tolerabler Streubreite liefert. Die zweite Untersuchung wurde 4 Tage nach oraler Einnahme von 3×1 Tabl. Fendilin à 50 mg, eine klinisch übliche Dosierung, durchgeführt.

Ergebnisse

Im Vergleich mit den Kontrollen waren unter Medikation *Herzfrequenz* (Abb. 1) und arterieller Blutdruck sowohl in Ruhe als auch bei Belastung unverändert. Da weder die *enddiastolische* noch die *endsystolische* Größe des linken Ventrikels beeinflußt wurden (Abb. 2), ergab sich auch für die *Verkürzungsfraktion* (Abb. 3) keine Veränderung. Bei Konstanz der Verkürzungsfraktion und Konstanz der herzfrequenzabhängigen Verkürzungszeit ergaben sich unter Medikation auch keine signifikanten Veränderungen der mittleren circumferentiellen *Faserverkürzungsgeschwindigkeit* (Abb. 4). Da keine Veränderung der Herzfrequenz und keine Veränderung der Ventrikeldimensionen eintrat, ergab sich auch keine Änderung der berechneten Volumengrößen (Schlagvolumen, *Herzminutenvolumen*).

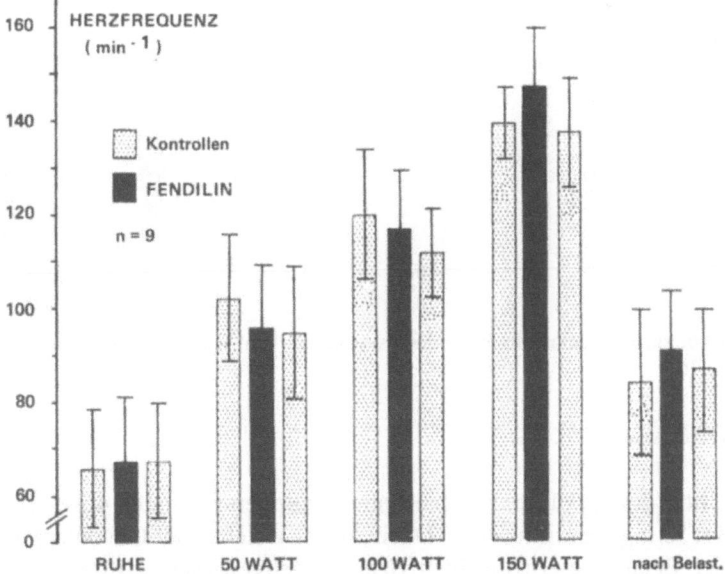

Abb. 1. Fendilin führt im Vergleich zu den Kontrollen zu keiner signifikanten Änderung der Ruhe- und Belastungsherzfrequenzen

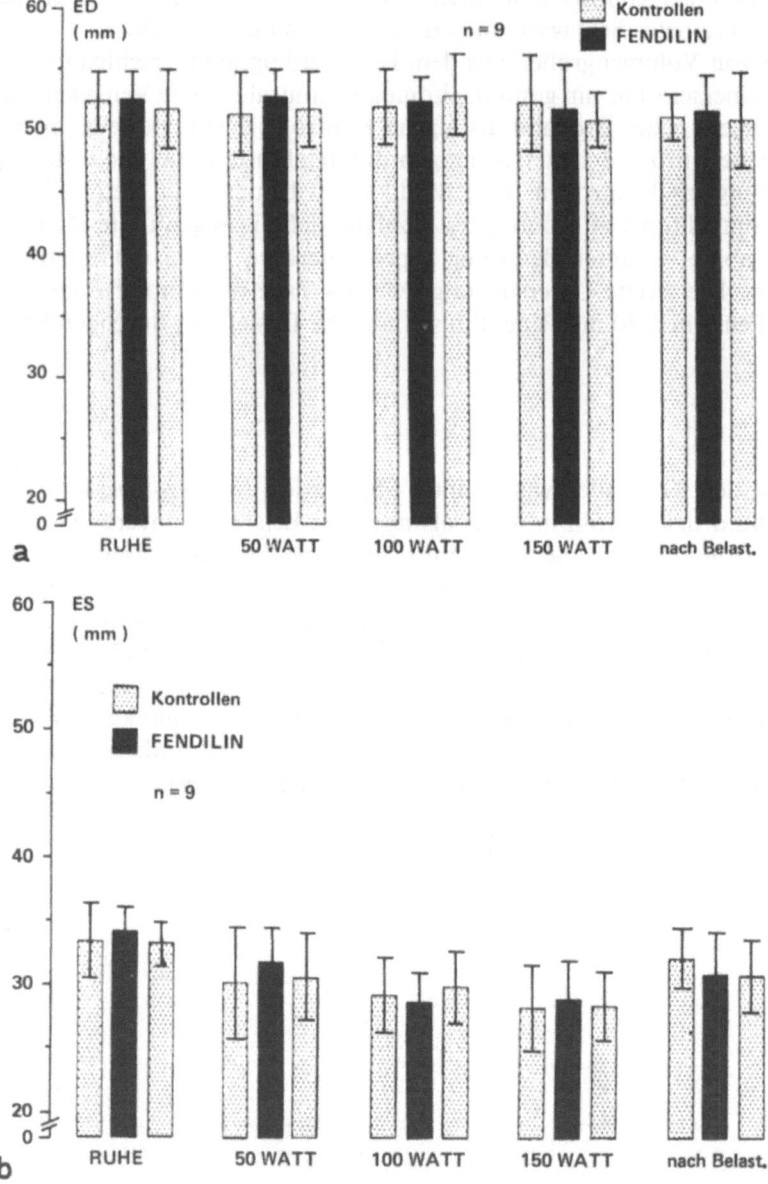

Abb. 2a, b. Enddiastolische und endsystolische Ventrikeldimensionen werden von Fendilin nicht beeinflußt

Diskussion

Unter den gewählten Versuchsbedingungen und nach 4tägiger oraler Einnahme von 3 × 50 mg Fendilin, einer Dosis, unter welcher bei Coronarpatienten eine Besserung der Belastungscoronarinsuffizienz nachgewiesen wurde, konnten wir am Herzgesunden weder Veränderungen der Hämodynamik noch der Kontraktilität feststellen. Wichtig erscheint uns für die eingangs gestellten klinischen Fragen, insbeson-

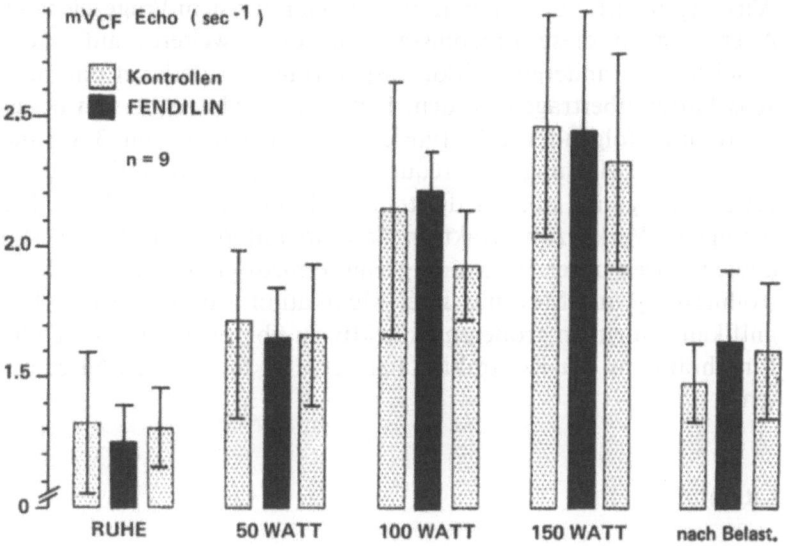

Abb. 3. Die Verkürzungsfraktion wird in Ruhe durch Fendilin nicht beeinflußt, auch ihr Anstieg unter Belastung bleibt voll erhalten

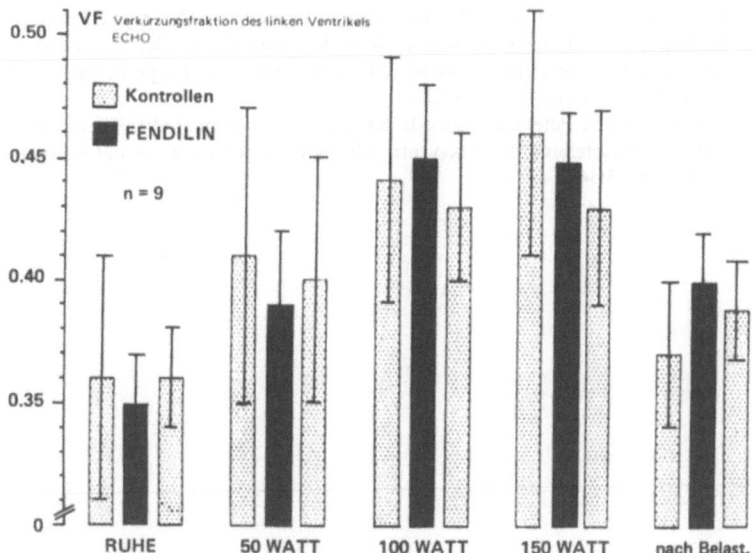

Abb. 4. Die mittlere circumferentielle Faserverkürzungsgeschwindigkeit nimmt unter Belastung stark zu. Diese Zunahme wird durch Fendilin nicht signifikant beeinflußt

dere die Tatsache, daß auch der Zuwachs an Kontraktilität unter Belastung, die Kontraktilitätsreserve, unter Fendilin keine Einbuße erfährt. Eine negativ-inotrope Wirkung kann somit am Menschen in klinischer Dosierung nicht nachgewiesen werden, entweder existiert sie überhaupt nicht oder sie ist so unbedeutend, daß sie sich der Messung mit den angewandten Methoden entzieht. Ob allerdings höhere Dosen dieses Medikamentes oder eine längere Behandlungsdauer doch negativ inotrope

Wirkungen entfalten könnten, muß noch mit einem Fragezeichen versehen werden. Auch können diese Ergebnisse nicht ohne weiteres auf andere Calcium-Antagonisten mit anderem Wirkungsspektrum und anderen pharmakokinetischen Eigenschaften übertragen werden. Unter Nifedipin zeigte sich bei gleicher Versuchsanordnung folgendes Bild (vorläufige Ergebnisse von 3 gesunden Probanden): Ruhe- und Belastungsherzfrequenzen blieben unverändert, der systolische Blutdruck sank gering ab, der diastolische Blutdruck blieb gleich. Die Kontraktilitätsparameter Verkürzungsfraktion und circumferentielle Faserverkürzungsgeschwindigkeit waren unter Belastung gering erniedrigt. Die Unterschiede zwischen Kontrollmessung und Messung unter Medikation waren jedoch so klein, daß deren Signifikanz an einem größeren Kollektiv zu überprüfen ist. Eine klinisch bedeutsame Einschränkung der Kontraktilitätsreserve ist auch durch Nifedipin nicht zu erwarten.

Literatur

1. Fleckenstein A, Kammermeier H, Döring HJ (1967) Zum Wirkungsmechanismus neuartiger Koronardilatatoren mit gleichzeitig Sauerstoff-einsparenden Myokard-Effekten, Prenylamin u. Iproveratril. Z Kreislaufforsch 56:839
2. Fleckenstein A (1971) Specific inhibitors and promotors of calcium action in the excitation-contraction coupling of heart muscle and their role in the prevention of production of myocardial lesions. In: Harries P, Opie L (eds) Calcium in the heart. Academic Press, London New York, p 169
3. Roskamm H, Skinner H, Lesch A, Wink K, Schnellbacher K, Schwendel V, Reindell H (1972) Die Kontraktilitätsreserve des gesunden linken Ventrikels bei körperlicher Belastung nach β-Rezeptorenblockade. Z Kreislaufforsch 61:802
4. Bubenheimer P, Petersen J, Pust B, Samek L, Roskamm H (1977) Ist Echokardiographie unter Belastung zur Beurteilung der linksventrikulären Funktion möglich und nützlich? Verh Dtsch Ges Kreislaufforsch 43:347

Der Einfluß von Fendilin als Monotherapie und in Kombination mit einem Beta-Rezeptorenblocker auf die Belastungshämodynamik Koronarkranker

W. Reiterer

Zusammenfassung

Bei 11 männlichen Patienten (mittleres Alter 52,5 a) mit deutlicher Leistungsminderung infolge Koronargefäßerkrankung (mittleres tolerierbares Belastungs-Steady-State 42 Watt; range 20 – 50 Watt) wurde die Auswirkung einer Kombinationstherapie zwischen dem Ca^{++}-Antagonisten Fendilin (Sensit®, 3 × 50 mg/die) und dem beta-Rezeptoren-Blocker Oxprenolol (Trasicor®, 3 × 40 mg/die) untersucht. Im Anschluß an eine Wash-out-Phase und nach 4wöchiger Behandlung wurden Meßwerte der zentralen Hämodynamik unter Ergometerarbeit im Liegen bestimmt (Mikroherzkatheterismus mit Ergospirometrie; direktes Ficksches Prinzip).

Voruntersuchungen mit einer 4wöchigen Monotherapie mit Fendilin (4 × 50 mg/die) bei einer anderen Patientengruppe (N = 7) hatten eine nitroglyzerinartige Drucksenkung im Lungenkreislauf mit fehlender Beeinflussung von Herzfrequenz und arteriellem Blutdruck gezeigt, wobei auch die Volumsleistung gering abgenommen hatte. In der Kombinationsbehandlung Fendilin-Oxprenolol zeigte sich die beta-Blocker-Wirkung in der Abnahme der Arbeitsherzfrequenz ($-7,8\%$; 2P $\leq$ 0,10) und in der Verminderung der Volumsleistung ($-8,8\%$; n.sig.; Leerwert als Bezugsgröße), wobei eine geringfügige Zunahme des linksventrikulären Füllungsdruckes (PAEDP; LW: 20,9 ± 2,2 mmHg; Therapie: 23,1 ± 1,5 mmHg) zu verzeichnen war. Es kann angenommen werden, daß ein weiteres Ansteigen des Füllungsdruckes durch venöses Pooling infolge des Ca^{++}-Antagonisten Fendilin hintangehalten wurde, da die zusätzliche Applikation von Nitroglyzerin (0,8 mg) zu einer geringeren Absenkung des unter Belastung erhöhten Füllungsdruckes führte als bei alleiniger Anwendung (17,1% versus 39,4%).

Einleitung

Ausmaß und Schweregrad der koronaren Herzkrankheit lassen sich durch einfache (Ergometrie, Ergospirometrie) oder aufwendige Funktionstests (Belastungshämodynamik) bestimmen, womit die beeinträchtigten Funktionsreserven und limitierenden Faktoren der körperlichen Leistungsfähigkeit erkannt und als Grundlage für Überlegungen zur therapeutischen Intervention hergezogen werden können [1 – 6]. Es ist naheliegend, daß eine enge Beziehung besteht zwischen der Funktionseinbuße und abnormer Reaktionen unter Belastung (Angina pectoris, Dyspnoe; EKG-Veränderungen, Herzrhythmusstörungen; Herzfrequenz- und Blutdruckregulation) und dem anatomischen Substrat der koronaren Herzkrankheit (Anzahl und Grad der Koronargefäßstenosen, reversibel ischämische Myokardareale mit gestörtem Kontraktionsverhalten, Narben) [7 – 10]. Während letztere Befunde vor allem für einen koronarchirurgischen Eingriff von Interesse sind, soll an Hand der leistungsphysiologischen Befunde die medikamentöse und somit symptomatische Therapie gezielt im Sinne einer Differentialtherapie Determinanten des myokardialen Sauerstoffbedarfes beeinflussen: Herzfrequenz, Nachlast (arterieller Blutdruck), Vorlast (Kapazität des Niederdrucksystems, Ventrikelfüllungsdruck), Herzgröße, Volumsleistung, Inotropiezustand [11, 12].

Sowohl für die Monotherapie als auch für die Kombinationsbehandlung der koronaren Herzkrankheit stehen drei Hauptgruppen von Medikamenten zur Verfügung: (1) Nitropräparate mit rasch oder protrahiert einsetzender Wirkung, (2) beta-Rezeptoren-Blocker und (3) Calciumantagonisten, wie Verapamil, Nifedipin, Perhexilin, Prenylamin und Fendilin. Der Wirkungsmechanismus der Ca^{++}-Antagonisten wurde als eine Hemmung des transmembranären Ca^{++}-Stromes und der Mobilisierung von Ca^{++} aus dem sarkoplasmatischen Retikulum beschrieben, wodurch die Muskelkontraktion als Reizantwort der elektrischen Erregung abgedämpft wird („elektromechanische Entkoppelung"). Für den Herzmuskel bedeutet dies einen negativen inotropen Effekt, hinsichtlich der Gefäßmuskulatur kann eine Vasodilatation (z. B. Koronargefäßerweiterung, Abnahme des peripheren Widerstandes, Erweiterung der Kapazitätsgefäße) beobachtet werden [13]. In bezug auf antianginösen Wirkungseintritt, Einfluß auf die Belastungsherzfrequenz und Arrhythmien sowie Veränderungen von Vor- und Nachlast weisen die aufgezählten Ca^{++}-Antagonisten jedoch deutlichst unterschiedliche Eigenschaften auf [14 – 23].

Zur Charakterisierung der Wirksamkeit von Fendilin (Sensit®) interessierten wir uns für den Effekt einer Langzeitbehandlung [19] auf die Belastungshämodynamik schwer limitierter Koronarkranker im Vergleich zur Akutwirkung von Nitroglyzerin [23]. Die untersuchten Patientengruppen waren unter Beachtung von Lebensalter, Leistungsvermögen und hämodynamischer Befunde als vergleichbar anzusehen. Nach vierwöchiger Behandlung mit Fendilin (4×50 mg/die p.o.) fand sich gleichgerichtet wie im Akutversuch mit Nitroglyzerin (0,8 mg; Spray) eine Normalisierung des linksventrikulären Füllungsdruckes (PAEDP) bei Konstanz der Herzfrequenz und des arteriellen Mitteldruckes im Vergleich zum Leerwert. Während die Volumsleistung bei hypozirkulatorischen Ausgangswerten sich nach Nitroglyzerin gering verbesserte (n.sig.), war unter Fendilin eine Abnahme zu verzeichnen.

In einer weiteren Studie wurde nun die Auswirkung einer Kombinationsbehandlung des Ca^{++}-Antagonisten Fendilin mit einem nicht kardioselektiven Beta-Rezeptorenblocker mit agonistischer Aktivität (Oxprenolol) auf die Belastungshämodynamik geprüft, wobei zusätzlich noch eine akute Intervention mit Nitroglyzerin erfolgte. Die Versuchsanordnung sollte die Frage beantworten, inwieweit die nitroglyzerinartige Drucksenkung von Fendilin trotz beta-Rezeptorenblockade nachweisbar bliebe und ob die zusätzliche Verabreichung von Nitroglyzerin zu einer weiteren Funktionsverbesserung führen könnte.

Krankengut und Methodik

15 Patienten nahmen aus freien Stücken an der Studie über die Kombinationsbehandlung Ca^{++}-Antagonist und beta-Rezeptoren-Blocker teil. Zur Auswertung gelangten die Daten von 11 Probanden (mittleres Alter 52,5 a, Körperoberfläche 1,90 m^2), bei denen die Diagnose einer koronaren Herzkrankheit durch Anamnese, ergometrische Untersuchung und in einzelnen Fällen durch Koronarangiogra-

phie gesichert war. Patienten mit einem St.p. Myokardinfarkt bzw. manifester Herzinsuffizienz und mit anderen Erkrankungen, die eine zusätzliche Medikation erforderten oder bei denen eine Einzelsubstanz der Kombinationsbehandlung indiziert wäre (Hypertonie), wurden nicht in die Studie aufgenommen.

Die Kontrollwerte wurden nach einer ca. 10tägigen Leerphase erhoben. Nach einer 4wöchigen Therapiephase mit 3×1 drg. Fendilin (Sensit, drg à 50 mg) und 3×1 tbl Oxprenolol (Trasicor, tbl à 40 mg) wurden die Untersuchungen 1,5 Std nach Einnahme der morgendlichen Dosis vorgenommen. Ca. 20 min nach Ende der Belastungsprüfung wurde 10 min nach Applikation zweier Hübe eines Nitroglyzerinsprays (Nitrolinqual®-Spray, 0,4 mg Nitroglyzerin pro Einzeldosis) der Leistungstest wiederholt.

Die invasive, rechnerunterstützte leistungsphysiologische Untersuchung bestand aus einer Volumsbelastung durch Hochlagerung der Beine (Lagerungsversuch) und aus einer Fahrradergometerarbeit im Liegen (dynamische Arbeit). Neben ergospirometrischen Daten (Sauerstoffaufnahme, Atemminutenvolumen u.a.) wurden die Druckwerte im kleinen Kreislauf mittels Einschwemmkatheter (F_4) und die Blutdruckwerte im großen Kreislauf auskultatorisch, in einzelnen Fällen auch blutig gemessen. Das Herzminutenvolumen und abgeleitete Größen der zentralen Hämodynamik wurden nach dem Fickschen Prinzip bereits während der Untersuchung mit Hilfe der Datenverarbeitungsanlage berechnet und neben ergospirometrischen Daten und Druckwerten als alphanumerischer Print-out und als Plotterdiagramm online dargestellt. Einzelheiten über die Untersuchungstechnik wurden an anderer Stelle berichtet [4, 24]. Während der hämodynamischen Untersuchung unter der Therapiephase wurde jene vergleichbare Belastungsstufe für das Steady-State eingestellt, die in der Leerwertsperiode gerade noch − nicht mehr symptomfrei − toleriert worden war (im Mittel 41,8 Watt, range 20−20 Watt).

Tabelle 1. Einfluß von *Nitroglyzerin, Fendilin, Fendilin-Oxprenolol* und *Fendilin-Oxprenolol-Nitroglyzerin* auf die Belastungshämodynamik Koronarkranker (verschiedene Patientenkollektive, vergleichbar nach Alter und Schweregrad der Leistungseinbuße: maximal toleriertes Steady-State 41 − 42 Watt)

Intervention Meßwerte	LW- beta-Sen	LW-Ni	NP	Ni	Sen	beta-Sen	beta-Sen- Ni
fh (min^{-1})	102	104	98	102	104	*94*[(*)]	*95* ($\bar{x}$)
CI (l/min/m²)	5,4	5,5	6,3	*5,7*	4,9**	5,0	*5,3**
BPpm (mmHg)	124	123	114	121	120	*117*	*117*
PAEDP (mmHg)	21	23,6	13	*14,3****	*14,5***	23,1	*17,4****
SWI (g · m/m²)	94	93	100	92	82	89	95
VO2 (l/min)	0,96	0,95	0,95	0,96	0,85**	0,92	0,98**
N	11	11	14	11	7	11	11

fh = Herzfrequenz, CI = Herzindex; BPpm = arterieller Mitteldruck; PAEDP = enddiastolischer Pulmonalarteriendruck als Index für den linksventrikulären Füllungsdruck; SWI = Schlagarbeitsindex; VO2 = Sauerstoffaufnahme; LW = Leerwert; NP = Normalpersonen; Ni = Nitroglyzerin (0,8 mg), Sen = Fendilin (Sensit; 4×50 mg/die durch 4 Wochen); beta-Sen = Fendilin (Sensit; 3×50 mg/die) und Oxprenolol (Trasicor; 3×40 mg/die) durch 4 Wochen; beta-Sen-Ni = zusätzliche Applikation von Nitroglyzerin (0,8 mg).
Die Klammern kennzeichnen die Anordnung für statistische Untersuchungen bei paarweiser Versuchsanordnung

Die statistische Analyse der erhobenen Daten erfolgte im Paarvergleich zwischen Leerwert und Meßwert (nur dynamische Arbeit). Zur Illustration sind in Tabelle 1 Normalwertsbereiche für hämodynamische Meßwerte (extrapoliert auf eine Steady-State-Belastungsstufe von 42 Watt) von herz-lungen-gesunden Probanden − mittleres Alter 47 a; Körperoberfläche 1,95 m² − angegeben, die zumindest eine Dauerleistung von 100 Watt tolerierten.

Ergebnisse

Die Daten aus Voruntersuchungen über die Akutwirkung von Nitroglyzerin (N = 11) [25] und über den Langzeiteffekt von Fendilin als Monotherapie (N = 7) [19] sind in den Abb. 1 und 3, sowie in der Tabelle 1 wiedergegeben und sollen das Wirkungsspektrum der Einzelsubstanzen hervorstreichen (s. Einleitung).

In Tabelle 2 sind die erhobenen Meßdaten von 11 Koronarkranken wiedergegeben, bei denen unter der Kombinationsbehandlung Fendilin-Oxprenolol auch eine hämodynamische Untersuchung unter körperlicher Belastung nach Nitroglyzeringabe durchgeführt wurde. Die Veränderungen von einzelnen Meßwerten in der untersuchten Patientengruppe sind in Abb. 2 graphisch dargestellt (rechnergesteuertes Plotterdiagramm).

Die Belastungsherzfrequenz vermindert sich unter der Kombinationsbehandlung (2P ≤ 0,10) und bleibt nach Nitroglyzerin unverändert. Die Volumsleistung (Herzindex) nimmt unter körperlicher Belastung im Liegen (mittleres Steady-state

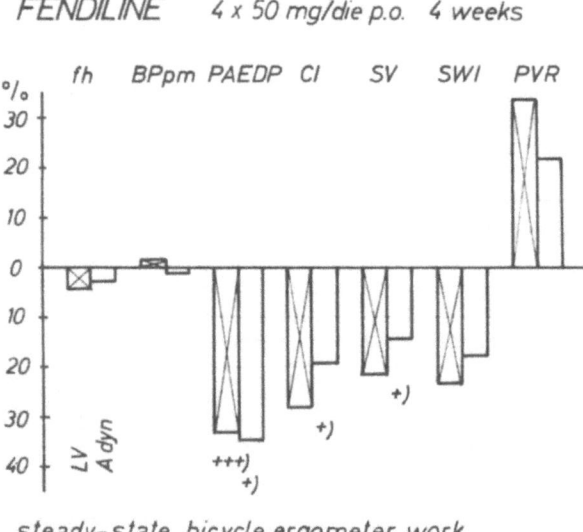

Abb. 1. Einfluß einer 4wöchigen Fendilin (Sensit®)-Therapie auf die zentrale Hämodynamik unter Volumsbelastung (Lagerungsversuch) und unter dynamischer Arbeit. Prozentuelle Abweichung vom Leerwert. LV = Lagerungsversuch: Volumsbelastung durch Anheben der Beine in liegender Position auf die Pedale der Tretkurbel [24]; A dyn = Fahrradergometrie im Liegen [19]

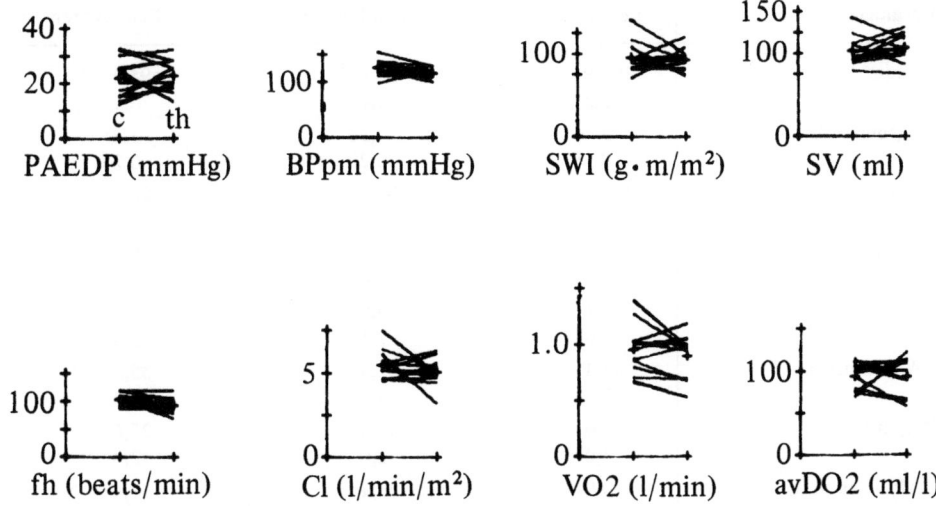

FENDILINE−OXPRENOLOL
Effects on Central Hemodynamics in CHD (N=11, mean load = 42W)

Abb. 2. Individuelle Veränderung von Meßwerten der zentralen Hämodynamik unter der 4wöchigen Kombinationstherapie von Fendilin (3 × 50 mg) mit Oxprenolol (3 × 40 mg). c = Leerwert; th = Kombinationsbehandlung; + = Mittelwert

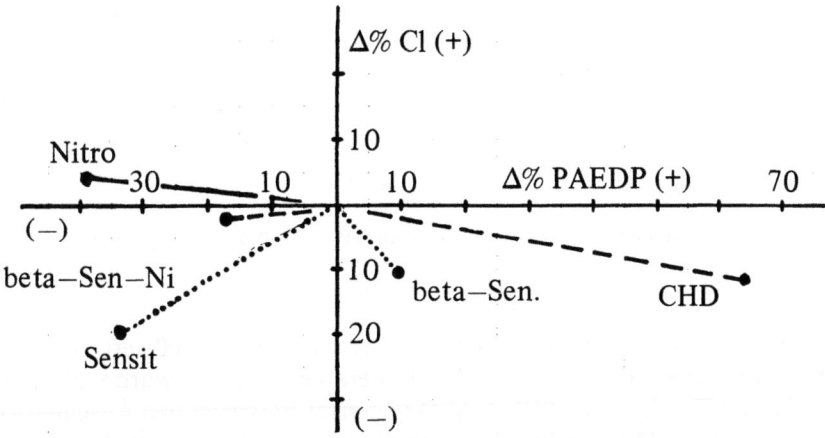

Abb. 3. Belastungshämodynamik bei koronarer Herzkrankheit. Prozentuelle Veränderungen im Herzfunktionsdiagramm (Volumsleistung gegen Füllungsdruck) durch verschiedene Interventionen. CHD = Abweichung von Pat. mit koronarer Herzkrankheit vom Normalverhalten (N = 11; Leerwert aus der Fendilin-Oxprenolol-Studie); Nitro = Akutwirkung von 0,8 mg Nitroglyzerin als Spray (N = 11; aus lit. 25); Sensit = Veränderung nach 4wöchiger Behandlung mit 4 × 50 mg Fendilin (N = 7; aus lit. 19); beta-Sen = Effekt einer 4wöchigen Kombinationsbehandlung von Fendilin (3 × 50 mg) und Oxprenolol (3 × 40 mg), N = 11; beta-Sen-Ni = Akuteffekt einer zusätzlichen Verabreichung von Nitroglyzerin als Spray; N = 11). Mittleres Belastungssteady-state 41 bis 42 Watt. CI = Herzindex l/min/m²; PAEDP = enddiastolischer Pulmonalarteriendruck als Index für den linksventrikulären Füllungsdruck mmHg (s. Tabelle 1)

Tabelle 2. Einfluß der Kombinationsbehandlung Ca^{++}-Antagonist-beta-Rezeptorenblocker auf die Belastungshämodynamik Koronarkranker. Interventionseffekt von Nitroglyzerin

Parameter	Leerwert	Fendilin-Oxprenolol	Fen-Oxpren-Nitro
fh min^{-1}	101,9	$94,4^{(+)}$	95,4 ($\bar{x}$)
	3,3	4,6	5,1 ($s_{\bar{x}}$)
CI $l/min/m^2$	5,44	4,96	$5,28^{+}$
	0,28	0,23	0,23
SV ml	100,5	101,5	$106,8^{(+)}$
	6,2	5,8	6,7
$\dot{V}O2$ l/min	0,96	0,92	$0,98^{++}$
	0,07	0,06	0,06
Dav ml/l	94,7	99,0	101,0
	4,6	7,1	5,4
PASP mmHg	45,4	47,9	$35,3^{+++}$
	3,5	3,2	3,3
PApm mmHg	33,0	35,4	$25,6^{+++}$
	3,0	2,0	2,4
PAEDP mmHg	20,9	23,1	$17,4^{+++}$
	2,2	1,5	1,7
BPpm mmHg	123,6	117,3	117,4
	4,7	3,9	3,5
PVR dyn · sec · cm^{-5}	1005	1032	965
	64	77	59
SWI g · m/m^2	93,8	88,5	$95,5^{+}$
	6,1	3,4	5,2
PulmVR dyn · sec · cm^{-5}	258	311	216^{+++}
	27	28	22
$S\bar{v}$ %	48,2	46,3	46,4
	2,3	3,5	3,1

N = 11; mittlere Belastungsstufe 41,8 Watt (s = 14,0); a = 52,5 (7,8); cm = 171,5 (4,6); kg = 77 (9,6); KO = 1,90 (0,12).
Die Klammer gibt den statistischen Vergleich an (2P: $+ \leq 0,05$; $++ \leq 0,01$; $+++ = 2P \leq 0,001$).

42 Watt) geringfügig ab ($-8,8\%$) und erreicht einen Meßwert, der auch in der Patientengruppe mit Fendilin als Monotherapie errechnet wurde. Nach Nitroglyzerin steigt der Herzindex an ($2P \leq 0,05$) und erreicht wieder den Ausgangswert der Leerwertsphase (5,44 $l/min/m^2$; Normalpersonen: 6,3 $l/min/m^2$). Die geringe Abnahme der Volumsleistung beruht zum Teil auf der Abnahme der Sauerstoffaufnahme und einer etwas deutlicheren Zunahme der arterio-venösen Sauerstoffsättigungsdifferenz ($+4,5\%$). Die Zunahme der Volumsleistung nach Nitroglyzerin beruht vorwiegend auf dem Anstieg der Sauerstoffaufnahme (Ficksches Prinzip).

Die Druckwerte im Lungenkreislauf, insbesondere der enddiastolische Pulmonalarteriendruck, zeigen, wenn auch geringgradig ansteigend, unter der Ca^{++}-Antagonist-beta-Rezeptoren-Blocker-Kombination keine gerichtete Veränderung. Die Akutwirkung von Nitroglyzerin führt zum hochsignifikanten Druckabfall im kleinen Kreislauf ($2P \leq 0,001$), jedoch werden nicht mehr jene „normalisierten" Werte gefunden wie bei alleiniger Applikation von Nitroglyzerin oder auch Sensit

(s. Tabelle 1 und Abb. 3). Die Kombinationsbehandlung Fendilin-Oxprenolol bewirkt eine unbedeutende Abnahme des arteriellen Mitteldruckes ($-5,1\%$ n.sig.) und des Schlagarbeitsindex ($-5,6\%$), der periphere Widerstand bleibt praktisch unverändert, der pulmonalvaskuläre Widerstand steigt an ($+20,5\%$ n.sig.). Unter der angewandten Nitroglyzerindosis (0,8 mg als Spray) bleibt der arterielle Mitteldruck unverändert, der Schlagarbeitsindex steigt an ($2P \leq 0,05$) und der pulmonalvaskuläre Widerstand fällt signifikant ab ($30,5\%$; $2P \leq 0,001$).

Bislang wurden 15 Probanden unter der Kombinationsbehandlung Ca^{++}-Antagonist-beta-Blocker untersucht. Die Symptomatik der koronaren Herzkrankheit blieb während des Beobachtungszeitraumes konstant. Abnorme Reaktionen wie die Entwicklung einer manifesten Herzinsuffizienz oder einer zunehmenden Leistungseinbuße wurden nicht gesehen.

Diskussion

Nach den Ergebnissen hämodynamischer Untersuchungen bei Koronarkranken mit schwerer Leistungseinbuße war die Auswirkung einer Langzeittherapie mit dem Ca^{++}-Antagonisten Fendilin als nitroglyzerinartiger Effekt hinsichtlich der Drucksenkung im Niederdruck-System anzusprechen: unter Volumsbelastung fehlte ein Druckanstieg im Lungenkreislauf wie nach Verabreichung von Nitroglyzerin, so daß bei Konstanz des arteriellen Mitteldruckes ein Wirkungsmechanismus im Sinne eines venösen Pooling anzunehmen ist [19]. Dies steht im Gegensatz zu einem anderen Ca^{++}-Antagonisten, wie Nifedipin, der durch Abnahme des peripheren Widerstandes die Nachlast vermindert und infolge des raschen Wirkungseintrittes zur Therapie des Angina pectoris-Anfalles eingesetzt werden kann [16]. Unter körperlicher Belastung bewirkte Fendilin eine gleichgerichtete Normalisierung des linksventrikulären Füllungsdruckes wie Nitroglyzerin, jedoch wurde im Gegensatz zu Nitroglyzerin eine Abnahme des Herzminutenvolumens gefunden.

Zur Steigerung der täglichen Belastungstoleranz von Koronarkranken erschien uns die Kombination von Fendilin mit einem beta-Rezeptoren-Blocker durchaus sinnvoll, da einerseits der Drucksteigerung im Lungenkreislauf durch den beta-Blocker entgegengewirkt und andererseits durch Absenken der Herzfrequenz die myokardiale Sauerstoffbilanz verbessert werden könnte. Zum anderen sollten aber auch Nebenwirkungen infolge additiver negativ inotroper Effekte bedacht werden.

In der klinischen Beurteilung des Effektes der Kombinationsbehandlung Ca^{++}-Antagonist-beta-Rezeptorenblocker blieb die Symptomatik bei unseren Koronarkranken unverändert im Vergleich zur Vorbehandlung, die zumeist aus der Verabreichung von beta-Blockern in Kombination mit langwirksamen Nitroglyzerinverbindungen bestand. Eine Zunahme der Belastungsdyspnoe, Angina-pectoris-Beschwerden oder gar Symptome einer manifesten Herzinsuffizienz wurden nicht beobachtet.

Unter Ergometerarbeit in liegender Position fanden wir nach 4wöchiger Behandlung mit Sensit® und Trasicor® eine Abnahme der Herzfrequenz ($-7,8\%$ $2P \leq 0,10$). Die erwartete Drucksenkung im Lungenkreislauf, insbesondere die Abnahme des linksventrikulären Füllungsdruckes (PAEDP), wurde nicht gesehen. Es kann aber angenommen werden, daß eine weitere Drucksteigerung über den Leerwert hinaus durch den beta-Blocker abgefangen wurde. Im Vergleich zum Leerwert findet sich eine geringe Abnahme der Volumsleistung, die im Mittel dem Meßwert unter der Monotherapie mit Fendilin entspricht. Die zusätzliche Verabreichung von Nitroglyzerin führt wohl wieder zur Anhebung der Volumsleistung auf den Vergleichswert (Leerwertsphase), jedoch ist die Verminderung des linksventrikulären Füllungsdruckes nicht mehr so deutlich wie bei alleiniger Verabreichung von Nitroglyzerin. Der Mechanismus des venösen Pooling dürfte durch die gleichzeitige Behandlung mit dem Ca-Antagonisten Fendilin bereits zum Großteil genutzt sein, zum anderen sind verstärkt negativ inotrope Einflüsse auf den Herzmuskel durch die Ca^{++}-Antagonist-beta-Rezeptoren-Blocker-Kombination in Betracht zu ziehen.

Erste Ergebnisse über die Kombinationsbehandlung von Nifedipine mit einem beta-Blocker [26, 27] sind nur bedingt vergleichbar, da die Hauptwirkung des Ca^{++}-Antagonisten Nifedipine in der Verminderung der Nachlast mit regulativem Anstieg der Herzfrequenz liegt. Wie in der Kombinationsbehandlung mit Fendilin kann die zusätzliche Erhöhung des Füllungsdruckes durch den beta-Rezeptorenblocker verhindert werden.

Durch die Kombinationsbehandlung zwischen Ca^{++}-Antagonist und beta-Blocker kann durchaus im Einzelfall eine Verbesserung der Belastungshämodynamik erzielt werden. Eine Entscheidung zu dieser Kombinationstherapie oder anderen, die den Einsatz von Nitroglyzerinpräparaten betreffen, sollte im Einzelfall und bevor nicht noch mehr Erfahrungswerte vorliegen nur auf Grund von Meßdaten aus aufwendigeren Funktionsprüfungen (Belastungshämodynamik) getroffen werden.

Literatur

1. Astrand PO (1976) Quantification of exercise capability and evaluation of physical capacity in man. Prog Cardiovasc Dis 19:51
2. Bruce RA (1977) Exercise testing for evaluation of ventricular function. N Engl J Med 296:671
3. Redwood DR, Epstein SE (1972) Uses and limitations of stress testing in the evaluation of ischemic heart disease. Circulation 46:1115
4. Reiterer W (1977) Kriterien der körperlichen Leistungsfähigkeit. Limitierende Faktoren und diagnostische Kriterien des Ausdauerleistungsvermögens. Wien Med Wochenschr [Suppl] 127:42
5. Urbaszek W, Schauer J, Günther K, Modersohn D, Pankau H, Achenbach H (1976) Zur Interpretation des pulmonalarteriellen Druckes bei ischämischer Herzkrankheit. Dtsch Gesundheitswes 31:195
6. Zohmann RL (1977) Exercise stress test interpretation for cardiac diagnosis and functional evaluation. Arch Phys Med Rehabil 58:235
7. Moraski RE, Russel RO, Smith M, Racklay C (1975) Left ventricular function in patients with and without myocardial infarction and one, two or three vessel coronary artery disease. Am J Cardiol 35:1
8. Rentrop P, Petersen J, Roskamm H (1976) Left ventricular function in relation to the severity of coronary artery disease. In: Roskamm H, Hahn C (eds) Ventricular function at rest and during exercise. Springer, Berlin Heidelberg New York, p 71
9. Roskamm H, Samek L, Zweigle K, Stürzenhofecker P, Petersen J, Prokoph J (1977) Die Beziehungen zwischen den Befunden der Koronarangiographie und des Belastungs-EKG bei Patienten ohne transmuralen Myokardinfarkt. Z Kardiol 66:273
10. Stürzenhofecker P, Schnellbacher K, Roskamm H (1976) Cardiac output and filling pressures at rest and during exercise. In: Roskamm H, Hahn C (eds) Ventricular function at rest and during exercise. Springer, Berlin Heidelberg New York, p 28
11. Bretschneider HJ (1972) Die hämodynamischen Determinanten des myokardialen Sauerstoffverbrauches. In: Dengler HJ (Hrsg) Die therapeutische Anwendung beta-sympathikolytischer Stoffe. 4. Rothenburger Gespräch. Schattauer, München, S 45
12. Greeff K (1973) Pharmakotherapie ischämischer Herzerkrankungen. Grundlagen der Physiologie, Pathophysiologie und Pharmakologie. Herz Kreisl 5:239

13. Fleckenstein A, Fleckenstein-Grün G, Byon YK, Courret G (1977) Fundamentale Herz- und Gefäßwirkungen des Ca^{++}-antagonistischen Koronartherapeutikums Fendilin (Sensit®). Arzneim Forsch 27:562
14. Kaltenbach M, Becker HJ, Krehan L, Schulz W (1978) Prüfung der antianginösen Wirksamkeit verschiedener Calzium-Antagonisten. Z Kardiol 67:196
15. König FK, Schneider B (1975) Sensit — ein koronarwirksamer Ca^{++}-Antagonist im Doppelblindversuch mit einem Standardkoronartherapeutikum. Herz Kreisl 7:593
16. Lichtlen P (1975) Coronary and left ventricular dynamics under nifedipine in comparison to nitrates, beta-blocking agents and dipyridamole. In: Lochner W, Braasch W, Krenebarg G (eds) New therapy of ischemic heart disease. Springer, Berlin Heidelberg New York, p 212
17. Lichtlen P, Engel HJ, Amende I, Rafflenbeul W, Simon R (1976) Mechanisms of various antianginal drugs. Relationship between regional flow behavior and contractility. In: Domingos A, Lichtlen PR (eds) New therapy of ischemic heart disease. Excerpta Medica, Amsterdam, p 14
18. Reiterer W (1976) Belastbarkeit Koronargefäßkranker unter Perhexilin (Doppelblindstudie). Herz Kreisl 8:132
19. Reiterer W (to be published) Effects of the Ca^{++}-antagonist fendiline on exercise performance in coronary heart disease evaluated by computer assisted ergospirometry in non-steady-state exercise and by central hemodynamics in steady-state exercise.
20. Singh BN, Roche AHG (1977) Effects of intravenous verapamil on hemodynamics in patients with heart disease. Am Heart J 94:593
21. Spiel R, Enenkel W (1976) Wirkung von Fendilin auf die Belastungsuntersuchung Koronarkranker. Wien Med Wochenschr 126:186
22. Streicher KA, Guckenbiehl W, Olbermann W (1976) Einfluß von Fendilinhydrochlorid (Sensit) im Belastungstest bei Patienten mit koronarer Herzerkrankung. Med Welt 27:1395
23. Vuori I, Kallio V, Hämäläinen H, Pietilä J (1977) Effects of nifedipine and glyzerylnitrate on the ergometric performance of patients after myocardial infarction. Curr Ther Res 20:435
24. Reiterer W, Nissel H, Czitober H (1975) Hämodynamik des Lungenkreislaufes im höheren Alter. Arbeitsgemeinschaft f klin Atemphysiologie, Arbeitstagung Graz, 1975, S 156
25. Reiterer W, Czitober H (1978) Der Einfluß von Nitroglyzerin auf die zentrale Hämodynamik im Lagerungsversuch und unter körperlicher Belastung bei Koronargefäßkranken. Wien Med Wochenschr 128:237
26. Koch G (1978) Kombinierte Beta-Rezeptor- und Calcium-Blockade bei Koronarinsuffizienz: Effekt auf Hämodynamik und Catecholamine. Z Kardiol [Suppl] 5:68
27. Krais T, Rutsch W, Paeprer H, Schmutzler H (1978) Zentrale Ruhe- und Belastungshämodynamik unter Kombinationstherapie mit Beta-Rezeptorenblocker und Calciumantagonist bei Koronarinsuffizienz. Z Kardiol [Suppl] 5:69
28. Reiterer W (1976) Evaluation of physical performance by rectangular-triangular bicycle ergometry and computer-assisted ergospirometry. Basic Res Cardiol 71:482
29. Schnellbacher K, Roskamm H, Reindell H (1974) Der Einfluß einer Beta-Rezeptoren-Blockade auf Leistungsfähigkeit, Hämodynamik und Herzgröße bei Normalpersonen. Herz, Kreisl 8:432

Hämodynamik während belastungsinduzierter Angina pectoris nach einmaliger Gabe von Fendilin und Nifedipin. – Ist die Nitroglycerinwirkung noch nachweisbar?

K. Schnellbacher, D. Kalusche und H. Roskamm

Durch medikamentöse Beeinflussung der Vor- und Nachbelastung des Herzens kann bei vielen Angina pectoris-Patienten die Leistungsfähigkeit angehoben werden. Während für Nitroglycerin eine Senkung der Vorbelastung des Herzens nachgewiesen ist, ist die Beeinflussung der Vorbelastung durch die beiden Calciumantagonisten Fendilin und Nifedipin noch umstritten: Von Interesse war daher für uns die Frage, ob Fendilin und Nifedipin nach einmaliger oraler Gabe die Senkung der Vorbelastung durch Nitroglycerin voll ausschöpfen oder ob durch zusätzliche Gabe von Nitroglycerin eine weitere symptomatische Verbesserung und Senkung des linksventrikulären Füllungsdrucks – als Indikator für die Vorbelastung – erreicht werden kann.

Zur Klärung dieser Frage führten wir bei jeweils 8 typischen Angina pectoris-Patienten, bei welchen meist eine 3- bzw. 2-Gefäßerkrankung des Herzens angiographisch nachgewiesen war, Belastungsuntersuchungen durch; im Leerversuch wurden die Patienten in liegender Position ergometrisch belastet, bis Angina pectoris-Beschwerden oder ein sehr starker Anstieg des Pulmonalkapillardruckes zum Abbruch der Belastung zwangen. Im Anschluß an den Leerversuch erhielten die Patienten 200 mg Fendilin bzw. 20 mg Nifedipin oral und wurden 90 min später unter gleichen Bedingungen ein zweites Mal belastet; auf der höchsten vergleichbaren Belastungsstufe, welche sowohl im Leer- als auch im Medikamentenversuch erreicht wurde, erhielten die Patienten zusätzlich 1 Kap. mit 0,8 mg Nitroglycerin; die Belastung wurde auf der gleichen Belastungsstufe um weitere 6 min verlängert. Da auf der Abbruchstufe des Leerversuchs nach Nifedipin-Gabe drei Patienten noch keine sichere Angina pectoris angaben, wurde bei diesen drei Patienten die Belastungsstufe vor der Nitroglycerin-Gabe nochmals um 25 Watt erhöht. Die Bewertung der Angina pectoris-Symptomatik erfolgte nach einem Punktsystem, wobei ein Punkt dem Beschwerdebeginn, zwei Punkte einer deutlichen Angina pectoris und drei Punkte einer schweren Angina pectoris entspricht, welche zum Abbruch der Belastung bzw. zur Nitroglycerin-Gabe zwingt.

Bei den nachfolgenden Versuchen sind die Effekte von Fendilin und Nifedipin nicht direkt miteinander vergleichbar, da es sich um zwei unterschiedliche Patientenkollektive handelt, wobei das Patientenkollektiv beim Nifedipin-Versuch sicherlich eine ausgeprägtere Belastungscoronarinsuffizienz hatte als das Kollektiv, bei welchem die Fendilin-Versuche durchgeführt wurden. Das Hauptgewicht unserer Untersuchungen liegt auf dem Vergleich der Untersuchungsbefunde zwischen alleiniger Gabe von Fendilin bzw. Nifedipin einerseits und der Kombinationstherapie mit Nitroglycerin andererseits.

Beim Fendilin-Versuch lag die maximale vergleichbare Belastungsstufe im Durchschnitt bei 62 Watt (Abb. 1); während sich unter Fendilin die Beschwerdesymptomatik nur minimal verbesserte, kam es nach Nitroglycerin-Gabe innerhalb von

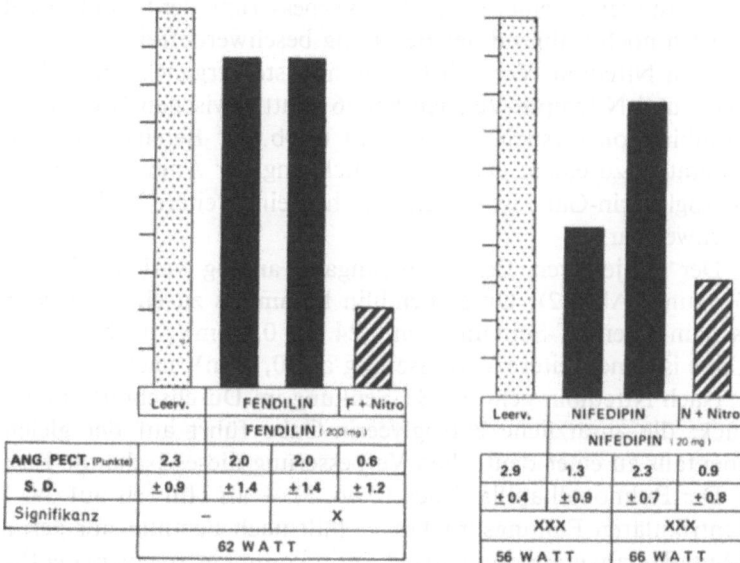

	Leerv.	FENDILIN		F + Nitro
		FENDILIN (200 mg)		
ANG. PECT. (Punkte)	2,3	2.0	2.0	0.6
S. D.	± 0.9	± 1.4	± 1.4	± 1.2
Signifikanz		–		x
	62 W A T T			

Leerv.	NIFEDIPIN		N + Nitro
	NIFEDIPIN (20 mg)		
2.9	1.3	2.3	0.9
± 0.4	± 0.9	± 0.7	± 0.8
	xxx		xxx
56 W A T T		66 W A T T	

Abb. 1. Das Verhalten der Angina pectoris auf der höchsten vergleichbaren Belastungsstufe im Leer- und Medikamenten-Versuch (Fendilin links, Nifedipin rechts) sowie in Kombination mit Nitroglycerin (Skalierung entspricht 100% des Leerwertes)

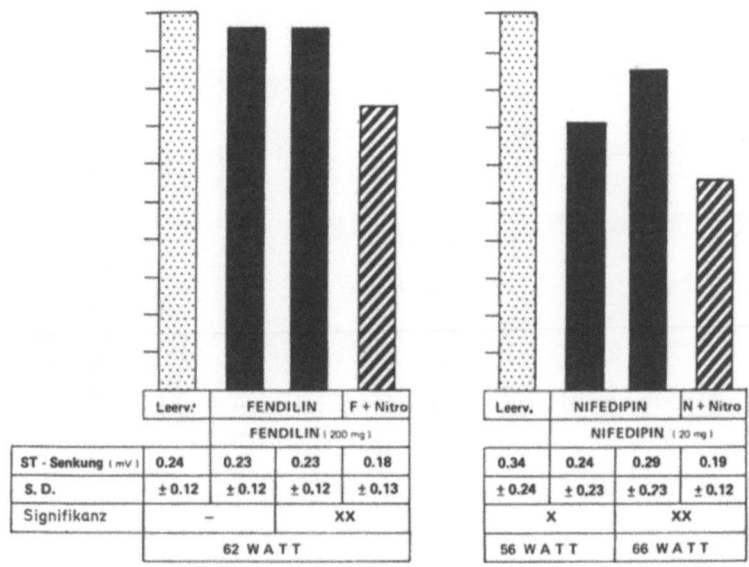

	Leerv.	FENDILIN		F + Nitro
		FENDILIN (200 mg)		
ST - Senkung (mV)	0.24	0.23	0.23	0.18
S. D.	± 0.12	± 0.12	± 0.12	± 0.13
Signifikanz		–		xx
	62 W A T T			

Leerv.	NIFEDIPIN		N + Nitro
	NIFEDIPIN (20 mg)		
0.34	0.24	0.29	0.19
± 0.24	± 0.23	± 0.23	± 0.12
x		xx	
56 W A T T		66 W A T T	

Abb. 2. Das Verhalten der ischämischen ST-Senkung auf der höchsten vergleichbaren Belastungsstufe im Leer- und Medikamenten-Versuch (Fendilin links, Nifedipin rechts) sowie in Kombination mit Nitroglycerin (Skalierung entspricht 100% des Leerwertes)

1 – 2 Minuten zu einer deutlichen Verbesserung der Symptomatik, 5 der 8 Patienten wurden noch während der Belastung beschwerdefrei.

Beim Nifedipin-Versuch lag die höchste vergleichbare Belastungsstufe zwischen Leer- und Nifedipin-Versuch bei 56 Watt, zwischen Nifedipin- und Nitroglycerin-Kombinationsversuch bei 66 Watt (Abb. 1). Bereits unter Nifedipin-Einwirkung kommt es zu einem deutlichen Rückgang der Angina pectoris-Beschwerden, nach Nitroglycerin-Gabe ist jedoch auch hier eine weitere Verbesserung der Symptomatik nachweisbar.

Der subjektiven Beschwerdeangabe analog verhält sich die ischämische ST-Senkung (Abb. 2): Unter Fendilin kommt es zu einer geringen Verbesserung der ischämischen ST-Senkung von 0,24 auf 0,23 mV, nach zusätzlicher Nitroglycerin-Gabe ist eine weitere Verbesserung auf 0,18 mV nachweisbar.

Nach Nifedipin geht die ST-Senkung im Durchschnitt von 0,34 auf 0,24 mV zurück; die zusätzliche Nitroglycerin-Gabe führt auf der gleichen Belastungsstufe ebenfalls zu einer deutlichen Verbesserung dieses Ischämie-Parameters.

Der Pulmonalkapillardruck (Abb. 3) – als Hinweis auf das Verhalten des linksventrikulären Füllungsdruckes – fällt nach Fendilin nur geringgradig von 25 auf 22 mmHg ab; erst unter Nitroglycerin kommt es zu einem deutlichen Abfall um weitere 9 auf 13 mmHg. Im Gegensatz zu Fendilin führt Nifedipin nach 90 Minuten zu einem deutlichen Rückgang des Pulmonalkapillardruckes von 34 auf 24 mmHg; nach zusätzlicher Gabe von Nitroglycerin zeigt der Pulmonalkapillardruck einen weiteren deutlichen Abfall von 26 auf 18 mmHg. Sowohl bei Fendilin- als auch bei Nifedipin-Vorbehandlung (Abb. 4) führt die zusätzliche Gabe von Nitroglycerin bei

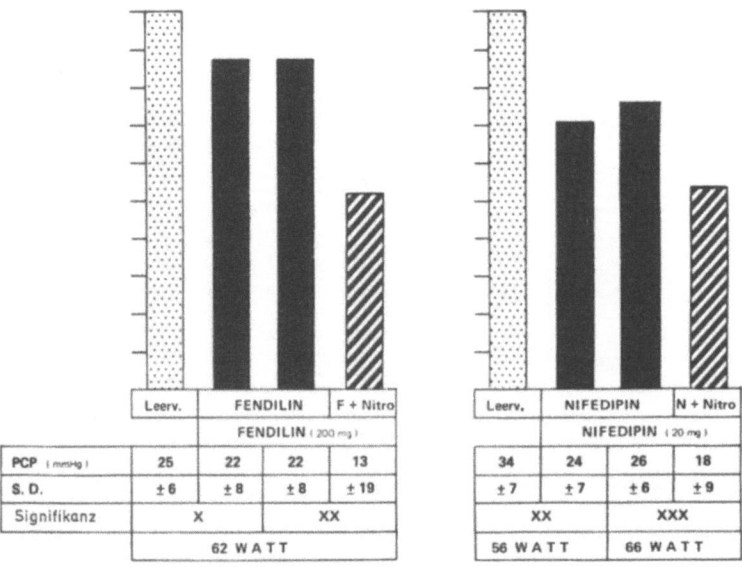

	Leerv.	FENDILIN	F + Nitro	Leerv.	NIFEDIPIN	N + Nitro
		FENDILIN (200 mg)			NIFEDIPIN (20 mg)	
PCP (mmHg)	25	22	22	13	34	24	26	18
S. D.	± 6	± 8	± 8	± 19	± 7	± 7	± 6	± 9
Signifikanz		X		XX		XX		XXX
		62 W A T T			56 W A T T	66 W A T T

Abb. 3. Das Verhalten des Pulmonalkapillardruckes auf der höchsten vergleichbaren Belastungsstufe im Leer- und Medikamenten-Versuch (Fendilin links, Nifedipin rechts) sowie in Kombination mit Nitroglycerin (Skalierung entspricht 100% des Leerwertes)

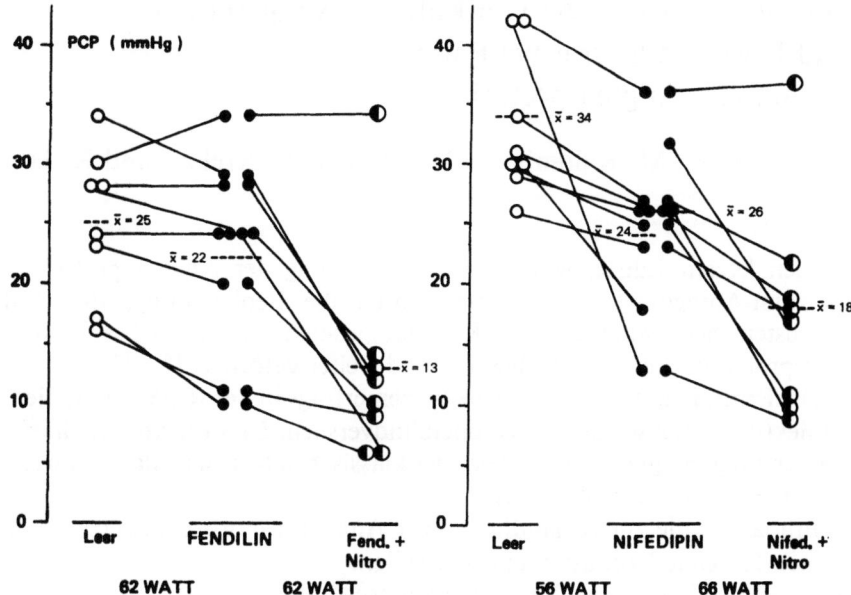

Abb. 4. Bei jeweils 7 von 8 Angina pectoris-Patienten kommt es nach Fendilin (links)- bzw. Nifedipin (rechts)-Vorbehandlung unter Nitroglycerin zu einer weiteren deutlichen Senkung des PC-Druckes auf gleicher Belastungsstufe

7 von 8 Patienten noch während der ergometrischen Belastung zu einem deutlichen Abfall des Pulmonalkapillardruckes in den oberen Normbereich.

Insgesamt sprechen unsere Befunde dafür, daß beide Calciumantagonisten die unter Nitroglycerin mögliche Senkung der Vorbelastung nicht voll ausschöpfen: Die zusätzliche Gabe von Nitroglycerin führt zu einem deutlichen Abfall des linksventrikulären Füllungsdruckes als Indikator für die Senkung der Vorbelastung des Herzens; dem entspricht auch die deutliche Verbesserung der Symptomatik und der ischämischen ST-Senkung. Inwieweit allerdings eine längere Vorbehandlung mit den beiden Calciumantagonisten den Wirkungsmechanismus des Nitroglycerins besser ausschöpft, vermögen wir aufgrund unserer Befunde nicht zu sagen.

Dosiswirkungsrelation von Kalzium-Antagonisten und Isosorbiddinitrat bei Patienten mit stabiler Angina pectoris

H.-J. Becker, M. Kaltenbach, H. Werner, L. Krehan und R. Hopf

In den letzten Jahren wurden zur Behandlung der Angina pectoris zunehmend Kalzium-Antagonisten eingesetzt. Durch die Beobachtung, daß Kalzium-Antagonisten bei Patienten mit Koronarspasmen besser wirksam sind als Beta-Rezeptorenblocker, wurde dieser Trend weiter gefördert [1 – 5].

Die Prüfung antianginöser Substanzen erfolgt in der Regel durch die Beurteilung subjektiver Beschwerden im Doppelblindversuch. Dies führte jedoch oft zu irreführenden Folgerungen, was die Aera der klassischen Koronardilatoren wie Carbochromen bzw. Dipyridamol beweist.

Präparate, die zur Behandlung einer Angina pectoris eingesetzt werden können, sollten folgende Voraussetzungen erfüllen:
1. Die Beseitigung oder Besserung der Ischämie.
2. Die Besserung der Belastbarkeit.
3. Die Beseitigung oder Besserung der Schmerzen.

Das wichtigste Kriterium zur Beurteilung der antianginösen Potenz einer Substanz ist die Beeinflussung der Ischämie. Die Beseitigung oder Besserung der Schmerzen steht erst an 3. Stelle, da eine Analgesie auch ohne Beseitigung der Ischämie möglich ist, was aber für den Koronarkranken fatal sein kann.

Der Parameter der ischämischen ST-Streckensenkungen im Belastungs-EKG eignet sich zur Prüfung der antianginösen Wirksamkeit einer Substanz, wenn folgende Vorsichtsmaßnahmen bzw. Forderungen erfüllt sind:
1. Es dürfen nur Patienten mit gesicherter Koronarsklerose in die Untersuchung einbezogen werden.
2. Die Patienten sollten frei von einer Begleitmedikation sein (Digoxin-Präparate müssen mindestens 14 Tage vorher, kurzwirkende Beta-Rezeptorenblocker 48 Std vorher und langwirkende Nitrate mindestens 24 Std vorher abgesetzt werden).
3. Durch mehrere Vorversuche muß festgestellt sein, daß die Ischämie reproduzierbar ist.
4. Es muß auch während der Belastung eine sorgfältige Ableitungstechnik erfolgen.
5. Neben Leer- und Medikamentenversuchen sind Auslaßversuche und Placebo-Versuche erforderlich.
6. Die Belastungen müssen jeweils zur gleichen Tageszeit vorgenommen werden [6].

Unter diesen strengen Richtlinien wurden von uns 5 verschiedene Kalzium-Antagonisten sowie Isosorbiddinitrat in verschiedenen Dosen geprüft [7 – 12].

Ergebnisse

Prenylamin

Prenylamin gehört zu den ältesten Kalzium-Antagonisten. Es zeigte bei 13 Patienten in einer Dosierung von 240 mg oral keine signifikante Änderung der ischämischen ST-Streckensenkung im Belastungs-EKG.

Verapamil

19 Patienten zeigten 10 min nach i.v. Gabe von 5 mg Verapamil eine Besserung der ischämischen ST-Streckensenkung um 40%.

90 min nach oraler Gabe von 240 mg betrug diese Besserung bei 18 Patienten 23% und nach Gabe von 320 mg bei 24 Patienten 50%.

Demnach handelt es sich hier um eine in hoher Dosierung sicher antianginös wirksame Substanz (s. Tabelle 1).

Nifedipin

Unter Nifedipin konnte akut wie chronisch eine deutliche Besserung der Ischämie nachgewiesen werden.

Bei 18 Patienten, bei denen die Belastung 30 min nach buccaler Applikation durchgeführt wurde, zeigten 17 eine Besserung der ischämischen ST-Streckensenkung von 48%.

Diese Besserung wurde in einer anderen Untersuchungsreihe bei 11 Patienten über 6 Wochen einer täglichen Behandlung mit 3×20 mg Nifedipin unverändert anhaltend nachgewiesen (Abb. 1). Im Auslaßversuch eine Woche nach Beendigung der Therapie mit Nifedipin entsprach die Ischämie der des Vorversuchs [7]. In Einzelfällen kann Nifedipin infolge starker sympathischer Gegenregulation des vasodilatie-

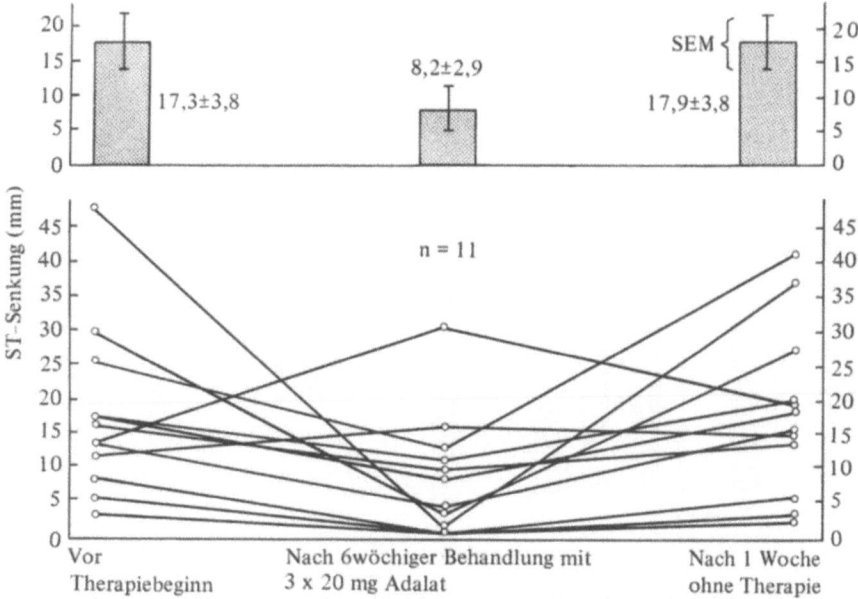

Abb. 1. Die Abbildung zeigt die Beeinflussung der Ischämie bei 11 Patienten unter chronischer Behandlung mit Nifedipin. Daraus ist zu entnehmen, daß auch nach 6 Wochen noch eine gute Wirksamkeit erkennbar ist. Im Auslaßversuch entspricht die Ischämie dem Vorversuch, so daß auf eine länger anhaltende Beeinflussung der Ischämie durch Kalzium-Antagonisten auch nach Absetzen nicht geschlossen werden kann

renden Effektes zu einer Tachykardie führen. Dadurch wird unter Umständen die antianginöse Wirkung überdeckt oder gar eine Angina ausgelöst.

Fendilin

Bei 20 Patienten konnte 135 min nach oraler Gabe von 300 mg Fendilin keine Besserung der ischämischen ST-Streckensenkung beobachtet werden. Auch nach einer 4wöchigen Behandlung mit 3 × 50 mg täglich ließ sich keine Besserung der ischämischen ST-Streckensenkung erkennen. Erst nach dieser chronischen Behandlung und zusätzlicher Gabe von 300 mg, also einer Gesamtdosis von 450 mg, war eine Besserung der ischämischen ST-Streckensenkung um 17% nachweisbar, die gegenüber dem Placeboversuch aber nicht signifikant war. Es muß offenbleiben, ob durch eine weitere Dosissteigerung ein antianginöser Effekt erzielt werden kann (Abb. 2 u. Tabelle 1).

Perhexilinmaleat

15 Patienten, bei denen eine 2wöchige Behandlung mit Perhexilinmaleat in einer Dosierung von 200 mg tgl. durchgeführt wurde, zeigten eine Besserung der ischämischen ST-Streckensenkung von 33%. Die gleichen Patienten zeigten nach 2wöchiger Gabe von 400 mg Perhexilinmaleat täglich eine Besserung von 36%. Eine Verdopplung der Dosis hatte somit nicht eine wesentliche Besserung der Ischämie bewirkt.

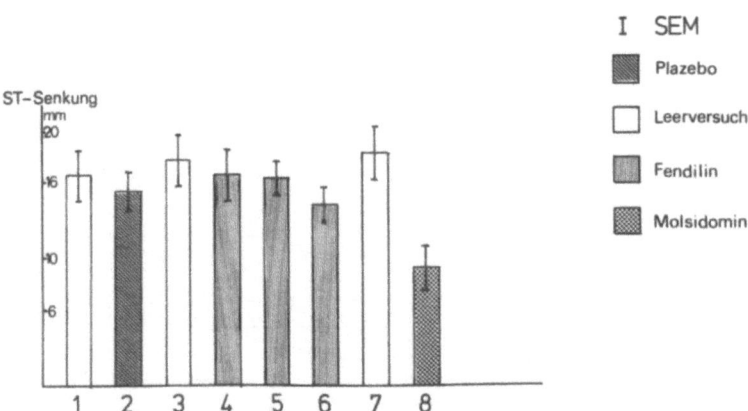

Abb. 2. Beim Vergleich der Wirkung von Molsidomin und Fendilin auf die ischämische ST-Streckensenkung bei 20 Patienten läßt sich erkennen, daß 135 min nach 300 mg (Säule Nr. 4) Fendilin keine Beeinflussung der Ischämie nachweisbar war. Auch nach einer 4wöchigen Behandlung mit 3 × 50 mg (Säule Nr. 5) konnte keine Besserung beobachtet werden. Erst nach zusätzlicher Gabe von 300 mg (Säule Nr. 6) war eine Besserung der ischämischen ST-Streckensenkung erkennbar, jedoch war diese Besserung gegenüber dem Placebo-Versuch nicht signifikant. Unter Molsidomin (Säule Nr. 8) war jedoch eine signifikante Besserung der Ischämie bei dieser Patientengruppe zu erkennen

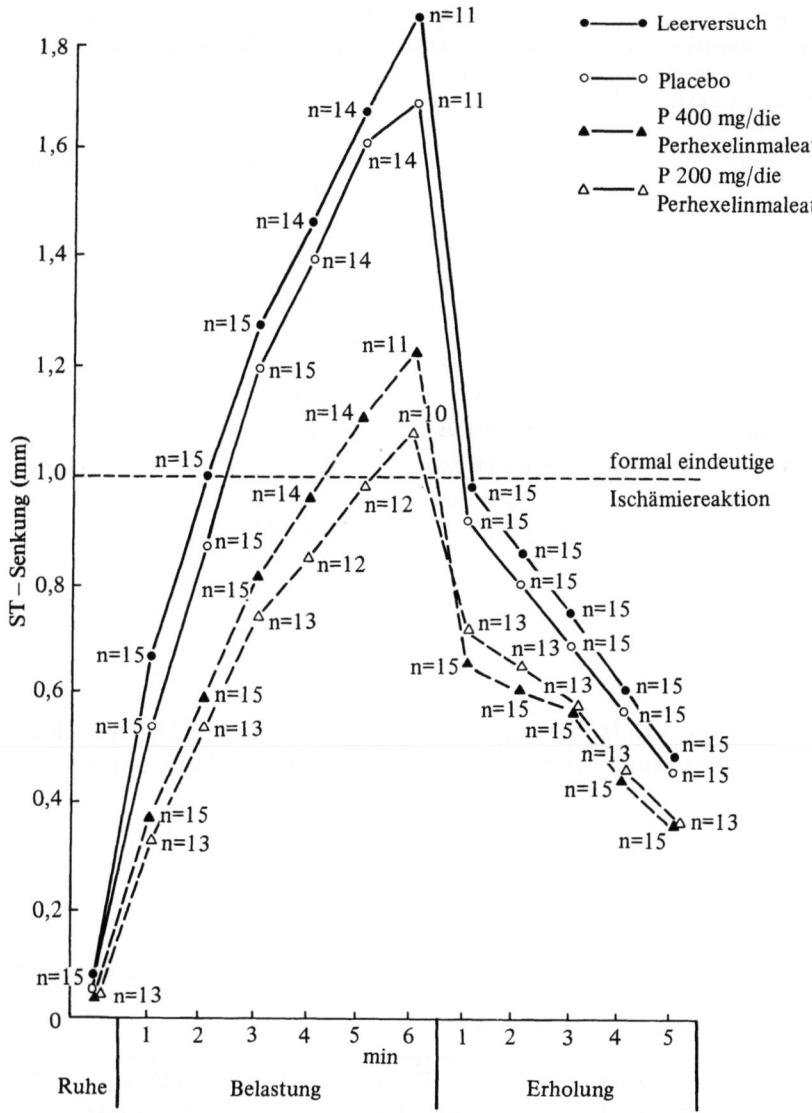

Abb. 3. Aus der Abbildung ist die deutliche Besserung der Ischämie unter Perhexilinmaleat gut erkennbar, wobei die Besserung von 400 mg Tagesdosis gegenüber 200 mg nicht bedeutsam ist

(Abb. 3 u. Tabelle 1) Es wurden aber unter der höheren Dosis wesentlich mehr Nebenwirkungen angegeben.

Tabelle 1. Aus der Tabelle ist die antianginöse Wirksamkeit geprüft am Parameter der ischämischen ST-Streckensenkung im Belastungs-EKG von verschiedenen Kalzium-Antagonisten zu entnehmen. Danach sind Verapamil, Nifedipin und Perhexilinmaleat gut wirksam, während Prenylamin und Fendilin weitgehend unwirksam sind

Substanz	Dosis	Untersuchungszeit nach Applikation (min)	antianginöse Wirkung		n
				%	
Prenylamin	240 mg per os	90	Ø	–	13
Verapamil	240 mg per os	90	+	23	18
	320 mg per os	90	+	50	24
	5 mg i.v.	10	+	40	19
Nifedipin	20 mg per os	30	+	48	18
Fendilin	300 mg per os	135	Ø	–	20
Perhexilinmaleat	200 mg per os	120 – 180	+	33	15
	400 mg per os	120 – 180	+	36	15

Isosorbiddinitrat

Unter Gabe von Isosorbiddinitrat war 120 min nach oraler Applikation je nach Dosis eine Besserung der ischämischen ST-Streckensenkung um 25 – 64% nachweisbar (Abb. 4).

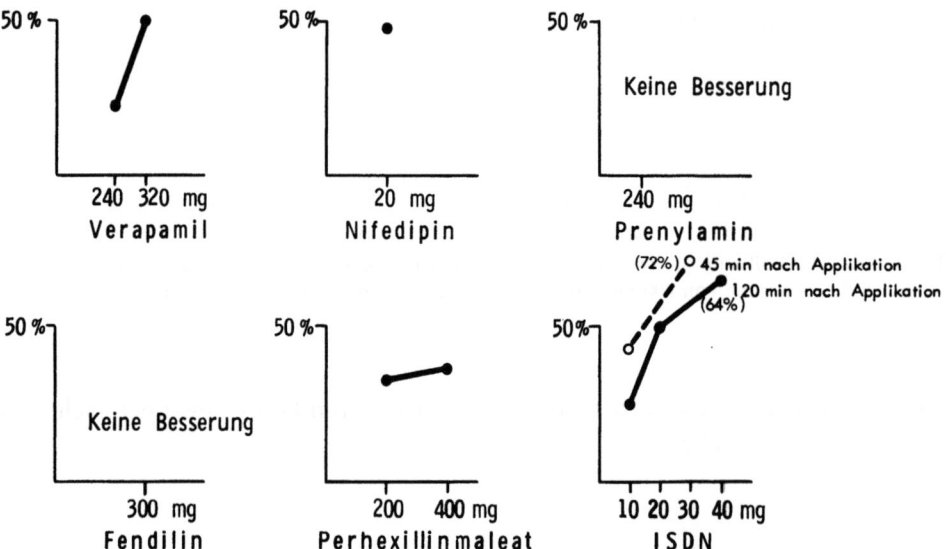

Abb. 4. Gegenüber Perhexilinmaleat ist unter Isosorbiddinitrat mit Steigerung der Dosis auch eine eindeutige Zunahme der Besserung der ischämischen ST-Streckensenkung nachweisbar, die 45 min nach Applikation stärker ist als nach 120 min. 320 mg Verapamil entsprechen in ihrer Wirkung etwa 20 mg Nifedipin

Bei 10 Patienten, bei denen die Belastungsuntersuchung 45 min nach 10 und an einem anderen Tag nach 30 mg Isosorbiddinitrat durchgeführt wurde, zeigten eine Besserung von 43% bei der niedrigeren Dosis und um 72% bei der höheren Dosis (s. Tabelle 2).

Tabelle 2. Hier ist die Beeinflussung der ischämischen ST-Streckensenkung im Belastungs-EKG bei Patienten mit koronarer Herzkrankheit unter verschiedenen Dosen oral applizierten Isosorbiddinitrats zu entnehmen. Danach wird die gute Dosiswirkungsbeziehung erkennbar

	Dosis (mg)	Zeit nach Applikation (min)	Besserung der ST-Senkung (%)	n
Isosorbiddinitrat	10	120	25	11
	20	120	50	24
	40	120	64	7
Isosorbiddinitrat	10	45	43	10
	30	45	72	10

Diskussion

Die Untersuchungsergebnisse machen deutlich, daß es sich bei den Kalzium-Antagonisten nicht um eine einheitliche Substanzgruppe wie etwa die Beta-Rezeptorenblocker handelt. Werden Beta-Rezeptorenblocker in vergleichbaren Dosen gegeben, erzielt man etwa die gleiche Besserung der Ischämie [13]. Enge Dosiswirkungsbeziehungen, wie sie beim Isosorbiddinitrat beobachtet wurden [11, 14, 15], scheinen bei den Kalzium-Antagonisten nicht nachweisbar. So wurde z. B. beim Perhexilinmaleat trotz Verdopplung der Dosis nur eine Wirkungsverbesserung um 3% beobachtet. Der unterschiedliche Wirkungsmechanismus der Kalzium-Antagonisten ist auch von Kaufmann [16] aufgrund seiner Untersuchungen über das Amplituden-Frequenzverhalten des isolierten Papillarmuskels der Katze unter den verschiedenen Wirkstoffen beobachtet werden. Auch Fleckenstein [17] hat auf die unterschiedliche Spezifität und Stärke hingewiesen. Danach ist Nifedipin als der stärkste Kalzium-Antagonist einzuordnen, während Prenylamin und Fendilin nur relativ schwach wirksam sind.

In der Literatur sind unterschiedliche Angaben über die Beeinflussung der ischämischen ST-Streckensenkung durch Fendilin zu finden [18 – 21]. So wurde von Gill und Schneider [19] eine signifikante Reduzierung der ischämischen ST-Senkung beschrieben. Diese Untersuchung ist jedoch nicht relevant, da während der Prüfung z. B. Digitalis-Glykoside zugelassen waren. Die Digitalisierung schließt aber eine Beurteilung der ischämischen ST-Streckensenkung aus.

Von Streicher u. Mitarb. [21] wurde bei 7 von 10 Patienten eine schwache Besserung der ischämischen ST-Streckensenkung unter Fendilin beobachtet. Auch Enenkel und Spiel [18] beobachteten eine Besserung der Ischämie unter Fendilin, jedoch hatten diese Patienten zusätzlich eine Begleitmedikation.

Von anderen Autoren wurden lediglich qualitative Eindrücke über die Wirkung des Fendilin wiedergegeben [20].

Der Einwand, daß die hier untersuchten Patienten, die keinen Effekt unter Fendilin zeigten, für eine Prüfung einer antianginösen Substanz nicht geeignet sind, läßt
sich damit entkräften, daß die gleiche Patientengruppe 60 min nach 2 mg Molsidomin eine signifikante Besserung der Ischämie um 50% aufwies. Auch die Patientengruppe, die Nifedipin erhalten hatte, war mit der, die Fendilin erhielt, vergleichbar
[7, 12].

Die antianginöse Wirksamkeit von Nifedipin wird in der Litertur einheitlicher
beurteilt [3, 4, 8, 11, 22, 23]. Für die Wirkungsweise des Nifedipin sind die Beobachtungen von Kober u. Mitarb. [24, 25] von Bedeutung, die zeigen konnten, daß nach
intrakoronarer Injektion von Nifedipin im Gegensatz zu Nitroglycerin eine deutliche Minderung der ischämischen ST-Streckensenkung im Belastungs-EKG nachzuweisen ist. Dies bedeutet, daß der periphere Effekt, der bei Nifedipin wie auch bei
Verapamil zweifelsohne vorhanden ist, nicht allein für diese Besserung verantwortlich gemacht werden kann. Die intrakoronar verwandte Dosis i.v. gespritzt führt dagegen zu keiner Besserung der Ischämie.

Die Befunde sprechen dafür, daß ein direkter myokardialer Angriffspunkt von
Nifedipin beim Menschen vorliegt. Für die antianginöse Wirkung nicht verantwortlich ist, daß es innerhalb weniger Minuten nach Applikation von Nifedipin zu einer
Koronarflußzunahme kommt, die aber sehr rasch innerhalb weniger Minuten wieder abklingt. Die Besserung der Ischämie wird noch zu einem Zeitpunkt beobachtet,
in dem die Erhöhung des Koronarflusses längst abgeklungen ist (5 Minuten resp. 60
Minuten). Die hier vorgelegten Ergebnisse nach Gabe von Perhexilinmaleat entsprechen denen der Arbeitsgruppe von Rudolph [26].

Zusammenfassung

Die Untersuchungen zeigen, daß die antianginöse Potenz der verschiedenen
Kalzium-Antagonisten sehr unterschiedlich ist.

Zu den gut wirksamen antianginösen Substanzen gehören Verapamil, Nifedipin
und das etwas schwächer wirksame Perhexilinmaleat.

Zu den weitgehend unwirksamen Substanzen gehören Prenylamin sowie
Prenylamin-Derivate.

Im Gegensatz zu Beta-Rezeptorenblockern können Kalziumantagonisten bei Patienten mit Koronarspasmus oder koronarspastischer Komponente unbedenklich
empfohlen werden.

Literatur

1. Cherrier F, Neimann J-L, Groussin P, Aliot E, Cuilliere M, Feisel J (1978) Prinzmetal angina: A
   study of 100 cases. In: Kaltenbach M, Lichtlen P, Balcon R, Bussmann WD (eds) Coronary heart
   disease. Thieme, Stuttgart, pp 191–198

2. Ekelund LG, Atterhög JH, Melin AL (1973) Effect of nifedipine on exercise tolerance in patients with angina pectoris. In: Hashimoto K, Kimua E, Kobayashi T (eds) I. International Nifedipine Adalat (R) Symposion Tokyo 1973. University Tokyo Press, Tokyo, pp 144 – 149

3. Hopf R, Schmidt H, Kaltenbach M (1978) Kombination von Isosorbiddinitrat mit Nifedipin bei der Behandlung der koronaren Herzkrankheit. Z Kardiol [Suppl] 5:67

4. Lichtlen P, Engel HJ, Wolf R (1978) Calcium-Antagonisten in der Therapie der Angina pectoris. Z Kardiol [Suppl] 5:66

5. Roskamm H (1978) Grundlage, Anwendung und Wirkung der Behandlung mit Beta-Blockern bei koronarer Herzkrankheit. Z Kardiol [Suppl] 5:58

6. Henkels U, Blümchen G (1977) Tageszeitliche Schwankungen der Belastungs-Koronarinsuffizienz. Münch Med Wochenschr [Suppl 1] 119:58 – 63

7. Becker H-J, Kaltenbach M, Kober G (1975) Comparison of the effects of nifedipine with other substances on the myocardial ischemia ander loading conditions. In: Lochner W, Braasch W, Kroneberg G (eds) II. International Adalat Symposion. Springer, Berlin Heidelberg New York, pp 156 – 163

8. Gräf V, Becker H-J, Kober G, Kaltenbach M (1971) Evaluation of different antianginal drugs. In: Kaltenbach M, Lichtlen P (eds) Coronary heart disease. Thieme, Stuttgart, pp 181 – 189

9. Hunscha H-G, Kaltenbach M, Schellhorn W (1966) Zur Therapie der Angina pectoris. Objektive Prüfung von Medikamentenwirkungen mit Hilfe von Arbeitsversuchen. Therapiewoche 16:1153

10. Kaltenbach M (1970) Medikamentöse Therapie der Angina pectoris. Arzneim Forsch 20:1304 – 1310

11. Kaltenbach M, Kober G, Schulz W, Becker H-J, Werner H, Hopf R (1978) Antianginal activity of calcium – inhibitive drugs and isosorbid dinitrate. In: Kaltenbach M, Lichtlen P, Balcon R, Bussmann WD (eds) Coronary heart disease. Thieme, Stuttgart, pp 301 – 307

12. Werner H (1978) Einfluß von Fendilin und Molsidomin auf Herzfrequenz, Blutdruck und ischämische ST-Streckensenkung im Belastungs-EKG bei Koronarkranken. Inaugural Dissertation, Frankfurt/M

13. Becker H-J, Kaltenbach M (to be published) Zur antianginösen Wirkung verschiedener Beta-Rezeptorenblocker bei Verwendung äquipotenter Dosen. Herz/Kreislauf

14. Becker H-J, Walden G, Kaltenbach M (1976) Gibt es eine „Tachyphylaxie" bzw. Gewöhnung bei der Behandlung der Angina pectoris mit Nitrokörpern. Verh Dtsch Ges Inn Med 82:1208 – 1210

15. Hennermann K-H (to be published) Vergleich von Isosorbiddinitrat in retardierter und nicht retardierter Form bei der Beeinflussung der ischämischen ST-Streckensenkung im Belastungs-EKG. Inaugural Dissertation, Frankfurt/M

16. Kaufmann R (1977) Differenzierung verschiedener Kalzium-Antagonisten. Munch Med Wochenschr [Suppl 1] 119:6 – 11

17. Fleckenstein A (1977) Specific pharmacology of calcium in myocardium, cardiac pacemakers an vascular smooth muscle. Annu Rev Pharmacol Toxicol 17:149 – 166

18. Enenkel W, Spiel R (1978, to be published) Effekt von Fendilin auf Belastungs-EKG und Belastungshämodynamik bei Koronarkranken. Calcium-Antagonismus Ffm. Springer, Heidelberg

19. Gill E, Schneider B (1977) Doppelblindstudie mit einem Calcium-Antagonist. Z Praeklin Klin Geriatr 6:77

20. Schmidt-Voigt J (1975) Therapie der Angina pectoris. Fortschr Med 93:1423 – 1429

21. Streicher KA, Guckenbiel W, Olbermann W (1976) Einfluß von Fendilinhydrochlorid (Sensit) im Belastungstest bei Patienten mit koronarer Herzerkrankung. Med Welt 27:1395 – 1397

22. Grandjean T, Valenti P, Cherifi MA (1977) Wirkung von Adalat auf die Belastungstoleranz und linksventrikuläre Funktion bei Patienten mit Angina pectoris. Munch Med Wochenschr [Suppl 1] 119:48 – 52

23. Wick E, Strodter D (1977) Die Angina pectoris Schwelle vor und nach Nifedipin. Munch Med Wochenschr [Suppl 1] 119:53 – 57

24. Kaltenbach M, Kober G, Schulz W, Bamberg E (1978) Cardiac and peripheral action of a calcium inhibitive antianginal drug. VIII. World Congress of Cardiology 1978 in Tokyo Congress-abstract

25. Schulz H, Kober G, Bamberg E, Kaltenbach M (1978) Antianginöse Wirkung des Calcium-Antagonisten Nifedipin bei intrakoronarer und intravenöser Applikation. Z Kardiol [Suppl] 5:66

26. Goebel G, Mannes GA, Kafka W, Fleck E, Rudolph W (1977) Behandlung der Angina pectoris mit Perhexilinmaleat. Herz 3:289 – 297

Effekt von Fendilin auf Belastungs-EKG und Belastungshämodynamik bei Koronarkranken

W. Enenkel und R. Spiel

Mit der Gruppe der Calcium-Antagonisten steht uns in der Therapie der Angina pectoris ein neues therapeutisches Prinzip zur Verfügung. Die Wirkung dieser Substanzgruppe im Tierexperiment wurde von Fleckenstein analysiert, andere Untersucher haben die Ergebnisse bestätigt.

Klinische Untersuchungen mit Calcium-Antagonisten bei Patienten mit stabiler Angina pectoris liegen derzeit noch in nicht sehr großer Zahl vor. Das liegt wohl zum Teil auch daran, daß die Wirksamkeit antianginöser Substanzen schwer objektivierbar und die Methodik der Objektivierbarkeit häufig umstritten ist.

Im folgenden soll der Versuch beschrieben werden, mit Hilfe von ergometrischen Arbeitsversuchen die Wirkung von Fendilin bei Patienten mit Angina pectoris zu objektivieren.

Patientengut und Methodik

Untersucht wurden 21 Patienten, 14 Männer und 7 Frauen, mit gesicherter Angina pectoris. Die Diagnose wurde aus belastungsabhängigen typischen Herzschmerzen und den typischen ST-Streckenveränderungen im Belastungs-EKG gestellt. Kein Patient erhielt während der Untersuchungsphase Digitalisglykoside. Alle Patienten waren in einer stabilen Phase der Erkrankung.

Als Ausschlußkriterien galten Myokardinfarkt in der Vorgeschichte, klinische Zeichen einer Herzinsuffizienz und Alter über 65 Jahre.

Bei allen Patienten wurden 2 Belastungsuntersuchungen ausgewertet und zwar eine nach einer mindestens 28 Tage dauernden Therapie mit Langzeitnitriten und eine zweite nach einer Behandlungsdauer von 28 Tagen mit Fendilin (200 mg/Tag per os).

Die ergometrischen Arbeitsversuche wurden in liegender Position mit einem drehzahlunabhängigen Ergometer in rektangulärer Belastung nach dem relativen steady state Prinzip durchgeführt. Die Untersuchungen erfolgten vormittags 2 Std nach Einnahme des Medikamentes.

Gemessen und registriert wurden in Abständen von 1 min vor, während und nach Belastung folgende Parameter:

12-Ableitungs-EKG	arterieller Blutdruck
Herzfrequenz	Pulmonalarteriendruck (Swan-Ganz-Katheter).

Beim ersten Arbeitsversuch wurde immer eine Ausbelastung angestrebt, international anerkannte Abbruchkriterien jedoch streng beachtet. Bei der zweiten Ergometrie wurde immer mindestens die höchste Belastungsstufe des ersten Tests erreicht, um dadurch Vergleiche der haemodynamischen Situation zu ermöglichen. Bei einigen Patienten war unter Fendilin eine höhere Belastungsstufe möglich.

Ergebnisse

1. *Herzschlagfrequenz.* Zwischen der Behandlungsphase mit Nitriten und der Behandlungsphase mit Fendilin zeigten die Mittelwerte der Herzfrequenz weder in Ruhe noch in den einzelnen Belastungsstufen einen statistisch signifikanten Unterschied (Abb. 1). Trotzdem fanden wir in Einzelfällen während der Fendilin-Therapie schon in Ruhe eine höhere Herzfrequenz, bei Belastung stieg die Frequenz auf höhere Werte an als während der Nitrittherapie. Die so reagierenden Patienten zeigten unter Fendilin auch zumeist einen etwas niedrigeren arteriellen Blutdruck.

2. *Arterieller Blutdruck.* Die arteriellen Blutdruckwerte zeigten ein ähnliches Verhalten. Sowohl die Ruhewerte als auch die Belastungswerte des systolischen und des diastolischen Druckes zeigten bei Vergleich der beiden Behandlungsphasen keinen statistischen Unterschied ihrer Mittelwerte (Abb. 2). Es muß jedoch darauf hingewiesen werden, daß bei einzelnen Fällen unter Fendilin die Blutdruckwerte niedriger lagen, was zumeist mit höheren Herzfrequenzen einherging. Auf einzelne Patienten, die während der Fendilin-Therapie höhere arterielle Blutdruckwerte aufwiesen als unter Nitrit-Therapie, wird später noch kurz eingegangen werden.

3. *Pulmonalarteriendrucke.* Die statistische Auswertung der enddiastolischen Pulmonalarteriendrucke (PADP) ergab, daß zwischen den beiden Therapiephasen kein signifikanter Unterschied bestand. Die Mittelwerte sowohl in Ruhe als auch in den einzelnen Belastungsstufen zeigten also keine signifikante Differenz (Abb. 3). Beim PADP traten jedoch die größten Streuungen auf, die Analyse dieser Einzelwerte ist hier aufschlußreicher als die Betrachtung der Mittelwerte.

In Ruhe hatten 9 Patienten unter Fendilin-Therapie einen niedrigeren PADP, 6 Patienten unter Nitrit-Therapie, bei 6 Patienten waren die Werte gleich hoch.

Unter Belastung waren die PADP-Werte während Fendilin-Therapie bei 13 Patienten niedriger, während Nitrit-Therapie bei 8 Patienten.

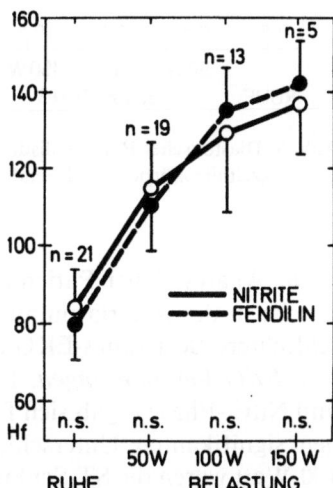

Abb. 1. Herzschlagfrequenz. Die geringfügigen Unterschiede erreichen in keiner Belastungsstufe statistisches Signifikanzniveau

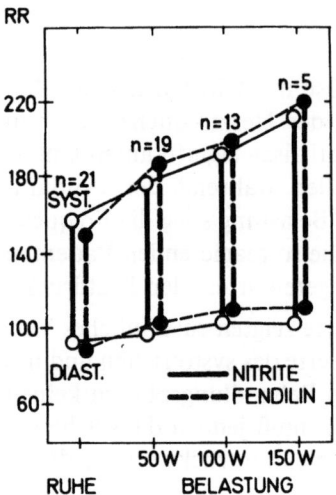

Abb. 2. Blutdruckverhalten. Weder in Ruhe noch bei dynamischer Belastung zeigen sich statistisch zu sichernde Unterschiede der gemittelten Blutdruckwerte

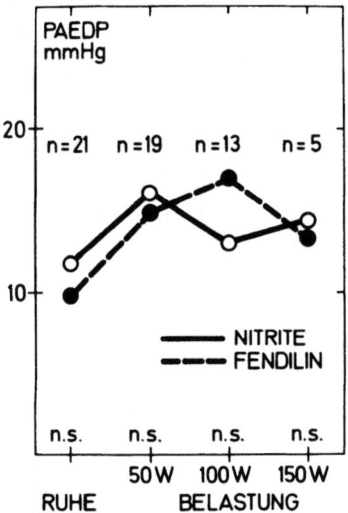

Abb. 3. Diastolischer Pulmonalisdruck. Kein wesentlicher Unterschied zwischen gemittelten Werten unter Langzeitnitrokörpern und Fendilin

Die Analyse jener Patienten, die während Fendilin-Therapie höhere Belastungsdrucke in der Arteria pulmonalis aufwiesen, ergab, daß diese Patienten auch das schlechtere Belastungs-EKG und die höheren arteriellen Blutdrucke zeigten.

4. *EKG-Veränderungen.* Beim Vergleich der ST-Senkung zwischen Sensit-Phase und Nitrit-Phase ergab sich folgendes: Die Ruhe-Elektrokardiogramme zeigten keinen signifikanten Unterschied. In den Belastungsstufen von 50 Watt und von 100 Watt waren die ST-Senkungen in der Sensit-Phase signifikant geringer als in der

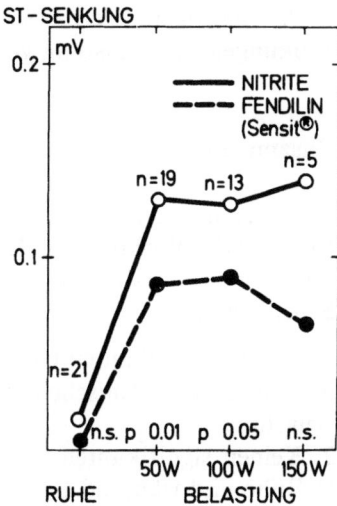

Abb. 4. Gemittelte ST-Streckensenkung. Keine Unterschiede in Körperruhe; während Belastung deutlicher Rückgang der ST-Senkung in der Fendilin-Phase (50 und 100 Watt p = 0,01 bzw. 0,05; 150 Watt nicht signifikant)

Nitrat-Phase. Bei 150 Watt war auf Grund der kleinen Fallzahl keine Signifikanz zu errechnen (Abb. 4). Beurteilt man den Einzelfall, findet man unter Fendilin-Therapie bei der Hälfte der Patienten eine Besserung der ST-Streckensenkung um mehr als 0,5 mm (= 0,05 mV), bei einem Viertel der Patienten eine Verschlechterung.

Diskussion

Der Vergleich der Wirkung von Fendilin gegen Nitrokörper wurde deshalb gewählt, weil Nitrite bzw. Nitrate als allgemein anerkanntes Therapieprinzip gelten und aus früheren Untersuchungen die Auswirkung von Langzeitnitriten auf den ergometrischen Arbeitsversuch bekannt ist.

Methodisch mag anfechtbar sein, daß es sich um eine offene Studie ohne crossover und ohne Leerversuch handelt. Wir haben daher derzeit eine Studie laufen, die diese Einwände berücksichtigt.

Trotzdem glauben wir aussagen zu können, daß Fendilin auf den ergometrischen Arbeitsversuch bei Patienten mit stabiler Angina pectoris gleich gut wirkt wie Langzeitnitrite. Nur bei wenigen Patienten stieg unter Fendilin der Belastungsdruck in der Pulmonalarterie stärker an als unter Nitriten, was praktisch immer mit einem schlechteren Belastungs-EKG und höheren arteriellen Blutdruckwerten verbunden war.

Die negativ inotrope Wirkung des Präparates scheint also nicht für den Anstieg des PADP verantwortlich zu sein. Eher muß man annehmen, daß bei den Patienten das Medikament nicht gleich gut imstande war wie Nitrite, das Herz während Belastung vor einer Ischaemie zu schützen. Das ausgeprägtere ischaemische Areal führte zu deutlicheren EKG-Veränderungen und zu einem stärkeren Anstieg des PADP.

Das häufigere Verhalten bestand jedoch darin, daß unter Fendilin die ST-Senkungen bei Belastung geringer und die PADP-Werte niedriger waren.

Zusammenfassung

Die Wirkung von Fendilin (Sensit®) wurde bei 21 Patienten mit stabiler Angina pectoris mit der Wirkung von Langzeitnitriten verglichen. Der Vergleich der ergometrischen Arbeitsversuche unter der Wirkung von Nitriten und unter der Wirkung von Sensit® ergab:

1. Keinen signifikanten Unterschied der Mittelwerte von Herzschlagfrequenz, systolischem und diastolischem arteriellen Blutdruck in Ruhe und während maximaler Belastung.
2. Keinen signifikanten Unterschied der enddiastolischen Pulmonalarteriendrucke in Ruhe und während Belastung.
3. Signifikant geringere ST-Senkungen während Belastung unter der Wirkung von Fendilin.
4. Veränderungen der Haemodynamik gehen mit einer Verbesserung bzw. Verschlechterung der ischaemischen ST-Veränderungen parallel.

Change in Exercise Tolerance in Patients with Angina Pectoris Induced by Administration of a Calcium-Blocker, Nifedipine (Adalat), Alone or in Combination with Beta-Blockers

L.-G. Ekelund

In an earlier study [1], nifedipine induced a significant increase in exercise tolerance after acute administration to patients with angina pectoris. As the effect of nifedipine (Adalat) during prolonged treatment is not sufficiently clear [2], the present subacute study was undertaken.

Material and Methods

Twenty-one patients, aged 53 – 68 years (mean 60,3), previously treated for at least 6 months with beta-blockers for angina pectoris entered the study. All had a classical history of angina pectoris of effort, mean duration 3.9 years, which had been stable for at least 6 months. All patients had performed 2 or more exercise tests before the study.

During the first period of 3 weeks the patients were treated with their ordinary beta-blocker. This was followed by two similar periods, each of 2 – 4 weeks, (usually 3 weeks treatment), with 10 mg Adalat 3 times daily or identical placebo tablets. Adalat and placebo were randomized. After the third period the patients were switched over to a combination of their ordinary beta-blocker and Adalat without any placebo administration. The Adalat and placebo capsules were given to the patients in the laboratory 30 min before the start of exercise tests and the beta-blocker 60 – 90 min earlier.

A diary card showing the number of nitroglycerine tablets taken each day, the number of anginal attacks, and the daily and weekly subjective assessments of angina pectoris symptoms was completed by the patient.

Exercise tests were performed in the sitting position on an electrically braked bicycle ergometer (EM 380, Siemens-Elema, Sweden) according to a standardized procedure with step-wise increasing work loads. The same bicycle was used throughout the study. All external influences were standardized and the patients were not allowed to smoke during the 2 h before the test. The electrocardiograms were monitored continuously and recorded intermittently.

The atrioventricular conduction time was measured from a resting electrocardiogram, using a magnifier taking the mean of 5 consecutive beats. The measurements were made without knowledge of the type of medication. Perceived exertion was estimated on a 16 point scale and corresponding scales were constructed for grading angina pectoris, dyspnea, and the sensation of fatigue in the legs [3].

Results

Clinical Assessments

There was a mean reduction in the number of attacks per week during Adalat treatment compared to placebo, but the difference was not significant. With the

combination (Adalat + beta-blocker), however, the reduction was highly significant ($p < 0.001$). The consumption of nitroglycerine was significantly reduced after
Adalat, $p < 0.05$, and after the combination $p < 0.001$ in comparison to the
placebo period. At the end of the study 18 patients preferred the combination, 2
patients either Adalat or the combination and one patient Adalat alone.
Disregarding the combination there was equal preference for Adalat and beta-
blocker.

Cardiovascular Effects

At rest there was a significant increase in heart rate, 5 beats/min, after Adalat
compared to placebo (Fig. 1). After Adalat + beta-blocker there was no significant
change in heart rate at rest. There were highly significant decreases in systolic and
diastolic blood pressure at rest after Adalat compared to placebo, 17 and 10 mmHg
respectively, and a more marked decrease after Adalat + beta-blocker, 29 and
16 mmHg, respectively (Fig. 2).

The atrioventricular conduction time was unchanged both after Adalat alone and
Adalat + beta-blocker compared to the placebo both in absolute values and after
correction for the variation induced by change in heart rate according to the
observed regression equation:

$$(PQ = 24.6 - 0.10 \times HR; \quad n = 21; \quad r = 0.41).$$

In standing position during the orthostatic test the difference in heart rate
between Adalat and placebo was about the same as in the supine position, but the
decrease in systolic blood pressure was somewhat smaller. After Adalat + beta-
blocker the orthostatic response was markedly diminished in respect to change in
heart rate but the response was unchanged in respect to systolic blood pressure.

During exercise at comparable loads there was no significant difference in heart
rate after Adalat compared to placebo, but a significantly lower heart rate after
Adalat + beta-blocker (20 beats/min, Fig. 3). Adalat alone gave a highly significant
decrease in systolic blood pressure of 18 mmHg but the combination with beta-
blocker gave a further decrease in systolic blood pressure, mean difference
37 mmHg (Fig. 4).

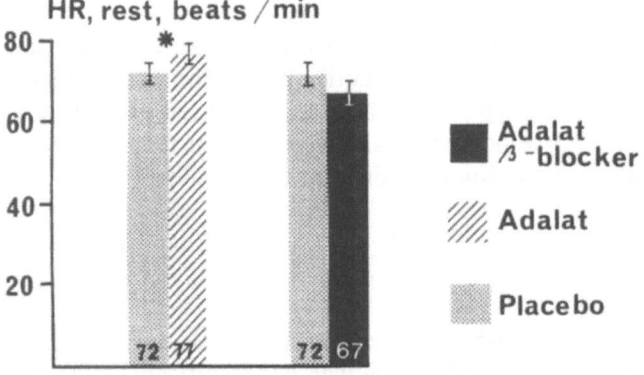

Fig. 1

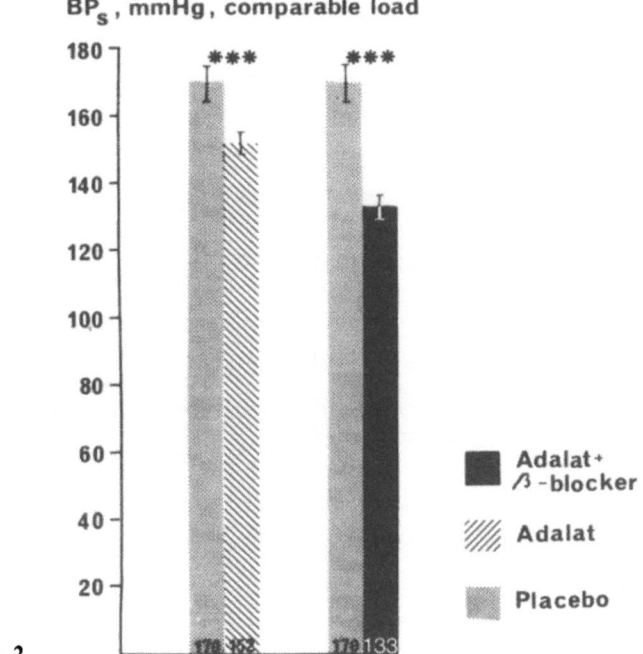

Fig. 2

At the end of the exercise at a higher load the heart rate was significantly higher, 6 beats/min after Adalat but significantly lower after Adalat + beta-blocker, 18 beats/min. In spite of the higher work load, the systolic blood pressure was still significantly lower after Adalat compared to placebo and further lower after Adalat + beta-blocker. The respiratory frequency at comparable load showed no significant variation between the different periods.

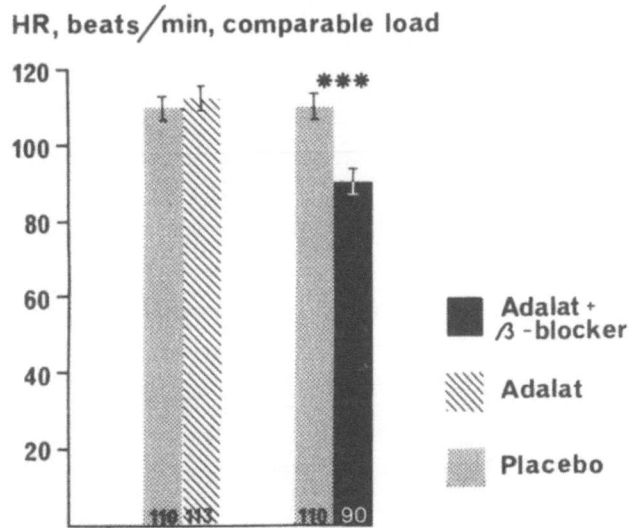

Fig. 3

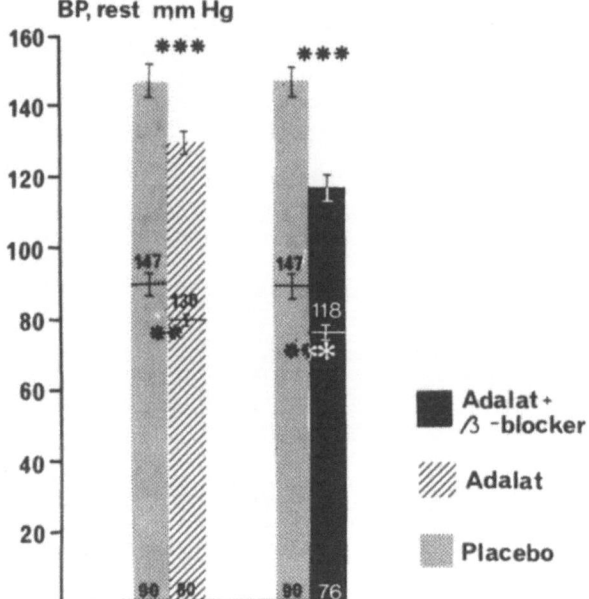

Fig. 4

Working Capacity

The exercise tolerance expressed as total work was significantly increased after Adalat compared to placebo and increased on an average by 20%, Fig. 5. The combination of Adalat + beta-blocker gave a mean increase of 41% in total work

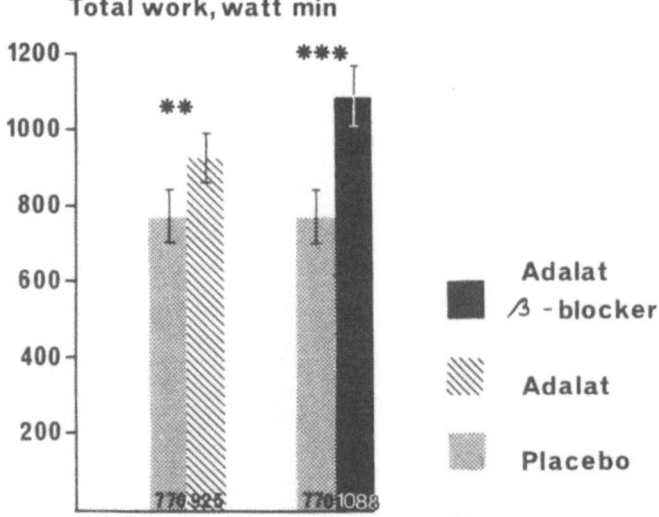

Fig. 5

(Fig. 5). Work load at break point, W_B, also increased significantly both after Adalat alone compared to placebo and Adalat + beta-blocker. The increase in total work after Adalat and Adalat + beta-blocker, respectively, was correlated positively to the systolic blood pressure at rest during the placebo period and also negatively to the change induced by Adalat and Adalat + beta-blocker, respectively, in systolic blood pressure during exercise at comparable loads.

The patients who increased their exercise tolerance expressed as total work by 15% or more were regarded as responders. Using this criterium 13 patients were responders to Adalat compared to placebo and 16 patients were regarded as responders to Adalat + beta-blocker.

Side-Effects

No serious side effects were observed with Adalat or the combination, only a slight facial reddening in three cases during Adalat alone but not during Adalat + beta-blocker. One patient developed ankle oedema after Adalat treatment and another patient had a slight tendency for the same type of ankle oedema.

Discussion

In the present investigation with a subacute study we found a fall in blood pressure after Adalat of the same magnitude at rest as in the earlier study by Atterhög et al. [1], but a more marked fall during exercise. The compensatory increase in heart rate was not so pronounced in the present study, with only a small increase at rest and no significant change during exercise at comparable loads. Adalat significantly increased exercise tolerance compared to placebo, the change being of the same order as in the acute study. The increase in exercise tolerance is certainly due mostly to the decrease in systolic blood pressure, with diminished heart work during exercise, which explains the correlation between change in systolic blood pressure during exercise and percentage change in exercise tolerance. The increase in exercise tolerance after Adalat compared to placebo was of the same magnitude as reported for beta-blockers and in the present study there was no significant difference between the period with Adalat and the period with the beta-blocker alone. The increase in exercise tolerance fits well with the subjective improvement rated from the decrease in nitroglycerine consumption and the decrease in daily attacks of angina. The combination of Adalat with the patients previous beta-blocker gave a further improvement in exercise tolerance which also was related to the initial systolic blood pressure at rest and to the drug-induced change in systolic blood pressure during exercise.

The Adalat induced decrease in systolic and diastolic blood pressure, both at rest and during exercise and specially that induced by the combination of Adalat and beta-blocker, indicates the use of these drugs in treatment of essential hypertension [4, 5].

A very interesting and important finding is the resistance of the atrioventricular conduction system to the influence of Adalat alone or even combined with a beta-blocker, as indicated by the unchanged atrioventricular conduction time. This is in marked contrast to the other calcium inhibiting drug, verapamil, which significantly prolongs the atrioventricular conduction time and which in combination with a beta-blocker may cause serious disturbances of the atrioventricular conduction.

References

1. Atterhög J-H, Ekelund L-G, Melin A-L (1975) Effect of nifedipine on exercise tolerance in patients with angina pectoris. Eur J Clin Pharmacol 8:125
2. Andersson K-E, Ekelund L-G, Johansson BW, Landmark K (1978) Calciumantagonists (Ca-blockers). Pharmacological, physiological and clinical aspects. Proc. from a meeting in Vedbaeck, Denmark 1977. Acta Pharmacol Toxicol (Kbh) 43:1
3. Borg G (1970) Perceived exertion as an indicator of somatic stress. Scand J Rehabil Med 2 – 3:92
4. Ekelund L-G, Orö L (1979) Antianginal efficiency of Nifedipine with and without a beta-blocker, studied with exercise test. A double-blind, randomized subacute study. Clin. Cardiology 2:203
5. Ekelund L-G, Ekelund C, Rössner S Antihypertensive effect of a calcium-blocker, nifedipine, alone and in combination with a beta-blocker, metoprolol, in patients with essential hypertension. A subacute study with exercise tests. In manuscript.

Der Stellenwert der Calcium-Antagonisten in der Angina pectoris-Therapie

H. Roskamm

Schlußbemerkung

Erlauben Sie mir bitte für die letzten Minuten dieses Symposiums ein paar abschließende Bemerkungen:

Es steht mir nicht zu, über den theoretischen Teil dieses Symposiums zusammenfassend oder ausblickend etwas zu sagen. Den überzeugenden Grundlagenuntersuchungen stehen noch viele Fragen und Unsicherheiten auf klinischem Gebiet gegenüber. Die einzelnen Calciumantagonisten zeigen doch große Unterschiede in ihren Wirkungen und in ihrer Wirksamkeit, jedenfalls bei den bislang empfohlenen Dosen. Ich möchte an dieser Stelle ein paar klinische Fragen beantworten, die sich mit dem Stellenwert dieser Substanzen innerhalb der Therapie der Angina pectoris befassen.

Hat die Einführung der Calciumantagonisten die Indikationsgrenze zwischen medikamentöser und chirurgischer Therapie der Angina pectoris zugunsten der Medikamente verschoben? Ich glaube, diese Frage muß man z. Zt. noch mit „nein" beantworten, zumal die vorwiegend vasospastische Angina pectoris ja auch bislang kaum zum Chirurgen geschickt wurde. Zu einer Zurücknahme der für uns heutzutage gültigen Indikationen für den aortenkoronaren Bypass könnte uns auch nur eine Substanz führen, welche die Symptomatik ganz entscheidend verbessert — um einen viel höheren Betrag als alle zur Zeit bekannten Medikamente — und gleichzeitig zu einer Prognoseverbesserung führt. Beta-Rezeptoren-Blocker reduzieren zwar die Häufigkeit des akuten Herztodes beim Post-Infarktpatienten [1, 2, 3] und verbessern selbstverständlich auch bei den meisten Patienten die Angina pectoris. Das Ausmaß der Verbesserung der Angina pectoris ist jedoch nicht vergleichbar mit der durch Koronarchirurgie erzielten. Während man mit den Beta-Blockern eine z. B. ungefähr 30%ige Erhöhung der Angina-pectoris-Schwelle erzielt, ist durch die Koronarchirurgie eine Verdoppelung bis Verdreifachung die Regel.

Ähnlich ist die Situation bei den Calciumantagonisten. Die Verbesserung der Angina pectoris-Symptomatik ist bei Patienten mit stabiler Angina pectoris während Belastung im Durchschnitt nicht größer als mit Beta-Blockern. Eine Prognoseverbesserung mit Calciumantagonisten ist bislang nicht bewiesen.

Weiterhin muß somit bei jeder schweren Angina pectoris die Indikation zur Koronarchirurgie geprüft werden; diese setzt eine Koronarangiographie voraus. Sie ist indiziert bei jeder Angina pectoris, die trotz ausreichender medikamentöser Therapie das Leben des Betroffenen stark beeinflußt. Bei Patienten mit schwerer Angina pectoris, z. B. einer 25-Watt-Angina pectoris, von der wir aus Erfahrung wissen, daß sie praktisch nie mit Medikamenten soweit gebessert werden kann, daß dem Patienten eine einigermaßen ausreichende Aktivität im täglichen Leben möglich ist, sollte möglichst bald angiographiert werden, ohne viel Zeit mit langfristigen medikamentösen Therapieverfahren zu verlieren. Hinzu kommt, daß die Häufigkeit von schweren morphologischen Befunden, wie linke Hauptstammstenose oder 3-Gefäßerkrankung – bei denen wir annehmen können, daß die Koronarchirurgie auch die Prognose verbessert – um so größer ist, je schwerer Angina pectoris und ischämische ST-Senkung während Belastung sind [4].

Medikamentöse Therapie bleibt für die überwiegende Zahl der Koronarpatienten die Therapie der Wahl; sie ist im einzelnen indiziert für folgende Gruppen:

1. Ohne vorliegende invasive Abklärung bei Patienten mit geringer Angina pectoris, verbunden mit geringer oder ohne ischämische ST-Senkung während körperlicher Belastung.
2. Nach erfolgter Koronarangiographie bei Patienten, die keine schwere Mehrgefäßerkrankung oder linke Hauptstammstenose haben, wenn der medikamentös erzielte Therapieerfolg dem Patienten ausreicht.
3. Nach erfolgter Koronarangiographie bei wegen diffuser Koronargefäßsklerose inoperablen Patienten.

Sind nun innerhalb der medikamentösen Therapie-Möglichkeiten die Calciumantagonisten nur eine Alternative zu den anderen Medikamentengruppen oder gibt es für sie spezielle Indikationen? Ich meine „ja", seit vor allem von Maseri u. Mitarb. [5, 6] die vasospastische Angina pectoris herausgestellt wurde. Vasospastische Angina pectoris bedeutet Verursachung der Koronarinsuffizienz durch einen Koronarspasmus entweder bei normalen Herzkranzarterien oder – wie meistens – bei vorliegenden mittelgradigen Stenosen, auf denen sich der Spasmus aufpfropft. Wann muß klinisch an eine vasospastische Angina pectoris gedacht werden? Je stärker die Diskrepanz zwischen schweren nächtlichen Angina pectoris-Anfällen oder solchen im Ruhezustand auf der einen Seite und einer guten Arbeitstoleranz auf der anderen Seite, desto häufiger wird eine vasospastische Angina pectoris vorkommen. Bei dieser vasospastischen Angina pectoris sind die Calciumantagonisten die Therapie der Wahl. Selbstverständlich kann man hier auch Nitropräparate verwenden. Wenn die nächtlichen Anfälle jedoch bevorzugt in den frühen Morgenstunden auftreten, ist ein über 8 bis 10 Std laufender Schutz durch Calciumantagonisten eher zu erzielen als durch eine abends zuvor eingenommene Tablette eines langwirkenden Nitrokörpers. Wir neigen dazu, bei allen Patienten, bei denen Ruhe-Angina pectoris besteht, die nicht eindeutig einer passageren Mehrarbeit des Herzens zuzuordnen ist, Calciumantagonisten zu verabreichen, dieses sind oft instabile Angina pectoris-Situationen.

Anders bei Patienten mit stabiler Angina pectoris, bei denen die Angina pectoris klar der Mehrbelastung des Herzens zuzuordnen ist und die im Ruhezustand niemals Beschwerden bekommen. Insbesondere bei denjenigen, bei denen eine hohe Herzfrequenz während körperlicher Belastung auf einen hohen Sympathikusdrive hinweist, ist der Beta-Rezeptoren-Blocker die Therapie der Wahl.

Sowohl Calciumantagonisten als auch Beta-Rezeptoren-Blocker können mit Nitropräparaten kombiniert werden.

Die Kombination von Nitrokörpern und Beta-Rezeptoren-Blockern hat sich seit langem als auch pathophysiologisch sehr sinnvoll erwiesen. Die Calciumantagonisten schöpfen den vorrangigen Wirkungsmechanismus der Nitrokörper nicht aus, auch diese Kombination ist somit sinnvoll [7]. Die Kombination von Calciumantagonisten mit Beta-Blockern ergibt eine deutliche Steigerung der Wirkung gegenüber der Monotherapie mit einer dieser Substanzen [8]. Die Kombinationstherapie scheint auch nicht problematisch zu sein; kontraindiziert ist wohl nur, bei bestehender Beta-Rezeptoren-Therapie, eine zusätzliche i.v.-Injektion von Isoptin zu verabreichen.

Bei Patienten mit schwerer Angina pectoris, die inoperabel sind, sehen wir häufig durch Anwendung einer Dreierkombination − Nitrokörper, Beta-Blocker und Calciumantagonisten − dann doch einen signifikanten Therapieerfolg.

Auf dem letzten amerikanischen Kardiologenkongreß in Dallas wurde gezeigt, daß sich auch bislang als organisch bezeichnete Stenosen im Koronarangiogramm nach Gaben von Nitroglyzerin erweitern [10].

Auch bei überwiegend organischen Stenosen scheint also in vielen Fällen eine erweiterungsfähige funktionelle Komponente vorzuliegen. Dieser Faktor wäre − neben der Senkung der Nachbelastung und vielleicht geringgradig auch der Vorbelastung − ein weiterer Ansatzpunkt nicht nur für die Therapie mit Nitrokörpern, sondern auch für die Calciumantagonisten. Durch weitere Untersuchungen muß geklärt werden, welche Art von Stenosen dies sind, ob das Alter des Patienten einen wesentlichen Einfluß hat, usw.

Viele Fragen bleiben offen. Gibt es eine Gewöhnung an Calciumantagonisten, wenn diese sehr lange gegeben werden? Nach 6 Monaten scheint es nach den Untersuchungen von Ekelund [8] noch keine zu geben. Kann mit einer Prognoseverbesserung gerechnet werden? Kann gar damit gerechnet werden, daß mit Calciumantagonisten eine primäre Prophylaxe des arteriosklerotischen Grundprozesses erreicht wird? Die aus dem Fleckensteinschen Arbeitskreis von Frey [9] vorgelegten Ergebnisse über die prophylaktische Wirkung bei artifizieller Mönckebergscher Arteriosklerose können dieses vielleicht hoffen lassen.

Entsprechend der universellen Bedeutung des Calciumstoffwechsels waren auch vielgestaltige Effekte der Calciumantagonisten zu erwarten. Die erfolgreiche Behandlung, insbesondere von supraventrikulären Arrhythmien mit Isoptin ist seit langem bekannt. Die Myokardprotektion bei Herzoperationen scheint sehr erfolgversprechend. Die Behandlung der hypertrophischen Myokardiopathien und die Behandlung der Hypertonie befinden sich sicherlich noch in einem Versuchsstadium. In der Zukunft ist wahrscheinlich mit einer Zunahme der Indikationen für diese Substanzgruppe zu rechnen. Wer hätte vor 10 Jahren daran gedacht, daß eines guten Tages Psychiater und Neurologen Angst und Tremor u. a. auch mit Beta-Blockern behandeln?

Ich darf diese Tagung abschließen mit einem Dank an Sie alle, an die Sponsorfirma, und an diejenigen hinter den Kulissen, die für Organisation und Simultanübersetzung verantwortlich waren.

Literatur

1. Ahlmark G, Saetre H (1976) Long-term treatment with betablockers after myocardial infarction. Eur J Clin Pharmacol 10:77
2. Multicentre International Study (1975) Improvement in prognosis of myocardial infarction by long-term β-adrenoreceptor blockade using practolol. Br Med J iii:735
3. Wilhelmsson C, Vedin JA, Wilhelmsen L, Tibblin G, Werkö L (1974) Reduction of sudden deaths after myocardial infarction by treatment with alprenolol. Lancet II:1157
4. Roskamm H, Samek L, Zweigle K, Stürzenhofecker P, Petersen J, Rentrop P, Prokoph J (1977) Die Beziehungen zwischen den Befunden der Koronarangiographie und des Belastungs-EKG bei Patienten ohne transmuralen Myokardinfarkt. Z Kardiol 66:273

5. Maseri A, Severi S, L'Abbate A, Pesola A (1977) Variant angina: One aspect of a continuous spectrum of vasospastic angina. Circulation 56:III – 33
6. Maseri A (1980) Application of calciumantagonists in patients with vasospastic angina pectoris. Calcium-Antagonism-Symposium p 243, Berlin Heidelberg New York: Springer 1980
7. Schnellbacher K, Kalusche D, Roskamm H (1980) Hämodynamik während belastungsinduzierter Angina pectoris nach einmaliger Gabe von Fendilin und Nifedipin. – Ist die Nitroglycerin-Wirkung noch nachweisbar? Calcium-Antagonismus-Symposium S 314, Berlin Heidelberg New York: Springer 1980
8. Ekelund LG (1980) Change in exercise tolerance in patients with angina pectoris induced by administration of a calcium-blocker, nifedipine (adalat), alone or in combination with beta-blockers. Calcium-Antagonismus-Symposium S 331, Berlin Heidelberg New York: Springer 1980
9. Frey M: Verhütung experimenteller Gefäßverkalkungen (Mönckebergs Typ der Arteriosklerose) durch Calciumantagonisten bei Ratten. Calcium-Antagonismus-Symposium, Frankfurt, Dezember 1978
10. Oravetz R, Lee G, Baker L, Titus P (1978) Prominent dilation of stenotic coronary artery lesions following sublingual nitroglycerin by quantitative arteriography. Circulation 58:25

Sachverzeichnis

Subject Index

Arterielle Hypertonie

Ätiopathogenese, Diagnostik
und Therapie

Herausgeber: J. Rosenthal
1980. 170 zum Teil farbige Abbildungen,
75 Tabellen. Etwa 600 Seiten
ISBN 3-540-08713-3
In Vorbereitung

Vom Belastungs-EKG zur Koronarangiographie

Ihre zentrale Bedeutung für zeitgemäße
Diagnose und Therapie der koronaren
Herzkrankheit

Herausgeber: M. Kaltenbach,
H. Roskamm
Mit Beiträgen von H.-J. Becker,
W.-D. Bussmann, M. Kaltenbach,
G. Kober, J. Petersen, H. Roskamm,
L. Samek, P. Stürzenhofecker
Unter Mitarbeit von P. Bubenheimer,
H.-J. Engel, A. Grüntzig, G. Hör,
P. Lichtlen, P. Rentrop, E. Sauer,
H. Schicha, H. Sebening
1980. 318 Abbildungen in 800 Einzeldar-
stellungen. Etwa 390 Seiten
Gebunden DM 148,-; approx. US $ 87.40
ISBN 3-540-09861-5

S. Effert, P. Hanrath, W. Bleifeld

Echokardiographie

Mit einem Beitrag „Echokardiographie
im Kindesalter" von J. Keutel
1979. 72 Abbildungen, 9 Tabellen.
X, 146 Seiten
Gebunden DM 68,-; approx. US $ 40.20
ISBN 3-540-09166-1

Cardiac Glycosides

Editors: G. Bodem, H. J. Dengler
1978. 125 figures, 70 tables. XI, 426 pages
(International Boehringer Mannheim
Symposia)
DM 58,-; approx. US $ 34.30
ISBN 3-540-08692-7

B. Lüderitz

Elektrische Stimulation des Herzens

Diagnostik und Therapie kardialer
Rhythmusstörungen

Unter Mitarbeit von D. W. Fleischmann,
C. Naumann d'Alnoncourt,
M. Schlepper, L. Seipel, G. Steinbeck
Korrigierter Nachdruck. 1980. 229 Abbil-
dungen, 46 Tabellen. XII, 398 Seiten
Gebunden DM 68,-; approx. US $ 40.20
ISBN 3-540-09164-5

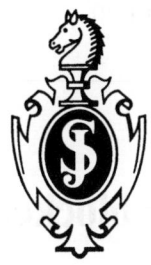

Springer-Verlag
Berlin
Heidelberg
New York

Cardiomyopathy and Myocardial Biopsy

Editors: M. Kaltenbach, F. Loogen,
E. G. J. Olsen
In cooperation with W.-D. Bussmann
With contributions by numerous experts
Corrected printing. 1978. 203 figures,
56 tables. XIV, 337 pages
Cloth DM 58,–; approx. US $ 34.30
ISBN 3-540-08474-6

Herzrhythmusstörungen

Herausgeber: H. Hochrein
Mit Beiträgen von O. A. Beck,
F. B. Everling, H.-U. Lehmann, E. Witt
1980. 108 Abbildungen, 57 Tabellen.
XV, 298 Seiten
(Kliniktaschenbücher)
DM 29,50; approx. US $ 17.40
ISBN 3-540-08714-1

B. E. Strauer

Das Hochdruckherz

Funktion, koronare Hämodynamik und
Hypertrophie des linken Ventrikels bei
der essentiellen Hypertonie
1979. 50 Abbildungen, 15 Tabellen.
V, 92 Seiten
DM 24,–; approx. US $ 14.20
ISBN 3-540-08966-7

Therapie mit Beta-Rezeptorenblockern

Herausgeber: H.-D. Bolte
Unter Mitarbeit von O. Benkert, J. Cyran,
E. Erdmann, H. Kuhn, K. O. Stumpe
1979. 20 Abbildungen, 31 Tabellen.
VIII, 121 Seiten
Gebunden DM 38,–; approx. US $ 22.50
ISBN 3-540-09465-2

Myocardial Failure

Editors: G. Riecker, A. Weber,
J. Goodwin
Co-Editors: H.-D. Bolte, B. Lüderitz,
B. E. Strauer, E. Erdmann
1977. 172 figures, 52 tables.
XII, 374 pages
(International Boehringer Mannheim
Symposia)
DM 48,–; approx. US $ 28.40
ISBN 3-540-08225-5
Distribution rights for Japan:
Nankodo Co. Ltd., Tokyo

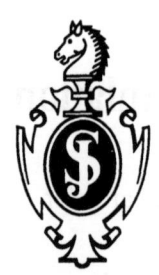

Springer-Verlag
Berlin
Heidelberg
New York

MIX
Papier aus verantwortungs-
vollen Quellen
www.fsc.org
FSC® C083411

If you have any concerns about our products,
you can contact us on:
ProductSafety@springernature.com

In case Publisher is established outside the EU,
the EU authorized representative is:
Springer Nature Customer Service Center GmbH
Europaplatz 3, 69115 Heidelberg, Germany

Printed by Libri Plureos GmbH
in Hamburg, Germany

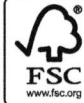